oxygen
WOMEN'S FITNESS

TOTAL
Women's
FITNESS

Releasing the
Inner You!

By Gerard Thorne and Phil Embleton

Published by MuscleMag International
5775 McLaughlin Road
Mississauga, ON
Canada L5R 3P7

10 9 8 7 6 5 4 3 2 Pbk

Canadian Cataloguing in Publication Data

Thorne, Gerard, 1963-
   Total women's fitness : releasing the inner you / by Gerard Thorne
and Phil Embleton.

Includes bibliographical references.
ISBN 1-55210-026-X

   1. Bodybuilding for women. 2. Physical fitness for women.
I. Embleton, Phil, 1963- II. Title.

GV546.6.W64T484 2002   646.7'5'082   C2002-904441-3

Designed by Jackie Thibeault
Edited by Sandy Wheeler

Distributed in Canada by
CANBOOK Services
c/o Pearson Canada
P.O. Box 335
195 Harry Walker Parkway N.
Newmarket, ON
L3Y 4X7
800-399-6858

Distributed in the U.S. by
BookWorld Services
1941 Whitfield Park Loop
Sarasota, FL 34243

Printed in Canada

Acknowledgments

Many authors might assume that, by their seventh book, they wouldn't need the assistance of others. Well, we have no intention of jumping to that conclusion. Writing and producing a book of this size takes more than the efforts of two humble authors.

To Jackie Thibeault and the staff at *Oxygen* and *MuscleMag International*, we once again offer our sincere thanks. To Bertha Thorne and John McCarthy, our continued thanks for keeping us on the financial straight and narrow. Our apologies to the IRS. Our thanks also go out to Melanie Hiscock for her input and advice. All the best on your future fitness career, Melanie.

Finally to Robert Kennedy, we say thanks for your faith in us and perhaps more important, for starting *MuscleMag International* all those years ago. We are just happy to be able to contribute in our own small way.

Gerard Thorne
Phil Embleton

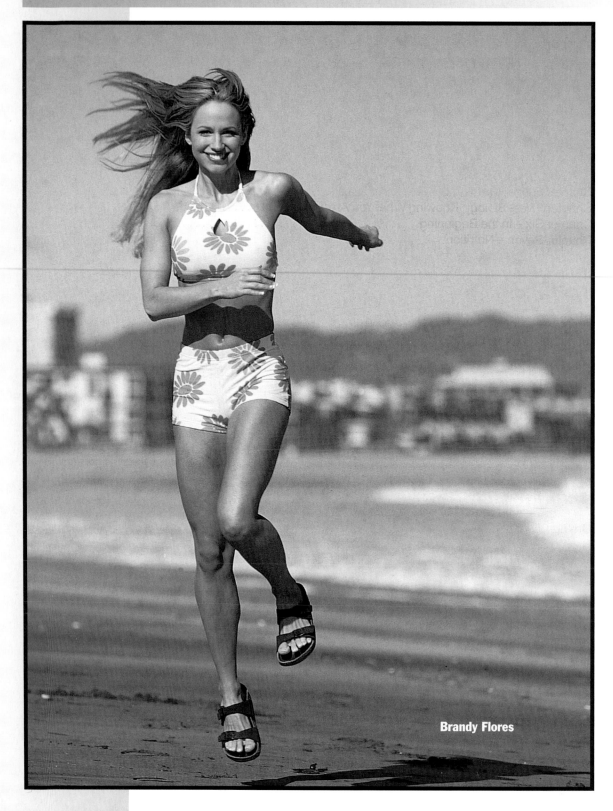

Brandy Flores

Table of Contents

Foreword by Robert Kennedy 6

Introduction – Debunking the Myths 8

Book One
Chapter One – Here, There, Everywhere. 16
Chapter Two – The Equipment. 34
Chapter Three – Exercise Fundamentals. 52
Chapter Four – Warming Up 58
Chapter Five – Biology, Knowing What You Are 62
Chapter Six – In the Beginning 82
Chapter Seven – Nutrition 86
Chapter Eight – The Intermediate Level. 152
Chapter Nine – Exercise Descriptions 166
Chapter Ten – Injuries. 200

Book Two
Chapter Eleven – Advanced Training Techniques and Principles 210
Chapter Twelve – Overtraining 226
Chapter Thirteen – Cardiovascular Training 232
Chapter Fourteen – Staying Motivated. 244
Chapter Fifteen – Getting "Back" At It 250
Chapter Sixteen – A Chest to be Proud Of 262
Chapter Seventeen – Shoulder-Training 268
Chapter Eighteen – Thighs and Glutes 276
Chapter Nineteen – Hamstrings 290
Chapter Twenty – Calves 295
Chapter Twenty-One – Biceps. 298
Chapter Twenty-Two – Triceps. 304
Chapter Twenty-Three – Abdominals 310
Chapter Twenty-Four – Getting in Shape Doesn't
    Have to be Boring 314

Book Three
Chapter Twenty-Five – Special Considerations. 340
Chapter Twenty-Six – Competition 352
Chapter Twenty-Seven – Supplements 382
Chapter Twenty-Eight – Thermogenesis 422
Chapter Twenty-Nine – Hair Care 432
Chapter Thirty – Cosmetics 444
Chapter Thirty-One – Fitness Money 460
Chapter Thirty-Two – Plastic Surgery 478
Chapter Thirty-Three – Questions and Answers. 492

Glossary. 524

Foreword – by Robert Kennedy

The most difficult thing to do with your own life is to change it. As a young artist in England I made a respectable living. I wasn't rich, but I had enough to pay my rent, go down to the pub with my mates, and occasionally escort an attractive lady to the movies.

But I wasn't content. Life was on cruise control, and I didn't have a goal. I wanted to start a magazine but most of my subjects lived in North America. Emigrating to the US is a long and arduous process, so I began to think about Canada. In those days it was very easy for British citizens to move there. You could even vote! (I didn't know who the Canadian politicians were or what they stood for, so I did the responsible thing and flipped a coin.) Emigrating meant I would have to leave my friends, and everything I was familiar with to start my life over in a new land.

Everyone tried to talk me out of it. My friends read me stories about the terrible Canadian winters. My father, a big fan of western movies, was worried about Indian attacks! I explained to him that that was just in the movies, and historically it was the settlers who had started most of the trouble. I tried to point out the positive aspects – the large forests, the open prairies, the Rockies. That last one was a mistake. Dad went down to the local library and asked for information about the Rocky Mountains. The librarian handed him a book about the Donner Party! That charming tale was about a group of settlers who got stranded in the mountains and resorted to cannibalism. They weren't even in the

"Where will I dwell in this new found land? What will I do in this new found land? Who will I love in this new found land?"
– part of an old song recounting the concerns of a new settler.

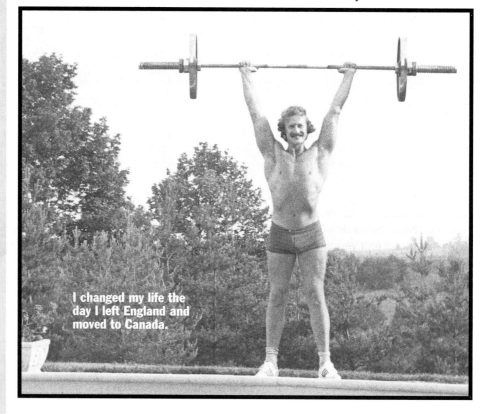

I changed my life the day I left England and moved to Canada.

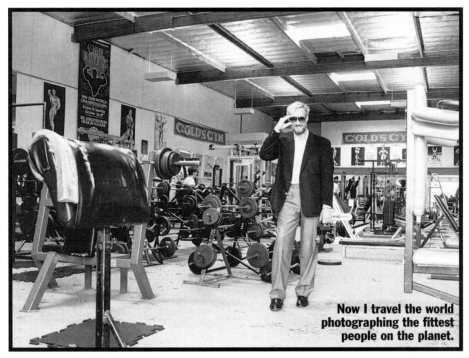

Now I travel the world photographing the fittest people on the planet.

Rockies! I had to bring home a number of books on the Rockies before Dad calmed down.

One of the most difficult times of my life was the day I left England for Canada. I wanted to cry, I wanted to say to everyone that I'd made a mistake, but mostly I wanted to be sick. I did none of those things. I held my head high, maintained a positive attitude, and reassured my friends and family that I'd be fine. I changed my life that day. In Canada I started a business and a family. I now travel the world photographing the fittest people on the planet!

There are other ways to change your life, and they're all just as difficult. And whether you make the difficult decision to change a job or end a relationship, the most important thing is to do it calmly, with respect and dignity for everyone involved.

Which brings me to this book, *Total Women's Fitness – Releasing the Inner You!* One of the most challenging decisions you can face is to change your lifestyle. Where do I find the strength to motivate myself to change? How do you correct years of bad habits? How do I train with less than perfect health? How can I improve myself? This book provides the answers to those questions and much much more.

We have choices in life. You can stay in your comfortable rut, or make a difficult decision and change your life. I sincerely hope this book helps you to make the right choice.

Robert Kennedy,
Publisher, *Oxygen, MuscleMag International*
and *American Health and Fitness.*

Debunking the Myths

Outdated beliefs and differences from men in absolute strength have resulted in misconceived approaches to strength training for women. It is true that their higher levels of testosterone explains men's superior absolute strength. But when other measures of strength are used, such as strength relative to cross-sectional area of muscle, men and women are nearly equal in strength. Those women who engage in the same strength-training programs as men benefit from increased bone and soft-tissue strength, increased lean body mass, decreased fat, and enhanced self-confidence. Convinced yet?

Although American women first began strength training for sports back in the 1950s to improve their performance, they have traditionally participated in strength training less than men have. Such forms of exercise were not considered feminine, and a lack of research and information regarding the effects of weight training on women made this a predominantly male activity. Women's participation was particularly limited until 1972, when federal laws mandated equal access to educational programs – including athletics – for men and women in schools that receive federal funding. Since then women's sports participation has boomed and strength training has grown in popularity among active women.

Nevertheless, the social stigma and lack of accurate information persisted and fed misconceptions that kept women away from engaging in any serious forms of strength training. Though gender differences regarding absolute strength do exist, women are just as capable as men of developing strength relative to total muscle mass. Consequently, women should strength train in the same ways as men, using the same program designs, exercises, intensities and volumes – relative to their body size and level of strength, of course – so they can achieve the maximum physiologic and psychological benefits.

Angie Chittenden

Respectable Women Shouldn't Do That Sort of Thing

Most cultures, particularly Western societies, have traditionally viewed strength as a masculine trait and promoted a small, frail body as feminine. Consequently, girls have been discouraged from participating in gross-motor-skill activities and strength development. Such sex role stereotypes, formed early in childhood, can influence behavior and prevent many women from realizing their full potential.

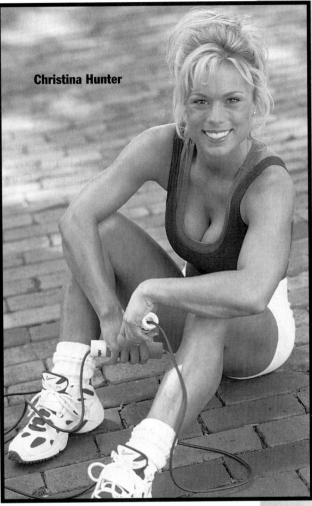

Christina Hunter

The advent of the women's movement in the 1970s allowed many women to overcome such traditional socialization and participate more freely in sports and strength training. However, change occurs slowly, and physical strength and strength training are still not as common or accepted for women as they are for men. Through the works of Joe Weider's *Shape* magazine, Robert Kennedy's *Oxygen* magazine and others, millions of women are hitting the gyms in record numbers, and a once traditionally male arena is now as co-ed as any tennis court or golf course.

Is There Really a Gender Gap?

Research on male and female strength potential reveals that the average female possess about two-thirds of the strength of the average male.[1,2] However, the measurement of strength in absolute terms fosters misconceptions about the strength of women, how women see themselves, and the way they exercise.

The Role of Hormones

Hormones, those dastardly little devils that poets and physiologists alike have studied for thousands of years, play a role in the development of absolute strength in men and women, but the exact influence is not clear. The most important hormone for strength development is testosterone.

The role of testosterone in strength development is complex and significantly more variable than that of other hormones. Though women on average have about one-tenth the testosterone of men,[4] the level varies greatly among women, and influences women's strength development more than is typical in men.[3] Women who have higher testosterone levels may have a greater potential for strength and power development than other women. This should come as no shock to readers who have followed the Olympics for the past couple of decades. Recent revelations from the former East German sport's program have outlined how thousands of women were given testosterone (and testosterone derivatives) injections to increase their muscular size and strength. In many cases the unsuspecting girls were masculinized to the point that their gender was in doubt.

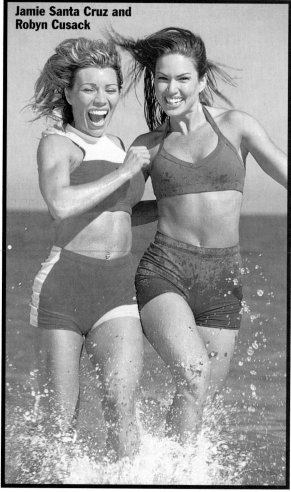

Jamie Santa Cruz and Robyn Cusack

We must add that women's testosterone levels naturally fluctuate from one woman to the next. A woman who is near the upper limit of her testosterone threshold may have an advantage in developing strength over other women. Though hormones may influence the potential for strength development among women, they most likely do not account for significant male-female differences in absolute strength.

Physiologic Factors

Another explanation for physiologic differences in strength between men and women is size and body structure. For example, the average American male is about 13 cm taller than the average female, and about 40 pounds heavier. Men average 40 to 50 pounds more lean body mass and 8 to 10 pounds less fat than women. Men typically also have a taller, wider frame that supports more muscle, as well as broader shoulders that provide greater leverage advantage. We see the same differences among male weightlifters and powerlifters. Few 180-pounders can hoist the same amount of weight as some 280 to 300-pound behemoth superheavyweights. In fact body size and strength difference is one of the primary reasons why most strength sports have weight class divisions.

The Stronger Sex!

Strength, however, should not be viewed in absolute terms. The gender differences in absolute strength, for example, are not consistent across all muscle groups. The average female possess about 40 to 60 percent of the upper-body strength and 70 to 75 percent of the lower-body strength of the average male.[3] Men may have an advantage in neuromuscular response time that results in greater force-production speed than women.[5] However, the distribution of muscle fiber types – fast and slow twitch – is similar in the two sexes, and women are able to use a greater portion of stored energy than men during activities in which muscle is prestretched.

More significantly, if the amount of lean body mass is factored into the strength equation, the relative strength difference between men and women is less appreciable. Based on a ratio of strength to lean body mass, women are about equal in strength to men, and when strength is calculated per cross-sectional area of muscle, no significant gender difference exists.

So, ladies, the old stereotypical belief that men are the stronger sex and women are weak and dainty is not as cut and dried as once thought.

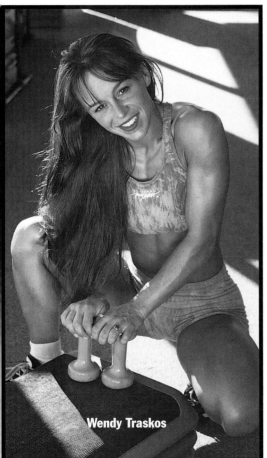

Wendy Traskos

10 Myths About Women And Strength Training

Myth #1 – Women can't get strong. Untrue. The average woman gains strength at a slightly faster rate than the average man.

Myth #2 – Strength training de-feminizes women. Strength training offers a wide array of potential benefits (functional, mental and physical health), and is as appropriate and available for women as for men.

Myth #3 – Lifting weights will cause women to develop relatively large muscles. Women don't have the genetic potential to develop large muscles because, except in very rare instances, they don't have enough of the hormone testosterone, which is necessary for the development of muscle tissue.

Myth #4 – Strength training will make a woman muscle-bound. Strength training increases flexibility and we know now that women can't develop large muscles.

Myth #5 – A woman's muscle will turn to fat when she stops training. Muscle doesn't turn to fat, and vice versa. If a muscle is not used it will shrink (atrophy).

Myth #6 – A woman can take protein supplements to enhance her physique.

Extra protein does not enhance a woman's physique. Excess amounts of protein are converted to fat and stored in the body.

Myth #7 – Rigorous strength training can help a woman rid her body of fat. Strength training can firm and tone muscle but it cannot directly burn fat. Strength training can increase a woman's metabolic rate, the rate at which calories are used, therefore more fat calories are likely to be utilized.

Myth #8 – Strength training increases the need for vitamins. Vitamins are not a source of energy and do not contribute to a woman's body structure. A woman who strength trains receives no benefit from taking an excessive dose of vitamins. Eat a diet of a variety of healthful foods to ensure adequate nutrition.

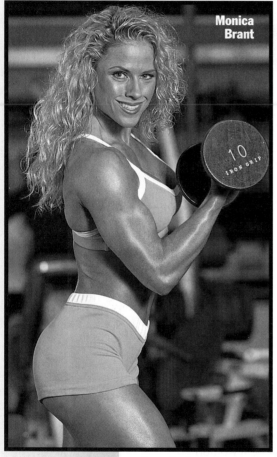

Monica Brant

Myth #9 – Strength training is for young women. No, it's never too late to improve your muscular fitness. Strength training can help extend a woman's functional life span.

Myth #10 – Strength training is expensive. Not true. A muscle doesn't know the cost of a machine it's using. Muscle responds to the stress being applied to it … a pair of dumbells or a barbell and plates can be just as effective as an expensive machine.

Strength Training Benefits For Women

The fact that you picked up this book is likely evidence enough that you intend to engage in some serious strength training. If not, then pay close attention to the following benefits of this endeavor. You'll notice the terms *record setting* and *bulking up* are mentioned nowhere. Weight training for women is one of the most beneficial forms of exercise there is.

Prevention of Osteoporosis

We sometimes laugh when we hear a comedian joke, "I've fallen, and I can't get up." But bone fractures among the elderly, especially women, are at an all-time high. The loss of calcium and other bone-building minerals from bones is called osteoporosis. Women, more than men, need to meet the minimal essential *strain* required for bone-modeling to occur and ultimately for reducing the risk of osteoporosis. Prevention of osteoporosis requires above-normal stressing of both the muscles and bones. One of the unknown benefits of strength training is that it causes the bones to absorb more calcium and other building minerals. And since bone-building is proportional to the degree of overload (the amount of stress applied beyond the normal load), the greater the overload – within limits – the greater the amount of bone-building. In simple terms, weightlifting and hence bone-building helps prevent fractures and helps ensure against osteoporosis.

We should add that cartilage, tendons and ligaments also have minimal essential "strain requirements." Optimal strength development requires loads and intensities that progressively increase the training stimulus or stress. Strong cartilage, tendons and ligaments are essential for joint integrity, stability and injury prevention.

Lean Body Mass and Fat

Strength training also increases lean body mass and decreases fat. This results in less nonfunctional fat to carry and a greater proportion of lean body mass, which can provide functional strength. Compared to fat, muscle is metabolically more active and increases metabolic rate, fat oxidation, and calorie consumption. Increased muscle mass and muscle cross-sectional area also correlate with increased strength. Participation in strength-training exercises will develop functional strength and most likely improve performance – whether it is an increased ability to spike a volleyball or pick up a child.

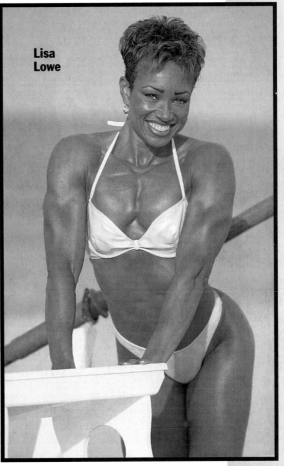

Lisa Lowe

Psychological Well-Being

With all the attention paid to the physiological benefits of strength training, we are happy to report there are psychological benefits as well. Studies have shown that women who engage in strength training benefit from improved self-esteem.[3] Female athletes appear to be able to balance strength and femininity. According to one survey, 94 percent of the participants reported that athletic participation did not lead them to feel less feminine. Such psychological benefits arise from the physiologic changes that occur as a result of strength training and from the process of encountering and mastering physical challenges. Thus, both *the process* and *the outcome* of strength training benefit women.[3]

REFERENCES

1. Hettinger J: *Physiology of Strength*, Springfield, IL, Charles Thomas, 1961
2. Holloway JB: Individual differences and their implications for resistance training, in Baechle TR (ed): Essentials of Strength Training and Conditioning, Champaign, IL, *Human Kinetics*, 1994, pp 151-162
3. National Strength and Conditioning Association: Position Paper: Strength Training for Female Athletes. National Strength and Conditioning Association, Colorado Springs, 1990
4. Hakkinen K, Pakarinen A, Kyrolainen H, et al. Neuromuscular adaptations and serum hormones in females during prolonged power training. *Int J Sports Med* 1990;11(2):91-98
5. Karlsson J, Jacobs I: Is the significance of muscle fiber types to muscle metabolism different in females than in males? in Borms J, Hebbelink M, Venerando A (eds): Women and Sport, an Historical, Biological, Physiological and Sports Medical Approach. Basel, Switzerland, S Karger, 1981

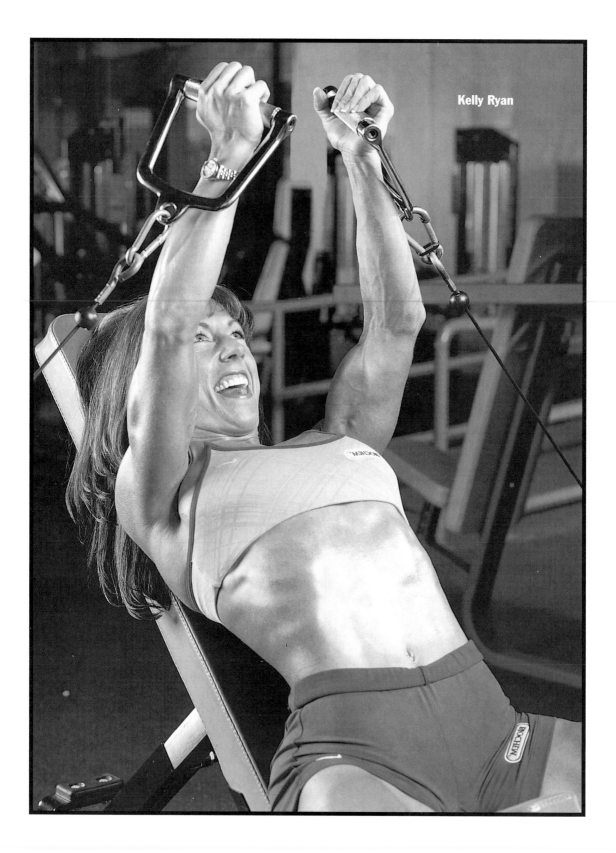

Kelly Ryan

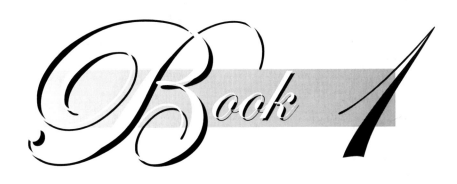

CHAPTER ONE

Here, There, Everywhere

One of the most fundamental decisions you'll ever have to make as you embark on the road to total fitness is where to train. Essentially you have two choices – at home or at a commercial gym. Both have advantages and disadvantages and a whole host of factors must be taken into account before you make your selection. We should add that, while the bulk of this book is aimed toward training at a commercial gym, many of the exercises and techniques could be utilized at home.

Home Alone 1

For many the ideal training facility is their house or apartment. No crowds, no fighting for parking space, no having to kick people off cardio machines. You can even adjust the music and temperature to your own desire.

The first obstacle you'll be faced with when training at home is equipment – in simpler terms, the lack thereof. Unless you have a friend or relative who was at one time into weight training, you'll have to make some purchases. The most basic items you'll need are a couple of sets of dumbells, a barbell and some weight plates, an adjustable bench, and a piece of cardio equipment. Let's take a look at each.

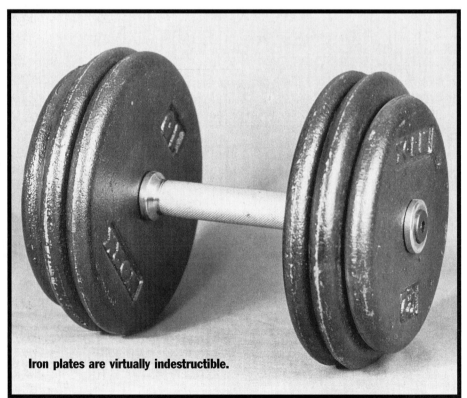

Iron plates are virtually indestructible.

Most of the top names in fitness and bodybuilding got their first taste of weightlifting from an old York or Weider barbell set left under the Christmas tree. Before rushing out to buy a set, look around. There's a good chance some relative or friend has an old set in the basement or attic. If you strike out, another option is to hit a few flea markets. Many private garage sales feature old weight training equipment. The typical scenario sees the kids all grown up and moved off and Mom and Dad decide to clean house. You could easily pick up a barbell set with a couple of hundred pounds of weight for a few dollars. If buying new is your only option, all is not lost. Most major department and hardware stores sell barbell sets. For a basic 110-pound set the price generally ranges from $75 to $150.

There are two basic types of weight plates. Iron plates are just that, solid iron. They come in these sizes: 2.5, 5, 10, 25, 35 and 45 pounds. The nice thing about iron plates is durability. Go into an older gym and odds are the plates there are older than you are! Iron plates are virtually indestructible.

For the home market, manufacturers have come up with plastic or vinyl plates. No, they are not made of plastic but instead consist of an outer shell or casing filled up with sand or cement. The nice thing about vinyl plates is that they don't rust, and they tend to be kinder to household floors. Iron plates rust from moisture buildup and can really do a number on your hardwood floor. If plastic plates have a downside it's their thickness. Because they are less dense than solid iron, the plates need to be much thicker to give the same weight, meaning you can stack fewer of them on a bar. But this probably won't be an issue unless you get into heavy powerlifting. Most people who get serious about powerlifting either join a gym or invest in an Olympic barbell set.

Besides a barbell you'll need a couple of sets of dumbells. For most readers dumbells in the 5 to 30-pound range will suffice. As with barbells, check around to see if you can buy them used. Most barbell starter sets also come with two short dumbell handles. A set of collars will allow you to add or remove plates to change the weight of the dumbells.

Another item you'll need is an adjustable bench. The heavy-duty commercial benches will set you back $500 or more, but most department stores sell home models for about $100 to $150. Some people build their own, but a few words of caution. Keep in mind the bench will be supporting your weight *plus* the weight you are lifting. This could easily work out to over 200 pounds. That's why most commercial benches are made out of metal. If your carpenter knows what he or she is doing then wood will suffice, but make sure it is of sturdy design. Here's another point to remember. It's virtually impossible to build a sturdy adjustable bench out of wood. You'd need to build both a flat and incline bench to do the same exercises as one metal adjustable bench.

Timea Majorova

To complete your home gym you'll need one final piece of equipment – some sort of cardio machine. For a couple of hundred dollars you can buy a home model treadmill or cycle. Of course such units come nowhere near the durability of the $5000-plus commercial models found at most gyms (much more on cardio equipment and cardiovascular conditioning in Chapter Thirteen).

Add it all up and you'll see that you can set up a nice little home gym for under $1000. Of course it all depends on your goals, available space, and finances. Some individuals have home gyms that rival small commercial gyms.

Even though the home gym we've described will enable you to perform a good workout, there's one more piece of equipment you might want to consider buying and that's a multistation. As the name implies, this large piece of equipment enables you to hit just about the entire body. Many readers may be familiar with the large Universal multistation found in most high school and university gyms. It's not surprising that equipment manufacturers have made available smaller versions of such units to target the home gym market. For $200 to $1000 or more you can buy a multistation that has attachments to target just about every major muscle in the body.

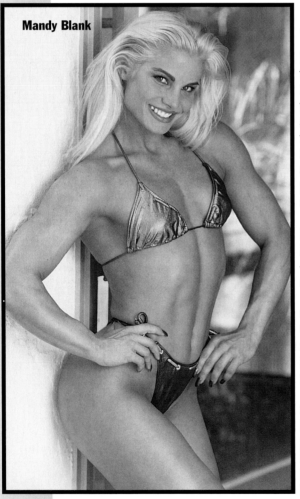

Mandy Blank

Home Alone 2

Despite the advantages of home training, there are some limitations. First of all, because it's so convenient you may never use it. We know this sounds contradictory but you'll quickly find that something you can easily do later often gets continuously put off. In short, later never comes. You need a great deal of discipline to make time and train at home.

Another drawback is distractions. Between the phone, the door, possibly kids, even the ever-beckoning fridge – all play a role in interfering with a quality workout.

A third consideration is equipment variety. Unless you have megabucks with the space to go with it, there's no way your home setup can come close to rivaling commercial gyms with regards to equipment selection.

A final downside to home gyms is the lack of what could be called "a knowledge pool." Gyms are filled with people who have spent many years building up their knowledge of fitness. From the certified instructors to the long-time members, gyms offer you instant access to virtually all the answers to your questions. At home you are limited to books and magazines. These are great sources, but let's face it, nothing beats the one-on-one interaction that only comes with a real person.

We hope by now you are beginning to seriously consider joining a gym. Great! Let's take a close look at the different types of gyms and what each has to offer.

The Health Spa

At one end of the training spectrum we find the health spa. This upscale facility caters more to high-powered executives than the mainstream population. The best term to describe the health spa is *posh*. Most have expensive memberships ($1000 or more per year) and spend as much money on improving the sauna or lounge as they do on adding a new piece of training equipment.

Health spas tend to contain only machines, with maybe a couple of sets of dumbells thrown in as an afterthought. Forget trying to do a barbell exercise. Health spas go out of their way to avoid barbells as such items only "attract body-builders and powerlifters, and my gosh we don't want those kinds of people in here." Seriously, though, while they don't say so in their ads or write it out on signs, most health spas are set up to keep hard trainers away. As such, the type of equipment that would attract bodybuilders, powerlifters, etc. is rarely found at health spas. Basically their philosophy is "if we don't have it, they won't come here."

Despite our negative introduction, health spas have a few advantages. For starters, most are kept in immaculate condition. *Spotless* is probably a better word. The machines gleam, and the change rooms are practically manicured. Another advantage to health spas is the uniformity of the clientele. Even though the authors find health spas have a stuffy atmosphere, we'll be the first to admit that some mainstream gyms are inhabited by a wide assortment of characters — some obnoxious, some polite. Of course this is what gives each gym its own unique flavor. But if you want a gym full of upscale clones, the health spa is the place to go. About all we can say is that, unless you don't have access to another type of facility, give it a pass.

Health spas cater more to high-powered executives than the mainstream population.

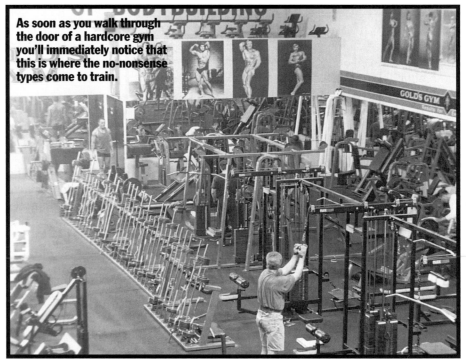

As soon as you walk through the door of a hardcore gym you'll immediately notice that this is where the no-nonsense types come to train.

Hardcore Gyms

It only makes sense to follow health spas with hardcore gyms as they are at the opposite end of the spectrum. Where health spas go out of their way to keep bodybuilders and powerlifters away, hardcore gyms are filled with such characters. As soon as you walk through the door of a hardcore gym you'll immediately notice that this is where the no-nonsense types come to train. You won't find many copies of the *Wall Street Journal* lying on the counter.

As the name implies, the hardcore gym is just that, a place for people to go and engage in some serious training. Perhaps the most famous hardcore facility was the original Gold's Gym in Venice Beach, California. Back in the late '60s and early '70s Gold's was the favorite haunt of Arnold Schwarzenegger and the other top bodybuilders of the era. The equipment and atmosphere alone is enough to keep the stock market crowd away from hardcore gyms. Chrome-platted equipment is not in abundance at such establishments. The barbell and dumbell reign supreme.

The primary advantage to hardcore gyms is their no-nonsense approach to training. Lounging around and discussing the stock market is pretty much frowned upon. We alluded to another advantage to hardcore gyms earlier. Such facilities are filled with members who regularly compete in bodybuilding, powerlifting or fitness contests. Whether or not you intend to compete some day is entirely up to you. The fact remains, to achieve success in any of these disciplines you need a great deal of dedication and knowledge. Bodybuilders are walking encyclopedias of information concerning bodyfat reduction. Likewise female fitness competitors know all the tricks for firming up stubborn bodyparts.

If it's pure strength you want, you need look no further than a competitive powerlifter. And readers, chivalry is not dead. Despite their sometimes crude and rough appearance, the guys you find training at a hardcore gym will be only too happy to answer your questions about exercise and nutrition. In fact they'll be flattered, it's a great boost to their ego. If there's one problem it will be that you may not be able to get them to stop talking about training!

Despite the authors' bias toward hardcore gyms, we'll admit there are a few disadvantages. Where some of the patrons can be positive resources, others can be downright offensive. Competitive bodybuilders, especially close to contest time, have been known to be a little on the "edgy" side. The combination of reduced calorie intake and copious amounts of performance-enhancing drugs often turns mild-mannered individuals into aggressive, belligerent Neanderthals. Just staring at such a character is enough to bring forth a wail of growls and grunts that would do one of the late Diane Fossey's mountain gorillas proud. Even in the off-season the atmosphere in hardcore gyms is serious and intense.

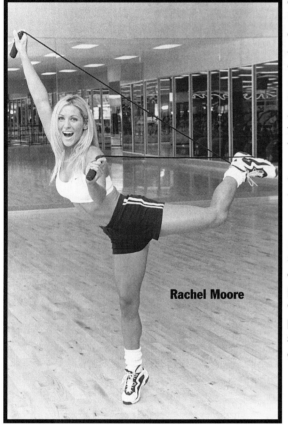

Rachel Moore

We must also point out that the membership in most hardcore gyms is predominantly male. In itself this is not such a bad thing, but a gym full of competitive males may not be the best place for you to take your first workout. On the other hand, if you have no problem working side by side with some zoo critters, then by all means give a hardcore gym a try.

Middle-of-the-Road: Straddling the Divide

Despite the appeal of health spas and hardcore gyms to a select few, most individuals prefer to work out at some sort of middle-of-the-road establishment (henceforth referred to as the fitness center). Despite their origins, most of the larger gym chains like World, Gold's and Powerhouse now fall in the category of mainstream. Likewise, most YMCAs and similar centers with fitness facilities fall right in the middle. There are numerous reasons why fitness centers are the most popular training establishments these days. At the top of the list is economics. The more people you can move through your doors the better your financial outlook. In short, the more of a given population you can attract the greater your profit margin. That's why you'll rarely find health spas or hardcore gyms in smaller centers. Occasionally someone who owns his or her own building will open a small gym, but it's primarily a place for the owner and friends to work out. Making big bucks is not a major goal. By and large you need a large population center to make the hardcore gym fly. The same goes for the health spa; the limited number of clientele available makes it difficult to survive economically. General fitness centers, however, cater to just about everyone, and as such have a much bigger potential membership pool to work with.

Fitness centers have numerous advantages over the other two categories. For starters they usually have the largest selection of equipment. Most have one or two complete lines of strength-training machines, a large selection of barbells, dumbells and racks, and a well-equipped cardio section. Fitness centers also tend to have the best atmosphere of the three categories. Odds are you won't have to listen to someone talking about the latest steroid cycle or stock investment. For the most part it's just average people talking about everyday topics. The final advantage to fitness centers is cost. Because they attract a larger percentage of the population, they can afford to offer cheaper membership fees.

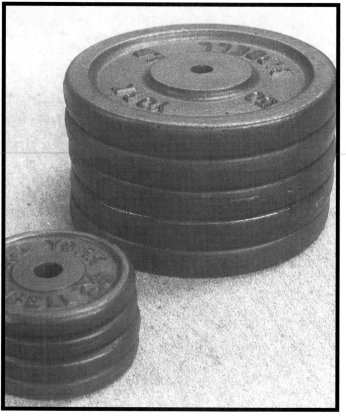

One Last Comment

Where you work out is entirely your decision. We hope we've given you some food for thought. Those readers in larger areas will no doubt have access to all three types of training facility. Most offer day passes, so experiment before you lay down $500 or more. In fact most gyms offer monthly passes as well. A month is long enough to get a feel for the place without the expenditure of a huge amount of money (most monthly fees fall in the range of $30 to $50). For variety you could switch gyms on a regular basis.

What to Wear

Granted you're not headed to a New Year's Eve ball, but there are dress codes at most gyms. Wear too much and you'll faint from heat exhaustion. Wear too little and you'll make the evening news! For most gyms a sweatshirt and track pants is the norm, but a T-shirt and shorts is also acceptable. You can be a bit more risky and wear spandex, but a few words of caution about this "revealing" form of gym wear. Spandex is designed to hug the body almost like a second skin. There'll be nothing left to the imagination. Every crevice, crease and fold will be highlighted in all its glory. If you have a few pounds in the wrong places, it will be there on display for all to see. Of course this can serve as motivation to get rid of it. The advantage to spandex is its comfort and thermoregulation. Spandex seems to adapt to the gym climate, keeping you warm when it's cold, and cool when it's warm.

Where to Buy

Just about any department or clothing store sells T-shirts and track suits. As for spandex you may need to check out a specialty store. You may not need to venture far to shop for your workout apparel. Many gyms these days have their own line of workout clothes. Some throw in a few freebies as a membership sales gimmick. Another option is to check out the latest issue of *MuscleMag International, Oxygen, Shape,* or other such magazine. Flip through and you'll see dozens of ads for workout clothes. Many of the top fitness and bodybuilding competitors have their own clothing line.

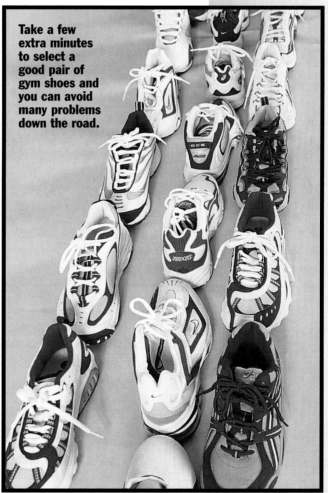

Take a few extra minutes to select a good pair of gym shoes and you can avoid many problems down the road.

Footwear

You probably have lots of experience buying shoes and high heels, but how many times in the past have you bought workout shoes? If you're like most newcomers to fitness, probably not often. Make the wrong choice and you run the risk of blisters, a lousy training experience, and possibly even an injury. It's that important. Take a few extra minutes to select a good pair of gym shoes and you can help avoid these problems down the road.

Cross-Trainers or Runners?

The best way to choose footwear is to define your primary form of fitness. If you are active in a variety of sports, a cross-trainer is your best bet. These shoes are versatile and provide average support for most foot motions. Cross-trainers are ideal for someone who combines weight training with aerobics classes and stationary machines.

If you participate in high-impact activities at least three times per week, you should purchase a shoe designed to handle that kind of heavy-duty stress, even if it means having more than one pair of gym shoes in your closet. Many people have natural imperfections in their landing or take-off. Constant repetition of such will take its toll.

Cross-trainers will provide some stability but are limited because they cover such a broad range of foot movements. Buying a sports-specific shoe will help counterbalance any naturally occurring problems.

For those who run more than twice a week, running shoes are an absolute must. This is a very high-impact activity that is laced with repetitive movements. Running shoes are designed to compensate for that wide variety in peoples' landing styles; many of which are anatomically incorrect.

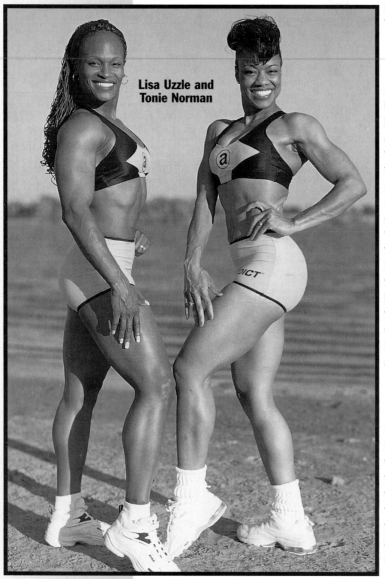

Lisa Uzzle and
Tonie Norman

The Feet Have It

Perhaps the first thing you should do before heading to the store is become better aquainted with your feet. There are three basic foot types – normal, flat and high-arched. The classification system is based on how your foot interacts with the ground. If you're unsure as to your foot type, a quick glance at an old pair of running shoes will give you an idea. If the center of the ball of your shoe is worn out, you have a normal foot and a neutral footstrike. If there is more wear behind the big toe, you likely have a flat foot and a tendency to pronate. Conversely more wear behind the little toe indicates a high arch and a supinator.

The Big Fix

If your primary form of aerobic activity is running, you have a lot to consider when choosing your shoe. Basically your feet perform three tasks when you run. They absorb shock, adapt to the ground, and assist in propelling you forward. If your feet lag behind in any of the three, it is up to your running shoes to help compensate. Most

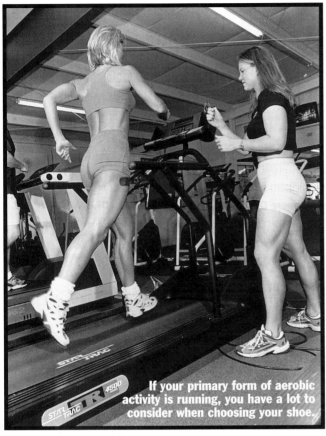

If your primary form of aerobic activity is running, you have a lot to consider when choosing your shoe.

runners land on their heels and roll inward in preparation for the foot to propel the body forward. The majority of problems occur with this inward roll.

If you roll to a vertical position, with the heel aligned directly under the lower leg, you are a neutral pronator. Therefore you want to choose a neutral shoe that combines cushioning with support.

If you roll too far or not far enough, extra stress is placed on the foot, which could lead to injuries if you don't buy footwear that will ease the problem. Over-pronators need to reduce the foot's inward roll, so they require motion-controlled or stability shoes. Motion-controlled footwear provides the most support and is best for severe over-pronators. Supinator's feet are poor shock absorbers and require a flexibility or cushioning shoe.

Shopping for a cross-trainer is less stressful. Your primary goals are comfort and ankle support. Since cross-trainers are designed to meet a wide variety of purposes, they will not adapt to make corrections for a specific foot type. If aerobics and racquet sports rank high, you need a cross-trainer with strong lateral support. If your workouts consist primarily of lifting weights and using stationary cardio equipment, lateral support is not as important.

Tips for Shopping

Armed with the previous information, it's now time to make that big purchase. Our first suggestion is to go to a specialty store. Most of the employees are active in sports and usually very knowledgeable about footwear. Clerks in large department stores tend to be more concerned about making the sale.

If possible try to avoid morning shopping. Your feet swell as the day goes on and if you buy shoes that fit early in the morning they will be too tight and uncomfortable later in the day. The one exception to this is if you work out early in the morning.

Here's another suggestion. Check the shoe fit wearing the same socks you will be wearing for your workouts. Again you want to mimic your workout habits.

The most important tip is to check and recheck the fit. The edge of your thumb should fit between your big toe and the top of your shoe. If not, the shoe is too tight. Conversely if your heels slide up and down when you walk or run, the shoe is too big. Many specialty stores now have treadmills for customers to test run their products. Hop on for a few minutes and alternate walking, jogging and running. If the shoe size or style is not right, your body will usually give you some warning signs.

A final suggestion is to invest a few extra dollars when buying your running shoes or cross-trainers. More expensive shoes usually have better material and will last far longer than the "$19.99 specials." Better quality shoes also tend to have better cushioning and support built in.

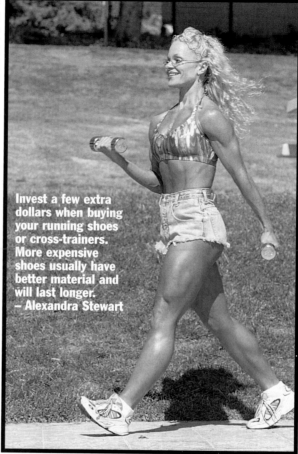

Invest a few extra dollars when buying your running shoes or cross-trainers. More expensive shoes usually have better material and will last longer.
– Alexandra Stewart

When to Train

The simplest answer to this question is "when it's convenient." Despite what you sometimes read or hear, there is no "best time" to train. For some 5:00 a.m. is the perfect time. For others, nothing ends a day like a good workout. The bottom line to any fitness program is consistency. As long as you are working out on a regular basis, it doesn't really matter what time you train, at least not from a physiological point of view. There is, however, one practical consideration. Most people train when it is most convenient. For many, especially those who work or attend classes, this time usually falls between 4:00 p.m. and 9:00 p.m. Go to any gym at 5:30 in the evening and it's a lesson in madness. Even before you walk into the gym you may have to fight for a parking space. Then you may have to take a number to get a piece of cardio equipment. The strength-training section is usually not as bad but you may have to modify your routine by changing exercises. Later in the book we'll be showing you different techniques and exercises to add variety to your workouts. Besides shocking the muscles, you will have a big selection to choose from when things get hectic in the gym.

Training Partners

Most things in life are more fun when done in a group. Weight training is no exception, and while many readers will opt for the solitary experience, others will find training with an accomplice more rewarding. What we are talking about here is training with a partner. It's great if you and your friend join the gym together – from day one you can work out side by side. Most readers, however, will need to recruit a training partner from the multitudes you meet.

There are numerous advantages to training with a partner. For starters a good training partner can *motivate* you on days when you just don't feel like training. You can then return the favor on her less than energetic days. Another advantage is *safety.* Although machines are safe, some free weight exercises are best done with a spotter nearby. You can rely on other members to help you out, but nothing beats a regular spotter who knows your every quirk and idiosyncrasy.

A third advantage to training partners is *intensity.* It's easy to get lazy when training alone. You'll save that extra rep or two to put the bar back on the rack, but a good training partner will make you do those couple of extra reps.

One less common benefit of training with a partner is the swapping of information. Unless one of you has been training for a much longer period of time, odds are you'll both know exercises and techniques that the other was unaware of. Within a few days of teaming up, you could both double your training knowledge.

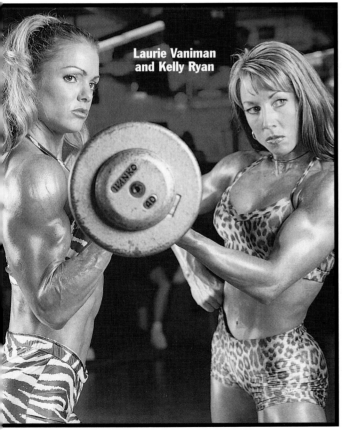

Laurie Vaniman and Kelly Ryan

"There aren't really any fitness competitors I can train with. And honestly, training with my boyfriend, because he's a man, makes me work harder to keep up. Of course we use different weights, but it pushes me harder."
– Michelle Brown, tenth-place Ms. Fitness USA competitor, offering her views on training partners.

Choosing a Good Training Partner

A whole list of variables must be addressed in order for a partnership to thrive. The most basic is *proximity.* If you train late in the evening and she prefers mornings, no matter how compatible you are, it just isn't gonna happen. You need to find someone whose daily schedule is very similar to your own. After a few weeks of training you'll notice the same faces arriving at the gym around the same time you do. From this pool you will choose your training partner.

Your next step is to make contact with someone who is following a similar training program to yours. Don't worry about a few exercise differences. One or both of you can modify your routine as things move along. Incidentally, some of the best gym partnerships happened by accident. Two people find they are constantly spotting one another on the same exercises and before they know it they are working out set for set.

One thing you may want to take into account is strength differences. Odds are most other women will fall within the same strength zone as you, but teaming up with a state or national powerlifting competitor might not be such a good idea. It won't create problems on machine exercises, as it's merely a matter of moving the pin to change the poundage. But having to constantly add and remove plates on barbell exercises can get annoying. It probably makes sense to team up with someone who is similar in strength to you (within 10 to 20 pounds on most exercises).

A final consideration is personality. Even though you may train at the same time, follow similar routines, and have similar strength levels, the two of you just may not click as partners because of personality differences. It's not that one of you is at fault. It's just that some personalities don't work well together, even though in all respects you are dealing with two normal people. Odds are you won't have to analyze this issue too closely as within one or two workouts you'll both realize that this partnership is not meant to be. Don't worry about it, it's a big pond.

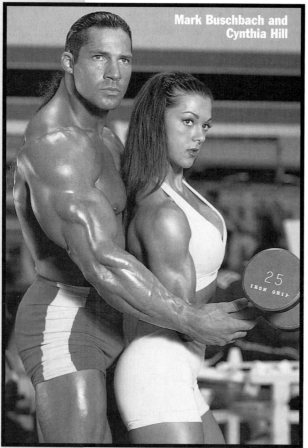

Mark Buschbach and Cynthia Hill

What About Him?

All of the previous may leave many readers wondering if a guy could make a good training partner. Well, the answer is – yes, why not! About the only negative aspect that might prevent a male-female training partnership from working is the strength differences. On average males are much stronger than females, particularly on upper-body exercises (although a few ladies these days can bury most guys in the gym!). That aspect alone should not end an otherwise productive partnership. The two of you can perform the exact same exercises and routines. You'll push yourself a tad harder to show him you're no slouch, and he's got the male ego of his to keep him motivated. The two of you can have your own battle of the sexes right then and there. And may we add, some of the best romantic relationships started right there at the squat rack!

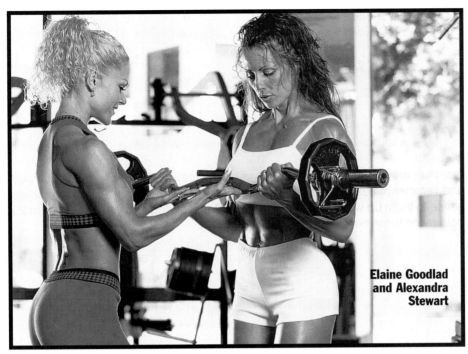

Elaine Goodlad
and Alexandra
Stewart

Tips for a Safe and Productive Workout

Before proceeding to the actual training section of this book, a few words on safety and etiquette are in order. Some may seem like common sense, but others may never have occurred to you. In any case adhering to the following will ensure your workouts are both safe and rewarding. If we start sounding like your parents, we apologize. But trust us, it's for your own good!

Hair

Learning by your own mistakes has its place, but not on this issue. Although most machines are designed to reduce this risk of getting your hair caught in a moving part, the risk is there nevertheless. The best example is the lat pulldown machine. Granted the pulley wheels are out of harm's way, but the same cannot be said for the bar itself – especially those bars that have the ends capable of swiveling around a center attachment. On numerous occasions the authors have observed individuals getting their hair caught in the bar as they pulled it down behind their head. Later we will be examining the merits and safety of behind-the-head pulldowns. Suffice to say, if you decide to perform the exercise in this manner, make sure your hair is tied out of the way.

Maxing Out

Maxing out is gym slang for trying to see how much weight you can hoist for one lift. The authors debated discussing the issue here as maxing out tends to almost exclusively practiced by the male species. We are after all the ones with the big egos to bruise! But given the importance of this issue we thought it couldn't hurt to at least comment on it.

There may come a point in your training when you start getting curious about just how much strength you have gained. In itself there's nothing wrong with this. In fact, where is it written that only males are allowed to test their strength? You've made great progress over the last few months so why not make a few tests. If you decide to test your strength on any of the primary lifts (squats, presses, deadlifts, etc.) always make sure you have a helper (called a spotter in gym jargon) on hand. That way if you miss the lift your partner can come to your rescue, so to speak. You

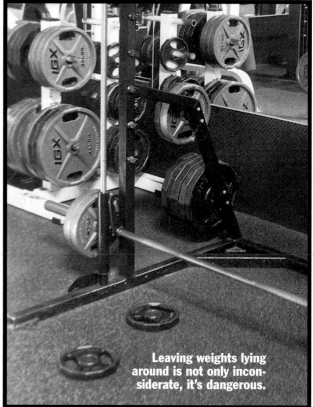

Leaving weights lying around is not only inconsiderate, it's dangerous.

have to ask yourself, however, if it's all worth it. Single max lifts don't do a whole lot for strength, size or conditioning. Even powerlifters usually practice singles only during the weeks leading up to a contest. Most of the year is spent in the 4 to 6 rep range. Attempting to lift a maximum weight places incredible stress on the joints, muscles, and associated structures and tissues. Even with proper technique the risk of injury is greatly increased.

House Cleaning

Nothing is as irritating to gym staff and members alike as someone who constantly leaves weights and equipment lying around. This practice is not only inconsiderate to other members, it's also downright dangerous. All it takes is for someone to step on a misplaced dumbell and you have a spinal injury or worse. The same goes for weight plates. They make excellent obstacles to trip over. Leaving barbells and plates on a rack is not as dangerous, but it's still being inconsiderate to the next person.

The best example here is the plate-loaded leg press. Every now and then some moron will leave 15 or 20 45-pound plates on the machine and go merrily on his way. If the next person needs only half that amount, he or she has to spend five minutes unloading plates. (Even if she *could* use all the weight, she'd still need to unload it for a couple of lighter warmup sets.)

Then there's the safety aspect to consider. Having to remove nearly a thousand pounds of weight is frustrating. You're in a pissed off mood to begin with and odds are you are going to try to do it as quick as possible. Sooner or later one of those 45-pound brutes will slip out of your hand and land on your foot. You'll end up with at least a blackened big toe, although numerous individuals have broken their toes or the foot itself.

At risk of sounding like your mother, *please clean up after yourself!* Not only will you reduce the risk of injury to the next person, but also the example you set can't but help rub off on other members.

Dropping Weights

Please refrain from dropping your weights onto the gym floor. The problem is not so much the noise but the damage you can cause to the floor or to the weights themselves. Granted there's not much risk of breaking an iron plate, but dumbells are another matter. If you drop a set of dumbells from any height (one foot or more), odds are both ends will not hit the floor at the same time. When one end strikes the floor first, it causes the handle to twist. At about $25 to $30 a shot, gym owners don't like to keep shelling out money for handle replacements because a few idiots keep dropping them. Besides the dumbells, there's the floor to consider. Many old gyms have wooden floors. In a contest between wood and iron, iron always wins. Even the new rubber athletic flooring can take only so much pounding before it starts to rip. Weight plates are especially dangerous as their edges are on the sharp side. When finished with your weights, *set* them down on the floor. There's no need to drop them from two or three feet up just to make a point.

Equipment Hogging

Equipment hogs rank right up there with those who leave their weights lying around. Most people who go to the gym have only a limited amount of time. There's nothing as bad as having to add an extra 15 to 20 minutes to your workout because a few individuals ahead of you decide to use the equipment as a place to socialize or take a nap. Even if someone wants to do more than 3 or 4 sets (groups of lifts) of a given exercise, there's no reason they can't let you work in. Conversely, if you are using a piece of equipment, always be mindful of others who may also want to use that machine.

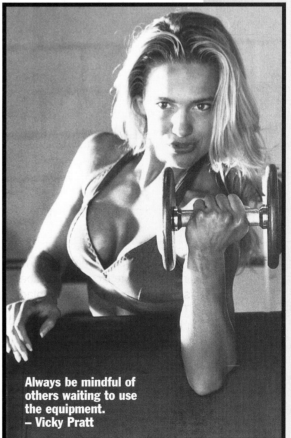

**Always be mindful of others waiting to use the equipment.
– Vicky Pratt**

Clean the Machines After You Use Them

Even in air-conditioned gyms most people work up a good sweat while training. As soon as the muscles start working, the body temperature goes up. This in turn causes the body to activate its cooling mechanisms. All would be nice if sweat went from the skin to the air, but things are not that neat. Many machines require you to sit, lie or hold on. The end result is a transfer of sweat to the machine. Most gyms have spray bottles and paper towels placed around for members to clean up after themselves. Nothing is as bad as going to the leg extension machine and seeing a river of sweat flowing down the backboard. Not only is it disgusting to look at but in this day and age it's downright unhealthy. Who knows what germs are contained in that liquid medium? As soon as you finish using any piece of equipment where your sweat gets left behind, please give it a wipe down for the next person.

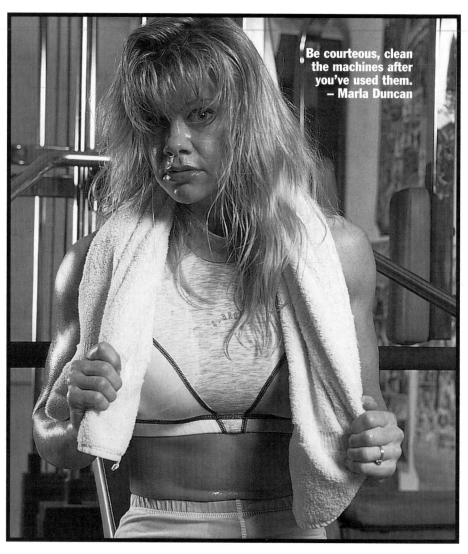

Be courteous, clean the machines after you've used them.
– Marla Duncan

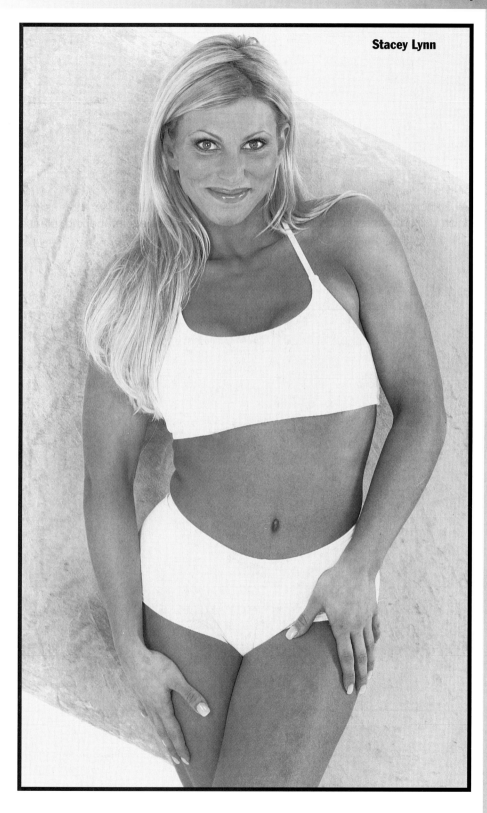

Stacey Lynn

CHAPTER TWO

*T*he Equipment

You may be surprised to learn that, like most other sports and forms of physical activity, weight training has a whole spectrum of equipment to choose from. Generally speaking these items can be divided into two categories, personal and gym. Although you will be required to use much of the gym equipment in your workouts, the use of personal equipment is not mandatory.

Personal Equipment

Belts

Perhaps the most well-known piece of personal equipment is the weightlifting belt. Contrary to popular belief, weightlifting belts won't allow you to hoist more weight, at least not physically. The primary function of a belt is to provide extra lower-back support on such exercises as presses, squats and rows. While being among the most effective exercises for working the muscles, these movements also put extra pressure on the lower spinal column. A belt acts as a brace and adds support to the region.

A lesser known benefit of belts is they keep the region warm. Like a blanket, a belt will keep the lower back a few degrees warmer, thus making it less susceptible to injuries.

We'd be remiss if we didn't point out the fact that there are mixed feelings within the world of weight training. Some experts argue that wearing a belt will only weaken the lower back by continuously keeping the stress away from it. They believe the old "use it or lose it" theory. The other argument is, some exercises place more stress on the lower back than it was designed to handle. Even with perfect technique, exercises such as squats, deadlifts and rows put stress on the lower spinal column.

Our view falls somewhere between the two. There's probably no need to wear a belt on every exercise, but on movements that bring the lower back into play, it's most likely a good idea.

Given all this, the next issue is how to select a good belt. As with most commercial goods these days there's a full spectrum of quality to choose from. At the lower end you have the $15 to $20 jobs that are mass produced and sold in

Monica Brant

most major department stores. As starter belts they are probably okay, but most belts in this price range tend to be flimsy. They are usually made out of very thin leather or imitation leather, and offer no more back support than if you had wrapped a towel around your waist. We should add that the price tag alone is not enough to judge a good belt. Some of the more expensive belts also fall victim to poor quality, especially some of those very colorful and stylish-looking Velcro belts. They may make you stand out in a gym, but most manufacturers don't even have the decency to use imitation leather, let alone the real deal. Some are nothing more than cloth or webbing material. In short, don't trade in lower-back support to make a fashion statement.

If you plan on making weight training a regular part of your life, we suggest you go out and buy a quality belt. Those made from thick leather are best, but some of the imitation leathers these days do come close. The best belts offer the advantage of stiffness, and hence good back support, while at the same time they conform to the shape of each individual's lower back. You can buy a good leather belt for between $30 and $50.

If money is no object, another option is to have a belt tailor-made. For a negotiated price ($50 to $70 seems to be the most common range) you can have a leather goods store custom make one for you. Of course you have to ask yourself if the extra expense is worth it. For most readers a middle of the road belt will probably suffice.

Gloves

Golfers have them, hockey players need them, and baseball players look stupid without them. Few sports these days can be played without some sort of hand protection, and weight training is no different. Most weightlifting exercises require you to grab and hold on to a bar, dumbell or handle. For those new to the activity a period of time will come when the skin on the hands will start to chafe and blister. When this happens you have two options; keep training and let the skin on the hands thicken and callous, or wear some sort of covering in the form of gloves. In fact it makes good sense to wear gloves from day one. Now some people view callusing as a right of passage, much the same as the old white-collar versus blue-collar hands look. But for others, having hands covered by layers of dead skin is nothing more than an annoyance. For musicians, models, and those who work with small objects (i.e. watchmakers), rough, callused hands are an impediment. What's the best solution? Wear a pair of weightlifting gloves.

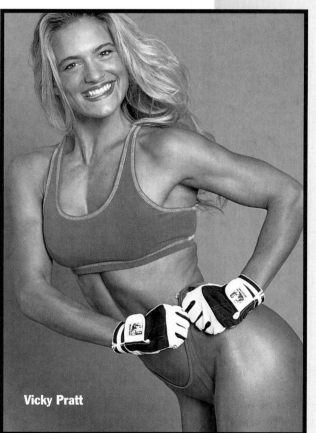

Vicky Pratt

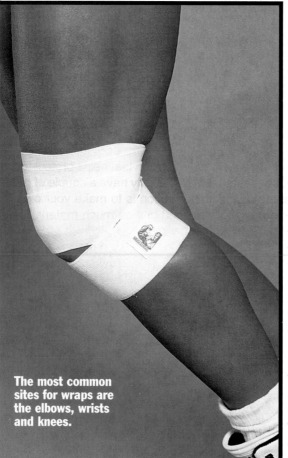

The most common sites for wraps are the elbows, wrists and knees.

Gloves come in many styles and makes, but most are made from leather or cloth. Many have the fingertips cut off to allow for a better grip. Most are tightened by either Velcro or a couple of metal fasteners.

While there's little debating the fact that gloves protect the hands, there are opposing viewpoints concerning the way they feel. Some argue that gloves prevent the user from getting as good a grip as with the bare hands. Others counter that they get a much better grip with gloves. During a workout it doesn't take long for the hands become very sweaty, making it difficult to hold on to a barbell or dumbell.

Before rushing out to buy a set of gloves, check around to see if someone will loan you a pair for a workout. After a few exercises you'll know if they are for you. If yes, look to spend about $15 to $20 for a good pair of gloves.

Wraps

Wraps fall into the same category as belts – you either swear by them or detest them. Wraps are pieces of bandage (2 to 5 inches wide) that are wrapped around joints to add extra support during exercises. The most common sites for wrapping are the elbows, wrists and knees. As with belts, wrapping has it desenters who argue that continuously wearing wraps takes too much stress away from the joints and never allows them to strengthen properly. The counter argument is that, despite perfect form, some exercises place abnormal amounts of stress on the joints, and wrapping serves as a sort of preventive medicine. Most top athletes these days believe in wearing wraps. Just take a close look the next time a sporting event comes on TV. You'll see 12-year-old gymnasts wrapped up like Egyptian mummies, and seven-foot basketball players wearing literally yards of bandage.

Most readers probably won't need to use wraps, but those who start going heavy on exercises such as squats, presses and rows, or have a pre-existing joint injury, may want to consider wrapping. Wraps are among the cheapest items of weight training equipment. You can pick up a set of wrapping bandages in most drug stores or sporting-goods stores for $5 to $10.

Straps

You'll soon discover that on certain movements your forearms tire out before the muscle you are trying to fatigue. On many exercises the forearms are the weakest link in the chain, so to speak. Even by performing direct forearm exercises to strengthen those particular muscles, there will be times when your grip gives out first. The best solution is to use a set of straps. Straps are narrow pieces of leather or webbing material (1 to 2 inches wide) that you wrap around the bar or handle, thus securing your hands in such a manner that the more you pull the tighter the straps get.

Straps are relatively cheap and can be purchased for $15 to $20. You can get more elaborate versions that have foam insulation that helps protect the wrists from chafing. We should add that most gyms usually have a couple of old sets kicking around for members to use. Another option is to make your own. For a few dollars you can go into a crafts store and buy as much material as you'll ever need. Cut the strips into 18 to 20-inch lengths and stitch a short loop at one end (just enough for one end of the strap to feed through). Some of the best straps we've seen were made from old martial arts belts.

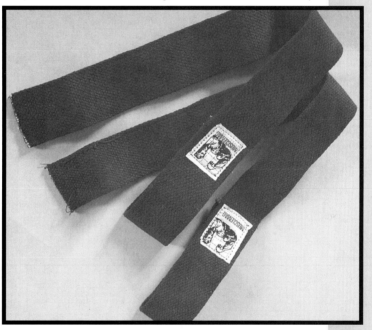

As with belts and wraps, the debate continues with regard to straps. You shouldn't use them on every exercise, as the forearms will never get a chance to strengthen on their own. But then again hand straps are invaluable on exercises such as pulldowns and rows.

Chalk

Chalk is another of those option where personal preference plays a big role. Gymnasts practically bathe in it. Likewise Olympic lifters go through copious amounts. Chalk is used to compensate for the moisture that builds up on the hands and makes holding on to a bar or handle difficult. In effect it's a drying agent. Chalk is relatively inexpensive and a couple of dollars will get you a large block of it. However, before rushing out and buying a block, check your gym's policy on chalk use. Health spas won't allow it through the door, while hardcore gyms often look like the White Cliffs of Dover. Fitness centers fall somewhere in between. Some will allow chalk, others ban it. A quick glance around the first time you go into the gym will answer the question. If in doubt, check with a staff member.

Headband

Laugh if you will, but there's a good reason for wearing a headband – sweat! Unless you've got glandular problems or the heart of a cold-blooded Republican, most readers are going to shed buckets of sweat during a typical workout. Nothing is as irritating as having to wipe the sweat from your face every few minutes. And for those with contact lenses or glasses the problem is compounded. Most sporting goods stores sell them for $5 to $10, or for mere pennies you can make a headband in any color, style or size you want.

Water Bottle

To replace the sweat, which you'll be continuously shedding, you have two options – the drinking fountain or a water bottle. A few words about water fountains. Depending on your gym, the fountain may be kept in good hygienic shape or it may be a cesspool of filth. Those who work out in older buildings have lead pipes to worry about. Now we are not trying to scare you away from water fountains, but do some quick math and you'll see that, on a typical day in a large gym, some thousand or more members will have their mouths in close proximity to the fountain. Some will cough, many will spit, and all will breathe on it. Given some of the diseases kicking around these days, it's probably a good idea to opt

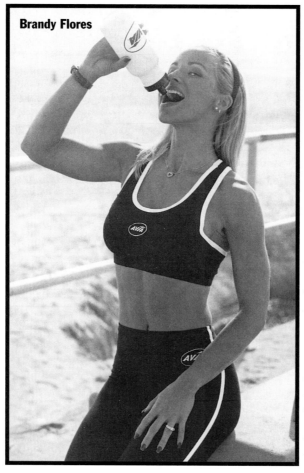

Brandy Flores

for the water bottle. For a couple of bucks you can pick up a 16- to 20-ounce plastic bottle that you'll only need to fill once or twice per workout. Even the container bottled water comes in can be reused. Many gyms will throw in a water bottle as a freebie for signing up. In our opinion, use your own water bottle. It's a small price to pay for preventing your body from becoming a breeding ground for bacteria or viruses.

Training Journal

One of the best ways to know where you are going is to know where you have been. Even though within a few weeks you'll probably memorize the exercises and weights you are using, it's still a good idea to write things down. For a few dollars you can pick

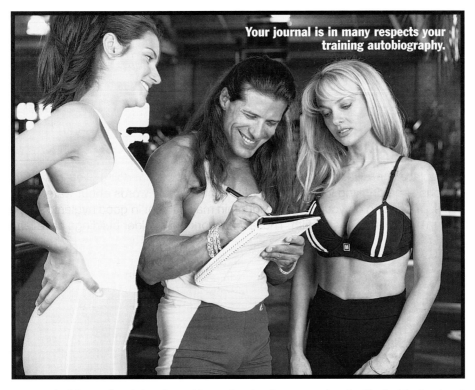

Your journal is in many respects your training autobiography.

up a spiral-bound notebook and keep track of your workouts. Probably the best reason for doing so is for comparison. Let's say in three months your progress has come to a halt. Flip through your notebook and see if anything jumps out at you. Are you using the exact same weights as when you started? Are you doing the same exercises? Have you done anything to shock your muscles? Is there a correlation between your workout energy and your eating habits that day? It's one thing to rely on memory, but having it all written down makes far more sense.

Another benefit of keeping a training journal is motivation. Let's say it's one of those days when you start questioning if it's all worthwhile. Simply flip back through your journal and take a look at how far you've come. Weights that you now warm up with were once your workout poundages. Your journal is in many respects your training autobiography.

Although you can record just about anything in your workout journal, here are a few suggestions:
1. Bodyweight (once a month)
2. Name of exercises
3. Poundages used on each exercise
4. Sets and reps for each exercise
5. How you felt that day
6. Your food intake that day
7. The time of the day you trained
8. The length of your workout
9. And of course, the date

"Ah ... excuse me, just one more thing."
– *television's lovable rain-coated Detective Columbo (Peter Falk) being his usual annoying self as he flips through his seemingly unorganized notebook.*

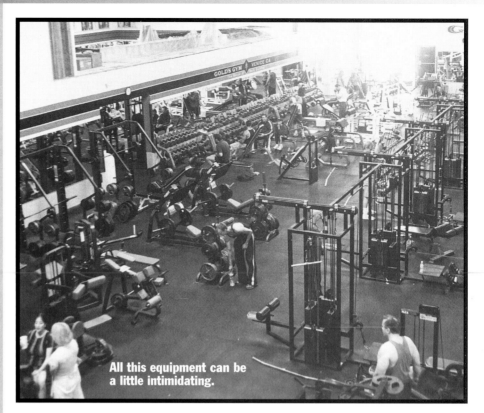

All this equipment can be a little intimidating.

Equipment – The Gym

Even though much of what we just discussed is optional, most of the items in the next section are mandatory if you hope to transform your physique. Your first day in the gym will be a combination of excitement and bewilderment. It's exciting because you are about to embark on a new quest; but it's also bewildering as where do you start? You have all this fancy chrome-plated equipment that seems to have no coherent function or purpose. Many people compare it to the torture machinery once popular in medieval castles. And you know something, depending on how you use it, you may do just that – torture yourself! Hopefully that's where we come in.

Machines

The most complex-looking equipment in any gym are the cardio and strength-training machines. As we'll be saying much more on cardio machines in the chapter on aerobic conditioning, we'll limit our discussion here to the strength machines.

Most gyms have the various machines arranged by upper and lower bodypart. Keep in mind the following is not meant to be an all-encompassing list. Nor will we go into great detail on exercise performance. Instead we'll simply give you a brief introduction to some of the machines you'll meet up with upon your first visit to the gym. Before long you'll realize that using them is as simple as riding a bike.

Leg Machines

Leg-training can be divided into three sections – thighs, hamstrings and calves. The two most common thigh exercises are the leg press and leg extension. With the leg press you are required to sit down straight or on a 45-degree angle and push a platform away from you. The leg extension consists of a chair where you place your feet under a set of rollers and lift upward. Virtually all gyms have at least one of each. Bigger gyms may also have a hack machine, in which you stand up but lean back on a slight angle, resting a set of pads on the shoulders. From that position you squat up and down.

The most common hamstrings machine in any gym is the lying leg curl. You lie face down on a flat pad with your legs stretched out behind you, heels hooked under a set of rollers. From there you bend the legs at the knees, curling your feet toward the butt. Some gyms have seated leg curls that are virtually opposite in appearance to the seated leg extension. Instead of starting the legs low and extending upward, you have the legs stretched out straight and curl down and back. Finally, your gym may have a standing leg curl machine. As the name implies, you stand up straight and with one knee resting on a support, curl the lower leg upward.

The two most common calf exercises are the standing and seated calf raises. The standing version consists of an upright machine with a platform and two pads that rest on your shoulders. Then it's simply a matter of keeping the legs straight and flexing up and down at the ankle while standing on the edge of the platform. For the seated calf machine you sit down and rest the pads on your knees. Again the movement consists of a simple up and down flexing at the ankle.

Upper Body

Even though the legs account for about 50 percent of the body's muscle mass, the greatest variety of exercise machines are for the upper body. The main reason is, the gripping ability of the hands allows for many different machine designs. The feet on the other hand can't hold on to bars or handles and must be either hooked under rollers (i.e. the leg extension and leg curl) or placed on a platform (leg press and calf raise).

The best example of upper body variety concerns the chest. There are flat pressing machines where you lie on your back and press straight upward. Incline machines have a pad usually angled at 30 to 45 degrees, enabling you to target the upper chest. Decline machines are just the opposite, targeting the lower

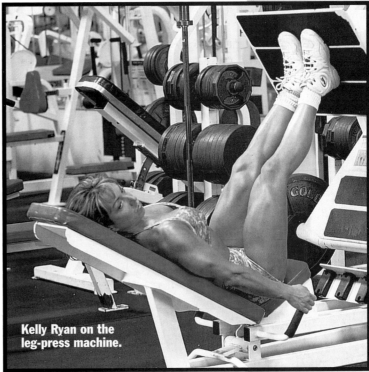

Kelly Ryan on the leg-press machine.

and outer chest. There are pec-dek machines that require you to sit up straight and by either holding a pair of handles or resting the forearms and elbows on pads push forward and inward in a hugging-type motion. Finally you have cable crossover machines that consist of two high cable pulleys. You stand between the pulleys and hold on to a set of handles which you draw forward and downward so they meet in front of your body.

We should add that, depending on the size of your gym, it may or may not have all these machines. Most gyms have a flat press, an incline press, and usually some sort of pec-dek and cable crossover machine. Items such as decline presses and vertical presses are usually found only in the biggest gyms.

Back-training consists of two primary pieces of equipment – the pulldown machine and the rowing machine. The lat pulldown is one of the most common types of apparatus you'll find in any gym. If yours doesn't have a lat pulldown, you might want to consider joining another gym. The machine consists of a long bar connected to an overhead cable and pulley system. You simply pull the bar down to the upper chest or behind the head (more on this later in the book).

Rowing machines come in three types – seated, vertical and T-bar. Seated rows consist of nothing more than a long flat bench that is resting on or just slightly above the floor. You sit down and grab a narrow handle attachment. With knees slightly bent, pull it into the lower rib cage. Vertical rows consist of a chair with an upright pad that you rest on the front of the body. Then it's just a matter of pulling a set of handles toward the body. T-bar rows are sort of in between seated and vertical rows. You lie face down on a pad (usually angled at 45 degrees) and pull a set of handles toward your upper body. Some gyms have older T-bars that don't have the bracing pad. For advanced trainers these may

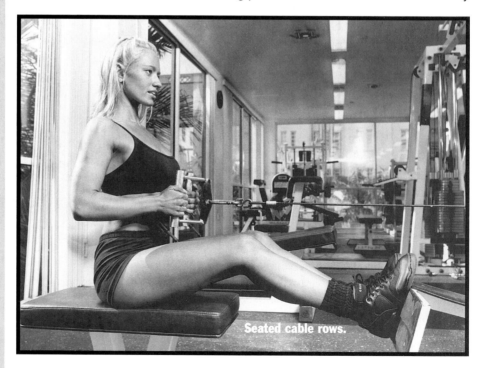

Seated cable rows.

be okay, but keep in mind that the absence of a pad means the lower back will take much of the strain. For some this helps strengthen the lower back muscles, for others it's a shortcut to traction therapy.

One final piece of equipment you may have access to is the assisted chinup machine. In this case you stand or kneel on a pad which is counterbalanced. That is it pushes upward as you pull yourself up to a bar or set of overhead handles. The theory behind this machine is that most people cannot do chinups using their entire bodyweight. Unlike most exercises where you can reduce the weight to complete a given number of lifts, chinups require you to hoist your entire bodyweight from day one. As most individuals can't do this, equipment manufacturers have designed machines that sort of act as helpers. Generally speaking whatever weight you put on the stack pushes upward with that much pressure. The goal is to use less and less weight as time goes on until you can lift your bodyweight. We should add that most people never get to the stage where they can do consecutive lifts with their entire bodyweight. And because of differences between the sexes with regard to upper body strength, women are at a disadvantage. Still the assisted chinup machines allow anyone regardless of strength to perform this great exercise.

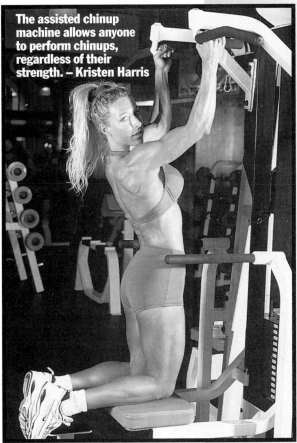

The assisted chinup machine allows anyone to perform chinups, regardless of their strength. – Kristen Harris

Shoulder machines can be divided into two groups – pressing and lateral raise machines. Shoulder press machines are similar to chest press machines in that you grab a set of handles and push away from the body, but instead of lying flat or on an incline, you sit up straight and push the arms above the head. Lateral raise machines also require you to sit or stand, but this time the arms are bent and resting beneath a set of pads, which you raise outward and upward.

Depending on your gym you may have access to biceps or triceps machines. Most designs require you to sit on a chair or bench and rest your arms on an incline pad. For biceps you grab a bar or set of handles with the arms stretched out, and curl the forearms toward you. For triceps it's just the opposite, you start with the arms close to the chest and push downward. We should add that, given their cost and relatively limited usage, most gyms don't have biceps and triceps machines.

The final category of machines your gym may have is abdominal and spinal erector (lower-back) machines. As with biceps and triceps, many gyms don't bother to make the financial investment in such equipment, preferring instead to let members do bodyweight exercises (crunches and back extensions).

Free Weights

Free weight is an all-encompassing term that refers to barbells and dumbells. Even though they have similarities, we'll discuss the two categories separately.

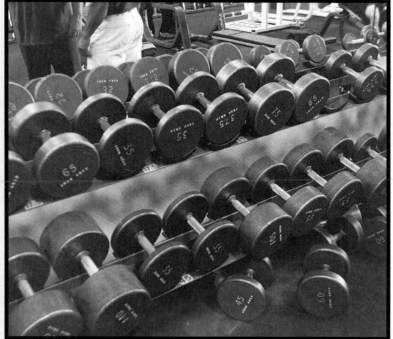

Dumbells

Dumbells are the junior member of the free weight family. They consist of a short bar that has one or more plates on each end. Any exercise that can be performed with a barbell can be duplicated with a pair of dumbells. Most dumbell exercises involve holding one in each hand, but a few can be performed with just one bell. The advantage of dumbells over a barbell is that they allow for a greater range of motion. In addition their small size enables you to move them in positions that would not be possible with the larger, bulkier barbell.

Dumbells come in many styles. The "professional" style is the familiar short bar with attached round plates. Many gyms also have one-piece dumbells that have the ends in a hexagon shape. Hexagon dumbells are great for gyms as they won't roll around on the floor, and their proportionally smaller ends make them more convenient for some exercises, particularly those done behind the head. The other popular type of dumbell is also one piece but the ends have the traditional round shape. Even though they are made in larger sizes, most gyms use the one-piece styles for weights of less than 50 pounds, and the professional style for everything over 50. Why is that? The primary reason is, the heavier dumbells have more stress placed on them, especially when they hit the floor. One-piece dumbells tend to break, whereas the professional styles are sturdier. Occasionally the handle will bend but then it's just a matter of removing the plates and loading them onto a new handle. Once a one-piece dumbell breaks or bends, it becomes just an oversize paperweight.

Barbells

Barbells are perhaps the most familiar piece of equipment in any gym and, like dumbells, they come in many different shapes and sizes. As they tend to be used for different exercises, we'll discuss them individually.

Olympic Barbells

These are the big brutes of the barbell fraternity. The next time you see some Bulgarian pocket Hercules hoisting three times his bodyweight over his head on

TV, the odds are good to excellent he's using an Olympic barbell. Olympic bars are the largest type of barbell. They are a little over seven feet in length and weight 45 pounds. They consist of two sections, the narrower but longer inner section you hold on to, and the two wider end pieces called sleeves. Olympic bars are designed to support enormous poundages and are usually rated for 750 or 1000 pounds. The plates that go on the ends of such bars have the holes cut out to exactly fit the diameter of the barbell sleeves. The plates come in six standard sizes, 2.5, 5, 10, 25, 35 and 45 pounds (some plates have the corresponding kilogram units marked on them as well). In large gyms, or

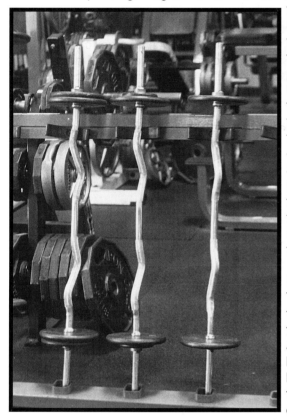

wherever a number of trainers may be lifting literally thousands of pounds, you may find 100-pound plates, but these are a rarity. Just hoisting a 100-pound plate from the rack to the bar is beyond the scope of the average trainer. (You'll see what we mean when you start adding a few 45-pounders to the leg press!) Olympic bars are used on such basic compound movements as squats, bench press, deadlifts, barbell rows and shoulder presses. A few hardy specimens may use them for curls, but for most people the length of the bar makes it too clumsy to work with.

EZ-Curl Bars
The awkwardness of the Olympic bar for many exercises has led manufacturers to produce smaller bars. In addition many individuals find straight bars hard on the wrists when doing biceps and triceps exercises. The solution to this problem is to use what's called an EZ-curl bar, which is shorter (about 3.5 feet long) and lighter than Olympic bars (20 to 25 pounds). EZ-curl bars also have four bends (two per side) that allow you to rotate the hands slightly inward. They are great for working the biceps and triceps and later in the book we'll be discussing their many uses.

Other Bars
Besides Olympic and EZ-curl bars most gyms have other types of bars that you can use for working out. To eliminate the inconvenience of having to add and remove plates, many gyms have fixed barbell sets. The bars are smaller than Olympic bars (4 to 5 feet long) and have the weight plates welded in place. The total weight of the bar plus plates is usually written on the ends and it's just a matter of selecting the poundage you want. These bars are usually found stacked in vertical or horizontal racks.

Less common but just as effective are similar bars that require you to add the weight plates yourself. To hold the plates in place, a set of metal collars or springs is used. Besides their shorter length, these bars have a smaller diameter than the Olympic bars, allowing you to get a better grip. Keep in mind the smaller diameter. The plates that fit on the Olympic bars won't fit on these bars, the hole in the plates is too large. Instead you'll need the specially designed plates that have the correspondingly smaller holes.

Benches

A simple movement like barbell curls or dumbell lateral raises can be performed without the assistance of any additional equipment. It's simply a case of grab it and go. But exercises such as squats, bench presses and shoulder presses necessitate the use of some sort of support rack.

The simplest piece of equipment to assist your free-weight workouts is a bench. Nothing complicated here, just a long support (four to five feet) that you can lie down on to work out. Benches come in many different styles. Fixed benches are those where the angle is preset and cannot be changed. They may be flat (horizontal to the floor), inclined or declined. The last two need a slight clarification. Inclined means the head is higher than the feet as you lie back on

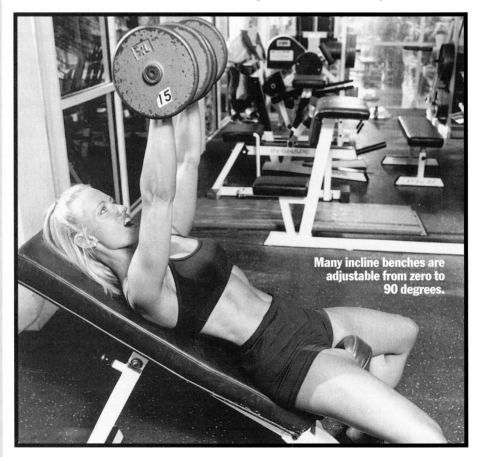

Many incline benches are adjustable from zero to 90 degrees.

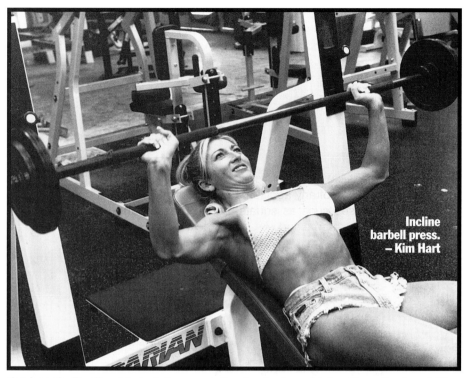

Incline
barbell press.
– Kim Hart

the bench. Declined is just the opposite, the feet are higher than the head. The angle may be the same (30 to 45 degrees being the most common) but the relative positions of the head and feet opposite. Keep in mind that incline and decline are relative terms and a decline bench can be used as an incline bench and vice versa. One thing to note is that, as you decline the body, there is a tendency to "fall" backwards (good old gravity). Properly designed decline benches usually have a set of rollers at the top so you can hook your feet in under to keep you from slipping off the bench. This is not an issue with incline benches as your feet are already on the ground and give you all the support you need.

Even though fixed benches have their place, most gyms complement them with adjustable benches. As the name suggests, adjustable benches allow you to change the angle from zero to 90 degrees. The advantage here is that most individuals have their favorite angles for doing exercises. For example many find 45 degrees too steep for hitting the upper chest. Instead the front deltoids do most of the work. The opposite is also true, anything less than 20 to 25 degrees tends to be too shallow for most when trying to stimulate the upper chest.

The next step up in complexity are benches with attached support structures commonly called racks. Let's use the flat barbell bench press as an example. If you try doing the exercise with just a flat bench you'll need to take the bar from the floor, position it on your thighs, and then lie back on the bench. After performing your set you do the reverse. You have to try to get the weight to your thighs, sit up and then place the bar back on the floor. You may be able to struggle through all this for the first couple of weeks, but the day quickly comes when you'll be using more weight than you can comfortably lift from the floor. Wouldn't it be nice if you could lie back on a bench and have the bar already positioned above you? Well guess what, virtually all gyms have what are called bench-press racks. They consist of a long, flat bench with a pair of uprights welded to one end. The uprights usually have a series of pegs so you can load your barbell on them and then lie down on the bench underneath. From there it's just a simple matter of grabbing the bar, doing your set, and then placing it back on the rack. As a safety precaution most bench racks have a set of pegs set down low, just above the average person's chest height. If you fail on your last rep and can't extend your arms back out full, you can "rack" the bar on the low pegs.

As you might imagine, incline barbell presses present the same problems as flat presses and there is a similarly designed bench that also allows you to rack the barbell above your head. Likewise shoulder presses also have their own rack, with the "bench" in this case being vertical. Less common are decline racks.

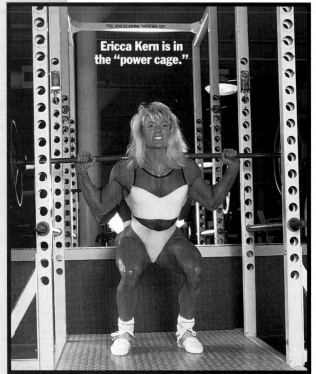

Ericca Kern is in the "power cage."

If bench pressing requires the use of a support rack, then for squatting a rack is mandatory. Most women squat with between 100 and 200 pounds, and the average guy goes 250 or 300. But there's no way you could hoist that much weight from the floor and lay it on your shoulders. Squat racks are very similar to bench-pressing racks but without the bench. Some are nothing more than a pair of upright bars with a hollow depression on the top to support the bar. Others are more elaborate and are sloped toward you with a series of catch pegs running down the front supports. If you get stuck in the down position it's just a matter of falling forward until the bar comes up against the closest pegs.

The safest squat racks are what are commonly called "power cages." These are large racks that consist of four thick iron uprights connected by a series of crossbeams. In effect you have to get inside an iron box. Besides the usual pegs to place the bar onto (often one set of movable pegs), there are usually two long bars that you can place horizontally from front to back on the sides. The plan is to set the bars a couple of inches below your maximum squat depth. That way if you get stuck it's only down a few inches to safety.

We should add that power racks could be used for just about any barbell exercises that require a support rack. Don't let the size and location of the power rack scare you either. Yes, we know it tends to be inhabited by a few colorful characters, but women have just as much right to it as guys. Now it's probably not a good idea to use the power rack for an exercise that could be done just as easily somewhere else (i.e. barbell curls), but for squats, shrugs, presses, etc. it's fair game. Odds are, once you demonstrate that you're capable of training just as hard as the guys train, you'll quickly be accepted as one of the "fraternity." You may even get guys coming up to you during workouts and asking you to give them a spot!

The Scott Bench or Preacher Bench

The preacher bench is a specially designed piece of equipment that is almost exclusively used for training the biceps. It consists of a small bench or stool connected to an inclined pad on which you rest your elbows and upper arms. The preacher bench is great for targeting the lower biceps and the pad prevents you from swinging the upper body. Up until the mid to late 1960s the bench was exclusively called the preacher bench, but then along came the world's first Mr. Olympia, Larry Scott. When word got around that Larry relied heavily on the bench to build his great biceps, the name "Scott bench" became just as common.

What's Best?

Up to this point we've only touched the surface with regard to equipment. Most gyms also have an assortment of cable machines and plate-loaded machines (machines where you add round plates as opposed to selecting the weight with a pin). Despite the variations in design, most machines work in essentially the same manner. And despite what sales people claim, most lines of equipment are comparable in terms of effectiveness. Some brands may have a better warranty and track record, but don't feel that because your gym has brand A and the gym down the street has brand B, you are missing out on something. Unless you make it to the elite athletic level and need a specific piece of apparatus to isolate a small muscle group, your gym's line of equipment will work just fine.

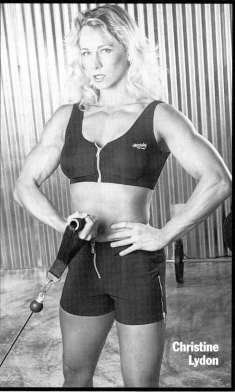

Christine
Lydon

Having said all that, the question that frequently gets asked by beginners (and many confused intermediate and advanced trainers as well) is – which is better, machines or free weights? The answer is – *it all depends!*

Machines and free weights both have advantages and disadvantages. The nice thing about machines is safety. With few exceptions most machines won't allow you to get "trapped" underneath. If you can't lift the handles or bar to the starting position you simply let go and walk away. Try doing that on a set of squats or barbell presses and you'll have a much bigger problem on your hands. Individuals have been found dead in their basements with a barbell across their necks. Collapsing on a set of squats without the benefit of a power rack could put you in therapy for six months. Not that we are trying to scare you away from free weights, but they do require a tad more concentration and care. They don't give you the same margin of error as machines do.

Besides safety, machines have another advantage. There are a number of movements that just cannot be duplicated with barbells and dumbells. The lat pulldown is a fine example. The free weight version of this exercise is the chinup. Now most people are not capable of lifting their entire bodyweight up to an overhead bar. Unless there's an assisted chinup machine in the gym (not high on the priority list of many gym owners), a great exercise must be eliminated from the routine. The lat pulldown, however, is a close second in terms of effectiveness. Instead of grabbing a bar and hoisting the body up, the body stays stationary and the bar comes down. There's no way to duplicate this exercise with a barbell or set of dumbells.

Another example is the leg curl (all versions). You may be able to hold a dumbell or weight plate between the feet and work the hamstrings, but it's very awkward. The leg-curl machine, however, has a set of padded rollers that fit neatly under your heels and allow you to do the exercise in comfort. Even die-hard free weight proponents spend most of their time using machines to hit the hamstrings.

A final benefit of machines is their simplicity. Even though we suggest asking an instructor when in doubt, most machines have their operating instructions posted on the top. In most cases it's fairly easy to figure out how to use the machine. Free weight exercises on the other hand require much more skill. A careful study of the instructions and photos throughout this book is a good way to start, but we'll admit it makes good sense to check with a qualified instructor for the finer points.

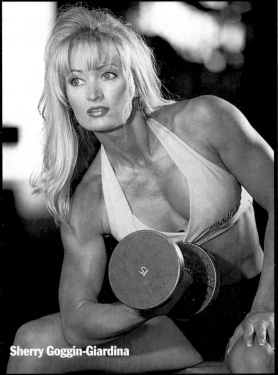

Sherry Goggin-Giardina

So far it sounds like we're trying to steer you clear of barbells and dumbells in favor of machines, but the old free weights have much to offer. Let's start with effectiveness. Even though some of the newer lines like Atlantis and Hammer Strength come close, few machines can duplicate a free weight exercise. Yes, it's possible for a machine to effectively target the larger muscle groups, but there's more to lifting a weight than using a primary muscle – you have all those secondary or stabilizing muscles to consider. Most machines only require you to lift the weight; they don't require you to balance the weight. But barbells and dumbells require you to *lift and balance.* This is why they are called free weights – they are not connected to cables, pulleys, or any other form of support. As soon as you start lifting a free weight both the primary and secondary muscles come into play. Most strength-training experts believe that free weights have the edge when it comes to effectiveness.

Another advantage to free weights is their versatility. Most machines can be used to hit only one or two muscle groups, while a barbell or set of dumbells can be adapted to hit the whole body. With the exception of the previously mentioned hamstrings (and perhaps the calves) free weights can be utilized to hit any muscle.

And finally a practical advantage to free weights – they are usually fairly easy to get at. With the exception of the large gyms, most facilities have only one or two of each machine. Unless you work out at down times, you may have to wait around to get at that pec-dek or shoulder-press machine. Most gyms, however, have two or three sets of each dumbell weight. And even if you can't get the 10s, it's no big deal going up to the 12s or back to the 8s for once. The same goes for benches, as most gyms have literally dozens of flat, incline and adjustable benches.

So which will it be, free weights or machines? Our suggestion is to use both. Every top fitness star, bodybuilder and elite athlete includes both forms of training in their routines. Later in the book we'll suggest numerous examples of mixed, free weight-only and machine-only routines. The nice thing about being comfortable with both types of exercise is that you'll be able to add much more variety to your workouts. Not only will this make your training time more effective but it will also be more fun, and in the opinion of the authors that's half the battle.

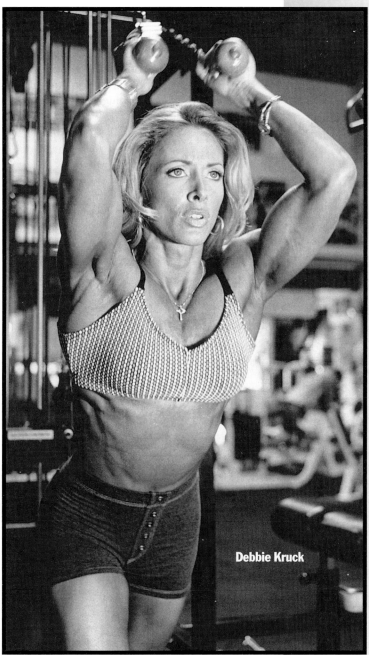

Debbie Kruck

CHAPTER THREE

Exercise Fundamentals

In some respects you've got 50 percent of the battle won; you're at the gym. Most of the population (over 90 percent by most estimates) do little or no exercise, so give yourself a pat on the back for taking those first steps toward a healthier lifestyle.

This chapter is in many respects the cornerstone for everything that follows. Before diving into the actual principles of strength training, we need to lay down a sort of vocabulary foundation. Just as most forms of exercise and athletics have their own terminology, so too do strength trainers like to communicate in their unique jargon. It won't be long, however, before you'll be talking "sets and reps" as a second language.

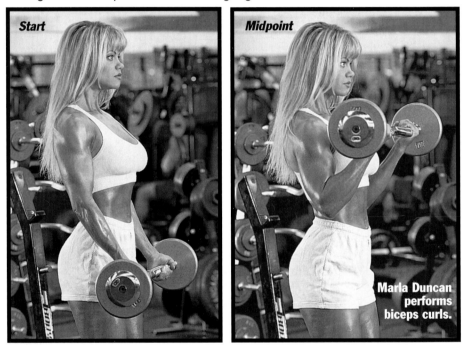

Start

Midpoint

Marla Duncan performs biceps curls.

Reps

The term *rep* can be considered the atom of strength training. It is perhaps the most basic word you'll need to know. In simple terms a rep is one complete movement of a given exercise. If for example you were doing biceps curls, you raise the bar up to the midpoint (positive portion of the rep), and then back down to the starting position (negative portion) – that is considered one rep. We know a few people who cut corners and consider the up and the down as two separate reps, but they are the exception.

Tempo

Tempo is just a fancy word to describe the speed at which you perform reps. Go into any gym and you'll see people hoisting and dropping weights in all sorts of haphazard ways. Hopefully most readers can see the folly of such practices. Just think about it for a moment. In the space of a couple of seconds the weight makes a complete 180-degree change in direction. The faster you go the more momentum is built up and placed on the joints. In effect the ligaments, cartilage and other soft tissue surrounding the joints are being used as elastic bands. Sooner or later these areas start fighting back in the form of injuries. That's why so many athletic careers are cut short. Most sports require rapid starts and sudden stops, which places more stress on the joints than they were designed to handle. Weight training can be a life-long activity – provided you follow safety guidelines.

Generally speaking one rep takes about five seconds to complete. This breaks down into two seconds to raise the weight, a one-second pause at the top, and another two seconds to lower the weight back down. Of course this is just one of the rep schemes you can follow. Up until about ten years ago rep tempo referred to the total time it took to perform one rep. Nowadays strength researchers and writers actually break the rep down into individual phases (up, pause and down). As expected exercising has become so precise that the topic of reps can now be represented in mathematical terms. The previous example could be expressed in the following manner: 2-1-2. Other rep schemes could be written as: 1-1-3, 1-1-5, 1-0-2.

In all cases the first number represents the time it takes to raise the weight, the middle number is the pause (if any), and the third number is the time it takes to lower the weight. Unless stated, the rep tempo used in this book is the standard 2-1-2 scheme. What's nice about this scheme is that it's fairly easy to do without having to count numbers. Basically, take a couple of seconds to raise the weight and an equal number to lower it. This will ensure you are doing the exercise in a safe and productive manner.

How Many Reps Per Set?

One of the most contentious issues in strength training is the number of consecutive reps to perform. Even though you hear different viewpoints, generally speaking the best rep range for strength and conditioning is 8 to 12. Lower reps (4 to 6) are best for pure strength, while anything higher is more of a cardio workout (and a poor one at that). We should add that 8 to 12 is the average range. Some individuals need to go lower than that with a heavier weight to get adequate

Jamie Santa Cruz

muscle stimulation. Others find just the opposite and anything less than 15 to 20 reps per set is useless for them. Despite what you'll read in this book and others, the bottom line is *experimentation.* Everyone is different and it takes time to discover what works best for you.

Sets

If reps are the atoms of the strength-training world, then sets are the molecules. As we mentioned earlier, reps are put together in consecutive groups. A set is simply a name for a group of continuous reps. The typical numbers of sets per exercise is 3 but some individuals do as many as 10 and as few as one.

The length of time to rest between sets is also debatable, but here's a good rule of thumb. Rest long enough to recover your breath but not long enough for the muscles to cool down. For most people this works out to about 60 seconds. On a larger muscle group like the legs, particularly thighs, you may need to rest 90 seconds to two minutes, while on a smaller muscle you might recover in 30 seconds. It's going to take you a few workouts to get a feel for your individual recovery system, but don't be surprised if 60 seconds feels about right.

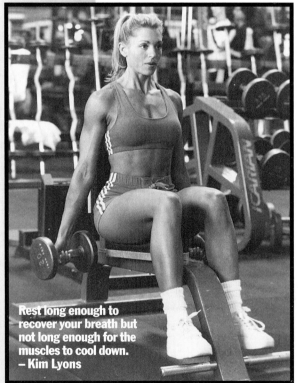

Rest long enough to recover your breath but not long enough for the muscles to cool down. – Kim Lyons

Breathing

It may seem strange to talk about something as basic as breathing, but even this life-giving procedure stirs up controversy. Some writers and personal trainers make a big deal and insist you pay special attention to your breathing. They are correct but only to a certain extent. Yes, you must breathe while doing reps, preferably on every rep, but there's probably no need to count breaths. You've been breathing since the day the doctor smacked your behind and said to your mom, "It's a girl." In over 20 years of strength training, neither of the authors has ever seen anyone pass out because she forgot to breathe. You have enough to concentrate on without worrying about something the body does automatically.

The one exception here is for those who have a habit of holding their breath. A few individuals will hold their breath for 3 or 4 reps before inhaling. Although rare, it is possible to put the body into oxygen debt and you could faint. Holding for 1 or 2 reps is no big deal, and in fact on heavy exercises like squats and leg presses it's almost impossible not to hold your breath. But if you are one of those who breathe two or three times per set, you may want to concentrate on exhaling as you lift or press. In simple terms you "blow the weight up."

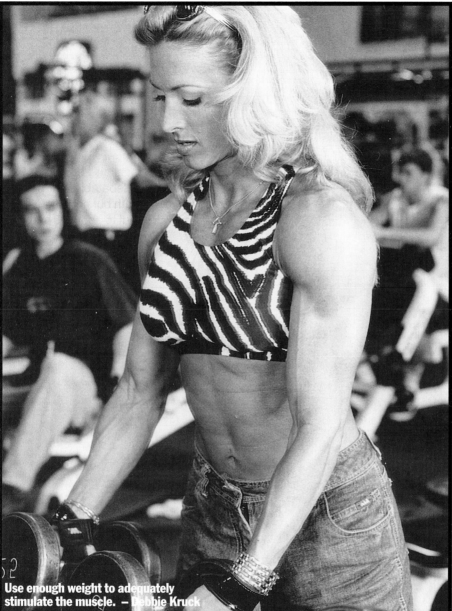

Use enough weight to adequately stimulate the muscle. — Debbie Kruck

Choosing Your Weight

One of the prevailing myths about weight training is that light weights and high reps increase the muscle tone and definition of a given area. Even many TV shows and magazine articles promote the theory "spot reducing is possible." It would be great if we could selectively target an area and shrink it, but the body doesn't work that way. The word *tone* does not mean to shrink, increase definition in the area, or change the shape.

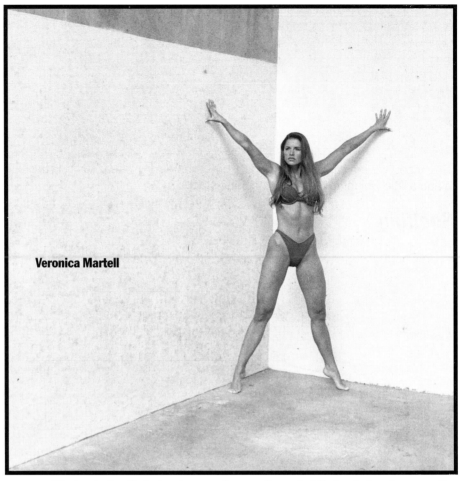

Veronica Martell

Toning is the first step in muscle growth and at its basic level means the muscles becomes firmer and harder. Doing high reps on, say, your triceps exercises won't increase the separation in that area. It won't cause the fat deposits there to suddenly disappear. The body is not selective when it converts stored fat into usable energy. It takes fat from all over the body. Actually five minutes of cardio training will probably do more for increasing the definition of the triceps than 15 or 20 high-rep sets of direct triceps exercise.

What does all this have to do with choosing your poundage? It means you must use enough weight to adequately stimulate the muscle. Strength training is just that – *strength* training. It's not cardio training, at least not in the traditional sense. Doing 15 or 20 reps with a really light weight will do virtually nothing to increase muscle strength or tone. The weight you select should be sufficient to bring the muscle to failure by the end of the set. If you are doing a set of 12 reps, the muscle should start tiring around rep 8 or 9. Then you have to work (but not strain) to get the last 3 or 4 reps. It's no use picking a weight that would allow you to get 20 reps but stopping at 12. The goal is to force the muscle to do some serious work so that during the recovery phase it rebuilds itself a little bigger and stronger.

Again we must stress the following: While women are capable of proportionally gaining as much strength as men gain, there's no way females will build the same degree of muscle mass as males. This is one of the biggest fears women have when it comes to strength training. Personal trainers are constantly hearing their female clients say, "Now I don't want to bulk up, just some muscle tone." It probably doesn't help matters when the first thing many women see upon entering the gym for the first time is some steroid-laced female bodybuilder sporting a physique that would win the Mr. America, 30 years ago. All we can say is, trust us. You won't sprout 20-inch biceps and a 50-inch chest a few months down the road. That is what many of the guys are aiming for and even most of them can't accomplish it. You have nothing to fear so don't hesitate to add a little weight to the bar or machine stack.

Spotting

Spotting is just gym jargon for lending a helping hand. On many exercises, particularly free-weight movements, the possibility exists that you could get stuck under the weight. For example losing control on a bench press leaves you looking a tad foolish with the bar across your chest. Squats are worse as you could literally collapse and do some serious damage to the spine. Having a helper or spotter handy ensures that if ever you get into difficulty she will come to your aid.

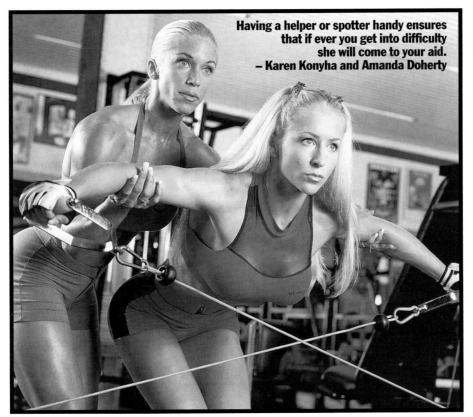

Having a helper or spotter handy ensures that if ever you get into difficulty she will come to your aid.
– Karen Konyha and Amanda Doherty

CHAPTER FOUR

Warming Up

Why Warm Up?

Although there are many benefits to warming up, most individuals spend little or no time getting ready for exercise. As the name implies, warming up raises body temperature. This temperature elevation reduces the risk of muscle and connective tissue injuries. In addition, increased blood flow to the muscles aids in the delivery of fuels required for muscle performance.

Those of you living in northern climates know how your car behaves on a cold winter's morning. Although most cars will let you turn the key and drive away, it's a good practice to let the car warm up for a few minutes. This helps circulate the various fluids that are essential to your car's running well. Cold fluids don't flow as easily as warm fluids, and that bucking, sputtering and coughing noise a car makes on a frigid day is a classic symptom of poor circulation.

Please excuse the previous introduction to auto-mechanics, but your body works much the same way. It operates more efficiently when it's properly warmed up. Your workouts will not only be more productive, they'll be safer. Think of your muscles as elastic bands. Throw an elastic in the fridge for a few hours and then try to stretch it. It will probably only stretch part way, but more than likely it will break. The body's muscles are in some ways like giant elastic bands; they stretch better when warm.

Warming up for a few minutes before a workout or a game is good preparation for both mind and body. Warming up sends your brain a wake-up signal and gets your body ready for more strenuous exercise. It's also a good way to avoid pulling a muscle, which can easily happen if you exert yourself suddenly. Many injuries can also be avoided with proper conditioning before the workout. A good way to start your warm up is with a series of stretching exercises. But remember, stretching should always be done slowly and carefully.

Mocha Lee

Light jogging and easy calisthenics reduce muscle tightness which limits mechanical efficiency and muscle power. Earlier onset of sweating promotes evaporative heat loss and as a result decreases the amount of heat stored by the body, helping to prevent body temperature from rising to dangerously high levels during more strenuous exercise. A proper warmup also prepares the cardiovascular and muscular systems for the upcoming physical activity and provides a transition from rest to strenuous exercise. This precaution may reduce the likelihood of excessive muscular soreness from strenuous activity.

Studies have also shown that warming up increases the speed of nerve impulses to muscles, enabling faster reaction times. This is one reason why professional athletes spend more time warming up compared to many recreational athletes. They know it will prevent injuries and help them compete better.

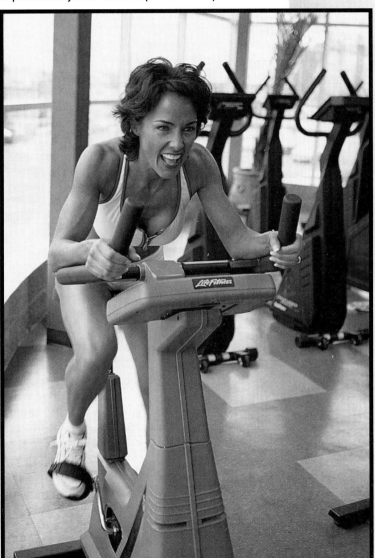

There is no secret to a good warmup. Any of the cardio machines in your gym will suffice. Begin by exercising slowly for three to five minutes or until a light sweat starts to form. Then slowly stretch the muscles you will be using. Each stretch should be held for 15 to 30 seconds without bouncing.

The primary goal of stretching exercises is to improve flexibility. Flexibility, combined with aerobic conditioning and strength training are the three broad objectives on which to focus as you maintain your body for the rigors and enjoyment of exercising. Proper stretching actually lengthens the muscle tissue, making it less tight and therefore less prone to trauma and tears. Oh, and did we tell you a proper stretching routine also feels good and can be the most relaxing period of your day?

There is no secret to a good warmup. Any of the cardio machines in your gym will suffice. – Colleen Sauvé

Stretching Hamstring Muscles

Stretching this muscle will help lessen the chance of knee injury.

Hamstring stretch – Sit on the floor and place the leg you wish to stretch straight out in front of you.

Then bend the other leg alongside to make a triangle with your legs. With a straight back, bend from your hips and reach for the toe of your straight leg with both hands. Hold for 20 seconds.

Achilles stretch – Stand facing a wall with one leg in front of the other. The front knee is bent, hands are on the wall. The back leg is straight with the heel flat on the floor. Lean toward the front knee, keeping the back foot and heel flat. Hold for 15 to 20 seconds. Relax. Repeat with the other leg.

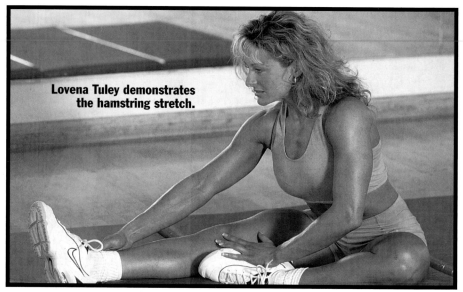

Lovena Tuley demonstrates the hamstring stretch.

Stretching Groin Muscles

The groin stretch will improve flexibility and allow the legs a larger range of motion. Here are two ways to stretch the groin, which is the muscle in the fold between the lower part (the trunk) of your body and your upper thigh.

Groin stretch – Sit on the floor or ground. Put the soles of your feet together, with your knees as close as possible to the floor and pointed outward. Grasp your ankles and hold that position for a count of 10. Relax and repeat three times.

Spread groin stretch – Start in a sitting position with your legs spread apart. Place your hands on the insides of your legs, and try to reach the insides of your ankles. Bend forward from the hips, keeping your knees flat. Hold until you feel tightness on the insides of your legs. Relax and repeat.

Stretching Calf Muscles

Calf stretch – Get in a push-up position, but with one knee on the ground. Put your weight on the toes of your other foot, then push the heel down until you feel a slight pull. Hold that position for a count of 10. Relax and repeat three times for each leg.

Calf raise – This stretch is used to strengthen the lower leg and ankle. Stand with your hands on your hips or on the back of a chair for balance. Spread your feet six to 12 inches apart and slowly raise your body up on the toes, lifting the heels. Return to the starting position and repeat 10 to 15 times.

Stretching Back Muscles

Back stretch – Here's how to stretch the back muscles. Lying on your back, raise one leg, grab the leg right below the knee, and slowly bring it up to your chest. Keep your other leg straight and your head on the ground. Hold this position for a count of 10. Repeat three times with each leg.

Stretching Shoulder Muscles

Shoulder stretch #1 – Move one arm across your body, almost as if you were going to take a backhand swing. Grasp the elbow of the arm in motion with your other hand and gently pull the arm further across your body. Hold for a count of 10 and repeat three times for each arm.

Shoulder stretch #2 – Interlace your fingers above your head. With the palms facing up, push your arms up and back gently. Hold for 15 seconds.

Shoulder stretch #3 – With your arms over-head, hold the elbow of one arm with the hand of the other arm. Gently pull your elbow behind your head, creating a stretch. Hold for 15 seconds.

Shoulder stretch #4 – With your arms extended overhead, hold the outside of your left hand with your right hand. Keeping your arms as straight and comfortable as possible, pull the left arm to the right side. Hold this stretch for 15 seconds on each side.

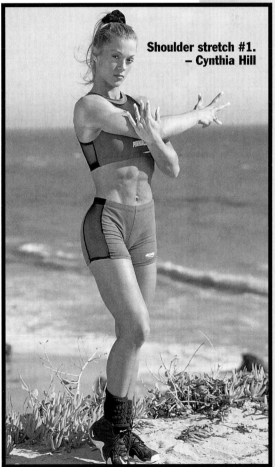

Shoulder stretch #1.
– Cynthia Hill

Biology – Knowing What You Are

Much of the following may bring back memories of high school biology class, so there is a use for what you learned in the lab after all. Chapter Five is only meant as a brief introduction to human biology. We have no intention of reproducing *Gray's Anatomy,* nor do we wish to bore you with topics that have little or no relevance in your life. Instead we included a few choice topics that we felt related specifically to fitness and aging. Our sincere apologies to the academics among you!

Exercise and Biology – The Inseparable Twosome

In addition to psychological and emotional benefits, exercise is essential for physical health. Physical benefits to the cardiovascular, respiratory system and musculoskeletal system are well documented. Understand the ways in which the body responds to exercise, and why, and you will understand the rationale behind the training techniques presented in this book. Until recently medical studies would arbitrarily select one sex for clinical trials and extrapolate the results to both. Differences in basic biology are now recognized as medically important in the pathology and treatment of disease. Consider the following examples:

- Men and women display different symptoms of heart attack. Chest pain is most common in men while women's symptoms are subtle, often being generalized fatigue, abdominal pain and nausea.
- Women with irritable bowel syndrome will respond better to a serotonin receptor antagonist than men.

Stacey Lynn

"When choosing between two evils, I always like to try the one I've never tried before."
– Mae West (1892-1980)

• Ibuprofen is not as effective as a pain reliever in women as in men.

• Nicotine replacement therapy is more effective in men than women.

• Women metabolize alcohol more slowly than men do because they make less gastric alcohol dehydrogenase. Therefore, less alcohol intake is required in women to reach the same blood alcohol level.

• Some language functions are active in both sides of a woman's brain but only in one hemisphere in men.

• Women experience depression two to three times more often than men, which may be due, in part, to a much lower rate of serotonin synthesis in women. (Some women claim it's due to living with men!)

• A new herpes virus vaccine is ineffective in men but works in some women.[1]

Clearly female and male physiology differs significantly. We have kept that point in mind throughout this chapter and the writing of this book.

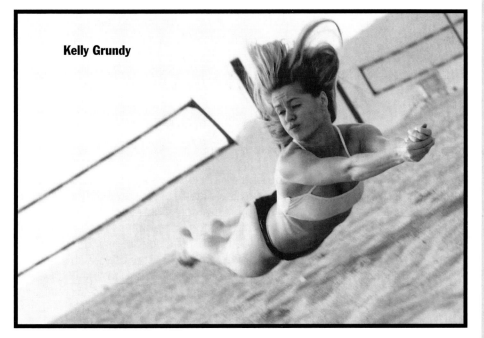

Kelly Grundy

"The only way to get rid of a temptation is to yield to it."
– Oscar Wilde (1854-1900)

Exercise Physiology

As you start to warm up for your first exercise of the workout, the muscles immediately begin to increase their need for energy, which is released from energy-rich compounds such as glycogen (a storage form of glucose). For the first few minutes the muscles will burn glycogen. This process is a form of anaerobic (without oxygen) metabolism because the heart and circulatory system have not yet increased blood flow to the exercising muscles. During this time there may be a burning sensation in the muscle due to the formation of lactic acid. This sensation will soon diminish as increased blood flow provides the oxygen needed for aerobic (with oxygen) metabolism of glycogen. In strenuous exercise (when oxygen needs outweigh oxygen delivery), an "oxygen debt" is built up within the muscles. The muscles are forced to use glucose for energy without oxygen (anaerobically), inefficiently leaving behind the metabolite lactic acid that must be broken down later. The oxygen required to return the muscle to normal after exercise is called the oxygen debt. The rate of breathing does not return to normal after exercise until the oxygen debt is repaid.

Once the stores of glycogen are used up, which usually occurs after about 20 minutes, the body will start to burn fat stores to produce the blood sugar it needs. The longer the exercise continues, the more fat is burned.[4]

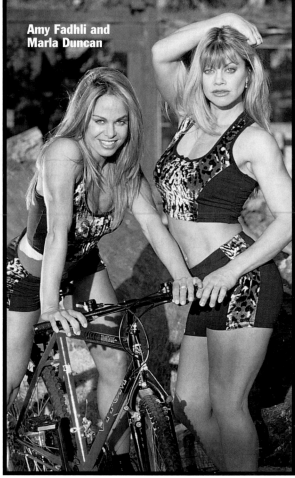

Amy Fadhli and
Marla Duncan

Muscles

Muscle is stimulated to produce an action potential. An action potential is an electrical charge across a cell membrane due to changes in the conduction of ions across the membrane. Muscle cells contain a contractile mechanism that is activated by the action potential. About 40 percent of the body is skeletal muscle, 5 to 10 percent is cardiac and smooth muscle.

Contraction by a Whole Muscle

Isometric versus Isotonic Contractions

Isometric muscle contractions occur when the muscle doesn't shorten. Isotonic contractions are those when the tension on a muscle remains constant but the muscle shortens, as in lifting a static amount of weight. Isometric contraction differs from isotonic in that the myofibrils don't slide over each other much as force is developed. Sliding does occur in isotonic contractions when external work is performed.

Motor Unit

The motor nerve and all the fibers it innervates are called the motor unit. The number of fibers is dependent on the necessity for fine control. In general, small muscles that react rapidly with fine control have one nerve and only a few muscle fibers. Those muscles that do not require fine control, such as the gastrocnemius (calf muscle), may have several hundred muscle fibers per motor unit.

Summation

The contraction of individual muscle fibers is an all-or-none affair. Any graded response must come from the number of motor units stimulated at any one time. Summation is the adding together of individual muscle twitches to make a whole muscle contraction. This can be accomplished by increasing the number of motor units contracting at one time (spatial summation) or by increasing the frequency of contraction of individual muscle contractions (temporal summation). These processes almost always occur simultaneously within normal muscle contraction. Individual motor units usually fire asynchronously.

All motor units are not created equal. Therefore one motor unit within a particular muscle may be as much as 50 times stronger than another. Smaller motor units are much more easily excited than larger ones because they are innervated by smaller nerve fibers that have a naturally lower threshold for excitation. In spatial summation, motor units are recruited by increasing the strength of the stimulus thereby increasing the strength of the contraction.

In temporal or wave summation the rapidity of each motor units contraction increases such that one contraction isn't completely over when the stimulus for the next arrives. So the force generated in the first is added to that generated by the second, third and so on. When a muscle is stimulated at progressively greater frequencies, a frequency is finally reached at which the successive contractions fuse together and cannot be distinguished one from the other.

"I don't know why we are here, but I'm pretty sure that it is not in order to enjoy ourselves."
– Ludwig Wittgenstein (1889-1951)

Muscle Fatigue

Prolonged contractions lead to muscle fatigue. The nerve continues to function properly passing the action potential on to the muscle fibers, but the contractions become weaker and weaker due to the lack of ATP (the supplement creatine can increase the length of time before muscle fatigue sets in).

Hypertrophy

Muscle hypertrophy (increase in muscle mass) is caused by forceful muscular activity. The diameters of individual fibers increase, nutrient and metabolic substances increase, mitochondria may increase, and the myofibrils also increase in size and number. Muscular hypertrophy increases the power for muscle contraction. Forceful muscle activity *above 75 percent of maximum* is necessary to produce hypertrophy – that's why isometric exercise even for short periods of time can have profound effects on muscle mass. However, prolonged light exercise increases endurance,

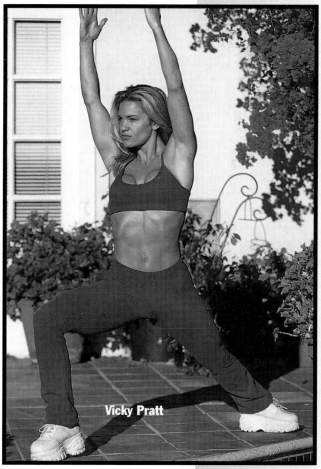
Vicky Pratt

causing increases in oxidative enzymes, myoglobin, and even blood capillaries. The important point here is, when a woman works out she *will not* become huge and bulky like a man. Professional female bodybuilders use anabolic steroids (which are testosterone derivatives), resulting in their manly physiques. This will not happen to you if you stay away from these drugs.

Atrophy

Muscle atrophy results when a muscle is not used for a length of time or is used for only weak contractions. For instance, atrophy occurs when limbs are put in casts. As little as one month of nonuse can sometimes decrease the muscle size to one-half normal. Damage to the nerve to a muscle results in atrophy as well. If the damage is repaired in the first three to four months the muscle will regain full function. After four months muscle fibers will have degenerated to fibrous and fatty tissue.

Muscle Types

"He who hesitates is a damned fool."
– Mae West (1892-1980)

Skeletal Muscle

Skeletal muscle makes up most of the body's muscle and does not contract without nervous stimulation. It is under voluntary control and lacks anatomic cellular connections between fibers. The fibers (cells) are multinucleate and appear striated due to the arrangement of actin and myosin protein filaments. Each fiber is a single cell, long, cylindrical and surrounded by a cell membrane. The muscle fibers contain many myofibrils that are made of myofilaments. These myofilaments are made of the contractile proteins. The key proteins in muscle contraction are myosin, actin, tropomyosin and troponin.

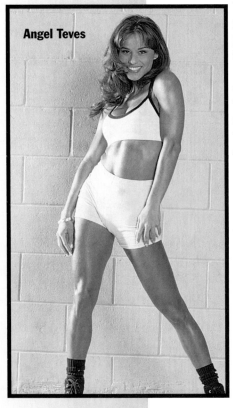

Angel Teves

Skeletal muscle fibers have differences in metabolic and contractile properties. Type I fibers are mostly found in the muscle for posture, as in the long muscles of the back. These are also called red muscles because the fibers contain many mitochondria that give the muscle more of a dark reddish hue. White muscles contain mostly Type II fibers and are specialized for fast, fine movements as in the muscles that move the eye or some hand muscles. The differences in fiber type occur because of differences in amino acid composition of the skeletal proteins without a change in biologic activity. Various forms of the proteins can be expressed, thus determining the functional characteristics of each muscle. Changes in muscle function can be caused by alterations in activity (training), hormonal environment or innervation.

Muscle fibers are classified by contractile and metabolic characteristics. Having a concentration of one type of fiber will make an athlete better suited for one type of sport. Ten to 20 years ago muscle fiber biopsies for athlete classification were common practice. Today we can perform exercise tests to determine what type of activities an athlete will excel at. There has been limited evidence to suggest that with chronic training an athlete will convert from one type to another.

Fast-twitch fibers (Type II) have a high capability for the electrochemical transmission of action potentials, a high activity level of myosin ATPase, a rapid level of calcium release and uptake by the sarcoplasmic reticulum, and a high rate of crossbridge turnover. They have a well-developed short-term glycolic system activated in short-term sprint activities as well as other forceful muscular contractions that depend almost entirely on anaerobic metabolism for energy. Some examples would be linemen, bobsledders and baseball athletes.

Slow-twitch fibers (Type I) are used for long-term synthesis of ATP from mainly aerobic metabolism. They are distinguished by a low level of myosin-ATPase, slow speed of contraction, and a glycolic capacity less well developed than fast-twitch fibers. Slow-twitch fibers have a high number of relatively large mitochondria. Slow-twitch fibers have high levels of myoglobin, making them appear red. This makes them much more fatigue resistant and well suited for prolonged aerobic exercise, such as riding a bicycle.

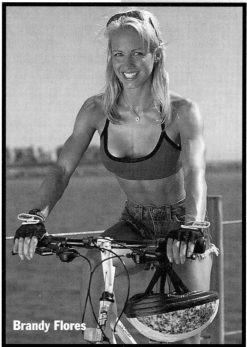
Brandy Flores

Contractile Proteins

Skeletal muscle is composed of cells, called fibers, that are specialized to contract or shorten in length. Each fiber is made of smaller subunits called myofibrils, composed of contractile proteins called myosin and actin, which are in turn responsible for muscle contraction at the molecular level. These contractile protein filaments are also called thick (myosin) and thin (actin) filaments. These protein filaments can interact. The myosin filaments have crossbridges that stick out from the filament to interact with the actin filaments during contraction. This structure allows the myosin filament to pull the actin filaments from both directions, thus shortening the fiber.

The actin filaments are composed of two strands of protein woven together. The actin filaments are anchored to Z-lines that make the boundaries of the functional unit of muscle contraction called the sarcomere. There are many sarcomeres in a muscle fiber and Z-lines are continuous across muscle fibers.

Sliding Filament Theory

Muscle contraction occurs by a sliding filament mechanism. The sarcomeres shorten (the Z-lines come closer together) because the actin filaments slide over the myosin filaments. The force behind muscle contraction is the ratchet movement of the tiny myosin heads toward the center of their sarcomere. This ratchet movement occurs many times during a muscle contraction.

The functional unit of the muscle cell is the sarcomere. The Z-lines have thin actin filaments connected to each end of the sarcomere. The thick myosin filaments contain the crossbridges to the actin. A thin filament called the tropomyosin is located along the actin filaments covering the binding sites with troponin.

During depolarization, calcium ions are released into the tubules and attached to the troponin. This action enables the crossbridge to bind to actin with ATP. When ATP is hydrolyzed to ADP + P + E, the action is the firing of the crossbridge. This happens many times and results in the two Z-lines being moved toward the center of the sarcomere.

Sequence of Events in Muscle Contraction

1. The muscle action potential depolarizes the transverse or T-tubules causing Ca++ to be released into the sarcoplasmic reticulum.
2. Ca++ ions bind to troponin on the tropomyosin in the actin filaments. This releases the actin so it can bind to the myosin filament crossbridge.
3. Actin combines with the myosin-ATP. Actin also causes the release of ATPase, which splits ATP.
4. Tension is created because energy from this reaction is used to produce movement of the myosin crossbridge.
5. ATP binds with the myosin bridge. This breaks the actin-myosin bond and allows the crossbridge to dissociate from the actin.
6. There is a slight difference in charges between a recently fired site and the crossbridge, which allows the crossbridge to be attracted to a new actin site. This charge quickly disappears.
7. All this happens very quickly and repeatedly, and is also responsible for the shortening of the filaments.

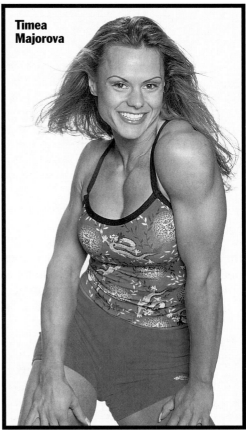

Timea Majorova

Muscle contraction requires a great deal of energy. Energy is required to break the bond between the myosin head and the actin-active sites as well as for removal of calcium from the cytoplasm by the use of a special pump within the sarcoplasmic reticulum. When the myosin head is tilted forward, after the power stroke, a binding site for ATP (the chief energy currency of the cell) is exposed. The breakdown of ATP to ADP releases the head from the actin filament and cocks it for the next ratchet power stroke.

Energy Sources

A great deal of energy is required for muscle contraction. At rest and during light exercise, muscles use lipids as their energy source. The use of carbohydrate becomes more important as the intensity of exercise increases. The breakdown of glucose to water and carbon dioxide generates energy that is transferred to regenerate phosphorylcreatine and ATP. ATP is only stored in small quantities in the muscle fibers (cells). Because ATP cannot be supplied by the bloodstream it must be resynthesized in the cell.

When oxygen supplies are inadequate this process is short-circuited and a metabolite (lactic acid) of one of the products builds up in the muscle. This process is called anaerobic metabolism (glycolysis) and is a normal function that can occur prior to the oxidative breakdown of glucose. Creatine phosphate is a substance that exists in limited quantities within the cells. This substance is hydrolyzed to form creatine, energy and phosphate. The energy that is liberated from this action is not mechanical energy. It is used to resynthesize the phosphate onto the ADP complex to form ATP. (Remember, when the crossbridge fires it hydrolyzes ATP to form ADP + P + energy.)

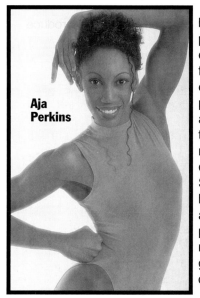

Aja
Perkins

Energy transfer in the form of phosphate bonds is termed phosphorylation. Energy from phosphorylation is ultimately generated by the oxidation of carbohydrates, fats and protein. This form of energy does not require the presence of oxygen so it is termed anaerobic. During this process lactate builds up in the muscles, causing a change in pH that inhibits enzyme activity. After the exercise an oxygen debt exists in that oxygen must be used to convert the lactate into carbon dioxide and water, and replenish energy stores. Short intense exercise utilizes anaerobic metabolic mechanisms more than more sustained activities. For example, in a 100-meter dash 85 percent of the energy is derived from anaerobic means while in a mile run only 20 percent is generated anaerobically. There is only one currency for mechanical work.

Excitation-Contraction Coupling

Contraction in skeletal muscle begins with an action potential in the muscle fiber. This causes the release of calcium from the sacroplasmic reticulum. The action potential in the muscle fiber begins after it is excited by interaction with a large insulated (myelinated) nerve fiber. The point of contact of the nerve and muscle is called the neuromuscular junction, which is normally located in the middle of the muscle fiber. Therefore an action potential initiated here spreads toward the ends of the fiber, making it possible for all sarcomeres to contract at the same time. Skeletal muscle has an adaptation that allows the action potential to spread deep within the fiber. The T or transverse tubules are internal extensions of the sarcolemma that penetrate through the fiber such that action potentials in the T-tubules cause the release of calcium from the nearby sarcoplasmic reticulum in the immediate vicinity of the myofibrils.

The sarcoplasmic reticulum contains calcium ions in very high concentration that are released when the adjacent T-tubule is excited. Pumps within the walls of the sarcoplasmic reticulum return the calcium within the cytoplasm to levels below those needed to activate the contractile process.

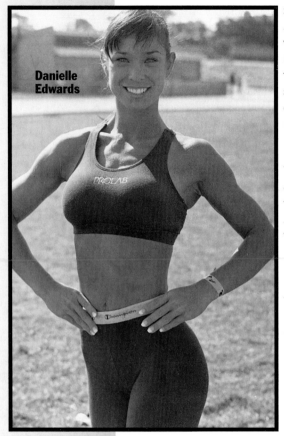

Danielle Edwards

Smooth Muscle

Smooth muscle is found in the walls of blood vessels, tubular organs such as the stomach and uterus, in the iris, and is associated with the hair follicles. It exists in the body as multiunit or visceral smooth muscle. It is not under voluntary control, each cell has one nucleus and it is displayed automatically in the visceral form. In multiunit smooth muscle each cell exists as a discreet independent unit that is innervated by a single nerve ending. Visceral smooth muscle exists as a sheet or bundle of fibers that are intimately connected by junctions that allow ions to flow freely and it therefore performs as a syncytium. Therefore, when one portion of visceral smooth muscle is stimulated, the action potential spreads to all other fibers.

Most of the same contractile proteins are present and active in smooth muscle contraction but they are not arranged as microscopically visible parallel myofilaments as in skeletal muscle. The contractile mechanism is very similar to skeletal muscle except that the myosin of smooth muscle only interacts with actin when it has been phosphorylated. In smooth muscle calcium binds to a protein called calmodulin and the complex then interacts with an enzyme that adds a phosphate group to myosin, thus activating it.

In smooth muscle T-tubules are absent, the sarcoplasmic reticulum is poorly developed, and the calcium pump is present but it is slower acting. Because of these differences in the contractile mechanism and machinery, smooth muscle takes about 30 times as long to contract and relax as does skeletal muscle – and it does so using much less energy. Elaborate neuro-muscular junctions are not present in smooth muscle. Often neurotransmitter is released only in close proximity to the muscle such that the neurotransmitter, which may be acetylcholine or norepinephrine, must diffuse to the muscle cells to interact with receptors on the cell membrane. Either of these neurotransmitters may be excitatory or inhibitory, depending on the receptors present on that particular smooth muscle cell. Because smooth muscle has spontaneous activity, neuronal input only serves to modify that activity rather than initiating it as in skeletal muscle. Local tissue factors, hormones and mechanical stretch can cause action potentials and thus contraction in smooth muscle. Unlike cardiac muscle, smooth muscle is capable of active regeneration after injury.

Cardiac Muscle

The heart is made of specialized muscle tissue with some similarities to both smooth and skeletal muscle. It is involuntary and mononucleate as is smooth muscle. Cardiac muscle is striated like skeletal muscle, which means it has microscopically visible myofilaments arranged in parallel with the sarcomere structure described above. These filaments slide along each other during the process of contraction in the same manner as occurs in skeletal muscle.

Cardiac muscle fibers branch and have a single nucleus per cell. Another difference in cardiac muscle is the presence of intercalated discs that are specialized connections between one cardiac muscle cell and another. These tight connections allow for almost completely free movement of ions so that action potentials can freely pass from one cell to another. This makes cardiac muscle tissue a functional syncytium. When one cell is excited the resultant action potential is spread to all of them. This is an important feature in that it allows the atrial or ventricular muscle to contract as one to forcefully pump blood. Action potentials in cardiac muscle are also specialized to maximize the pumping function of the heart. They last 10 to 30 times as long as those of skeletal muscle and cause a correspondingly increased period of contraction. Cardiac muscle has no regenerative capacity beyond early childhood.[3,4,5,6]

Artificial Muscle

Scientists in Germany have reported progress with experiments which they say could eventually lead to the manufacture of artificial human muscles. According to the journal *Science,* the artificial muscles can expand and contract in response to an electric charge just like human tissue. The process involves millions of tiny tubes (called carbon nanotubes), each one-millionth of a millimetre across. Like natural muscles, providing an electrical charge causes the individual fibers to expand and the whole structure to move.

However, any application of this work in replacing biological muscles is "nearer the dream factory than reality." Nanotubes are cylindrical molecules made of carbon atoms and are only a millionth of a millimetre in diameter. Their strength, flexibility and electrical properties have fascinated scientists. The tiny tubes expand and contract their length by about 1 percent when an electrical charge is applied and then removed.[7,8]

Naming the Skeletal Muscles

There are numerous ways to name muscles, but keep this in mind: The human body did not evolve to be neatly classified and characterized. Some muscles are easily named using basic terminology; others require combinations of different naming procedures. Here are some examples of muscles and how they are named.

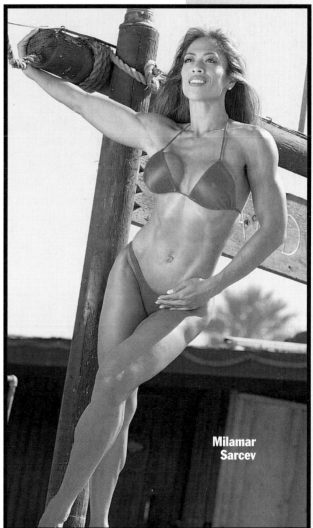

Milamar
Sarcev

Size – The largest muscle within a group is usually distinguished from the rest of the muscles within the same group.

Example – The gluteus maximus is the largest muscle in the buttocks.

Shape – The shape that a particular muscle resembles may be a factor in naming it.

Example – The deltoid is shaped like a delta or triangle.

Direction of fibers – The direction of the muscular fibers within a muscle (longitudinal vs. lateral) may be a consideration when naming a muscle.

Example – The rectus abdominus is the longitudinal muscle within the abdomen that comes from rectus, meaning straight.

Location – The location of a muscle in relationship to another bodypart may affect the naming of the muscle.

Example – The frontalis overlies the frontal bone. The latissimus dorsi lie on the dorsal region (back) of the body. (Think of a shark's dorsal fin.)

Number of attachments – Some muscles have more than one point of origin and/or attachment, which may factor into naming it.

Example – The biceps brachii has two attachments or origins. The triceps has three.

Action – The manner in which the muscle moves the bodypart for which it is responsible may be considered when naming the muscle.

Example – The extensor digitorum extends digits.

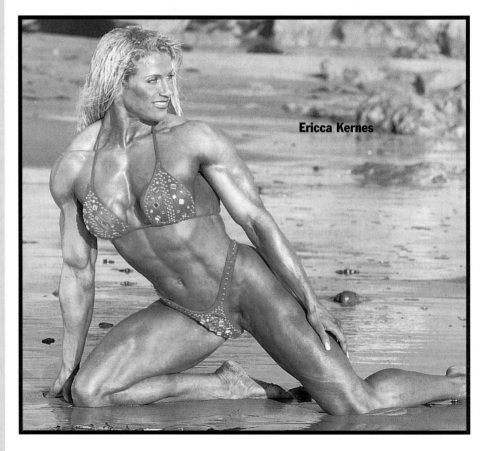

Ericca Kernes

The Menstrual Cycle

The average menstrual cycle is 28 days. However, only a very small percentage of cycles are exactly 28 days – most range from 25 to 36 days. Menstrual cycles usually start between the ages of 12 and 15 and continue until about the age of 45 to 50 when menopause occurs.

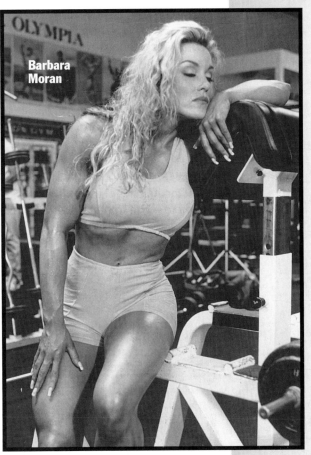

Barbara Moran

The female body involves four major hormones in the menstrual cycle: follicle-stimulating hormone (FSH), luteinizing hormone (LH), estrogen (estradiol) and progesterone. FSH and LH are protein hormones produced by cells of the anterior pituitary within the brain, in response to small peptide hormones from the hypothalamus (hypothalamic releasing factors). These pituitary hormones travel in the blood to the ovaries, where they stimulate the development of one or more eggs, each within a follicle. A follicle consists of an ovum surrounded by cells responsible for the growth and nurturing of the ovum. As the cycle progresses, one follicle becomes dominant and all others regress.

The menstrual cycle can be divided into three phases: the follicular (proliferative) phase, the ovulatory phase, and the luteal (secretory) phase. The follicular phase begins with the first day of menses (menstrual flow) and continues to approximately day 13 or 14 when ovulation takes place. During the follicular phase, FSH and LH are slowly rising in preparation for the LH surge (very high level of LH) at the time of ovulation. FSH is stimulating the growth of follicles in the ovaries. Estrogen and progesterone are relatively low throughout this time but slowly begin to rise toward the end of this phase. Estrogen, and progesterone to a lesser degree, are steroid hormones produced by cells of the developing ovarian follicle. Estrogen causes the endometrium to increase in thickness and vascularization (i.e. blood supply). At the end of the proliferative (follicular) phase, the endometrium is 2 to 3 mm thick and the glands are straight tubules with narrow lumens.

LH surges and peaks during the ovulatory phase (around day 14) and estrogen peaks at the same time. These peaks trigger ovulation. The ovum lives about 72 hours after ovulation, but it is fertilizable for only about 36 hours. Just before ovulation, progesterone levels begin to rise rapidly. Changes in cervical mucous accompany ovulation. The amount of mucous increases and it becomes clear and thin. This lubrication facilitates conception by aiding the passage of sperm through the cervical canal. Sperm can live for up to 72 hours

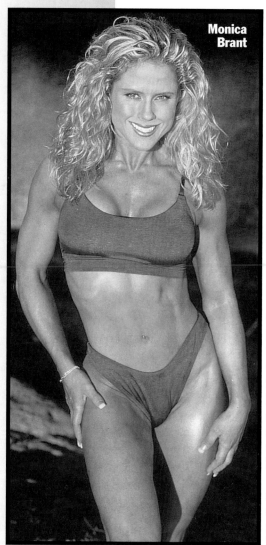

Monica Brant

in the female reproductive system. Therefore, the fertile period during a 28-day cycle is only about four to five days.

After ovulation (at the midpoint of the cycle), under the influence of LH, the ovarian follicular cells shift to the production of progesterone, becoming a yellowish structure called the corpus luteum (luteal phase). The corpus luteum remains intact for the remainder of the cycle. Progesterone causes the endometrial lining to become secretory and nutritive in anticipation of implantation of a fertilized egg. The uterine glands become very coiled and the endometrial lining reaches maximum thickness of about 5 mm during the luteal (secretory phase). Progesterone also inhibits the contractions of smooth muscle cells of the myometrium. The breast swelling, tenderness and pain experienced by some women is most likely due to the effects of progesterone on breast tissue.

In the luteal phase progesterone levels are very high – progesterone is important during this phase because, if the egg is fertilized and implanted in the uterus, progesterone keeps the uterus intact so that the pregnancy is maintained. The continued health of the corpus luteum (progesterone secretion) is assured by the production of human chorionic gonadotropin (HCG) by the implanted embryo, until the placenta develops and can take over. The detection of HCG in urine is the basis of laboratory and home pregnancy tests.

If fertilization and implantation have occurred, the corpus luteum will then be stimulated by HCG to continue its production of estrogen and progesterone to maintain the pregnancy. This aspect is important because the corpus luteum dies within 14 to 22 days of ovulation if fertilization and implantation do not occur. At the end of the secretory (luteal) phase, blood levels of estrogen and progesterone drop rapidly. The coiled arteries serving the endometrial lining contract, causing ischemia leading to tissue death in the functionalis. The blood vessels above the vasoconstriction rupture and bleeding begins, resulting in the monthly menstrual flow that normally lasts about five days.

Premenstrual Syndrome (PMS)

PMS is the name given to the common symptoms that accompany the onset of the monthly period. Symptoms include headache, mood changes, breast tenderness, bloating, edema, weight gain, backache, irritability, depression and anxiety. Treatment is symptomatic and includes analgesics, diuretics, tranquilizers and sedatives.

Dysmenorrhea

More commonly referred to as cramps, dysmenorrhea is the painful menstruation caused by abnormal uterine contractility that effects some 50 percent of menstruating women. Primary dysmenorrhea is that which is not related to an obvious physical cause. Sharp cramps are experienced the first couple days of the menses. Headache, nausea, vomiting, diarrhea and fatigue also may be symptoms of dysmenorrhea and are thought to be caused by the liberation of prostaglandins in the endometrium. Treatments include analgesics, anti-prostaglandins and hormones. Nonsteroidal anti-inflammatory drugs such as aspirin, indomethacin and ibuprofen inhibit prostaglandin synthesis and act as analgesics. In severe cases, hormone therapy is initiated to prevent ovulation as anovulatory cycles are usually painless.

Amenorrhea

Physiologic amenorrhea, or the cessation of menstrual periods, normally occurs in pregnancy, lactation, adolescence and menopause. Pathologic amenorrhea may be caused by endocrine disorders such as dysfunction of the hypothalamus, pituitary, ovary, thyroid or adrenal glands. Metabolic and psychogenic causes include malnutrition, obesity, chronic stress, drug addiction, diabetes, anorexia nervosa and anemia. Removal of the underlying cause will usually result in the resumption of normal periods. If hormone deficiencies are found, substitutional therapy is recommended.

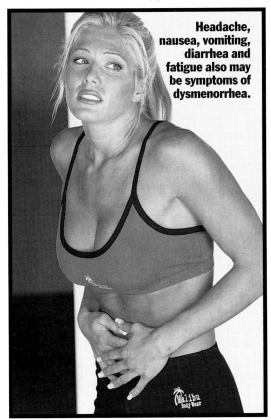

Headache, nausea, vomiting, diarrhea and fatigue also may be symptoms of dysmenorrhea.

A shift in body composition or weight loss can cause amenorrhea – as in anorexia nervosa, ballet dancers, long-distance runners or malnutrition. There seems to be a bodyfat threshold for the maintenance of normal cycles that is in the neighborhood of 18 percent. In many of these cases, if the patient gains weight normal cycles will resume. In obesity, weight loss and the concomitant decrease in stress on the body will enable a resumption of normal function. Amenorrhea may also result from psychogenic causes such as depression or chronic emotional stress.[11]

Hormones

Hormonal communication systems augment the nervous communication systems within the body. Hormones are chemical-signaling molecules (peptides, proteins or steroids) produced in one site of the body and then travel to another site to have an effect. In this way one cell can affect other distantly located cells. The endocrine system displays an elegant series of checks and balances in the form of feedback loops to facilitate the normal functioning of all bodily systems. Hormones may be made and have an action locally or may be made in one endocrine gland and have an effect at a distant site. Glands are functional units of hormone-secreting cells located in various regions of the body, making up the endocrine system. Each gland has specific functions that help to maintain the normal internal environment and promote the survival of the organism.

The Ovaries

The ovaries produce the steroid hormones (estrogens and progesterone) that cause the development of secondary sexual characteristics and develop and maintain the reproductive function in the female. Specifically the estrogens are secreted by the ovarian follicle, the corpus luteum and the placenta. LH from the anterior pituitary binds to receptors on the internal or granulosa cells to cause the production of estradiol from cholesterol or a downstream precursor androstenedione that is passed from the thecal cells to the granulosa cells. Progesterone is secreted mostly by the corpus luteum and the placenta but some is made by the developing follicle. Negative feedback from progesterone decreases LH secretion and large doses can prevent ovulation.

Estrogens in the bloodstream inhibit the release of FSH and LH, in some circumstances, via negative feedback. At other times, as in the preovu-

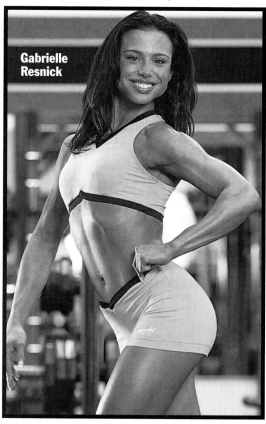

Gabrielle Resnick

latory LH surge, estrogens increase the release of LH via positive feedback. Estrogen also increases the excitability of uterine smooth muscle, myometrial sensitivity to oxytocin and increases the libido in women by a direct action on hypothalamic neurons.

Estrogens lower plasma cholesterol, inhibit atherogenesis (plaque formation in blood vessels), and are protective against myocardial infarction as suggested by the lower incidence of heart attacks and atherosclerosis in premenopausal women.

Progesterone has the principal targets of the uterus, breasts and the brain. It promotes the development of breast tissue, causes changes in the endometrial lining during the luteal phase of the cycle, decreases the excitability of myometrial cells and decreases uterine sensitivity to oxytocin.

Cells of the developing follicle also produce the polypeptide hormone inhibin, which inhibits FSH secretion by a direct action on the pituitary.

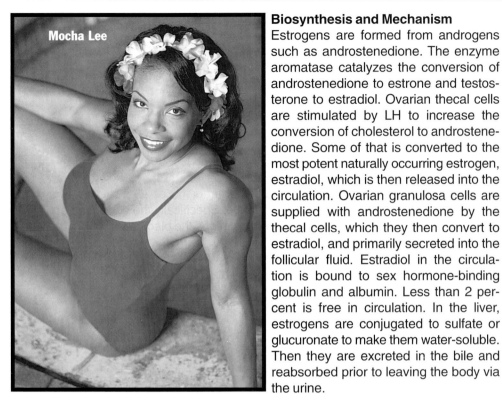

Mocha Lee

Biosynthesis and Mechanism

Estrogens are formed from androgens such as androstenedione. The enzyme aromatase catalyzes the conversion of androstenedione to estrone and testosterone to estradiol. Ovarian thecal cells are stimulated by LH to increase the conversion of cholesterol to androstenedione. Some of that is converted to the most potent naturally occurring estrogen, estradiol, which is then released into the circulation. Ovarian granulosa cells are supplied with androstenedione by the thecal cells, which they then convert to estradiol, and primarily secreted into the follicular fluid. Estradiol in the circulation is bound to sex hormone-binding globulin and albumin. Less than 2 percent is free in circulation. In the liver, estrogens are conjugated to sulfate or glucuronate to make them water-soluble. Then they are excreted in the bile and reabsorbed prior to leaving the body via the urine.

Physiological Effects

Normal development and maturation of the female is dependent on estrogens. Besides stimulating development of the reproductive structures and secondary sexual characteristics, estrogens are necessary to the cyclic endometrial changes necessary for reproduction, development of the breasts, health of the skin and vascular system, and bone homeostasis. Estrogen also affects intestinal motility, blood coagulation, cholesterol metabolism, female libido, and sodium and water conservation by the kidneys. Estrogens increase the uterine muscle mass, excitability and responsiveness to oxytocin. FSH secretion is negatively inhibited by estrogens, but LH may be either positively or negatively affected dependent on the hormonal milieu. Estrogens have an anabolic effect and have been used in animal husbandry to increase the weight of domestic animals. Estrogens increase libido in humans and are responsible for estrous behavior in animals. Plasma cholesterol is lowered by estrogens, which are protective against atherosclerotic disease.[12,13]

Puberty

Girls grow faster than boys do in early adolescence and it takes up to three years for boys to catch up. Girls' hip bones widen and flatten and the space in the middle opens enough for a baby's head to fit through.

In childhood the blood concentration of sex hormones is very low. At puberty the pulsatile release of GnRH begins causing a major increase in LH,

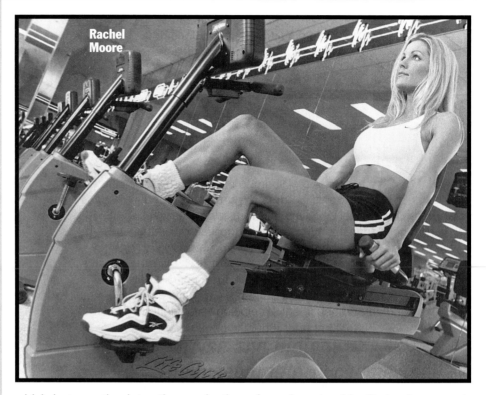

Rachel Moore

"Teenagers, God's revenge for making sex pleasurable."
– Phil, the bar owner, on the TV show Murphy Brown.

which in turn stimulates the production of ovarian steroids. Body changes at puberty include breast, uterine and vaginal development, and are due in part to estrogens. But they are also due to the lack of testosterone. The new female body configuration, distribution of fat, and hair growth are the result of the lower levels of testosterone in women. The female larynx retains its prepubertal dimensions, causing the voice to remain high-pitched. Estrogens have an anabolic effect that causes a rapid growth spurt and the closing of the epiphyseal plates of the long bones during puberty. Estrogens cause development of the glandular elements and stroma of the breast, as well as pigmentation of the nipples and areolas.

In response to hormone stimulation, the breasts enlarge with the growth of ductal and alveolar tissues and an increase in fat deposits. The nipple and areola also enlarge and become more sensitive to touch. When the teenager begins to menstruate, the breasts undergo a periodic premenstrual phase that varies with the individual but can include an increase in size, swelling and tenderness. The symptoms subside within a few days of the onset of bleeding.

Both boys and girls have to suffer extra hair growth in puberty – underarm hair, pubic hair and, for boys, chest hair. Pubic hair is short and curly because it grows sideways and its life span is only six months. And as if all that were not bad enough, puberty also brings emotional problems as teenagers learn to be more independent, discover that there are few black and white certainties in life, and cope with having sex on the brain. Hormones affect the center of the brain, which controls feelings and desires, but the body develops at a faster pace than the mind.

The worst aspect of adolescence for many is the curse of acne. Just as you are beginning to try to attract sexual attention, pimples coat your body. Hormones cause a rush of oil to the skin which blocks the skin ducts and traps bacteria.[13,14,15]

Pregnancy

Pregnancy causes changes in every system in the body. However, these changes generally revert back to prepregnancy state about six months after the baby is born. One of the most common and uncomfortable changes takes place in the kidneys. The hormones, particularly progesterone (which the body produces during pregnancy), cause the ureters (tubes that carry urine from the kidneys to the bladder) to dilate, allowing a greater amount of urine to make its way into the bladder in a shorter period of time. This larger amount of urine combined with the pressure the baby is putting on the bladder results in a frequent need to urinate.

Another often noticed change occurs in the stomach. As the uterus enlarges, it compresses the stomach, slowing the speed at which the stomach empties. Hormones also cause the sphincter at the base of esophagus (which keeps food in your stomach) to relax. The combined result of both of these changes is that belching and heartburn may occur. Melasma, the "mask of pregnancy" refers to a blotchy pigmented area on the forehead and sides of the face. This is possibly due to the placenta producing a melanocyte-stimulating hormone. The mask will usually fade away over time after the pregnancy.

During the pregnancy the mother may experience nausea and vomiting, especially in the first trimester. No medications have been approved for treatment of this problem. If "morning sickness" occurs, a physician may have some suggestions. Eating and drinking frequently and in small amounts may help alleviate the problem. Many other symptoms may be noticed. A physician should be consulted – that is the best source of information about the changes going on in the body.

Endocrine control of pregnancy: The embryo makes HCG (human chorionic gonadotropin) to signal the mother that it is present. HCG is similar to LH. It maintains the corpus luteum and endometrium. In later pregnancy, the placenta takes over the function of the

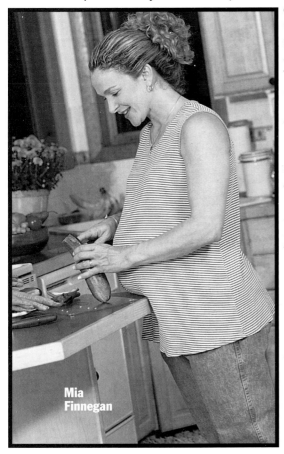

Mia
Finnegan

"Don't worry about pregnancy. We now know what causes it. "
– some anonymous smart-ass.

corpus luteum. HCG levels then fall. Estrogen and progesterone promote development of lactation tissue.

Birth and lactation occurs through contraction of the myometrium in response to oxytocin. Three stages are: dilation of the cervix, delivery of the fetus, delivery of the placenta. Lactation is stimulated by prolactin (milk formation) and oxytocin (milk let-down) in response to suckling.[16,17]

Menopause

The menopause signals the end of a woman's fertile life, and results from decreasing production of sex hormones by the ovaries. It normally occurs between the mid-40s and late 50s, although it can occur much earlier, and in extreme cases even in childhood. Certain types of chemotherapy treatment for cancer can also bring on the menopause. It is currently possible to freeze eggs in advance of chemotherapy treatment or surgery, but the chances of a successful pregnancy are low.[18]

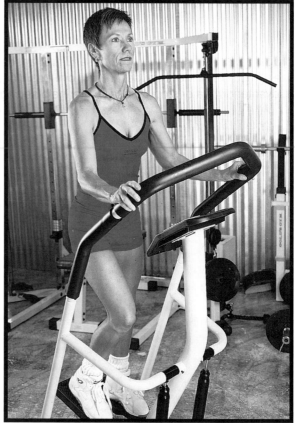

The menopause signals the end of a woman's fertile life, and results from decreasing production of sex hormones by the ovaries.

As well as the loss of the ability to bear children, women can suffer unpleasant symptoms such as the supply of sex hormones stops. Once the supply of hormones has fallen off, a woman will eventually cease to have a monthly menstrual cycle. Symptoms that may occur during menopause are hot flashes, changes in reproductive organs, cardiovascular disease, osteoporosis, nervousness and depression. Hot flashes are the most common symptom and are associated with estrogen withdrawal. Reproductive organ changes include vaginal dryness, thinning of the vaginal lining, and a decrease in size of the uterus and cervix. These changes are also a result of estrogen withdrawal and account for complaints such as vaginal itching and stress incontinence. There is an increased incidence of high blood pressure, stroke and heart disease following menopause probably due to the removal of the protection estrogen affords. Osteoporosis is also a risk when estrogen decreases, making postmenopausal women more at risk for fractures. The breasts become less glandular and are composed of more fat tissue than in reproductive years.

Treatment includes low-dose estrogen administration with some progesterone therapy and calcium supplementation. This therapy is protective of the breasts and uterus against cancer, deters the loss of bone, and increases HDL (high-density lipoproteins, the good ones) and lowers LDL (low-density lipoproteins, the bad ones) in the blood. Sometimes a topical vaginal estrogen cream is used to restore the vagina and external genitalia to a premenopausal state.[19]

Hormone-Replacement Therapy

Estrogens should be administered intermittently, or in combination with a progestin, at the lowest effective dose. Estrogens may be administered to relieve the symptoms of menopause, prevent ovulation, or suppress ovarian function as in dysmenorrhea or stop excessive uterine bleeding.

Postmenopausal

Estrogens can alleviate some of the systemic symptoms of estrogen deficiency in menopause and after menopause. These include hot flashes, sweating and atrophic vaginitis. Estrogens are also helpful in the treatment and prevention of osteoporosis. The smallest dose that will relieve the symptoms should be used. Local administration of estrogen to relieve the symptoms of atrophic vaginitis is very effective.

Adverse Effects

Hormone replacement therapy can cause breast tenderness, nausea and abnormal postmenopausal bleeding. These adverse effects can be avoided or minimized by using the smallest dose possible. Estrogen therapy also is associated with hyperpigmentation, migraine headaches, hypertension and gallbladder disease. There is evidence of an increased risk of endometrial cancer associated with estrogens and there may be some increased risk of breast cancer in at-risk patients.[13]

REFERENCES

1. www.e-womenshealth.net/
2. www.jockrash.com/physiology.html
3. www.e-muscles.net/
4. www.geocities.com/HotSprings/5484/mphysiology.htm
5. www.geocities.com/HotSprings/5484/mfiber.htm
6. www.geocities.com/HotSprings/5484/atp-pc.htm
7. news.bbc.co.uk/hi/english/sci/tech/newsid_348000/348915.stm#top
8. news.bbc.co.uk/hi/english/world/europe/newsid_351000/351057.stm#top
9. www.e-uterus.net/
10. www.e-hormone.com/
11. www.e-estrogens.com/
12. news.bbc.co.uk/hi/english/special_report/1998/05/98/the_human_body/newsid_110000/110183.stm#top
13. info.med.yale.edu/caim/bme350/lec981207.html
14. info.med.yale.edu/caim/bme350/lec981207.html
15. www.e-gynecologic.com/pregnant.html
16. news.bbc.co.uk/hi/english/health/medical_notes/newsid_455000/455393.stm
17. www.e-gynecologic.com/menopaus.html

CHAPTER SIX

In the Beginning

Well, you've made it. You're about to take your first step into the great unknown. Hopefully by the time you finish reading this chapter you'll be better prepared to embark on that great fitness adventure. Enough said. Let's get at it!

Whether your goal is international competition or just to get in shape, you must first condition and prepare the body. Nothing will set you back like diving in too hard and too fast. First we crawl, then we walk, and then we run – in that order. The same holds true for strength training. You want to first lay a good foundation so the body is able to handle the more advanced techniques and routines that come later. Please resist the urge to add sets and exercises to the following routines. It's great to have all that enthusiasm built up, but try to release it gradually over time, not all in one workout.

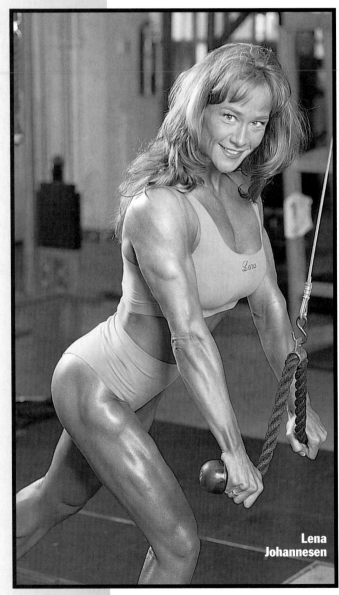

Lena
Johannesen

The Routines

Your first program will consist of a full-body workout. By this we mean you do one exercise for each major muscle group all in one session. Even though you may have the energy and desire to do more, limit your workouts to three or four per week. The best approach would be to alternate a day working out with a day off. After a period of a few weeks you can add an extra session or two of cardio on your day off, but for now, do both your cardio and strength training on the same day.

We suggest starting off with 2 sets of each exercise for somewhere between 8 and 12 reps. Then starting about the third week you can increase to 3 sets of each exercise. The same approach goes for cardio. Start with 15 to 20 minutes, and over a period of a few weeks increase it to 25 to 30 minutes. As most of the exercises we have chosen are called compound movements versus isolation, this is probably a good point to explain the difference between the two.

Compound vs. Isolation Exercises

Compound exercises are those that use more than one muscle group at one time. A good example is the bench press. The specific target of the bench press is the pectorals, or chest muscles. But the bench press also stimulates the triceps and deltoids as well. Isolation exercises are those that almost exclusively target the desired muscle, with little secondary assistance from other muscles. Even though 100 percent isolation is almost impossible, for practical purposes we say they are isolated.

Another way of looking at the two is to compare the number of joints being articulated. In a compound exercise two or more joints are involved, whereas isolation exercises usually involve just one joint.

In training terms, particularly at the beginning level, the use of more than one muscle group has numerous advantages in strength development. We are not saying isolation exercises which target a specific muscle are worthless. They have their place in weight training, and later programs will employ them. We will use them as a finisher, after our primary compound exercise, in order to bring additional blood and nutrients to the area being worked. This technique will help facilitate the healing process as well give you that nice pumped up feel and look. However, isolation exercises take a back seat to compound movements, which is where the following programs place their primary emphasis.

Compound exercises are very useful in strength development because of the heavier weight that can be lifted. The heavier the weight the more muscle tissue being stimulated. When you combine the pectorals, triceps and deltoids and have them work in conjunction in the bench press, you will obviously be able to lift more than using just the pectorals alone. That is why you can use far more weight on the bench press than dumbell flyes, or any other pectoral isolation exercise. Compound exercises are also more efficient. You will be working two or more muscles with one exercise. This means you are working more muscle in less time. Imagine if you had to work each muscle individually. You would have to be in the gym for hours at a time. Most people do not have that kind of time. That's

Laura Mak

where compound exercises are so beneficial. You will save huge amounts of your valuable time by focusing on the compound exercises. For detailed descriptions of all the following exercises, please see Chapter Nine.

Sample Routines

ROUTINE A	Sets	Reps
1. Leg press	2	10-12
2. Lying leg curl	2	10-12
3. Standing calf raise	2	10-12
4. Flat dumbell press	2	10-12
5. Lat pulldown	2	10-12
6. Machine shoulder press	2	10-12
7. Seated dumbell curl	2	10-12
8. Triceps pushdown	2	10-12
9. Crunch	2	15-20

Kim Lyons demonstrates the leg press.

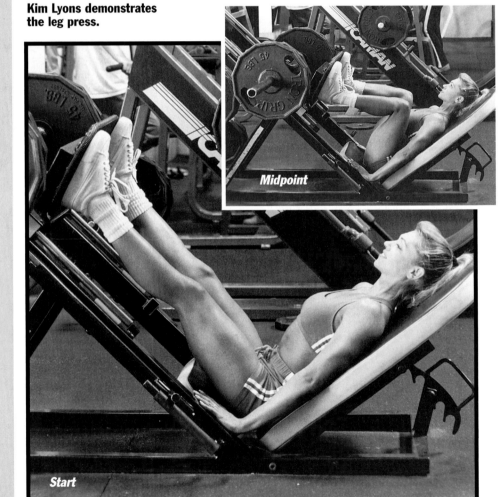

Midpoint

Start

ROUTINE B	Sets	Reps
1. Squat	2	10-12
2. Seated leg curl	2	10-12
3. Seated calf raise	2	10-12
4. Incline machine press	2	10-12
5. Assisted chinup	2	10-12
6. Dumbell press	2	10-12
7. Cable curl	2	10-12
8. Dumbell extension	2	10-12
9. Reverse crunch	2	15-20

ROUTINE C	Sets	Reps
1. Lunge	2	10-12
2. Standing leg curl	2	10-12
3. Toe press	2	10-12
4. Incline barbell press	2	10-12
5. Supported T-bar row	2	10-12
6. Front barbell press	2	10-12
7. Standing barbell curl	2	10-12
8. Lying EZ-bar extension	2	10-12
9. Lying leg raise	2	15-20

ROUTINE D	Sets	Reps
1. Hack squat	2	10-12
2. Stiff-leg deadlift	2	10-12
3. Donkey calf raise	2	10-12
4. Flat barbell press	2	10-12
5. Seated cable row	2	10-12
6. Upright row	2	10-12
7. Standing dumbell curl	2	10-12
8. Rope extension	2	10-12
9. Hanging leg raise	2	15-20

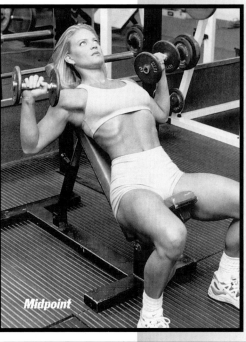

Midpoint

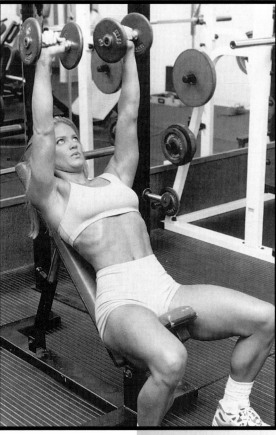

**Incline dumbell press.
– Jenny Johnson**

Start

Nutrition

No matter how many sets you perform in the gym or the variety of exercises in your routine, there is a limit to the quality of physique you can develop if you don't have your "kitchen behavior" under control. By this we mean your eating habits. All the exercise in the world is practically useless if you take in too many empty calories. And it's not just future fitness competitors we are talking about either. Healthy eating habits are pertinent to everyone. Here in Chapter Seven we introduce you to the various food groups, and suggest ways to modify your eating patterns so that your body receives the full spectrum of nutrients.

> *"The carp was dead, killed, assassinated, murdered in the first, second and third degree. Limp, I fell into a chair, with my hands still unwashed reached for a cigarette, lighted it and waited for the police to come and take me into custody."*
> *– Alice B Toklas*

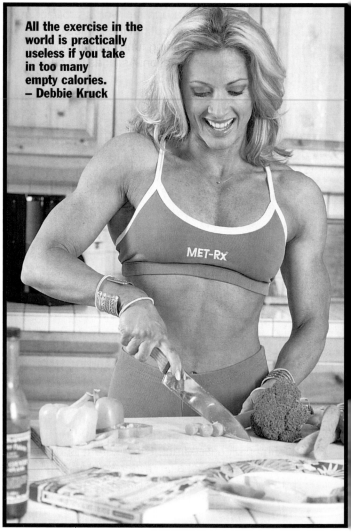

All the exercise in the world is practically useless if you take in too many empty calories.
– Debbie Kruck

Another Reason to Blame Your Ancestors

It has been dietary dogma for many years that a diet including a wide variety of foods, with plenty of fruit and vegetables, and modest amounts of fat and alcohol, combined with regular activity, will help maintain a healthy weight. And yet half the American population is overweight, a quarter is obese, and obesity is becoming a worldwide health problem. Why?

Basically we can blame our ancient ancestors. They ate like pigs. Literally. They ate anything – grubs, worms, roots, seeds – and any animal they could sink their teeth into. Of course, these hunter-gatherers were continually on the move, so calories were burned quickly. Food preservation is recent technology. Our ancestors had to gorge on whatever was available because they did not know how to store food. This gorge and starve cycle (practiced by numerous supermodels) has resulted in modern humans who must struggle daily with survival instincts that kept our ancestors chasing wooly mammoths. We don't need fat in the amounts we consume, and yet our bodies crave it because our instincts tell us that fat means the difference between life and death. Consciously we know that's not true for us, but we are only the third generation that has benefited from an abundance of food. If you or someone you know is overweight, it is not because of personal weakness. People do not choose to be obese. They are the victims of an ancient survival instinct as powerful as the drive to reproduce. Would you condemn a drowning man for swimming to shore? You wouldn't sneer at a burning woman rolling on the ground, trying to put out the flames.

There's nothing funny about being in a life-threatening situation. As far as the obese are concerned, their bodies are preparing for the next famine. It's not about low self-esteem, a lack of self-control or past victimization. It's about a couple of million years of evolutionary strategy that produced modern humans. We're hunter-gatherers who drive BMWs and go to fast-food restaurants. We carry cell phones instead of spears, we smell of soap instead of animal grease and wood smoke, but genetically we are no different than the people who hunted cave bears during the ice age. As a species, we've evolved the instinct to hunt down and ingest fat, and we do it with gusto.[1] A diet based exclusively on seeds and vegetables is not optimal; a diet based predominantly on a wide variety of seeds, roots, vegetables and nuts, with a small amount of animal or seafood is certainly one of the optimal ways of meeting our evolutionarily determined nutritional needs, and an excellent basis for planning your diet.

Fiber

Dietary fiber is the portion of plants that cannot be digested by the human digestive tract. The different kinds of plant fiber are divided into two classifications – *water-soluble fiber* consists of pectin, gums, mucilages, and some hemicelluloses; and *insoluble fiber* consists of lignin, cellulose and the remaining hemicelluloses. The primary action of fiber is in the gastrointestinal tract, but different forms of fiber have different physiological effects and health benefits.

Soluble fiber delays gastric emptying and intestinal transit. Viscous soluble fiber sources also slow the appearance of glucose in the blood and decrease serum cholesterol. Soluble fibers are rapidly broken down (fermented) by bacteria in the large bowel and do not

Tina Rigdon

have a laxative effect, with the exceptions of oats (which contains up to 50 percent soluble fiber as beta-glucan) and psyllium seed husks. Major food sources of soluble fiber include oats, beans, dried peas and legumes.

Insoluble fibers speed up intestinal transit and increase stool weight. They have a laxative effect. However, insoluble fibers have no effect on serum cholesterol. Major food sources of insoluble fiber include wheat bran, whole grain products and vegetables. Fruits, vegetables and barley are sources of both insoluble and soluble fiber. Nearly all fiber-containing foods have more insoluble than soluble dietary fiber. About two-thirds to three-quarters of the dietary fiber in typical mixed-food diets is insoluble fiber.

"When my mother had to get dinner for 8 she'd just make enough for 16 and only serve half."
– Gracie Allen

Americans presently consume 14 to 15 grams of dietary fiber daily. Recommendations for dietary fiber for adults are usually in the range of 20 to 35 grams per day or 10 to 13 grams of dietary fiber per 1000 calories. Many studies have shown the beneficial effect that soluble fiber has on plasma cholesterol and lipoprotein levels. In general, LDL decreases and HDL is unchanged. The magnitude of the cholesterol reduction is related to the person's initial cholesterol level – individuals with higher cholesterol levels respond more to soluble fiber than individuals with lower cholesterol levels.

Oat fiber is easily added to the diet, and is well tolerated by most people, producing very little gastrointestinal distention, bloating or gas. In response to a health claim petition filed by the Quaker Oats company in 1995, the Food and Drug Association (FDA) reviewed more than 37 studies that investigated the effects of oatmeal and oat bran on total cholesterol and LDL levels. Based on this extensive body of research, in 1997 the FDA approved the first food-specific health claim for oatmeal and heart disease: "Soluble fiber from oatmeal, as part of a low saturated fat, low-cholesterol diet, may reduce the risk of heart disease."

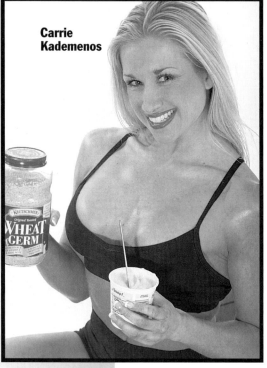

Carrie Kademenos

Small amounts of beans are also readily incorporated into the diet, and will lower plasma total cholesterol and LDL. Although some people note increased flatulence initially, adding beans to the diet gradually helps to decrease this complaint. There are also supplements to help prevent flatulence (Beano). The following cooking tips will also help: canned beans should be rinsed before use. Dried beans should be boiled, then allowed to soak for four hours, then drained and cooked with fresh water.

Fiber supplements made from pectin, guar gum, locust bean gum and pysllium seed husks may also reduce total cholesterol and LDL. However, viscosity, taste characteristics, and gastrointestinal side effects may be deterrents to long-term use.

How does soluble fiber lower serum cholesterol? Several theories have been proposed. The predominant theory involves the process by which soluble fiber affects bile acid circulation. In the liver, cholesterol is converted into bile acids, which are used to emulsify fats in the intestine for digestion and absorption. When

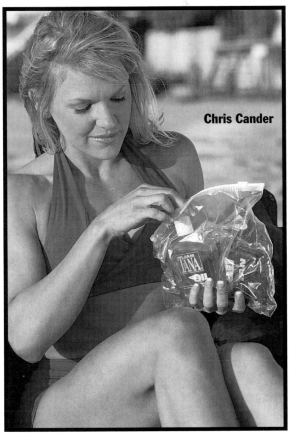

Chris Cander

bile acids are reabsorbed and come back to the liver (via the portal blood flow from the intestines), they block further production of bile acids, because the body doesn't need to produce more. This leaves more cholesterol in the intestines, which is dumped into the blood in the form of LDL cholesterol. This process, called the enterohepatic circulation of bile, is very effective in conserving bile.

Soluble fiber interferes with this process – it tends to bind with and increase the excretion of bile acids. When the excretion of bile acids is increased, the liver converts more LDL cholesterol into bile acids. This additional cholesterol is most easily obtained from the intestines, leaving less available for absorption. By causing more cholesterol to be used for bile acid production, soluble fiber helps take cholesterol out of circulation in the bloodstream. This is the major way in which soluble fiber is thought to lower serum cholesterol.

Other compounds in fiber sources may also affect cholesterol. The gamma analog of tocotrienol found in oats, barley and bran is a potent inhibitor of endogenous cholesterol biosynthesis and lowers blood cholesterol concentrations. An American Heart Association Science Advisory recommends a total dietary fiber intake of 25 to 30 grams per day from food (not supplements) to ensure nutritional adequacy and accentuate the lipid-lowering effects of a reduced-fat diet. Adding a fiber supplement to a diet otherwise high in saturated fat and cholesterol provides questionable cardiovascular benefits. However, the soluble fiber found in oats, barley, beans, soy products and pectin-rich fruits and vegetables provides additional cholesterol-lowering benefits that are beyond those achieved with reductions in total and saturated fat.[2]

People have been advised to consume high-fiber foods rather than load up on oat bran or psyllium, because fiber-rich foods also provide nutrients and phytochemicals. Some people with hypercholesterolemia may benefit from fiber supplements when diet modification is not sufficient or practical.

There is concern that dietary fibers may bind with certain minerals and decrease their bioavailability. This binding is unlikely to occur unless fiber intake is excessive and mineral intake inadequate. Excessive fiber intake may cause abdominal distress, gas and diarrhea. Dietary fiber should be increased gradually and accompanied by an adequate fluid intake. This allows the digestive system to adapt to the physiologic actions of the fiber.[18]

Whole grains have a lot of "woody" (for want of a better description fibre in their seed coat which helps regulate bowel activity. Less well known is the fact that many whole grains also contain soluble fibre, which also has positive health benefits. The soluble and insoluble fiber in seeds is known to be helpful in preventing constipation and diseases of the digestive tract such as diverticulitis. Fiber is also suspected to have a protective effect against colon cancer. Oats contain quite high amounts of soluble fiber, as does barley, and to a lesser extent wheat. Legumes high in soluble fiber are lentils, pinto beans and black beans. Legumes are also an excellent source of insoluble fiber. The fiber content of legumes slows the digestion of their carbohydrates content, regulating blood sugar levels.

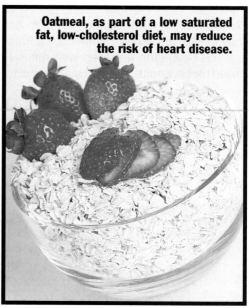

Oatmeal, as part of a low saturated fat, low-cholesterol diet, may reduce the risk of heart disease.

Oils

Despite the bad publicity fat receives in the media (and justly deserved, we might add), two kinds of fats – omega-3 and omega-6 – are essential for various body functions. They have to be obtained from the food we eat, as the human body can't synthesize them from other dietary fats. While omega-6 fatty acids are quite pervasive in the Western diet, omega-3 are not. Linolenic acid, an omega-3 fat, is found in flaxseeds, soya beans and pumpkin seeds. Flaxseed (linseed) is a very rich source of omega-3 fatty acids, with about 18.1 percent omega-3 content. The oils in oily seeds are an excellent energy source, and when eaten as part of the whole seed are slowly parceled out into the bloodstream over a period of hours. While oily seeds are a concentrated source of fuel, like any calorie-containing (or convertible) food, their calories are stored as fat only when we eat more calories than we need for energy. Otherwise the oils and carbohydrates are burned as fuel.

Estrogenic Effects

Naturally occurring plant substances, particularly in legumes, have been shown to have a weak estrogenic effect. Given our long evolutionary association with legumes, one must wonder if this effect hasn't become integrated into our biochemical background. Flax oil in particular is said to be estrogenic and may be helpful for postmenopausal women showing signs of hormone deficiency (such as atrophy and thinning of the vaginal walls). Soybeans also have a weak estrogenic effect.

Whole grains in general are suspected to help regulate estrogen levels in the body through their natural plant estrogens content (phytoestrogens), and through an effect of their fiber content. The fibre "lignan" in grains has been found to be weakly estrogenic.

Hormonally potent forms of estrogen (estradiol and estrone) are naturally metabolized in the liver to a less active form (estriol). This metabolite is eliminated into the bile, which empties into the digestive tract. The fibre in seeds binds to this estrogen, and it is removed from the body. There is some suggestion that without sufficient fibre, this estriol is altered by gut bacteria to the more potent forms and reabsorbed, altering the ratios of the forms of estrogen in the blood. There is some suggestion that such imbalances of the "estrogen profile" may tend to predispose women to various health problems.

Soybeans are filled with natural plant estrogens (or phytoestrogens) called bioflavonoids. Certain bioflavonoids are weak estrogens, having 1/50,000 the potency of a dose of synthetic estrogen. As weak estrogens, these compounds bind to estrogen receptors and act as a substitute form of estrogen in the body. They compete with the more potent estrogens made by a woman's body for these cell receptor sites. As a result, bioflavonoids can help to regulate estrogen levels.

After menopause estrogen levels drop and dietary sources of estrogen may have an important role in the female body. In Japan, where phytoestrogen-rich soybeans are a common part of the diet, only 10 to 15 percent of women experience menopause symptoms, whereas 80 to 85 percent of European and North American women (and those who eat a standard Western diet) experience symptoms at menopause.

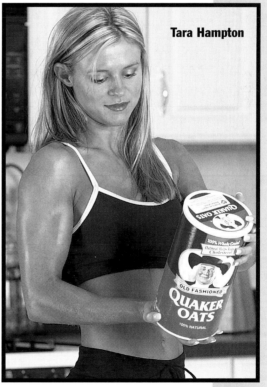

Tara Hampton

Some people assert that the early onset of puberty in girls in the West is "caused by" the soya component of food. However, Asian girls who eat similar or higher amounts of soy do not have early puberty. The much simpler and more obvious explanation is that the calorie-rich Western diet brings the body mass up to the critical 45 kg that allows the onset of menstruation.

In a recent study menopausal women were asked to supplement their diet with a phytoestrogen-containing food – soy flour, flax seed oil or red clover sprouts. The soy flour and flax oil (only) significantly prevented the vaginal mucosa from thinning and drying; but the effect of eliminating these foods reversed the situation.

Perhaps older women were good legume gatherers in our evolutionary past, resulting in modern menopausal women being biologically dependent on external sources of estrogen from legumes.

Protective Effects

Eating substantial amounts of soybeans and soybean products has been linked to a lower incidence of breast cancer in Japanese women, and in Japanese men lower mortality from prostate cancer. A recent study in USA of diet and heart disease in older women showed that one daily serving of whole grains – cereal or whole-grain bread – cut the risk of death from ischemic heart disease by nearly a third. Eating refined grains (for example white bread) didn't have a protective effect. When the protective effect of fiber, phytic acid and vitamin E were factored out, there was still a protective effect. The researchers speculate that it may be due to an as yet undiscovered phytochemical in grains, perhaps working together synergistically with the other protective plant compounds and forms of vitamin E in the seed.

The most important antioxidant we normally think of is vitamin E, yet there may be other antioxidants in some grains that are just as powerful. Oat flour, for example, has long been known for its antioxidant properties – to the extent it was once used as a component of such things as ready-mix cakes, in order to slow oxidative deterioration of the mix.

Women eating a diet that included 1.3 servings of whole grains had about a 30 to 40 percent lower risk rate of ischemic stroke, relative to the women whose normal intake was a half a serving of whole grains per day. So boosting intake of natural grains to even one serving per day has a powerful stroke-preventative effect. The particular attribute of grains responsible isn't known, but some useful chemical constituents have been identified:

Plants also contain a class of chemicals called *isoprenoids.* They help regulate such things as seed germination, and plant growth. Grain seeds contain an isoprenoid called *gamma-tocotrienol,* chemically somewhat similar to vitamin E. Laboratory experiments on the growth of human leukemia and breast cancer cell lines demonstrated that cancer cell growth was three times slower compared to a normal human cell culture which received the same dose of isoprenoid. The experiment used a dose of isoprenoids that anyone might be able to be obtain from eating a standard natural diet.

Recent research has shown that nitric oxide in the body has a protective effect on the integrity of the blood vessels. The amino acid arginine is the main source of nitric oxide in the body. Peanuts, sesame seeds and sunflower seeds are the richest sources of arginine, along with meat and nuts.

The natural phytochemicals known as *phenols* and *polyphenols* are hypothesized to be responsible for reducing the risk of cancers in people who eat sufficient fruit and vegetables. The various kinds of polyphenols have

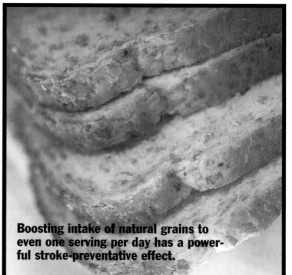

Boosting intake of natural grains to even one serving per day has a powerful stroke-preventative effect.

a variety of protective modes of action – carcinogen compound blocking, anti-oxidant and free radical scavenging, and tumor repression. While the phenols in fruit, black tea, red wine and vegetables are well known, few people know that in fact barley, at 1200 to 1500 mg per 100 gms, and some forms of sorghum (at up to 10,260 mg per 100 grams), have by far the highest amounts of any foods – other than dried figs (around 1000 mg per 100 grams of product).

Cultural Factors and Seed Consumption

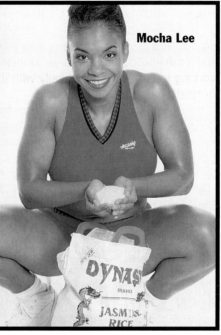

Mocha Lee

Throughout our evolutionary past much depended on cultural beliefs and practices (still does). Maize is deficient in the B group vitamins. In Central and South America the Indians ate maize with B vitamin-rich fish, avocadoes, tomatoes, peppers, and green leafy plants such as Malva (depending on the region). In North America, prior to the arrival of the colonizers, maize was steamed with clams, cooked with beans and meat, and generally used as a staple of a mixed diet. In some parts of Africa, once introduced, maize, overtook some of the original grains and became heavily relied upon. With the pressure of increasing population, it became almost the sole food, and pellagra (vitamin B deficiency) appeared.

In the West, flour has to be stored in bulk to meet the logistics of feeding massive city populations. Whole grains contain wheat-germ oil. Outside the protection of the whole seed, it quickly oxidizes and becomes rancid. The solution was to separate out the embryo (germ) with its oils and protein, remove the outer coat, and keep and mill only the carbohydrate store. The result: *white flour,* with the major natural oils, minerals and vitamins removed by milling. About the only advantage is that it keeps well.

Similarly rice is stripped of its nutrient-rich outer coat (bran) in the interests of a softer, whiter product, albeit a nutritionally gutted product our ancestors did not have the technology to create. The main vitamin lost is B1 (thiamin) – white rice has ten times less of this vitamin than the whole seed (brown rice). And what nutrient factor is absolutely essential for carbohydrate metabolism – thiamin.

Culturally, people in the West don't make or use flat breads. The seed an overwhelming number of us eat, the wheat seed, is turned into a "biological foam" by fermenting it with carbon dioxide-producing yeasts. The biofoam is then stabilized with heat. The result is the stabilized biofoam of wheat-seed carbohydrate that we call *bread.* Of the 200 pounds of grain seeds eaten annually by the average American, an estimated 95 percent is nutrient-stripped (and artificially "refortified" with a few of the originally stripped nutrients), and only 5 percent is derived from the whole grain our ancestors used to eat.

Why is wheat-seed biofoam more common than most other seed biofoams? Because wheat seed has a particular kind of protein in it called *gluten*, which can form a light springy mass when fermented with yeast. Removing the bran makes it even softer and "melt in the mouth." Most other grass seeds either don't have this protein or don't have much of it (oats and rye have some gluten), and their biofoams are not very foamy – they are dense and solid.

Gluten Intolerance

Some people are allergic to gluten. "Gluten intolerance" is more prevalent in women than men, and because it is genetically determined, its prevalence varies between about one person in 300 in western Ireland to one in 2000 for Europe in general. The gassiness, fatigue, depression and stomach discomfort, however, can be quickly eliminated by eating other grass seeds such as rice or millet, which contain no gluten.

The seeds we eat are chosen more for convenience and because of cultural norms, not because we must eat any one particular seed to have a healthy diet. Most of us are tolerant of most foods, including grass seeds of all kinds. Some have food allergies of greater or less importance (one estimate is 10 percent of the population). These allergies traverse virtually all foods, from beef to wheat, peanuts to oranges. The consequences range from mild gut disturbance to, in a tiny minority of cases, anaphylactic allergy reaction and death. But 90 percent or more of us have no food allergy. (Not all digestive effects are caused by allergy – beans cause gas, but that certainly doesn't equate to allergy!)

By choosing freshly ground whole seeds, sprouted seeds, biofoams with soaked whole seeds, boiled whole seeds, or freshly roasted/parched whole seeds, you are eating the foods humanity evolved to digest. And you will obtain the oils, vitamins, minerals and fiber you require for a healthy lifestyle.[12]

Fundamentals of Human Nutrition

"I was too old for a paper route, too young for Social Security, and too tired for an affair."
– Erma Bombeck, on why she started writing a humor column.

The food you eat is composed of hundreds of different kinds of materials, but mostly it is made up of three main nutrients – protein, carbohydrates and fat. These are commonly referred to as *macronutrients.* The science of nutrition is the study of the nutrients in foods and the body's ability to handle those nutrients. You metabolize many different nutrients, such as vitamins and minerals. However, you can only derive energy from these three macronutrients. They are vital to life. Without continual replenishment of the energy you expend you would soon die. When oxidized in the body, the energy nutrients break down, and some of their components bind with other compounds and form waste materials. As they are broken down they release energy. Some of this energy is released as heat and some is used as fuel for our activities.

This energy that is released by the macronutrients can be measured in *calories,* a word familiar to everyone as a measure of food energy and of the energy the body expends in large quantities during heavy exercise. Both carbohydrates and protein contain 4 calories per gram, whereas fat contains 9 calories per gram. Just by looking at these numbers we can see that it takes more than twice the amount of energy to burn a gram of fat than it does to burn a gram of protein or carbohydrate. Carbohydrates are your body's primary fuel source, because it is easier for your body to break down a gram of carbohydrate for energy than it is to break down a gram of fat. In order for your body to use fat as energy, you either have to be doing something aerobic for at least 15 minutes, or be completely depleted of carbohydrates so your body has no other choice but to use stored bodyfat for energy. The energy content of a food is determined by how much protein, carbohydrates and fat it contains. If you don't use these nutrients immediately after you eat them, your body will store them in the form of fat. Here's a simple rule: If you consume more than you use, you will gain weight. It doesn't matter if the excess is in the form of protein, carbohydrates or fat.

"If you drink, don't drive. Don't even putt."
– the late entertainer Dean Martin.

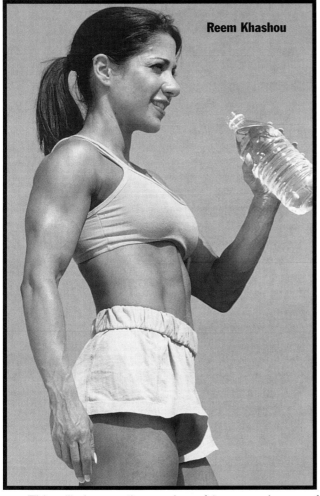

Reem Khashou

Water

Water forms the major part of every tissue within the body. The amount of water you actually need is about two to three liters per day. That's 2000 to 3000 grams. Water is a very important nutrient in that it provides the medium for which most of the body's activities are conducted. It also participates in most of the metabolic reactions that occur in the body and helps transport vital materials to the cells. One very important function of water is that it serves as the vehicle in which glycogen is transported into muscle cells. Glycogen is often referred to as *muscle fuel,* it powers muscle contraction. A simple calculation for determining your water requirement is to multiply your bodyweight by .6 and divide that by 12. This will give you the number of 8-ounce glasses of water you need. Example: If you weigh 140 pounds, calculate as follows: 140 x .6 ÷ 12 = 7. You need seven 8-ounce glasses of water per day.

Here are some "cold, hard facts" from the American Institute for Cancer Research about why increasing your water intake is important.[15]

1. Water helps you get moving by helping to relieve dry mouth and by refreshing the rest of your body.

2. Water plays a major role in preventing constipation. It encourages bowel movement and softens the stools.

3. Water moves food's nutrients through the body and ensures that nutrients are available when they are needed.

4. Instructions for many medicines say to "take with water." Water helps to hurry medicine to where it is needed.

5. Plenty of water keeps your skin in good shape from the inside.

6. The kidney system depends on water to help it work properly.

7. Athletes and coaches have long recognized that even mild dehydration can produce cramps and result in poor performance.

8. More water is the first and foremost treatment when kidney stones occur. Drinking sufficient amounts of water can help prevent them.

9. Dehydration can be avoided by monitoring your water intake. Both mental and physical performance may be impaired with even mild dehydration.

10. Water helps in regulating temperature and in balancing electrolytes.

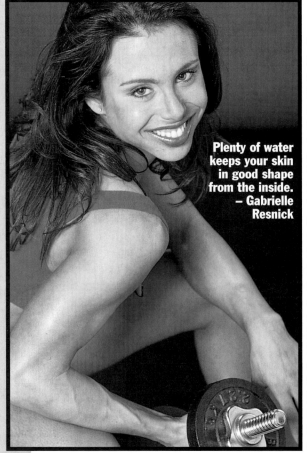

Plenty of water keeps your skin in good shape from the inside.
– Gabrielle Resnick

Vitamins

We cannot derive usable energy from vitamins, instead they serve as catalysts, making it possible for other nutrients to be digested, absorbed and metabolized into the body. There are 13 different vitamins and each one has a special role to play in the body. Vitamins A, D, E and K are known as fat-soluble vitamins. Vitamins B1, B2, B6, B12 and C are known as water-soluble vitamins. *Water*-soluble vitamins are for the most part carried in the bloodstream, excreted in the urine, needed in small doses, and are unlikely to be toxic. *Fat*-soluble vitamins are found in the fat and oily parts of foods. They tend to move into the liver and adipose (fat) tissue and remain there, rather than being excreted like most water-soluble vitamins. Storage of fat-soluble vitamins in the body makes it possible to survive long periods of time without having to supplement them in the diet. Because they are stored in the body, there is a risk of toxicity with fat-soluble vitamins.[16]

RDA vs. DV

Manufacturers of vitamin supplements in the United States are in the process of switching to a new label format that resembles the "Nutrition Facts" labels that Americans have been seeing on food packages for the past several years. The new label lists the percentages of *daily values* for various vitamins, rather than using the outdated term *US RDA*. You need not be concerned about this change – as far as vitamins are concerned, the two terms mean pretty much the same thing. The label on your supplement will still give you the information you need about the types and amounts of nutrients contained in the product. You may even find the new labels easier to use than the old ones because they're so similar to the familiar labels on food packages.

Vitamin A

Vitamin A is a family of fat-soluble vitamins. Retinol is one of the most active, or usable, forms of vitamin A, and is found in animal foods such as liver and eggs. It can be converted to retinal and retinoic acid, other active forms of the vitamin A family. Some plant foods contain orange pigments called *provitamin A carotenoids* that the liver can convert to retinol. Beta-carotene is a provitamin A carotenoid found in many foods.[1,2,3] Lycopene, lutein and zeaxanthin are also carotenoids commonly found in food, but your body cannot convert them to vitamin A.

Vitamin A plays an important role in vision, bone growth, reproduction, cell division and cell differentiation. It also maintains the surface linings of the eyes and respiratory, urinary and intestinal tracts.[8] When those linings break down, bacteria can enter the body and cause infection. Vitamin A also helps the body regulate its immune system. The immune system helps prevent or fight off infections by making white blood cells that destroy harmful bacteria and viruses. Vitamin A may help lymphocytes, a type of white blood cell that fights infections, function more effectively. Vitamin A also may help prevent bacteria and viruses from entering your body by maintaining the integrity of skin and mucous.

In addition to serving as a source of vitamin A, some carotenoids have been shown to function as antioxidants in laboratory tests. However, this role has not been consistently demonstrated in humans. Antioxidants protect cells from free radicals, which are potentially damaging byproducts of the body's metabolism that may contribute to the development of some chronic diseases.

What Foods Provide Vitamin A?

Whole eggs, whole milk and liver are among the few foods that naturally contain vitamin A. Vitamin A is present in the fat portion of whole milk, so it is not found in fat-free milk. Most fat-free milk and dried nonfat milk solids sold in the US are fortified with vitamin A. There are many other fortified foods such as breakfast cereals that also provide vitamin A.

There is no separate RDA for beta-carotene or other carotenoids. The Institute of Medicine (IOM) report suggests that consuming 3 to 6 mg of beta-carotene daily will maintain plasma B-carotene blood levels in the range

"Protect your bagels, put lox on them."
– sign at Bagel Connection, New Haven CT.

associated with a lower risk of chronic diseases.[13] This concentration can be achieved by a diet that provides five or more servings of fruits and vegetables per day.

When Can Vitamin A Deficiency Occur?

Vitamin A deficiency rarely occurs in the United States, but it is still a major public health problem in the developing world. It is most often associated with protein/calorie malnutrition and affects over 120 million children worldwide.[7] It is also a leading cause of childhood blindness. In countries where immunization programs are not widespread and vitamin A deficiency is common, millions of children die each year from complications of infectious diseases such as measles.[8]

What is the Association Between Vitamin A, Beta-Carotene and Cancer?

Surveys suggest an association between diets rich in beta-carotene and vitamin A and a lower risk of many types of cancer. There is evidence that higher intake of green and yellow vegetables or food sources of beta-carotene and/or vitamin A decreased the risk of lung cancer. A number of studies have tested the role of beta-carotene supplements in cancer prevention. Unfortunately, recent intervention studies have not supported a protective role for beta-carotene in cancer prevention. In a study of 29,000 men, incidence of lung cancer was greater in the group of smokers who took a daily supplement of beta-carotene. The Carotene and Retinol Efficacy Trial, a lung cancer chemoprevention trial that provided randomized subjects with supplements of beta carotene and vitamin A, was stopped after researchers discovered that subjects receiving beta carotene had a 46 percent higher risk of dying from lung cancer. The IOM states that "B-carotene supplements are not advisable for the general population," although they also state that this advice "does not pertain to the possible use of supplemental B-carotene as a provitamin A source for the prevention of vitamin A deficiency in populations with inadequate vitamin A nutriture."[17]

What is the Health Risk of Too Much Vitamin A?

Hypervitaminosis A refers to high storage levels of vitamin A in the body that can lead to toxic symptoms. Toxicity can result in dry, itchy skin, headache, fatigue, hair loss, loss of appetite, vomiting and liver damage. When toxic symptoms arise suddenly, which can happen after consuming very large amounts of vitamin A over a short period of time, signs of toxicity include dizziness, blurred vision, and loss of muscular co-ordination.

Although hypervitaminosis A can occur when very large amounts of liver are regularly consumed, most cases of vitamin A toxicity result from an excess intake of vitamin A in supplements. A generally recognized safe upper limit of intake for vitamin A from diet and supplements is 1600 to 2000 RE (8000 to 10,000 IU) per day. The Institute of Medicine is currently reviewing the scientific literature on vitamin A. They are considering revising the RDAs and establishing an upper limit (UL) of safe intake for vitamin A.

Vitamin A toxicity also can cause severe birth defects. Women of child-bearing age are advised to limit their total daily intake of vitamin A (retinol) from foods and supplements combined to no more than 1600 RE (8000 IU) per day.

Retinoids are compounds that are chemically similar to vitamin A. Over the past 15 years, synthetic retinoids have been prescribed for acne, psoriasis, and other skin disorders. Isotretinoin (Roaccutane or Accutane) is considered an effective antiacne therapy. At very high doses, however, it can be toxic, which is why this medication is usually saved for the most severe forms of acne. The most serious consequence of this medication is birth defects.

What is the Health Risk of Too Many Carotenoids?

Nutrient toxicity traditionally refers to adverse health effects from a high intake of a particular vitamin or mineral. For example, as we have outlined above, large amounts of the active form of vitamin A (naturally found in animal foods such as liver but also available in dietary supplements) can cause birth defects.

Provitamin A carotenoids such as beta-carotene are generally considered safe because they are not traditionally associated with specific adverse health effects. The conversion of provitamin A carotenoids to vitamin A decreases when body stores are full, which naturally limits further increases in storage levels. A high intake of provitamin A carotenoids can turn the skin yellow, but this is not considered dangerous to health.

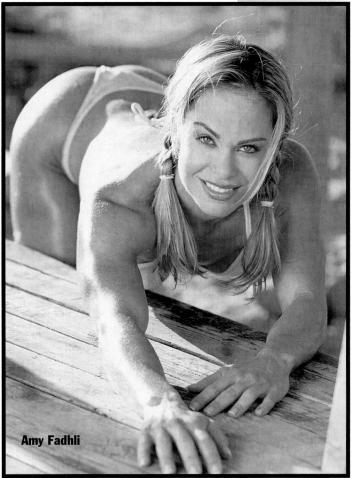

Amy Fadhli

The Institute of Medicine did not set a Tolerable Upper Intake Level (UL), the highest level of daily nutrient intake that is likely to pose no risk of adverse health effects, for B-carotene or carotenoids. Instead, they concluded that B-carotene supplements are not advisable for the general population. As stated earlier, however, they may be appropriate as a provitamin A source or for the prevention of vitamin A deficiency in specific populations.[3]

Vitamin B6

Vitamin B6 is a water-soluble vitamin that exists in three major chemical forms: pyridoxine, pyridoxal and pyridoxamine. It performs a wide variety of functions in your body and is essential for your good health. For example, vitamin B6 is needed for more than 100 enzymes involved in protein metabolism. It is also essential for red blood cell metabolism. The nervous and immune systems need vitamin B6 to function efficiently, and it is also needed for the conversion of tryptophan (an amino acid) to niacin (a vitamin).

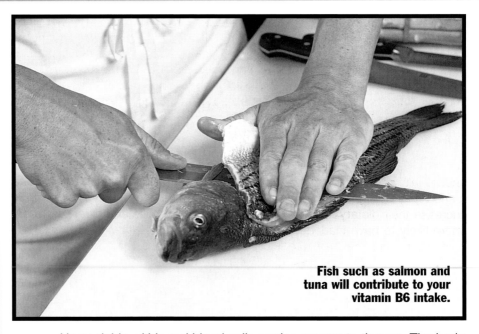

Fish such as salmon and tuna will contribute to your vitamin B6 intake.

Hemoglobin within red blood cells carries oxygen to tissues. The body needs vitamin B6 to make hemoglobin. Vitamin B6 also helps increase the amount of oxygen carried by hemoglobin. A vitamin B6 deficiency can result in a form of anemia similar to iron deficiency anemia.

An *immune response* is a broad term that describes a variety of biochemical changes that occur in an effort to fight off infections. Calories, protein, vitamins and minerals are important to the immune defenses because they promote the growth of white blood cells that directly fight infections. Vitamin B6, through its involvement in protein metabolism and cellular growth, is important to the immune system. It helps maintain the health of lymphoid organs (thymus, spleen and lymph nodes) that make your white blood cells. Animal studies show that a vitamin B6 deficiency can decrease the antibody production and suppress the immune response.

Vitamin B6 also helps maintain the blood glucose (sugar) within a normal range. When caloric intake is low the body needs vitamin B6 to help convert stored carbohydrates or other nutrients to glucose to maintain normal blood sugar levels. While a shortage of vitamin B6 will limit these functions, supplementation of B6 does not enhance them in well-nourished individuals.

"The bagel, an unsweetened donut with rigor mortis."
– Beatrice and Ira Henry Freeman

What Foods Provide Vitamin B6?
Foods such as fortified breakfast cereals, fish such as salmon and tuna fish, meats such as pork and chicken, bananas, beans and peanut butter, and many vegetables will contribute to your vitamin B6 intake.

When Can a Vitamin B6 Deficiency Occur?
Clinical signs of vitamin B6 deficiency are rarely seen in the United States. Many older Americans, however, have low blood levels of vitamin B6, which may suggest a marginal or suboptimal vitamin B6 nutritional status. Vitamin B6

deficiency can occur in individuals with a poor-quality diet who are deficient in many nutrients. Symptoms occur during later stages of deficiency, when intake has been very low for an extended time. Signs of vitamin B6 deficiency include dermatitis (skin inflammation), glossitis (a sore tongue), depression, confusion and convulsions. Vitamin B6 deficiency can also cause anemia. Some of these symptoms can also result from a variety of medical conditions other than vitamin B6 deficiency. It is important to have a physician evaluate these symptoms so that appropriate medical care can be given.

Who May Need Extra Vitamin B6 to Prevent a Deficiency?

Individuals with a poor-quality diet or an inadequate B6 intake for an extended period may benefit from taking a vitamin B6 supplement if they are unable to increase their dietary intake of vitamin B6.[1,15] Alcoholics and older adults are more likely to have inadequate vitamin B6 intake than other segments of the population because they may have limited variety in their diet. Alcohol also promotes the destruction and loss of vitamin B6 from the body.

Asthmatic children treated with the medicine theophylline may need to take a vitamin B6 supplement. Theophylline decreases body stores of vitamin B6, and theophylline-induced seizures have been linked to low body stores of the vitamin. A physician should be consulted about the need for vitamin B6 supplementation when theophylline is prescribed.

What Are Some Current Issues and Controversies About Vitamin B6?

Vitamin B6 is needed for the synthesis of neurotransmitters such as serotonin and dopamine. These neurotransmitters are required for normal nerve cell communication. Researchers have been investigating the relationship between vitamin B6 status and a wide variety of neurologic conditions such as seizures, chronic pain, depression, headache and Parkinson disease.

Lower levels of serotonin have been found in individuals suffering from depression and migraine headaches. So far, however, vitamin B6 supplements have not been proven effective for relieving these symptoms. One study found that a sugar pill was just as likely as vitamin B6 to relieve headaches and depression associated with low-dose oral contraceptives.

Alcohol abuse can result in neuropathy, abnormal nerve sensations in the arms and legs. A poor dietary intake contributes to this neuropathy and dietary supplements that include vitamin B6 may prevent or decrease its incidence.

Vitamin B6 and Carpal Tunnel Syndrome

Vitamin B6 was first recommended for carpal tunnel syndrome almost 30 years ago. Several popular books still recommend taking 100 to 200 milligrams of vitamin B6 daily to treat carpal tunnel syndrome, even though scientific studies do not indicate it is effective. Anyone taking large doses of vitamin B6 supplements for carpal tunnel syndrome needs to be aware that the Institute of Medicine recently established an upper tolerable limit of 100 mg per day for adults. There are documented cases in the literature of neuropathy caused by excessive vitamin B6 taken for treatment of carpal tunnel syndrome.

Vitamin B6 and Premenstrual Syndrome

Vitamin B6 has become a popular remedy for treating the discomforts associated with premenstrual syndrome (PMS). Unfortunately, clinical trials have failed to support any significant benefit.[23] One recent study indicated that a sugar pill was as likely to relieve symptoms of PMS as vitamin B6.[24] In addition, vitamin B6 toxicity has been seen in increasing numbers of women taking B6 supplements for PMS. One review indicated that neuropathy was present in 23 of 58 women taking daily vitamin B6 supplements for PMS whose blood levels of B6 were above normal. There is no convincing scientific evidence to support recommending vitamin B6 supplements for PMS.

Vitamin B6 and Interactions With Medications

There are many drugs that interfere with the metabolism of vitamin B6. Isoniazid, which is used to treat tuberculosis, and l-dopa, which is used to treat a variety of neurologic problems such as Parkinson disease, alter the activity of vitamin B6. There is disagreement about the need for routine vitamin B6 supplementation when taking isoniazid. Acute isoniazid toxicity can result in coma and seizures that are reversed by vitamin B6, but in a group of children receiving isoniazid, no

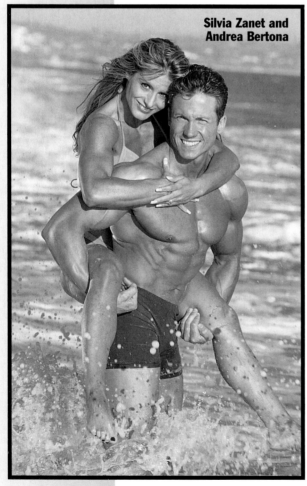

Silvia Zanet and Andrea Bertona

cases of neurological or neuropsychiatric problems were observed, regardless of whether or not they took a vitamin B6 supplement. Some doctors recommend taking a supplement that provides 100 percent of the RDA for B6 when isoniazid is prescribed, which is usually enough to prevent symptoms of vitamin B6 deficiency. It is important to consult with a physician about the need for a vitamin B6 supplement when taking isoniazid.

What's the Relationship Between B6, Homocysteine and Heart Disease?

A deficiency of vitamin B6, folic acid or vitamin B12 may increase your level of homocysteine, an amino acid normally found in your blood. There is evidence that an elevated homocysteine level is an independent risk factor for heart disease and stroke. Evidence suggests that high levels of homocysteine may damage coronary arteries or make it easier for blood clotting cells called platelets to clump together and form a clot. However, there is currently no evidence available to suggest that lowering homocysteine levels with vitamins will reduce your risk of heart disease. Clinical intervention trials are needed to determine whether supplementation with vitamin B6, folic acid or vitamin B12 can help protect you against developing coronary heart disease.

What is the Health Risk of Too Much Vitamin B6?

Too much vitamin B6 can result in nerve damage to the arms and legs. This neuropathy is usually related to high intake of vitamin B6 from supplements, and is reversible when supplementation is stopped. According to the Institute of Medicine, "Several reports show sensory neuropathy at doses lower than 500 mg per day." As previously mentioned, the Food and Nutrition Board of the Institute of Medicine has established an upper tolerable intake level (UL) for vitamin B6 of 100 mg per day for all adults.[4]

Vitamin B12 is naturally found in animal foods including fish, milk and milk products, eggs, meat and poultry.

Vitamin B12

Vitamin B12, also called cobalamin, helps maintain healthy nerve cells and red blood cells, and is also needed to make DNA, the genetic material in all cells. Vitamin B12 is bound to the protein in food. Hydrochloric acid in the stomach releases B12 from protein during digestion. Once released, B12 combines with a substance called intrinsic factor (IF) before it is absorbed into the bloodstream.

What Foods Provide Vitamin B12?

Vitamin B12 is naturally found in animal foods including fish, milk and milk products, eggs, meat and poultry. Fortified breakfast cereals are an excellent source of vitamin B12 and a particularly valuable source for vegetarians.[5,6,7] The table of selected food sources of vitamin B12 suggests dietary sources of vitamin B12.

"If rich food can kill, people live dangerously here."
– Alice Furland

What is the Recommended Dietary Allowance of Vitamin B12 for Adults?

The RDA is the average daily dietary intake level that is sufficient to meet the nutrient requirements of nearly all (97 to 98 percent) healthy individuals in each life-stage and gender group.[7] The 1998 RDAs of vitamin B12 (in micrograms) for adults are:

Life Stage	Men	Women
Ages 19+	2.4 mcg	2.4 mcg
All ages	2.6 mcg	2.8 mcg

When is a Deficiency of Vitamin B12 Likely to Occur?

Diets of most adult Americans provide the recommended intake of vitamin B12, but deficiency may still occur as a result of an inability to absorb B12 from food. It can also occur in individuals with dietary patterns that exclude animal or fortified foods. As a general rule, most individuals who develop a vitamin B12 deficiency have an underlying stomach or intestinal disorder that limits the absorption of vitamin B12. Sometimes the only symptom of these disorders is anemia resulting from B12 deficiency.

Characteristic signs of B12 deficiency include fatigue, weakness, nausea, constipation, flatulence (gas), loss of appetite, and weight loss. Deficiency can also lead to neurological changes such as numbness and tingling in the hands and feet. Additional symptoms of B12 deficiency are difficulty in maintaining balance, depression, confusion, poor memory, and soreness of the mouth or tongue . Some of these symptoms can also result from a variety of medical conditions other than vitamin B12 deficiency. It is important to have a physician evaluate these symptoms so that appropriate medical care can be provided.

Who May Need B12 Supplementation to Prevent a Deficiency?

Pernicious anemia is a form of anemia that occurs when there is an absence of intrinsic factor, a substance normally present in the stomach. Vitamin B12 binds with intrinsic factor before it is absorbed and used by the body. An absence of intrinsic factor prevents normal absorption of B12 and results in pernicious anemia.

Anyone with pernicious anemia usually needs intramuscular (IM) injections of vitamin B12. It is very important to remember that pernicious anemia is a chronic condition that should be monitored by a physician. Anyone with pernicious anemia has to take lifelong supplemental vitamin B12.

Individuals With Gastrointestinal Disorders

Individuals with stomach and small intestinal disorders may not absorb enough vitamin B12 from food to maintain healthy body stores. Sprue and celiac disease are intestinal disorders caused by intolerance to protein in wheat and wheat products. Regional enteritis, localized inflammation of the stomach or small intestine, also results in generalized malabsorption of vitamin B12. Excess bacteria in the stomach and small intestine also can decrease vitamin B12 absorption.

Surgical procedures of the gastrointestinal tract such as surgery to remove all or part of the stomach often result in a loss of cells that secrete stomach acid and intrinsic factor. Surgical removal of the distal ileum, a section of the intestines, can result in the inability to absorb B12. Anyone who has had either of these surgeries usually requires lifelong supplemental B12 to prevent a deficiency.

Older Adults

Vitamin B12 must be separated from protein in food before it can bind with intrinsic factor and be absorbed by your body. Bacterial overgrowth in the stomach and/or atrophic gastritis, an inflammation of the stomach, contribute to vitamin B12 deficiency in adults by limiting secretions of stomach acid needed to separate vitamin B12 from protein in food. Adults 50 years of age and older with these conditions are able to absorb the B12 in fortified foods and dietary supplements. Health care professionals may advise adults over the age of 50 to get their vitamin B12 from a dietary supplement or from foods fortified with vitamin B12 because 10 to 30 percent of older people may be unable to absorb vitamin B12 in food.

Vegetarians

Vegetarians who do not eat meats, fish, eggs, milk or milk products, or B12 fortified foods, consume no vitamin B12 and are at high risk of developing a deficiency of vitamin B12. When adults adopt a vegetarian diet, deficiency symptoms can be slow to appear because it usually takes years to deplete normal body stores of B12. However, severe symptoms of B12 deficiency, most often featuring poor neurological development, can show up quickly in children and breast-fed infants of women who follow a strict vegetarian diet.

Fortified cereals are one of the few plant food sources of vitamin B12, and are an important dietary source of B12 for vegetarians who consume no eggs, milk or milk products. Vegetarian adults who do not consume plant foods fortified with vitamin B12 need to consider taking a supplement containing B12. Vegetarian mothers should consult with a pediatrician regarding appropriate vitamin B12 supplementation for their infants and children.

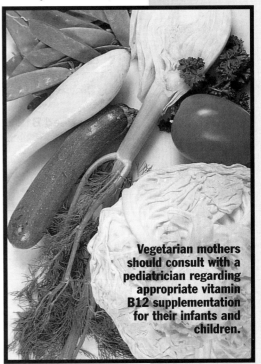

Vegetarian mothers should consult with a pediatrician regarding appropriate vitamin B12 supplementation for their infants and children.

What is the Relationship Between B12, Homocysteine and Heart Disease?

A deficiency of vitamin B12, folate, or vitamin B6 may increase your blood level of homocysteine, an amino acid normally found in your blood. There is evidence that an elevated blood level of homocysteine is an independent risk factor for heart disease and stroke. The evidence suggests that high levels of homocysteine may damage coronary arteries or make it easier for blood clotting cells called platelets to clump together and form a clot. However, there is currently no evidence available to suggest that lowering homocysteine level with vitamins will actually reduce your risk of heart disease. Clinical intervention trials are needed to determine whether supplementation with vitamin B12, folic acid or vitamin B6 can help protect you against developing coronary heart disease.

What is the Health Risk of Too Much Vitamin B12?

Vitamin B12 has a very low potential for toxicity. The Institute of Medicine states that "no adverse effects have been associated with excess vitamin B12 intake from food and supplements in healthy individuals." The Institute recommends adults over 50 years of age get most of their vitamin B12 from supplements or fortified food because of the high incidence of impaired absorption of B12 from unfortified foods in this population.[5]

Vitamin D

Vitamin D, calciferol, is a fat-soluble vitamin found in food, but also can be made in your body after exposure to ultraviolet rays from the sun. Vitamin D exists in several forms, each with a different activity. Some forms are relatively inactive in

"They used to have a fish on the menu ... that was smoked, grilled and peppered ... They did everything to this fish but pistol-whip it and dress it in Bermuda shorts."
– William E Geist

the body, and have limited ability to function as a vitamin. The liver and kidneys help convert vitamin D to its active hormone form.

The major biologic function of vitamin D is to maintain normal blood levels of calcium and phosphorus. Vitamin D aids in the absorption of calcium, helping to form and maintain strong bones. It promotes bone mineralization in concert with a number of other vitamins, minerals and hormones. Without vitamin D, bones can become thin, brittle, soft or misshapen. Vitamin D prevents rickets in children and osteomalacia in adults, which are skeletal diseases that result in defects that weaken bones.

What Are the Sources of Vitamin D?

Fortified foods are the major dietary sources of vitamin D. Prior to the fortification of milk products in the 1930s, rickets (a bone disease seen in children) was a major public health problem in the United States. Milk in the US is fortified with 10 micrograms (400 IU) of vitamin D per quart, and rickets is now uncommon in the US.

One cup of vitamin D fortified milk supplies about one-fourth of the estimated daily need for this vitamin for adults. Although milk is fortified with vitamin D, dairy products made from milk (such as cheese, yogurt and ice cream) are generally not fortified with vitamin D. Only a few foods naturally contain significant amounts of vitamin D, including fatty fish and fish oils.

Exposure to Sunlight

Exposure to sunlight is an important source of vitamin D. Ultraviolet (UV) rays from sunlight trigger vitamin D synthesis in the skin. Season, latitude, time of day, cloud cover, smog, and sunscreens affect UV ray exposure. Individuals with limited sun exposure should definitely include good sources of vitamin D in their diet.

Is There a Recommended Dietary Allowance of Vitamin D for Adults?

The 1998 RDA of vitamin D for adults, in micrograms (mcg) and International Units (IUs) are:

Life Stage	Men	Women
Ages 19-50	5 mcg (200 IU)	5 mcg (200 IU)
Ages 51-69	10 mcg (400 IU)	10 mcg (400 IU)
Ages 70+	15 mcg (600 IU)	15 mcg (600 IU)

(1 mcg vitamin D = 40 IU)

Estimates of intake in the United States are not available because dietary surveys do not assess vitamin D. Dietary intake of vitamin D is largely determined by the intake of fortified food.[4]

When Can Vitamin D Deficiency Occur?

A deficiency of vitamin D can occur when dietary intake of vitamin D is inadequate, when there is limited exposure to sunlight, when the kidney cannot convert vitamin D to its active form, or when someone cannot adequately absorb vitamin D from the gastrointestinal tract.

The classic vitamin D deficiency diseases are rickets and osteomalacia. In children vitamin D deficiency causes rickets, leading to skeletal deformities. In adults, vitamin D deficiency can lead to osteomalacia, which results in muscular weakness in addition to weak bones.

Who May Need Extra Vitamin D to Prevent a Deficiency?
Older Americans (over age 50) are thought to have a higher risk of developing vitamin D deficiency. The ability of skin to convert vitamin D to its active form decreases as we age. The kidneys, which help convert vitamin D to its active form, sometimes do not work as well when people age. Therefore, some older individuals may need vitamin D from a supplement.

Individuals with limited sun exposure should certainly include good sources of vitamin D in their diets. Homebound individuals, people living in northern latitudes such as in New England, Canada and Alaska, women who cover their body for religious reasons, and those working in occupations that prevent exposure to sunlight are all at risk of a vitamin D deficiency. If these people are unable to meet their daily dietary requirement, they may need supplemental vitamin D.

Individuals who have reduced ability to absorb dietary fat (fat malabsorption) may need extra vitamin D because it is a fat-soluble vitamin. Some causes of fat malabsorption are pancreatic enzyme deficiency, Crohn disease, cystic fibrosis, sprue, liver disease, surgical removal of part or all of the stomach, and small bowel disease. Symptoms of fat malabsorption include diarrhea and greasy stools.

Vitamin D supplements are often recommended for exclusively breast-

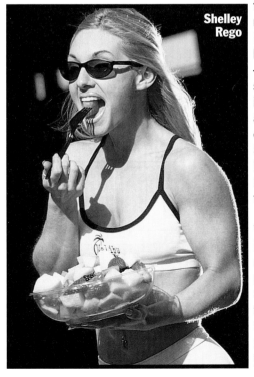

Shelley Rego

fed infants because human milk may not contain adequate vitamin D. The Institute of Medicine states that "With habitual small doses of sunshine breast – or formula-fed infants do not require supplemental vitamin D." Mothers of infants who are exclusively breastfed and have limited sun exposure should consult with a pediatrician on this issue. Since infant formulas are routinely fortified with vitamin D, formula-fed infants usually have adequate dietary intake of vitamin D.

Vitamin D and Osteoporosis
It is estimated that over 25 million adults in the United States have or are at risk of developing osteoporosis. Osteoporosis is a disease characterized by fragile bones. It results in increased risk of bone fractures. Having normal storage levels of vitamin D in your body helps keep your bones strong

and may help prevent osteoporosis in elderly, nonambulatory individuals, in postmenopausal women, and in individuals on chronic steroid therapy.

Researchers know that normal bone is constantly being remodeled (broken down and rebuilt). During menopause the balance between these two systems is upset, resulting in more bone being broken down (reabsorbed) than rebuilt. Estrogen replacement, which limits symptoms of menopause, can help slow down the development of osteoporosis by stimulating the activity of cells that rebuild bone.

Vitamin D deficiency, which occurs more often in postmenopausal women and older individuals, has been associated with greater incidence of hip fractures. A greater vitamin D intake from diet and supplements has been associated with less bone loss in older women. Since bone loss increases the risk of fractures, vitamin D supplementation may help prevent fractures resulting from osteoporosis.

In a group of women with osteoporosis hospitalized for hip fractures, 50 percent were found to have signs of vitamin D deficiency. Treatment of vitamin D deficiency can result in decreased incidence of hip fractures, and daily supplementation with 20 mcg (800 IU) of vitamin D may reduce the risk of osteoporotic fractures in elderly people with low blood levels of vitamin D.

Vitamin D and Cancer

Laboratory, animal and epidemiological evidence suggest that vitamin D may be protective against some cancers. Some dietary surveys have associated increased intake of dairy foods with decreased incidence of colon cancer. Another dietary survey associated a higher calcium and vitamin D intake with a lower incidence of colon cancer. Well-designed clinical trials need to be conducted to determine whether vitamin D deficiency increases cancer risk, or if an increased intake of vitamin D is protective against some cancers. Until such trials are conducted, it is premature to advise anyone to take vitamin D supplements to prevent cancer.

Vitamin D and Steroids

Corticosteroid medications are often prescribed to reduce inflammation from a variety of medical problems. These medicines may be essential for a person's medical treatment, but they have potential side effects, including decreased calcium absorption. There is some evidence that steroids may also impair vitamin D metabolism, further contributing to the loss of bone and development of osteoporosis associated with steroid medications. For these reasons, individuals on chronic steroid therapy should consult with their physician or registered dietitian about the need to increase vitamin D intake through diet and/or dietary supplements.

Vitamin D and Alzheimer Disease

Adults with Alzheimer disease have increased risk of hip fractures. This may be because many Alzheimer patients are homebound, and frequently sunlight deprived. Alzheimer's disease is more prevalent in older populations, so the fact that the ability of skin to convert vitamin D to its active form decreases as we age may also contribute to increased risk of hip fractures in this group. One study of women with Alzheimer disease found that decreased bone mineral density was associated with a low intake of vitamin D and inadequate sunlight exposure. Physicians evaluate the need for vitamin D supplementation as part of an overall treatment plan for adults with Alzheimer disease.

What is the Health Risk of Too Much Vitamin D?

There is a high health risk associated with consuming *too much* vitamin D. Vitamin D toxicity can cause nausea, vomiting, poor appetite, constipation, weakness and weight loss. It can also raise blood levels of calcium, causing changes in mental status such as confusion. High blood levels of calcium can cause heart rhythm abnormalities. Calcinosis, the deposition of calcium and phosphate in soft tissues like the kidney, can be caused by vitamin D toxicity.

Consuming too much vitamin D through diet alone is not likely unless you routinely take large amounts of cod liver oil, but much more likely to occur from high intake of vitamin D in supplements. The Food and Nutrition Board of the Institute of Medicine considers an intake of 25 mcg (1000 IU) for infants up to 12 months of age and 50 mcg (2000 IU) for children, adults, pregnant and lactating women to be the tolerable upper intake level (UL). A daily intake above the UL increases the risk of adverse health effects and is not advised.[6]

Vitamin E

E is a fat-soluble vitamin that exists in eight different forms. Each form has its own biological activity, the measure of potency or functional use in the body. Alpha-tocopherol is the most active form of vitamin E in humans, and is a powerful biological antioxidant. Antioxidants such as vitamin E act to protect your cells against the effects of free radicals, which are potentially damaging by-products of the body's metabolism. Free radicals can cause cell damage that may contribute to the development of cardiovascular disease and cancer. Studies are under way to determine whether vitamin E might help prevent or delay the development of those chronic diseases.

What Foods Provide Vitamin E?

Vegetable oils, nuts and green leafy vegetables are the main dietary sources of vitamin E. Fortified cereals are also an important source of vitamin E in the United States. The table of selected food sources of vitamin E suggests foods that contain vitamin E.[4]

What is the Recommended Dietary Allowance for Vitamin E for Adults?

The year 2000 RDA for vitamin E for adults, in milligrams (mg) and International Units (IUs) are:[5]

Life Stage	Men and Women	Pregnancy
Ages 19+	15 mg (22 IU)	
All ages	15 mg (22 IU)	19 mg or 28 IU

1 mg alpha-tocopherol equivalents = 1.5 IU

The RDA for vitamin E is based on the alpha-tocopherol form because it is the most active (usable) form. Unlike other vitamins, the form of alpha-tocopherol made in the laboratory and found in supplements is not identical to the natural form, and is not quite as active as the natural form.

The year 2000 Institute of Medicine (IOM) report on vitamin E states that intake estimates of vitamin E may be low because energy and fat intake is often under reported in national surveys and because the kind and amount of fat added during cooking is often not known. The IOM states that most North American adults get enough vitamin E from their normal diets to meet current recommendations. However, they do caution individuals who consume low-fat diets because vegetable oils are such a good dietary source of vitamin E. "Low-fat diets can substantially decrease vitamin E intakes if food choices are not carefully made to enhance alpha-tocopherol intakes."

> *"As for butter versus margarine, I trust cows more than chemists."*
> – Joan Gussow,
> Assistant Professor of Nutrition and Education, Teachers College, Columbia University.

When Can Vitamin E Deficiency Occur?

Vitamin E deficiency is rare in humans. There are three specific situations when a deficiency is likely to occur. It is seen in persons who cannot absorb dietary fat, has been found in premature, very low birth weight infants (birth weights less than 1500 grams, 3-1/2 pounds), and is seen in individuals with rare disorders of fat metabolism. A vitamin E deficiency is usually characterized by neurological problems due to poor nerve conduction.

Who May Need Extra Vitamin E to Prevent a Deficiency?

Individuals who cannot absorb fat may require vitamin E supplementation because some dietary fat is needed for the absorption of vitamin E from the gastrointestinal tract. Anyone diagnosed with cystic fibrosis, individuals who have had part or all of their stomach removed, and individuals with malabsorptive problems such as Crohn disease may not absorb fat and should discuss the need for supplemental vitamin E with their physician. People who cannot absorb fat often pass greasy stools or have chronic diarrhea.

Very low birth weight infants may be deficient in vitamin E. These infants are usually under the care of a neonatologist, a pediatrician specializing in the care of newborns, who evaluates and treats the exact nutritional needs of premature infants.

Abetalipoproteinemia is a rare inherited disorder of fat metabolism that results in poor absorption of dietary fat and vitamin E. The vitamin E deficiency associated with this disease causes problems such as poor transmission of nerve impulses, muscle weakness, and degeneration of the retina that can cause blindness. Individuals with abetalipoproteinemia may be prescribed special vitamin E supplements by a physician to treat this disorder.

Vitamin E and Heart Disease

Preliminary research has led to a widely held belief that vitamin E may help prevent or delay coronary heart disease. Researchers are fairly certain that oxidative modification of LDL-cholesterol (sometimes called "bad cholesterol") promotes blockages in coronary arteries that may lead to atherosclerosis and heart attacks. Vitamin E may help prevent or delay coronary heart disease by limiting the oxidation of LDL-cholesterol. A 1994 review of 5133 Finnish men and women aged 30 to 69 years suggested that increased dietary intake of vitamin E was associated with decreased mortality (death) from heart disease. But even though these observations are promising, randomized clinical trials raise questions about the role of vitamin E supplements in heart disease. The Heart Outcomes Prevention Evaluation (HOPE) study followed for 4.5 years almost 10,000 patients who were at high risk for heart attack or stroke. In this intervention study the subjects who received 265 mg (400 IU) of vitamin E daily did not experience significantly fewer cardiovascular events or hospitalizations for heart failure or chest pain when compared to those who received a sugar pill. The researchers suggested it is unlikely that the vitamin E supplement provided any protection against cardiovascular disease in the HOPE study. This study is continuing, to determine whether a longer duration of intervention with vitamin E supplementation will provide any protection against cardiovascular disease.

Vitamin E and Cancer

Antioxidants such as vitamin E help protect against the damaging effects of free radicals, which may contribute to the development of chronic diseases such as cancer. Vitamin E also may block the formation of nitrosamines, which are carcinogens formed in the stomach from nitrites consumed in the diet. It also may protect against the development of cancers by enhancing immune function. Unfortunately, human trials and surveys that tried to associate vitamin E with incidence of cancer have been generally inconclusive.

Some evidence associates higher intake of vitamin E with a decreased incidence of prostate cancer and breast cancer. There is evidence that vitamin E may reduce the size of cysts in women with fibrocystic breast disease, which is a risk factor for breast cancer. However, an examination of the effect of dietary factors, including vitamin E, on incidence of postmenopausal breast cancer in over 18,000 women from New York State did not associate a greater vitamin E intake with a reduced risk of developing breast cancer.

A study of women in Iowa provided evidence that an increased dietary intake of vitamin E may decrease the risk of colon cancer, especially in women under 65 years of age. On the other hand, vitamin E intake was not statistically associated with risk of colon cancer in almost 2000 adults with cancer that was compared to controls without cancer. At this time there is limited evidence to recommend vitamin E supplements for the prevention of cancer.

Vitamin E and Cataracts

Cataracts are growths on the lens of the eye that cloud vision. They increase the risk of disability and blindness in aging adults. Antioxidants are being studied to determine whether they can help prevent or delay cataract growth. Observational studies have found that lens clarity (used to diagnose cataracts), was better in regular users of vitamin E supplements, and in persons with higher blood levels of vitamin E. A study of middle-aged male smokers did not demonstrate any effect from vitamin E supplements on the incidence of cataract formation. The effects of smoking, a major risk factor for developing cataracts, may have overridden any potential benefit from the vitamin E, but the conflicting results also indicate a need for further studies before researchers can confidently recommend extra vitamin E for the prevention of cataracts.

"As life's pleasures go, food is second only to sex ... except for salami and eggs. Now that's better than sex, but only if the salami is thickly sliced."
– Alan King

What is the Health Risk of Too Much Vitamin E?

The health risk of too much vitamin E is low.[23] A recent review of the safety of this vitamin in the elderly indicated that taking vitamin E supplements for up to four months at doses of 530 mg (800 IU) – 35 times the current RDA – had no significant effect on general health, bodyweight, levels of body proteins, lipid levels, liver or kidney function, thyroid hormones, amount or kinds of blood cells, or bleeding time. Even though this study provides evidence that taking a vitamin E supplement containing 530 mg for four months is safe, the long-term safety of vitamin E supplementation has not been tested. The Institute of Medicine has set an upper tolerable intake level for vitamin E at 1000 mg (1500 IU) per day and for any form of supplementary alpha-tocopherol because the nutrient can act as an anticoagulant and increase the risk of bleeding problems. Check upper tolerable intake levels.[7]

Folate

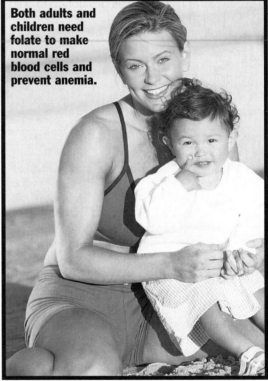

Both adults and children need folate to make normal red blood cells and prevent anemia.

Folate and folic acid are forms of a water-soluble B vitamin. Folate occurs naturally in food. Folic acid is the synthetic form of this vitamin that is found in supplements and fortified foods. Folate gets its name from the Latin word for leaf, *folium*. A key observation of researcher Lucy Wills nearly 70 years ago led to the identification of folate as the nutrient needed to prevent the anemia of pregnancy. Dr. Wills demonstrated that the anemia could be corrected by a yeast extract. Folate was identified as the corrective substance in yeast extract in the late 1930s and was extracted from spinach leaves in 1941. Folate is necessary for the production and maintenance of new cells. This is especially important during periods of rapid cell division and growth such as infancy and pregnancy. Folate is needed to make DNA and RNA, the building blocks of cells. It also helps prevent changes to DNA that may lead to cancer. Both adults and children need folate to make normal red blood cells and prevent anemia.

What Foods Provide Folate?

Leafy greens such as spinach and turnip greens, dry beans and peas, fortified cereals and grain products, and some fruits and vegetables are rich food sources of folate. Some breakfast cereals (ready-to-eat and others) are fortified with 25 percent or 100 percent of the daily value (DV) for folic acid. The table of selected food sources of folate and folic acid suggests dietary sources of this vitamin. In 1996 the Food and Drug Administration (FDA) published regulations requiring the addition of folic acid to enriched breads, cereals, flours, corn meals, pastas, rice and other grain products. This ruling took effect January 1, 1998, and was specifically targeted to reduce the risk of neural tube birth defects in newborns. Since the folic acid fortification program took effect, fortified foods have become a major source of folic acid in the American diet. Synthetic folic acid that is added to fortified foods and dietary supplements has a simpler chemical structure than the natural form of folate, and is absorbed more easily by the body. After digestion and absorption, however, the two forms are identical and function in exactly the same manner.

What is the Adult Recommended Dietary Allowance for Folate?
The 1998 RDAs for folate are expressed in a term called the Dietary Folate Equivalent. The DFE was developed to help account for the differences in absorption of naturally occurring dietary folate and the more bioavailable synthetic folic acid. The 1998 RDAs for folate expressed in micrograms (mcg) of DFE for adults are:

Life Stage	Men	Women
Ages 19+	400 mcg	400 mcg
All ages	600 mcg	500 mcg

1 mcg of food folate = 0.6 mcg folic acid from supplements and fortified foods

When Can Folate Deficiency Occur?
A deficiency of folate can occur when your need for folate is increased, when dietary intake of folate is inadequate, or when your body excretes (or loses) more folate than usual. Medications that interfere with your body's ability to use folate may also increase the need for this vitamin. Some situations that increase the need for folate include: pregnancy and lactation (breastfeeding), alcohol abuse, malabsorption, kidney dialysis, liver disease and certain anemias.

Signs of Folate Deficiency
Signs of folic acid deficiency are often subtle. Diarrhea, loss of appetite and weight loss can occur. Additional signs are weakness, sore tongue, headaches, heart palpitations, irritability and behavioral disorders. Women with folate deficiency who become pregnant are more likely to give birth to low birth weight and premature infants, and infants with neural tube defects. In adults anemia is a sign of advanced folate deficiency. In infants and children folate deficiency can slow growth rate. Some of these symptoms can also result from a variety of medical conditions other than folate deficiency. It is important to have a physician evaluate these symptoms so that appropriate medical care can be given.

Who May Need Extra Folic Acid to Prevent a Deficiency?
Women of childbearing age, people who abuse alcohol, anyone taking anticonvulsants or other medications that interfere with the action of folate, individuals diagnosed with anemia from folate deficiency, and individuals with malabsorption, liver disease, or who are receiving kidney dialysis treatment may benefit from a folic acid supplement.

Folic acid is very important for all women who may become pregnant. Adequate folate intake during the periconceptual period, the time just before and just after a woman becomes pregnant, protects against a number of congenital malformations including neural tube defects. Neural tube defects result in malformations of the spine (spina bifida), skull and brain (anencephaly). The risk of neural tube defects is significantly reduced when supplemental folic acid is consumed in addition to a healthful diet prior to and during the first month following conception. Women who could become pregnant are advised to eat foods fortified with folic acid or take supplements in addition to eating folate-rich foods to reduce the risk of some serious birth defects. Taking 400 micrograms of synthetic folic acid daily from fortified foods and/or supplements has been suggested. The RDA for folate equivalents for pregnant women is 600 micrograms.

Folate deficiency has been observed in alcoholics. A 1997 review of the nutritional status of chronic alcoholics found low folate status in more than 50 percent of those surveyed. Alcohol interferes with the absorption of folate and increases excretion of folate by the kidney. In addition, many alcohol abusers have poor-quality diets that do not provide the recommended intake of folate. Increasing folate intake through diet, or folic acid intake through fortified foods or supplements, may be beneficial to the health of alcoholics.

Anticonvulsant medications such as dilantin increase the need for folate. Anyone taking anticonvulsants or other medications that interfere with the body's ability to use folate should consult with a medical doctor about the need to take a folic acid supplement.

Anemia is a condition that occurs when red blood cells cannot carry enough oxygen. It can result from a wide variety of medical problems, including folate deficiency. Folate deficiency can result in the formation of large red blood cells that do not contain adequate hemoglobin, the substance in red blood cells that carries oxygen to your body's cells. Your physician can determine whether an anemia is associated with folate deficiency and whether supplemental folic acid is indicated.

Several medical conditions increase the risk of folic acid deficiency. Liver disease and kidney dialysis increase excretion (loss) of folic acid. Malabsorption can prevent your body from using folate in food. Medical doctors treating individuals with these disorders will evaluate the need for a folic acid supplement.

Caution About Folic Acid Supplements

Beware of the interaction between vitamin B12 and folic acid. Folic acid supplements can correct the anemia associated with vitamin B12 deficiency. Unfortunately, folic acid will not correct changes in the nervous system that result from vitamin B12 deficiency. Permanent nerve damage can occur if vitamin B12 deficiency is not treated. Intake of supplemental folic acid should not exceed 1000 micrograms (mcg) per day to prevent folic acid from masking symptoms of vitamin B12 deficiency.

Older adults must be made aware of the relationship between folic acid and vitamin B12 because they are at greater risk of having a vitamin B12 deficiency. If you are 50 years of age or older, ask your physician to check your B12 status before you take a supplement that contains folic acid.

Folic Acid and Heart Disease

A deficiency of folate, vitamin B12 or vitamin B6 may increase your level of homocysteine, an amino acid normally found in your blood. There is evidence that an elevated homocysteine level is an independent risk factor for heart disease and stroke. The evidence suggests that high levels of homocysteine may damage coronary arteries or make it easier for blood clotting cells called platelets to clump together and form a clot. However, there is currently no evidence available to suggest that lowering homocysteine with vitamins will reduce your risk of heart disease. Clinical intervention trials are needed to determine whether supplementation with folic acid, vitamin B12 or vitamin B6 can lower your risk of developing coronary heart disease.

Folic Acid and Cancer

Some evidence associates low blood levels of folate with a greater risk of cancer. Folate is involved in the synthesis, repair and functioning of DNA, our genetic map, and a deficiency of folate may result in damage to DNA that may lead to cancer. Several studies have associated diets low in folate with increased risk of breast, pancreatic and colon cancer. Findings from a study of over 121,000 nurses suggested that long-term folic acid supplementation (for 15 years) was associated with a decreased risk of colon cancer in women aged 55 to 69 years of age. However, associations between diet and disease do not indicate a direct cause. Researchers are continuing to investigate whether enhanced folate intake from foods or folic acid supplements may reduce the risk of cancer. Until results from such clinical trials are available, folic acid supplements should not be recommended to reduce the risk of cancer.

Folic Acid and Methotrexate for Cancer

Folate is important for cells and tissues that rapidly divide. Cancer cells divide rapidly, and drugs that interfere with folate metabolism are used to treat cancer. Methotrexate is a drug often used to treat cancer because it limits the activity of enzymes that need folate. Unfortunately, methotrexate can be toxic, producing side effects such as inflammation in the digestive tract that make it difficult to eat normally. Leucovorin is a form of folate that can help "rescue" or reverse the toxic effects of methotrexate. Whether or not folic acid supplements can help control the side effects of methotrexate without decreasing its effectiveness in chemotherapy is not known. Anyone receiving methotrexate must follow the advice of a medical doctor on the use of folic acid supplements.

Folic Acid and Methotrexate for Noncancerous Diseases

Low-dose methotrexate is used to treat a wide variety of noncancerous diseases such as rheumatoid arthritis, lupus, psoriasis, asthma, sarcoidoisis, primary biliary cirrhosis, and inflammatory bowel disease. Low doses of methotrexate can deplete folate stores and cause side effects that are similar to folate deficiency. Both high-folate diets and supplemental folic acid may help reduce the toxic side effects of low-dose methotrexate without decreasing its effectiveness. Anyone taking low-dose methotrexate for the health problems listed above should consult with a physician about the need for a folic acid supplement.

What is the Health Risk of Too Much Folic Acid?

The risk of toxicity from folic acid is low. The Institute of Medicine has established a tolerable upper intake level (UL) for folate of 1000 mcg per day for adult men and women, and a UL of 800 mcg for pregnant and lactating (breastfeeding) women under 18 years of age. Supplemental folic acid should not exceed the UL to prevent folic acid from masking symptoms of vitamin B12 deficiency.[8]

Vitamin K

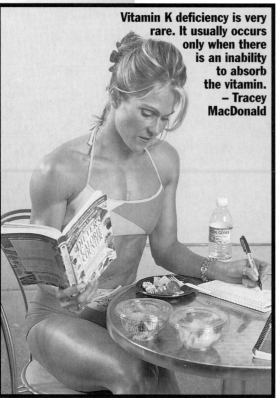

Vitamin K deficiency is very rare. It usually occurs only when there is an inability to absorb the vitamin.
– Tracey MacDonald

Vitamin K comes in several forms. It is known by the names *phytonadione, meadione,* and vitamins *K1, K2* and *K3.* Vitamin K is fat-soluble and that plays an important role in blood clotting. K converts protein called fibrinogen to its active form, fibrin, which helps to form a network over the injured tissue to trap the red blood cells. Without it you could bleed to death from even a minor wound. Under normal circumstances, very few adults are deficient in vitamin K. Vitamin K also has other important functions – although they're not as well understood as its role in blood coagulation. For example, K appears to be necessary for the formation of normal, healthy bone tissue. Scientists are currently investigating the possibility that supplementation with vitamin K may be helpful in the treatment of osteoporosis – the bone-thinning disease that is the cause of so many hip fractures in older adults.

Vitamin K is found in cabbage, cauliflower, spinach, and other green leafy vegetables, cereals, soybean and other vegetables. Vitamin K is also made by the bacteria lining the gastrointestinal tract. You can also find dietary sources of Vitamin K in most fruits and seeds. Additionally, it can be obtained through the consumption of cow's milk, dairy products and yogurt. Vitamin K deficiency is very rare. It usually occurs only when there is an inability to absorb the vitamin.[19]

Even though it is so important to blood clotting factors in the human organism, vitamin K deficiency does occur, and leads to hypoprothrombinemia, which is a fancy name for low levels of prothrombin in the human body. Vitamin K deficiency can result in delayed blood clotting and excessive bleeding. This can manifest in the form of bloody noses, excessive wound bleeding from minor cuts, and bleeding from the gums when brushing teeth. An individual experiencing vitamin K deficiency may also have uncontrolled bleeding in the intestine and urinary tract. Very rarely, vitamin K deficiency can also cause a brain bleed.[22]

Recommended sources of vitamin K vary, and typically it is obtained through the normal diet, but professionals seem to agree that an intake of approximately 300 mcg is adequate. Excess vitamin K intake has no known side effects. However, synthetic versions of the supplement have been known to cause liver damage. Before starting any form of supplementation you should, of

"You are about to have your first experience with a Greek lunch. I will kill you if you pretend to like it."
– Jacqueline Kennedy Onassis

course, consult your health-care practitioner. Vitamin K is best absorbed if taken with a fatty food (salad dressing on spinach, for example). Most people have adequate amounts of vitamin K (the body can produce its own) and don't need to supplement (the exception being those who have cystic fibrosis).[20]

Substance Interactions

These medications decrease the anticoagulant effect of this vitamin: antibiotics, cholestyramine, colestipol, coumarin, mineral oil, quinidine, salicylates, sucralfate, and sulfa drugs. Vitamin K with primaquine increases potential for toxic side effects. Antibiotics may destroy the normal beneficial bacteria in the intestinal tract, the same bacteria which produces vitamin K. Anyone taking antibiotics may want to increase intake of leafy vegetables.[21]

Vitamin K Overdose

There is no evidence of toxicity at doses up to 500 times the recommended daily allowances.

Minerals

Minerals are much smaller than vitamins and occur in much simpler forms. Like vitamins, minerals do not provide energy. There are dozens of minerals found in nature, and exactly 21 are essential for human nutrition. Minerals are just like vitamins in that they act as helpers in delivering nutrients and aiding in certain functions in the body. They are different in that they are used as physical building blocks – but unlike vitamins, minerals are indestructible. When you prepare your food you need to be concerned about overcooking because it is very easy to destroy vitamins. This is not the case with minerals.

Magnesium

Magnesium is a mineral needed by every cell of the body. About half of the body's magnesium stores are found inside cells of body tissues and organs, and half are combined with calcium and phosphorus in bone. Only 1 percent of the magnesium in the body is found in blood. The body works very hard to keep blood levels of magnesium constant.

Magnesium is needed for more than 300 biochemical reactions in the body. It helps maintain normal muscle and nerve function, keeps heart rhythm steady and bones strong. It is also involved in energy metabolism and protein synthesis.

What Foods Provide Magnesium?

Green vegetables such as spinach provide a good source because the center of the chlorophyll molecule contains magnesium. Nuts, seeds, and some whole grains are also good sources of magnesium.

Although present in many foods, magnesium usually occurs in small amounts. As with most nutrients, daily needs for magnesium cannot be met from a single food. Eating a wide variety of foods, including five servings of fruits and vegetables daily and plenty of whole grains, helps to ensure against an inadequate intake of magnesium.

Water can provide magnesium, but the amount varies according to the water supply. "Hard water" contains more magnesium than "soft water." Dietary surveys do not record estimated magnesium intake from water, which may lead to underestimating total magnesium intake and its variability.

What is the Recommended Dietary Allowance for Magnesium?

The 1999 RDAs for magnesium for adults in milligrams (mg) are: [4]

Life Stage	Men	Women	Pregnancy	Lactation
Ages 14-18	410 mg	360 mg	400 mg	360 mg
Ages 19-30	400 mg	310 mg	350 mg	310 mg
Ages 31+	420 mg	320 mg	360 mg	320 mg

> *"Dinner possessed only two dramatic features – the wine was a farce and the food a tragedy."*
> *– Anthony Poole*

Results of two national surveys, the National Health and Nutrition Examination Survey (NHANES III-1988-91) and the Continuing Survey of Food Intakes of Individuals (1994 CSFII) indicated that the diets of most adult men and women do not provide the recommended amounts of magnesium. The surveys also suggested that adults age 70 and over eat less magnesium than younger adults, and that non-Hispanic black subjects consume less magnesium than either non-Hispanic white or Hispanic subjects.[8]

When Can Magnesium Deficiency Occur?

Even though dietary surveys suggest that many Americans do not consume magnesium in recommended amounts, magnesium deficiency is rarely seen in the United States in adults. When magnesium deficiency does occur, it is usually due to excessive loss of magnesium in urine, gastrointestinal system disorders that cause a loss of magnesium or limit magnesium absorption, or a chronically low intake of magnesium.

Treatment with diuretics, some antibiotics, and some medicine used to treat cancer (such as cisplatin) can increase the loss of magnesium in urine. Poorly controlled diabetes increases loss of magnesium in urine, causing a depletion of magnesium stores. Alcohol also increases excretion of magnesium in urine, and a high alcohol intake has been associated with magnesium deficiency.

Gastrointestinal problems such as malabsorption disorders can cause magnesium depletion by preventing the body from using the magnesium in food. Chronic or excessive vomiting and diarrhea may also result in magnesium depletion.

Signs of magnesium deficiency include confusion, disorientation, loss of appetite, depression, muscle contractions and cramps, tingling, numbness, abnormal heart rhythms, coronary spasm and seizures.

What is the Best Way to Get Extra Magnesium?

Doctors will measure blood levels of magnesium whenever a magnesium deficiency is suspected. When levels are mildly depleted, increasing dietary intake of magnesium can help restore blood levels to normal. Eating at least five servings of fruits and vegetables daily, and choosing dark-green leafy vegetables often, as recommended by the Dietary Guidelines for Americans, the Food Guide Pyramid, and the Five-a-Day Program, will help adults at risk of having a magnesium deficiency consume recommended amounts of magnesium. When blood levels of magnesium are very low, an intravenous drip (IV drip) may be needed to return levels to normal. Magnesium tablets may also be prescribed, but some forms, in particular magnesium salts, can cause diarrhea. Your medical doctor or qualified health-care provider can recommend the best way to get extra magnesium when it is needed.

Magnesium and Blood Pressure

Evidence suggests that magnesium may play an important role in regulating blood pressure. Diets that provide plenty of fruits and vegetables (good sources of potassium and magnesium) are consistently associated with lower blood pressure. The DASH (Dietary Approaches to Stop Hypertension) study suggested that high blood pressure could be significantly lowered by a diet high in magnesium, potassium and calcium, and low in sodium and fat. In another study, the effect of various nutritional factors on incidence of high blood pressure was examined in over 30,000 US male health professionals. After four years of follow-up, it was found that a greater magnesium intake was significantly associated with a lower risk of hypertension. The evidence is strong enough that the Joint National Committee on Prevention, Detection, Evaluation and Treatment of High Blood Pressure recommends maintaining an adequate magnesium intake as a positive lifestyle modification for preventing and managing high blood pressure.

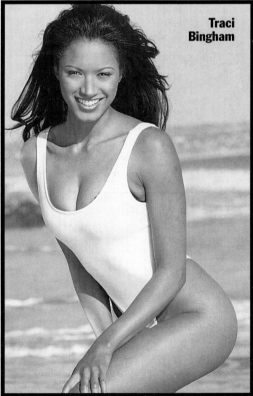

Traci Bingham

Magnesium and Heart Disease

Magnesium deficiency can cause metabolic changes that may contribute to heart attacks and strokes. There is also evidence that low body stores of magnesium increase the risk of abnormal heart rhythms, which may increase the risk of complications associated with a heart attack. Population surveys have associated higher blood levels of magnesium with lower risk of coronary heart disease. In addition, dietary surveys have suggested that a higher magnesium intake is associated with a lower risk of stroke. Further studies are needed to understand the complex relationships between dietary magnesium intake, indicators of magnesium status, and heart disease.

Magnesium and Osteoporosis

Magnesium deficiency may be a risk factor for postmenopausal osteoporosis. This may be due to the fact that magnesium deficiency alters calcium metabolism and the hormone that regulates calcium. Several studies have suggested that magnesium supplementation may improve bone mineral density, but researchers believe that further investigation on the role of magnesium in bone metabolism and osteoporosis is needed.

Magnesium and Diabetes

Magnesium is important to carbohydrate metabolism. It may influence the release and activity of insulin, the hormone that helps control blood glucose levels. Elevated blood glucose levels increase the loss of magnesium in the urine, which in turn lowers blood levels of magnesium. This explains why low blood levels of magnesium (hypomagnesemia) are seen in poorly controlled Type-I and Type-II diabetes.

In 1992 the American Diabetes Association issued a consensus statement that concluded: "Adequate dietary magnesium intake can generally be achieved by a nutritionally balanced meal plan as recommended by the American Diabetes Association." It recommended that "... only diabetic patients at high risk of hypomagnesemia should have total serum [blood] magnesium assessed, and such levels should be repleted [replaced] only if hypomagnesemia can be demonstrated."

What is the Health Risk of Too Much Magnesium?

Dietary magnesium does not pose a health risk, however, very high doses of magnesium supplements (which may be added to laxatives) can promote adverse effects such as diarrhea. Magnesium toxicity is more often associated with kidney failure, when the kidney loses the ability to remove excess magnesium. Very large doses of laxatives also have been associated with magnesium toxicity, even with normal kidney function. The elderly are at risk of magnesium toxicity because kidney function declines with age and they are more likely to take magnesium-containing laxatives and antacids.

"See that bivalve social climber, Feeding the rich Mrs. Hoggenheimer, Think of his joy as he gaily glides, Down to the middle of her gilded insides. Proud little oyster."
– Cole Porter

Signs of excess magnesium can be similar to magnesium deficiency and include mental status changes, nausea, diarrhea, appetite loss, muscle weakness, difficulty breathing, extremely low blood pressure, and irregular heartbeat.

The Institute of Medicine of the National Academy of Sciences has established a tolerable upper intake level (UL) for supplementary magnesium for adolescents and adults at 350 mg daily. As intake increases above the UL, the risk of adverse effects increases.[9]

Selenium

Selenium is an essential trace mineral in the human body. This nutrient is an important part of antioxidant enzymes that protect cells against the effects of free radicals produced during normal oxygen metabolism. The body has developed defenses

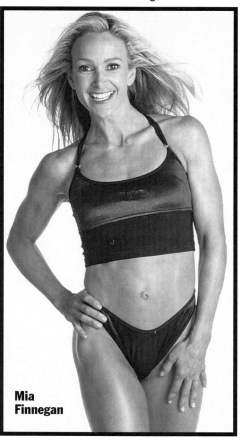

Mia Finnegan

such as antioxidants to control levels of free radicals that can damage cells and contribute to the development of some chronic diseases. Selenium is also essential for normal functioning of the immune system and thyroid gland.

What Foods Provide Selenium?

Plant foods are the major dietary sources of selenium in most countries throughout the world. The amount of selenium in soil, which varies by region, determines the amount of selenium in the plant foods that are grown in that soil. Researchers know that soils in the high plains of northern Nebraska and the Dakotas have very high levels of selenium. People living in those regions generally have the highest selenium intake in the United States. Soils in some parts of China and Russia have very low amounts of selenium and dietary selenium deficiency is often reported in those regions.

Selenium also can be found in some meats and seafood. Animals that eat grains or plants grown in selenium-rich soil have higher levels of selenium in their muscle. In the United States, meats and bread are common sources of dietary selenium. Some nuts, in particular Brazil nuts and walnuts, are also very good sources of selenium. The table of food sources of selenium suggests many dietary sources.

What is the Recommended Dietary Allowance of Selenium for Adults?

The year 2000 RDAs for selenium for adults in micrograms (mcg) are:[9]

Life Stage	Men	Women
Ages 19+	55 mcg	55 mcg
All ages	60 mcg	70 mcg

When Can Selenium Deficiency Occur?

Selenium deficiency is most commonly seen in parts of China where the selenium content in the soil, and therefore selenium intake, is very low. Selenium deficiency is linked to Keshan disease. The most common signs of selenium deficiency seen in this disease are an enlarged heart and poor heart function. Keshan disease has been observed in low-selenium areas of China, where dietary intake is less than 19 mcg per day for men and less than 13 mcg per day for women – significantly lower than the current RDA for selenium.

Selenium deficiency may also affect thyroid function because selenium is essential for the synthesis of active thyroid hormone. Researchers believe selenium deficiency may worsen the effects of iodine deficiency on thyroid function, and that adequate selenium nutritional status may help protect against some of the neurologic effects of iodine deficiency.

Who May Need Extra Selenium?

Gastrointestinal disorders such as Crohn disease can impair selenium absorption. Most cases of selenium depletion or deficiency are associated with severe gastrointestinal problems, such as in individuals who have had over half of their small intestines surgically removed. A physician will determine the need for selenium supplementation, and evaluate individuals who have gastrointestinal disease and depleted blood levels of selenium.

Selenium and Cancer

Some studies indicate that mortality (death) from cancer, including lung, colorectal and prostate cancers, is lower among people with higher selenium blood levels or intake. Also, the incidence of nonmelanoma skin cancer is significantly higher in areas of the United States with low soil selenium levels.

The effect of selenium supplementation on the recurrence of these types of skin cancers was studied in seven dermatology clinics in the US from 1983 through the early 1990s. Supplementation with 200 mcg selenium daily did not affect recurrence of skin cancer, but significantly reduced total mortality and mortality from cancers. In addition, incidence of prostate cancer, colorectal cancer, and lung cancer was lower in the group given selenium supplements.

However, not all studies have shown a relationship between selenium status and cancer. In 1982 over 60,000 participants of the Nurses Health Study with no history of cancer submitted toenail clippings for selenium analysis. Toenail analysis is thought to reflect selenium status over the previous year. After three and one-half years, researchers compared the toenail selenium levels of nurses with and without cancer. They did not find any apparent benefit of higher selenium levels.

Selenium and Heart Disease

Selenium is one of a group of antioxidants that may help limit the oxidation of LDL cholesterol and thereby help to prevent coronary artery disease. Currently there is insufficient evidence available to recommend selenium supplements for the prevention of coronary heart disease.

Selenium and Arthritis

The body's immune system naturally makes free radicals that can help destroy invading organisms and damaged tissue, and can also harm healthy tissue. Selenium, as an antioxidant, may help control levels of free radicals and help to relieve symptoms of arthritis. Current findings are considered preliminary, and further research is needed before selenium supplements can be recommended for individuals with arthritis.

Selenium and HIV

HIV/AIDS-related malabsorption can deplete levels of many nutrients. Selenium deficiency is commonly associated with HIV/AIDS, and has been associated with a high risk of death from this disease. Of 24 children with HIV who were observed for five years, those with low selenium levels died at a younger age – which may indicate faster disease progression. An examination of 125 HIV-positive men and women also associated selenium deficiency with mortality. Researchers believe that selenium may be important in HIV disease because of its role in the immune system and as an antioxidant. Selenium may also be needed for the replication of the HIV virus, which could deplete host levels of selenium. Researchers are actively investigating the role of selenium in HIV/AIDS, and see a need for clinical trials that evaluate the effect of selenium supplementation on HIV disease progression.

What is the Health Risk of Too Much Selenium?

There is a moderate to high health risk of too much selenium. High blood levels of selenium can result in a condition called selenosis. Symptoms include gastrointestinal upsets, hair loss, white blotchy nails, and mild nerve damage. Selenium toxicity is rare in the United States and the few reported cases have been associated with industrial accidents and a manufacturing error that led to an excessively high dose of selenium in a supplement. The Institute of Medicine has set a tolerable upper intake level for selenium at 400 micrograms per day for adults to prevent the risk of developing selenosis.[10]

Zinc

Zinc is an essential mineral. It is found in almost every cell in the body and is contained within more than 200 enzymes, substances needed for biochemical reactions. Zinc is important for a healthy immune system, for healing wounds, and for maintaining the sense of taste and smell. Zinc also supports normal growth and development during pregnancy, childhood and adolescence.

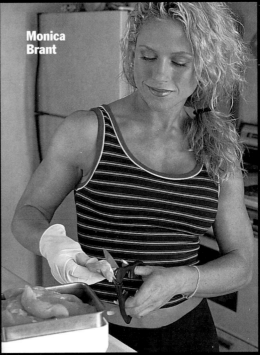

Monica Brant

What Foods Provide Zinc?

Meat and poultry provide the majority of zinc in the American diet. Other food sources include beans, nuts and dairy products. Oysters are the food containing the most zinc by weight, but beef is a more common source in the US diet. The zinc found in meat and oysters is easily absorbed by the body. Dietary phytates, which are found in whole-grain cereals and unleavened bread, may significantly decrease the body's absorption of zinc.

What is the Recommended Dietary Allowance for Zinc?

The 1989 RDAs for zinc for adults in milligrams (mg) are:

Life Stage	Men	Women
Ages 19+	15 mg	12 mg
All ages	15 mg	19 mg (first six months)
		16 mg (second six months)

Results of two national surveys, the National Health and Nutrition Examination Survey (NHANES III 1988-91) and the Continuing Survey of Food Intakes of Individuals (1994 CSFII) indicated that the diets of many adults, especially older Americans and women, do not provide the recommended amounts of zinc.

When Can Zinc Deficiency Occur?

Zinc deficiency can occur when zinc intake is inadequate, when there are increased losses of zinc from the body, or when the body's requirement for zinc

"The biggest seller is cookbooks and the second is diet books – how not to eat what you've just learned how to cook."
– Andy Rooney

increases. There is no specific deficiency disease associated with zinc. Instead, many general signs of zinc deficiency can appear, including poor appetite, weight loss, delayed healing of wounds, taste abnormalities and mental lethargy. As body stores of zinc decline, these symptoms worsen and are accompanied by diarrhea, hair loss, recurrent infection, and a form of dermatitis, a skin disorder. Zinc deficiency has also been linked to poor growth in childhood.

Who May Need Extra Zinc?

There is no single laboratory test available to determine nutritional zinc status. Instead, dietary intake is typically used to estimate the risk of a zinc deficiency. People who may benefit from a zinc supplement include those who do not consume enough calories, vegetarians, the elderly, pregnant and lactating women, and people who suffer from alcoholism or digestive diseases that cause diarrhea.

Anyone with a low caloric intake is at higher risk for having a low zinc intake and for developing a zinc deficiency. Vegetarians who consume a variety of legumes and nuts will probably meet their zinc requirement, but otherwise a vegetarian diet may be inadequate in zinc. Since the zinc from plant sources is absorbed less readily, the concern about zinc status increases in vegetarians who do not consume legumes and nuts.

Dietary surveys suggest that many Americans aged 51 and older, pregnant women and breastfeeding mothers do not consume recommended amounts of zinc. Therefore, to decrease their risk for developing a zinc deficiency, it is important for individuals in these groups to include sources of zinc in their daily diet. Zinc supplementation has been found to improve the growth rate in children with mild zinc deficiency and mild to moderate growth failure. Maternal zinc deficiency can delay fetal growth, and mothers who give birth to small for gestational age babies have been found to have lower zinc intakes during pregnancy. Breastfeeding increases the risk of depleting nutritional zinc status when dietary zinc intake is chronically low because of the greater need for zinc during lactation.

Zinc deficiency is frequently associated with alcoholism, which is often due to a lower intake of food. The need for a supplement as part of an overall treatment plan is usually evaluated by a physician in this situation.

Diarrhea causes a loss of zinc. Therefore, digestive diseases or gastrointestinal surgery that result in diarrhea are often associated with zinc deficiency. Individuals who experience chronic diarrhea should make sure they include sources of zinc in their daily diet (see table of food sources of zinc). A medical doctor can evaluate the need for zinc supplementation if diet alone fails to maintain normal zinc levels in the body.

Zinc, Infections and Wound-Healing

The immune system is adversely affected by even moderate degrees of zinc deficiency. People who are zinc-deficient have a more difficult time resisting infections. T-cell lymphocytes, white blood cells that help fight infection, do not function efficiently when zinc stores are low. When zinc supplements are given to individuals with low zinc levels, the numbers of T-cell lymphocytes circulating in the blood increase and the ability of lymphocytes to fight infection improves.

Studies show that poor, malnourished children in India, Africa, South America and Southeast Asia experience shorter courses of infectious diarrhea after taking zinc supplements. Zinc supplements are often used to treat skin ulcers or bedsores, but they do not increase the rate of wound-healing when zinc levels are normal.

Zinc and the Common Cold
A study of over 100 employees of the Cleveland Clinic indicated that zinc lozenges decreased the duration of colds by one-half. Some of the participants reported fewer days of congestion and nasal drainage, but no differences were seen in how long their fevers lasted or in the level of muscle aches they experienced. However, this study has been criticized by some researchers who believe that since zinc lozenges often have a bad taste, the participants may have known the difference between the supplement and placebo, which would compromise the results. Also, since other studies have shown no benefit, the debate continues on the true value of zinc supplements for cold symptoms.

Zinc and Iron Absorption
Iron deficiency anemia is considered a serious public health problem in the world today. Iron fortification programs were developed to prevent this deficiency and they have been credited with improving the iron status of millions of women, infants and children. Some researchers, however, have raised concern about the effects of iron fortification on other nutrients, including zinc. Iron taken in solution can inhibit the absorption of zinc, but foods fortified with iron do not.

What is the Health Risk of Too Much Zinc?
The health risk of taking too much zinc is moderate to high. Zinc toxicity has been seen in both acute and chronic forms. Intakes of 150 to 450 mg of zinc per day have been associated with low copper status, altered iron function, reduced immune function, and reduced levels of high-density lipoproteins (the good cholesterol). One case report cited severe nausea and vomiting within 30 minutes after the person ingested four grams of zinc gluconate (570 mg elemental zinc). The 1989 RDA committee stated that "chronic ingestion of zinc supplements exceeding 15 mg/day is not recommended without adequate medical supervision." The National Academy of Sciences is currently reviewing recent research and considering new recommendations on zinc intake and risk.[11]

Carbohydrates

Carbohydrates, as a class, are the most abundant organic compounds found in nature. They are produced by green plants and by bacteria using the process known as photosynthesis, in which carbon dioxide is taken from the air by means of solar energy to yield the carbohydrates as well as all the other chemicals needed by the organisms to survive and grow.

The carbohydrate group consists principally of sugar, starch, dextrin, cellulose and glycogen, substances that constitute an important part of the human diet and that of many animals. The simplest of them are the simple

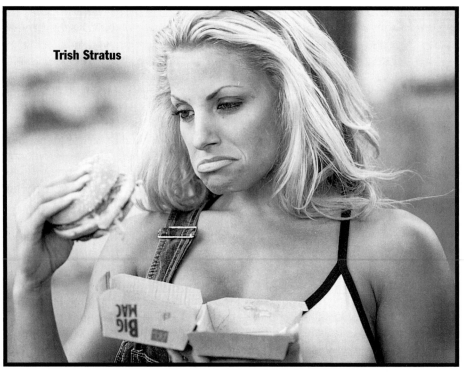

Trish Stratus

sugars, or monosaccharides, which contain either an aldehyde or a ketone group. The most important is glucose. Two monosaccharide molecules joined together by an oxygen atom, with the elimination of a molecule of water, yield a disaccharide, of which the most important are sucrose (ordinary cane sugar), lactose and maltose. Polysaccharides have enormous molecules made up of one type or several types of monosaccharide units – about 10 in glycogen, for example, 25 in starch, and 100 to 200 in cellulose.

Within living organisms, carbohydrates serve both essential structural and energy-storage functions. In plants, cellulose and hemicellulose are the main structural elements. In invertebrate animals, the polysaccharide chitin is the main component of the exoskeletons of arthropods. In vertebrate animals, the cell coatings of connective tissues contain carbohydrates. Cell membranes are rich in glycoproteins, and so forth. Plants use starch and animals use glycogen to store energy. When the energy is needed, the carbohydrates are broken down by enzymes.[25]

How Much Carbohydrate is Healthy to Eat?
If you look near the bottom of the Nutrition Facts panel on a food label, you'll see the recommended daily amount (RDA) of carbohydrate listed as 300 grams. That figure is based on a goal of 60 percent carbohydrate in a theoretical 2000-calorie/day diet. This is a reasonable ballpark for many adults, although the label also notes that those who eat 2500 calories per day should get 375 grams of carbohydrate.

The diet recommended in the most recent report on nutrition and cancer risk, published by the American Institute for Cancer Research, derives

55 to 75 percent of its calories from carbohydrate. People with lower calorie needs – those who are less active, older or trying to lose weight – may meet this goal with as little as 220 grams of carbohydrate.

These figures aside, when it comes to overall health, where you get your carbs is probably more important than exactly how much you eat. To get all the beneficial nutrients and phytochemicals you need, concentrate on high-fiber vegetables, fruits, beans and whole grains (like whole-wheat bread and brown rice).

Carbohydrate from refined grains (white bread, low-fiber cereals) should play a smaller role in your diet, and sweets should provide only a fraction of the day's carbohydrate.[24]

The Glycemic Index

The glycemic index ranks foods on how they affect our blood sugar levels. This index measures how much your blood sugar increases in the two or three hours after eating. The glycemic index is about foods high in carbohydrates. Foods high in fat or protein don't cause your blood sugar level to rise much.

Many people still think it is plain table sugar that those with diabetes need to avoid. The experts used to say that, but the glycemic index shows that even complex carbohydrates, like baked potatoes, can be even worse.

When you make use of the glycemic index to prepare healthy meals, you help keep your blood sugar levels under control. This rating is especially important for people with diabetes, although athletes and those who are overweight also stand to benefit from knowing about this relatively new concept in good nutrition.

Recent studies of large numbers of people with diabetes show that those who keep their blood sugar under tight control best avoid the complications that this disease can lead to. The experts agree. What works best for people with diabetes – and probably the rest of us as well – is regular exercise, little saturated fat, and a high-fiber diet. That is excellent advice – as far as it goes.

The real problem is carbohydrates. The official consensus remains that a high-carbohydrate diet is best for people who have diabetes. However, some experts, led by endocrinologists like Dr. Richard K. Bernstein, recommend a low-carbohydrate diet, because carbohydrates break down quickly during digestion and can raise blood sugar to dangerous levels.

Many high-carbohydrate foods have high glycemic index ratings, and certainly are not good in any substantial quantity for diabetics. Other carbohydrates break down more slowly, releasing glucose gradually into the blood stream, and are said to have a lower glycemic index rating. Does a substantial quantity of these foods with a lower glycemic index belong in your diet? Only your personal experience can answer that question.

Before the development of the glycemic index beginning in 1981, scientists assumed that our bodies absorbed and digested simple sugars quickly, producing rapid increases in the blood sugar level. This was the basis of the advice to avoid sugar, a proscription recently relaxed by the American Diabetes Association and others. Now we know that simple sugars don't make your blood sugar rise any more rapidly than some complex carbohydrates do. Of course, simple sugars are simply empty calories, and still should be minimized for that reason.

What About Portion Size? And How is GI Determined?

The glycemic index is about the *quality* of the carbohydrates, not the quantity. Obviously quantity matters too, but the measurement of the glycemic index of a food is not related to portion size. The GI rating remains the same whether you eat 10 grams of it or 1000 grams. To make a fair comparison, tests of the glycemic indexes of food usually use 50 grams of available carbohydrate in each food. You can eat twice as many carbohydrates in a food that, for example, has a glycemic index rating of 50 than one that has a glycemic index of 100 and have the same blood glucose response.

The glycemic index should not be your only criterion when selecting what foods to eat. The total amount of carbohydrate, the amount and type of fat, and the fiber and salt content are also important dietary considerations. The glycemic index is most useful when deciding which high-carbohydrate foods to eat. But don't let the glycemic index lull you into eating more carbs than your body can handle, particularly if you have diabetes. The number of grams of carbohydrates we consume is awfully important. Make sure you know the carbohydrate content of the foods you eat – study the nutritional information on the package.

First you need to decide the composition of your diet in terms of carbohydrates, fat and protein. Almost all the experts agree that we should minimize our intake of saturated and trans fat and eat a lot more fiber than we do. Some other fats, particularly those from cold-water fish and essential fatty acids such as found in large amounts in flax oil, seem to be beneficial. Beyond that, the battle rages between those who would have us eat more protein and those who say carbohydrates should provide most of our calories. We're no experts and we are genuinely puzzled, although we've begun to cut back on carbohydrates and eat more protein. Generally foods high in fat and protein have lower GI ratings than foods high in carbohydrate. In a real sense, the glycemic index is not applicable to high-fat and/or high-protein foods.

The problem is, even among the complex carbohydrates not all are created equal. Some break down quickly during digestion and can raise blood glucose to dangerous levels. These are the foods that have higher GIs. Other carbohydrates break down more slowly, releasing glucose gradually into the bloodstream and are said to have lower GI ratings.

As mentioned, before the development of the glycemic index scientists assumed that our bodies absorbed and digested simple sugars quickly and produced rapid increases in blood glucose levels. This was the basis of the advice to avoid sugar, a proscription recently relaxed by the American Diabetes Association and others.

To the contrary, the experts thought our bodies absorbed starches such as rice and potatoes slowly, causing only small rises in blood glucose. Clinical trials of the glycemic index have also proven that assumption to be false. In addition, the glucose response to a particular food may be somewhat individual. So it is probably a good idea to carefully watch your own blood glucose level after eating foods you have questions about and determine if they have high or low GI *for you personally.*

So, the concept of the glycemic index is very useful. But if you find a specific food produces an unexpected result, either high or low, take note and incorporate that reaction into your meal planning.[26]

Protein

We know that a gram of protein yields 4 calories of energy, but why is it so important in regard to building muscle. Amino acids are known as the building blocks of life. Each protein molecule may contain any of the 22 different amino acids, but in order for it to be a complete protein, it must contain the essential amino acids. There are nine amino acids that are considered essential because our bodies cannot produce them – they must be derived from dietary sources. When we consume a complete protein, it is broken down into amino acids. These amino acids have a variety of functions, one of the primary roles being that of repairing muscle tissue. Whenever you are in negative nitrogen balance, your body is in a catabolic state. That means it is breaking down your own muscle tissue to get the amino acids it needs for other functions. If you are not getting enough protein from your diet, your body will literally rob your own muscles of amino acids. This results in negative nitrogen balance and loss of lean muscle tissue. You're defeating the whole purpose of working out, because your body doesn't have the tools to repair the muscle tissue you just spent an hour in the gym breaking down. This will rapidly lead to being in an overtrained state (and some people wonder why they never make any gains in the gym). Studies reported that an intake of about 2 grams of protein per kg of bodyweight was required to maintain positive nitrogen balance in strength-training athletes. That's almost 1 gram of protein per pound of bodyweight, which far exceeds the recommended daily allowance.

Protein builds growing bodies, and protein is in turn made up of "building blocks" called amino acids. Our ancestors depended on grains that are low in the amino acid lysine, which makes their protein content less useful than it would otherwise have been. Wheat has about 8 to 15 percent protein, depending on the variety (ancient wheats had a higher protein content), rice has a low content of 7 percent. So grains in general are perhaps best regarded as primarily an energy and vitamin and mineral source.

Legumes on the other hand are very good sources of protein. Peanuts, for example, are protein-rich, with about 25 percent or more protein content (and a favorable amino acid profile). Lentils have about 25 percent, cowpeas have from 23 to 35 percent, and common beans about 22. Legumes tend to be low

> *"Goat cheese ... produced a bizarre eating era when sensible people insisted that this miserable cheese produced by these miserable creatures reared on miserable hardscrabble earth was actually superior to the magnificent creamy cheeses of the noblest dairy animals bred in the richest green valleys of the earth."*
> *– Russel Baker*

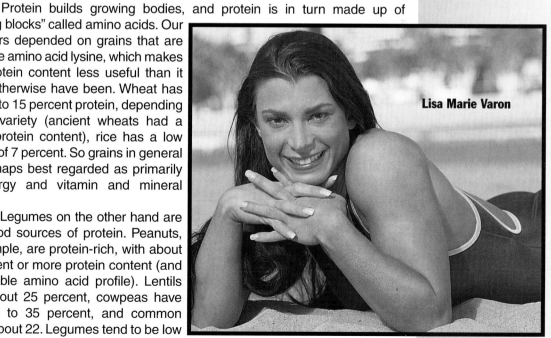

Lisa Marie Varon

in the amino acids methionine and cystine, but are high in the amino acid lysine. Lysine is low in grains, so eating the two together leverages the protein content of both. Co-incidentally, legumes such as lentils and peas tended to grow as weeds among wheat and other grains at the time they were being domesticated. In South America maize, a grain, was (and is) grown with beans, a legume. In Asia rice and soya beans complement each other.

In conjunction with tree seeds, and to a lesser extent meat/marrow, the protein and oils of wild African legumes may have been the deciding factor in allowing humans to develop and survive. Other seeds are also rich in protein. Sesame seeds are about 20 percent protein, but low in lysine. Mixing them with a legume such as the chickpea, Cicer arietum (e.g. in the middle Eastern dish "houmous") balances it out. Both sunflower seeds and pumpkin seeds are also high in protein.

Protein Testing

The simplest way to evaluate the protein quality of a food source is by "chemical scoring." This is where the amino acid composition of the protein itself is rated by comparing it to a reference protein. It is possible to determine the amino acid composition of any protein inexpensively, but unfortunately, chemical scoring does not always reflect accurately the way the body will use a protein.

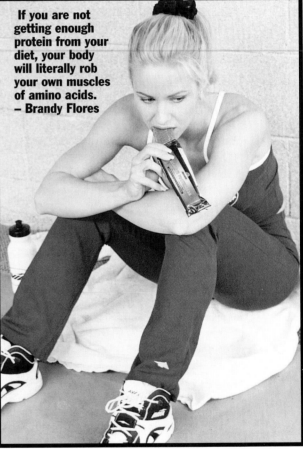

If you are not getting enough protein from your diet, your body will literally rob your own muscles of amino acids.
– Brandy Flores

The protein efficiency ratio (PER) is the best-known procedure for evaluating protein quality and is used in the US as the basis for regulations regarding food labeling. The PER has become outdated, primarily due to the fact that the ratio is based on the grams of weight gained by rats divided by the grams of protein they were fed. The biggest problem with the PER studies is that the need for amino acids in rats is not the same as that for human beings. Knowing a protein has a high PER is still a good indicator that it is a high-quality protein. Net protein utilization is a little more complex testing procedure, but has the same basic problem as PER in that it uses animals as test subjects.

The only way to determine the actual value of a protein as it is used by the human body, is to measure not only urinary but also fecal losses of nitrogen when the protein is actually fed to human beings under test conditions. This determines the biological value of the protein. The primary reason this method is so important in determining the bioavailability of protein is because it is done on actual humans, giving us a more accurate protein value, while determining exactly what the nitrogen retention is. This is very important because it lets us know how much of the protein we can assimilate (actually use) after we consume it.

Our ancestors obtained protein from grubs, meat, tubers, fish and plant foliage. While these can be eaten raw, all are physically easier to eat cooked, or cause indigestion and/or food poisoning if they are not cooked. And our ancestors were big on seeds.

While you *could* eat whole rice grass seeds (for example) without parching them first, only about 25 percent of the proteins are digestible. Cook the whole seed, and about 65 percent of the protein is available. Grinding raw rice seeds makes more than 25 percent of the protein available. Grinding and cooking rice seeds improves protein availability beyond 65 percent. The cultural evolution of both grinding and cooking seeds brought an evolutionary advantage in the form of greater access to protein.

Grass seeds in particular had to be "heat-parched" anyway, to get rid of the adherent woody chaff covering the seed (later, with domestication, this chaff became easy to remove by beating). So some degree of cooking was more out of necessity than by choice.

A few seeds have somewhat less protein digestibility after cooking, but they are the exception. You would have to cook grass seeds at 200-280°C (392-536°F) to reduce rather than improve their protein digestibility. Meat protein digestibility, in comparison, decreases when cooking is above only 100°C (212°F).

Seeds contain *antinutrients* – substances such as saponins, tannins, protein-splitting enzymes inhibitors and phytates. These compounds reduce the body's ability to access the nutrients in seeds. The type and amount of antinutrient varies both with the species of plant and the local variety of the species.

Most, but not all, antinutrients are destroyed or reduced by cooking. Soaking and leaching are necessary to reduce antinutrients, particularly in some varieties of bean and other legumes. Soaking and sprouting seeds also reduces phytates. Soybeans, for example, contain an inhibitor that interferes with the absorption of the amino acid tryptophan. The inhibitor can be neutralized both by cooking and by sprouting (the sprouted root must be three to four inches long for this to be largely complete).

A very low percentage of the starches in some seeds "resist" being digested (up to 7 percent for wheat and oats, and 20 percent for baked beans). These undigested starches are fermented by the microflora of the colon, producing variable quantities of gas.

Guided by the practices of recent African gatherer-hunters, it seems likely our African ancestors mainly dealt with antinutritional factors by roasting the seeds. Sometimes they were soaked as well, either before or after roasting (and grinding). These are classic techniques we use even today when preparing legumes.

Carbohydrates

The primary role of carbohydrates or sugars is to provide the body with energy. Their second role is to spare protein from being used as energy, so that it will always be available to build and repair muscle. This is why many times you will hear carbohydrates being referred to as protein-sparing. There are two kinds of carbohydrates, *simple* and *complex.* A simple carbohydrate is made up of only one sugar. When you eat a simple sugar your body uses it for energy immediately, resulting in a quick rise in blood sugar levels, prompting the hormone insulin to be released. Insulin is the most anabolic hormone in the body and serves as a regulator. Its purpose is to even out blood sugar levels by sending the sugars where they need to go. If your body doesn't use all of the simple sugar you have just eaten, it will store the excess in fat cells. The process is different for complex carbohydrates, which are composed of more than one sugar. When you eat complex carbohydrates, they are broken down into glucose, and insulin is again secreted to regulate where the sugar goes. However, this time if your body does not use all of the complex carbohydrates, the excess will be stored as glycogen in either the muscle cell or liver cell for later use.

> *"Human beings do not eat nutrients, they eat food. "*
> *– Mary Catherine Bateson*

Whole grains are made of a rich starch store (the endosperm) comprising from 60 to 80 percent of the seed (depending on the species and variety), the embryo plant (the germ) rich in protein, fats and vitamins, and comprising only about 3 percent of the seed, and the seed coat, the bran, which is where most of the B vitamins (and many of the minerals) are. At 80 percent carbohydrate, like tubers, seeds are an excellent fuel for daily activity. And whole seeds contain the B1 vitamin necessary for carbohydrate metabolism. Grains are relatively slow-burners, so they don't push up your blood sugar levels and then suddenly drop them. Seeds tend to keep blood sugars relatively stable.

Going Natural, Going Nuts

Our gorging and rather smelly ancestors ate every animal or plant that wasn't actually toxic (or died after eating the toxic ones). A seasonal food source of amazing variety was plant seed. Seeds are a rich store of energy, protein, vitamins (especially vitamin E), minerals and protective phytochemicals. Our ancestors gorged on wild seeds because they did not have the technology to store them. Seeds are difficult to keep from becoming moldy or insect infested. Unlike nuts, most grass seeds have no hard shell to deter birds and bugs. When the seasonal seed resource was depleted, our ancestors moved on to another food, and didn't eat seeds until the next harvest season a year later.

Today we can choose from a wide variety of seeds. But for historical and cultural reasons, Western peoples eat only a few kinds of seeds, and, with the exception of beans and peas, generally eat only the carbohydrate store of the seed, leaving the vitamin, oil and mineral-rich parts behind.

Investing the time to change our cultural mind set to include more whole seeds of all kinds, or using canned precooked whole seeds, can increase the amount of nutrients and protective plant chemicals consumed per calorie eaten, and help to displace unnatural, less nutrient dense, industrially modified foods. The result is a way of eating in harmony with the absolute needs of our ancient gene-determined biochemistry … and over time, the removal of one the most important barriers to good health.

Humans evolved in the forests, woodlands, and plains of Africa. The human animal spread into virtually all environments – from tropical rainforest to arid desert – because that animal which is you and me today had evolved the kind of guts that could digest most kinds of food – animal or plant (except woody twiglets and cellulosy grass blades). Our natural diet is everything edible. But in any given area of the world, we relied on starchy plants, nut and seed oils, or animal fat for fuel to burn for energy. Animals that know how dangerous humans are tend to run – fast, and in the opposite direction – and are fat only at certain times of year. Plants have the virtue of standing still, so underground storage tubers and carbohydrate-rich seeds are a reliable source of energy, and in some cases, fat and protein.

No reasonable energy source was ignored, and wild seeds were no exception. Of those wild African species worth collecting, probably the most important are the numerous species of wild millets native to West and East Africa. The term *millet* is a slightly confusing generic name to mean both millet (Panicum, Setaria, Echinochloa, Eleusine and Pennisetum spp.) and sorghum (Sorghum spp.).

Early humans exploiting the riches of marsh, delta and riverine environments had access to the seeds of a reed-like grass, Phragmites autralis (communis) ditch reed or water grass, which, although the yield was probably relatively poor (there is little literature on this subject to form a view), had the virtue of being both widespread and in thick stands. When our ancestors migrated out of Africa, they found this seasonal food source in damp and marshy places from the tropics to the temperate lands. These grass seeds were indeed our "evolutionary fellow travelers."

Numerous legume seeds were available to our African ancestors. As humans radiated out of Africa into all the regions of the world, they exploited all food sources they came across, grasses included. In parts of Australia the aboriginal people regularly harvested wild grass seeds, and it is likely that, given time, they would have domesticated them. Indigenous tribespeople of the grasslands of southern South America gathered grass seeds for food, and even brought one species of brome grass into cultivation. In Mexico one of the local "panic grasses" (Panicum spp., a kind of millet) was collected, and ultimately domesticated. Palaeanthropologists have found 19,000-year-old stone mortars for

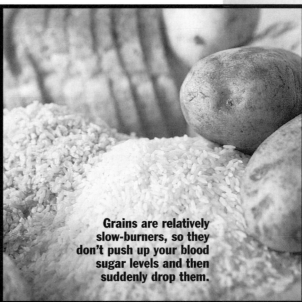

Grains are relatively slow-burners, so they don't push up your blood sugar levels and then suddenly drop them.

Avocado growers denied publicly and indignantly the insidious, slanderous rumors that avocados were an aphrodisiac. Sales immediately mounted.
– *Waverley Root*

grinding grain that show wild grains were not just parched but *processed,* at least since that time.

Our ancestors probably parched the whole grains on ember-heated stones (this would have burnt off the husks around the seed), and made a dough from the cooked flour. (Tibetan people today eat a dough from roasted barley flour mixed with tea and yak butter and formed into a ball – tsampa.) Such dough laid on hot stones or embers would have made the first unleavened bread. The roasted flour could perhaps have been mixed with water to make a thin porridge.

Fat

Fats are the ideal fuel for long-term energy. This is the reason you need to incorporate some sort of aerobic exercise into your program. If you don't, you can never effectively utilize fat stores. Fat is classified into three different groups, and the one we really need to be concerned about is simple fat, also known as triglycerides. This is the only group of fats we can derive energy from. There are saturated fats and unsaturated fats, and when we talk about fats in our diet, we want them to come from unsaturated fats. Unsaturated fats come from plants and vegetables, whereas saturated fats come from animals.

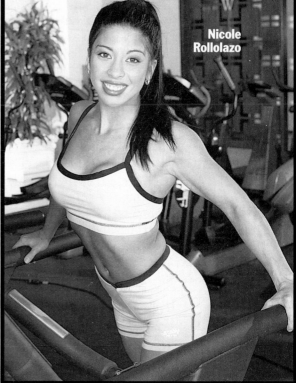

Nicole Rollolazo

Meat

For our African ancestors hunting big game was unproductive – the animal tended to disappear over the horizon as soon as it saw us – relative to spending the same amount of time and energy hunting small game, or gathering plant food. We evolved to eat everything that moved, but possibly mostly small animals.

As a result, "meat" for our distant ancestors was anything that moved – birds, rodents, lizards, turtles, grubs, and animals of all kinds. Once a large animal was killed, its carcass was regarded (even by today's hunter-gatherer societies) as a variably valuable resource. The internal organs, especially the liver, were of the highest value. The more choice and easily transportable muscle meats were next in value, and the tougher and more bony parts (bone is very heavy to carry) were least valued.

We eat only four animals now, and no small ones, although our genes are unchanged. Today, "meat" for us means virtually four animals – an animal so familiar it has no common name, the cattle beast; the sheep; the pig; and the domestic fowl (chicken). Most of us will rarely eat any other kind of animal in our lifetime. The word *meat* has come to mean muscles, not internal organs. In a wonderful cultural flip-flop, that which was once prized, the internal organs are now called *offal.* And in many households in the West the internal organs are now called "ugh" or "yuck."

Muscle meat by itself may raise levels of the amino acid *homocysteine* in the blood, and high levels of homocysteine have been associated with tendency to heart disease. But folic acid and B vitamins have been found to prevent elevated homocysteine levels. The liver is an excellent source of folic acid, so eating the whole animal keeps the balance of health. Folic acid is also high in some green vegetables, particularly spinach. Meat and vegetables go together.

The sources of fat and the kinds of fat we have today are completely different to those of our evolutionary history. As the World Health Organization Report points out, we have a much higher ratio of saturated to unsaturated fatty acids in our diet now. But it is a little misleading. The implication is that we are eating too much saturated fat. This is certainly true in absolute terms (we do overeat), but there are actually two significant points to be aware of.

First, we eat too much. We regularly overeat. Whether fat or carbohydrate, calories in excess of those needed to burn for energy are stored as fat. Carbohydrates (pasta, bread, potatoes – any carbohydrate, natural or not) in excess of our needs for energy are converted to fat. That's worth repeating. Excess carbohydrates are stored as fat.

Animal fat is a normal food for the human animal. It is a normal food and has been for countless millenia. Animal fat in itself is not dangerous, but large wild animals were only fat at certain times of year. Their muscle meats contained only about 4 percent fat. No part of the carcass was left uneaten, including the fat stores. However, on balance, in evolutionary terms we did not regularly eat "a lot of fat." Let's be clear. Excess calories from any source are dangerous – *very dangerous.*

Second, we have been eating saturated animal fat throughout all of our evolutionary history. Organ meats (especially brains) and nuts, seeds and green leafy plants provide the small amounts of essential polyunsaturated fatty acids our bodies aren't able to manufacture. Saturated fats are evolutionarily natural, whether derived directly from animal fat, or the body has to construct its saturated fats from the nuts, tubers and seeds that it eats. We ate the marrow of the larger bones – indeed, some scientists believe nutrient-rich marrow was a key factor in providing the very dense nutrients needed to build a baby with a very large and nutrient-demanding brain. Marrow contains about 75 percent of its fat as monounsaturated fats.

What we have almost *never* ever eaten before in our evolutionary history are *hydrogenated* fats. These are industrially extracted vegetable oils that are made solid and stable through an industrial/chemical process called hydrogenation. Tiny amounts occur naturally in the stomachs of grass-fed cows. They are excellent for deep-frying and for baked goods. They are stable, cheap, and ideally suited to industrial food production. But large-scale industrial hydrogenated vegetable fats did not exist ten generations ago, or at any time in

"Of all the peoples whom I have studied, from city dwellers to cliff dwellers, I always find that at least 50 percent would prefer to have at least one jungle between themselves and their mothers-in-law."
– anthropologist Margaret Mead

our evolutionary history, and there is some evidence that, in the quantities currently consumed in the West, they have a role in the development of cardiovascular disease.

The animals whose bodies we eat are either herbivores (cattle beasts and sheep) or more or less omnivores (pigs, chickens). The kinds of fats in their bodies to the greater degree reflect the kinds of fats the animals themselves eat. Only grass-fed domestic animals have a "fat profile" fairly similar to wild herbivores. When animals are fed supplements of grains or compounded feeds derived from a wide variety of plant and animal products and byproducts, their level of bodyfat tends to reflect the fats present in the grains and feeds they are fed.

For example, pigs in America are fed primarily a soya bean/maize-based feed. Their back fat, typical of the fat on pork chops, for example, has around 39 to 43 percent oleic acid and 19 to 23 percent palmitic acid. Adding sunflower oil (higher in monounsaturated fats, particularly oleic acid) to the standard feed increases the oleic acid component of the fat to about 60 percent and reduces the (somewhat undesirable) palmitic acid to 17 percent. Including ground up whole sunflower seeds of a high oleic type as a major part of the standard soya/maize feed changed the oleic acid content of the back fat to about 67 percent (olive oil, by way of comparison, is about 72 percent oleic acids), and the palmitic down to 12 percent. Pigs are omnivores (as we are), not grass-eaters (ruminants). Therefore their fat profile reflects the kinds of fats they are fed. Our bodyfat profile also reflects the kinds of fats we eat, and in part the kinds of fats the pigs we eat, eat! On the other hand, as grass-eaters for most of their lives, cattle are much less affected by "finishing" on meal; but are nevertheless still affected.

For practical purposes the end result is that corn-fed or feedlot-finished cattle have, relative to grass-fed animals, more of one kind of fatty acid (type of fat), namely omega-6 fatty acids, and less of another kind, omega-3, than they would if they had been totally grass-fed until the day of slaughter. (Corn/maize and soybeans, common ingredients in animal feeds, are particularly high in omega-6 fats.) Feedlot cattle may have almost no omega-3 in their fat after 196 days in the feedlot – whereas grass-fed animals have about 7 percent. Some wild game has about 4 percent. We need both omega-6 and omega-3 fats – they are vital to many bodily processes – but we need them in the right amounts and the right ratio of one to the other.

Currently it is thought that the ratio of omega-6 fatty acids to omega-3 should be 4 of omega-6 to 1 of omega-3. A more evolutionarily appropriate ratio of these two essential fatty acids has been linked to a greatly reduced risk of breast cancer and coronary heart disease. The average ratio in the USA today is around 17 omega-6 to 1 omega-3. But grain-fed beef consumption is responsible for only a very small part of the skewing of this ratio. (Recent research has shown that cattle fed with a particular variety of corn/zea mais bred to be high in corn oil, give meat with a very high marbling score, and are more likely of being graded "US choice." If *natural corn* is replaced with *high-oil corn* to get better prices, there may be a further increase in omega-6 fatty acids in US beef, although compared to some urban/processed food dietary loadings, it would still be relatively unimportant. Steers fed a diet with high levels of soya bean oil increased their percentage of desirable monounsaturated fats, whereas bulls on the same diet increased their polyunsaturated fats.)

Interestingly, one form of omega-6 linoleic acid, "conjugated linoleic acid," found primarily in grass-fed meat (and beef has the second highest amount in its fat of any domestic animal) and cheese, has now been found to help prevent the onset of adult-onset or noninsulin-dependent diabetes. Tests showed it also has the effect of reducing bodyfat – at least in laboratory rats! (The amount in a normal daily serving meat or cheese is only about one-quarter the amount needed to produce these effects.)

In addition, natural, grass-fed beef has a higher antioxidant capacity than feedlot beef, which means the grass-fed cuts of meat retain their red color longer. In fact, it has been proposed to add vitamin E (the alpha-tocopherol form) to the feedlot cattle diet to bring the shelf life of the meat up to match that of meat from grass-fed animals.

You might have inferred that the World Health Organization is suggesting we ought to eat more unsaturated fatty acids, such as various vegetable oils. In fact, in evolutionary terms we probably ate far fewer omega-6 unsaturated fatty acids than we do today, and more omega-3. Aside from being informed on safety issues, it is more important to eat meat, especially organ meat, than to be fixated on the particular pattern of fatty acids in the animals fat. In orders of magnitude, far greater benefit can be had by getting regular exercise, selecting natural food over processed food, and substituting fresh monounsaturated oils such as olive oil instead of high omega-6 vegetable oils. The naturally low omega-3 part of the modern diet can be bumped up by eating omega-3 rich fish such as sardines, or (if you object to "sardine breath") by taking omega-3 supplements regularly.

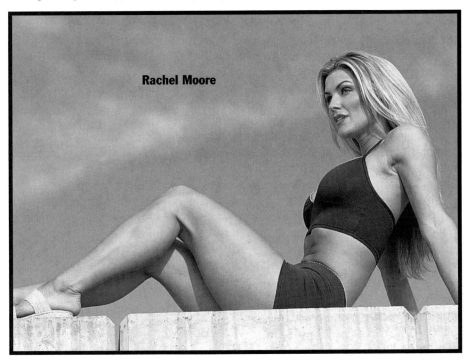

Rachel Moore

Even if we compensate for the unnaturally high omega-6 component of the modern diet by taking additional omega-3, the omega-3 oils must still have saturated animal fat present in order to make possible the protective antithrombitic metabolic process.

We sedentary Westerners need to reduce fat and carbohydrate intake, eat whole foods, and avoid processed foods. Today we believe we need to reduce our overall saturated fat intake by reducing our intake of industrial saturated fats, but still take in animal fat commensurate with our energy needs (or substitute whole grains, nuts and tubers so our body can make its own saturated fat). For most sedentary urbanites that means reducing animal fat intake as well. We need to obtain our essential polyunsaturated fats from whole natural sources such as organ meats, nuts, seeds and leafy green vegetables. We also need to reduce the excessive amount of omega-6 fats such as soya we eat by substituting with monounsaturated oils (such as olive oil). We need to eat more foods that contain omega-3 (such as fish) or take omega-3 supplements. This addition in itself will tend toward restoring a more evolutionarily natural balance. The easiest way overall is to eat natural foods – including meats – and skip highly processed foods.[13]

Types of Meat

Cattle

The prehistoric cave paintings of France show our (relatively) recent ancestors hunting this animal. Our evolutionary histories have long been intertwined. Forest-dwelling Guar, Bos frontalis, and Banteng, Bos javanicus would have likely been our prey as we radiated through India, and down into South East Asia; first as Homo erectus, then as Homo sapiens reradiating out of Africa and displacing H. erectus.

Types of Beef Products

Hormone-Free: Cattle in the United States, but not Europe, are often administered a natural growth hormone to make them grow faster and put on more weight – up to 20 percent more. The hormone used is an additional dose of exactly the same hormone the animal produces itself naturally, so there are no human health implications. About all that can be said is that implanted steers have been shown to have a higher saturated fatty acid to unsaturated fatty acid ratio than non-implanted animals, but total fat amount per steak was the same as non-implanted animals. Feedlot-finished steers have been shown to have up to a third more fat content in some cuts than a comparable grass-fed steer – they don't have as much carotene in the fat, with less vitamin E, and the omega-3 content declines the longer they are in the feedlot.

Antibiotic-Free: There appears to be no risk to human health from the breakdown products of antibiotics used to cure sick animals or prevent disease at critical stages of a calf's life. The same types of antibiotics are used in humans. The ethical issue is the over use of antibiotics to promote growth, and the concurrent creation of antibiotic-resistant bacteria.

"What is sauce for the goose may be sauce for the gander, but is not necessarily sauce for the chicken, the duck, the turkey or the guinea hen."
– Alice B. Toklas

Liver: The premium part of the animal, chock full of vitamins and minerals, especially B group vitamins. In virtually all hunter-gatherer societies, liver is the choice part of an animal.

Brains

Brains contain relatively large amounts of the essential w3 fatty acids EPA and DHA (beef fat is very approximately half saturated fat and half monounsaturated fat and with only a few percent polyunsaturated – but the fat in brains is about one-fifth polyunsaturated, with the rest somewhat evenly split between saturated and monounsaturated fats. These fatty acids are fairly unstable, and easily destroyed by heat. Luckily, brain is a delicate tissue, and needs only brief cooking. There is a huge food issue in Europe on the safety of eating brains. Bovine Spongiform Encephalopathy (BSE) is a transmissible, neurodegenerative, fatal brain disease of cattle. This disease has a long incubation period of four to five years, but ultimately is fatal for cattle within weeks to months of onset. BSE first came to the attention of the scientific community in November 1986 with the appearance in cattle of a newly recognized form of neurological disease in the United Kingdom (UK).

Studies conducted in the UK suggest that the source of BSE was cattle feed prepared from the carcasses of ruminants such as sheep. Speculation as to the cause of the appearance of the agent causing the disease has ranged from spontaneous occurrence in cattle, the carcasses of which then entered the cattle food chain, to entry into the cattle food chain from the carcasses of sheep with a similar disease, scrapie.

BSE is associated with a transmissible agent. The agent affects the brain and spinal cord of cattle and lesions are characterized by sponge-like changes visible with an ordinary microscope. The agent is highly stable, resisting freezing, drying and heating at normal cooking temperatures, even those used for pasteurization and sterilization. The nature of the BSE agent is still a matter of debate. According to the prion theory the agent is composed largely, if not entirely, of a self-replicating protein referred to as a prion. Another theory argues that the agent is virus-like and possesses nucleic acids, which carry genetic information. Strong evidence collected over the past decade supports the prion theory, but the ability of the BSE agent to form multiple strains is more easily explained by a virus-like agent.[23]

A newly recognized form of CJD, variant Creutzfeldt-Jakob disease (vCJD) was first reported in March 1996 in the UK. In contrast to the classical forms of CJD, vCJD has affected younger patients (average age 29 years, as opposed to 65 years), has a relatively longer duration of illness (median of 14 months as opposed to 4.5 months), and is strongly linked to exposure to BSE, probably through food. Recent studies have confirmed that vCJD is distinct from sporadic and acquired CJD.

From October 1996 to early December 2000, 87 cases of vCJD were reported in the United Kingdom (UK), three in France, and a single case in the Republic of Ireland. Insufficient information is available at present to make any precise prediction about the future number of vCJD cases.

Since few countries have surveillance systems, the geographical distribution of the incidence of vCJD needs to be better defined. Similarities

"After eating, an epicure gives a thin smile of satisfaction; a gastronome, burping into his napkin, praises the food in a magazine; a gourmet, repressing his burp, criticizes the food in the same magazine; a gourmand belches happily and tells everybody where he ate; a glutton embraces the white porcelain altar, or, more plainly, he barfs."
– William Safire

observed between the strain of the agent responsible for vCJD and those of BSE (and closely related agents transmitted naturally and experimentally to different animal species) are consistent with the hypothesis discussed during two 1996 WHO consultations. The hypothesis states that the cluster of vCJD cases is due to the same agent that caused BSE in cattle.[23]

Bone Marrow

Bone marrow is rarely eaten in the West (except in parts of France, and even there it is becoming uncommon). Marrow has monounsaturated fat (about 75 percent) as well as saturated fat. It is a very nutritionally dense source of food. In fact, one scientist has suggested that humans were able to survive and thrive in Africa in part due to the ability to scavenge bones and crack them open with stone hammers to extract the marrow. Some people eat marrow raw, when it has a firm texture, and some heat it until it has a butter-like consistency. Note: bone marrow is different from so-called spinal marrow, which is biologically a continuation of the brain tissue. Eating spinal marrow presents the same food safety dangers as eating brains (see previous heading).

Hamburger

Once the choice cuts have been removed from a cattle beast's carcass (usually grain-fed), there remains the fatty bits that have no real market. To make use of these parts, premier lean grass-ranged beef is imported, ground, and added to the fatty pieces. Range-fed beef has more of the beneficial "conjugated linoleic acid" content in its tissue (derived from grass) and this amount is, for some reason, increased when the meat is broiled or grilled. For very active people, hamburger is very good food.

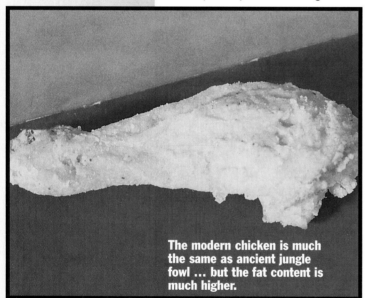

The modern chicken is much the same as ancient jungle fowl ... but the fat content is much higher.

Ground Beef

Ground beef is made from the cheaper, more fatty gristly cuts of feedlot or range-fed beef. There are usually regulations governing how much fat can be present in a product labeled "lean/premium mince." Mincing/grinding is a useful form of premastication. As stated, broiling/grilling seems to increase the beneficial conjugated linoleic acid content of meat.

Chicken, Poultry

Originally domesticated in China, the *red jungle fowl* has been associated with humans, and particularly with village life, for at least 4000 years. The male is a rooster, the female a hen, and the newly hatched babies are chicks. Selective breeding and scientific feed formulation means that today's newly hatched *Gallus gallus* will be heavy enough to be killed and eaten in only six or seven weeks. The chicken is pretty much an omnivore. It eats insects, seeds, leafy greens and fruits.

Birds in general have been a valuable food resource in all sorts of climates and environments. When we could catch them, these "reformed dinosaurs" provided a useful protein package, although their fat content was very low, except at certain times of year. The modern chicken is pretty much the same as the ancient jungle fowl, except it lays on muscle very much faster – the muscles are from a developing young bird, and so little-exercised that they are soft (tender) – and the fat content is also much higher.

The amount and type of amino acids which make up the protein content of eggs are considered to almost exactly match the amino acid profile the human body needs. In fact, other foods are measured against eggs, which is scored nationally at *100.* Compared to eggs, the flesh of the chicken that produced it comes in at 64, fish at 70, beef almost the same at 69, and so on.

Our African homeland has the greatest number of species of bird of any continent. These little oval protein packages don't run and don't fight, and children are skilled at finding them. Eggs have been a valuable resource for gatherer-hunters over the millenia of our evolution. The fat content of today's commercially produced eggs is about 21 percent essential fatty acids (the ones the human body can't manufacture but needs, so must obtain from food). In commercial battery-house eggs almost all this (20 percent) is omega-6, and only 1 percent is omega-3. It would be useful if the omega-3 content were higher (at least 4 times higher), or the omega-6 content lower.

The modern egg/cholesterol scare was started by a flawed 1965 study. Cholesterol expert Dr. John Allred, professor of nutrition at Ohio State University, points to the many clinical studies done on humans in the last ten years which have demonstrated that cholesterol in eggs has very little effect on a normal healthy person's blood cholesterol levels.

Sheep

Our ancestors first domesticated this wild animal about 10,000 years ago (400 human generations ago, if you count a new generation as occurring every 25 years), possibly in the uplands of present day Syria or Iraq. Along with the pig, this is probably one of the very first animals the human animal domesticated. Domesticated sheep are smaller than their wild ancestors. Most have lost their horns, and there have been changes in wool, color, ear shape, size, and so on.

Pig

Our ancestors have been eating species of pig in Africa and beyond since our own evolution as a species. Like all meats, pork is a good food. But as it cannot be solely grass-raised, maize and soya beans in the feed may create an overabundance of omega-6 fatty acids and a relative under supply of omega-3 fatty acids, relative to the ratio best suited to humans. Some cultures forbid the consumption of pork because its dietary habits make it an unclean animal. In the middle east pigs are known to carry parasites harmful to humans. There are accounts of cannibalism where the taste of human flesh is described as being reminiscent of "roast pork." The ban on pork may even be related to the almost universal taboo on cannibalism.

Turkey

The turkey was first domesticated in Mesoamerica from the flocks that roamed the North American continent and Mexico. All birds have been, and are, prey for humans. All the comments applying to chickens can be applied to turkeys, as they are raised essentially the same way. We don't regard the turkey as an egg-producing bird. And get this, in Turkey, the turkey is known as "the American bird."

Rabbit

The rabbit is the only rodent eaten regularly in the West. Yet bush rats and various Savannah rodents would have been far more likely to have been caught and consumed (along with other small game) by our ancestors than the big game animals. Accordingly, rabbits ought to be a prized component of a reconstructed, evolutionarily correct diet.

Presumably because they were so abundant in the wild, rabbits were not domesticated for food until the middle ages. Rabbits have extraordinarily ittle fat on them, about 2 percent. While domesticated rabbits are twice as fat, at about 5 percent, they are still lean eating. There are cases of trappers who starved to death while eating nothing but rabbit.

The only commercial meat rabbits are those that are caged and fed pellets. As the rabbit is a herbivore, the pellets are comprised chiefly of plant material. As the rabbit is so extraordinarily lean, there is unlikely to be much compositional difference between the wild and the farmed versions.

Duck

Ducks have been domesticated with less enthusiasm than jungle fowl, probably because they are "tied to water," and because harvesting wild ducks is relatively easy compared to keeping them. The Chinese were probably the first to domesticate ducks, but the date is uncertain. There is little doubt that our ancestors exploited the 100 or so duck species of the world, whether through taking eggs or adult birds. The duck has good amounts of nutritious yellow fat at the right time of year, and a substantial amount of protein in its breast meat.

Young ducks are grown for the market in a somewhat similar fashion to broiler chickens; and like chickens, they can have quite high fat content, especially under the skin. Again, the fat content (with a ratio of omega-6 fats to omega-3 of about 12:1) may not have the same fatty acid profile as the wild duck, but it is of no consequence as duck is such a passing small component of the average person's diet. Many people in North America and Australia are more likely to eat wild duck than domesticated duck anyway.

Quail

These small birds range right across Europe and Asia, South East Asia and Australasia. They have long been food for humans. These birds are so small that they don't make much of a meal, but because they form large groups, any effective trapping techniques caught useful numbers. Some species are migratory, and it is known that North Africans have found birds recently arrived from Europe to be easy prey. In fact, some exhausted birds literally fall out of the sky – a seasonal harvest for our North African ancestors.

Quail can only be farmed in low cages, usually stacked in tiers in a warm building, partly due to the need to maximize the number of birds per square meter, given their tiny size, and partly because quail that are disturbed have a defense mechanism of flying straight up – at speed. Birds raised in a high-roofed outside enclosure tend to be able to pick up enough speed to scalp themselves when they hit the roof netting. Quail are fed compounded feed, as are broiler chickens, with the adults needing more vegetation-based feed (such as alfalfa) than the young. Overall, farmed quail can probably be regarded as not very far removed in lipid profile from wild quail.

Geese

Wild geese are fatty, especially in the autumn season, but not as fatty as domestic geese. The reason, in part, is that most wild geese are migratory, and burn off the fat. Our ancestors would have been as fond of geese as of duck; and goslings are both fat and tender, in contrast to the adult bird, which is generally tough. Because of their grass-grazing habit, it is quite possible that their fats will include useful amounts of omega-3 fats and possibly the healthful conjugated linoleic acid.

There is effectively no commercial production of geese. They are a bird of a fast-disappearing peasant farming lifestyle. They are efficient converters of grain to meat, but most importantly they are grass-grazers. They can grow and fatten on grass and the insects they find for themselves without any supplementary feed. Apart from the geese force-fed on grains to create the fatty liver (foie gras) beloved by gourmets, most geese are still grass-fed with some supplemental grains. Accordingly, they are likely to have a similar nutritional profile to the wild geese our ancestors ate.

Goat

The goat was first domesticated about 10,000 years ago (400 human generations ago if you count a new generation as occurring every 25 years). Goats are of as ancient lineage as sheep, and were hunted for food in Ethiopia, North Africa, and in the Mediterranean and South West Asia. Goats are not raised for food in much number in the West, and those that are are often killed for export to Middle Eastern countries. Goats are invariably grass-fed, and are similar to their wild ancestors. An ideal food for the urban hunter-gatherer.

Deer

The approximately 41 deer species of the world have been hunted by humans ever since our ancestors radiated out of Africa into "deer country" – Eurasia and South East Asia. For example, in China the spotted deer was a commonly killed species; in the subarctic, *reindeer* was the prize (a subspecies, the North American caribou, is a form of the European tundra reindeer).

The *moose* (confusingly, known in Europe as elk) evolved in northern Eurasia (from a much larger animal), and was common in both Europe and Asia, its distribution varying with the climate and vegetation of the time. It wandered into North America across the land bridge only recently, maybe around 10,000 years ago. *Elk* (not to be confused with moose) evolved in the European landmass. It drifted into North America when the land bridge was present, and the remaining European population of elk drifted into several forms and subspecies we now know as the *red deer* – a common forest and upland browser.

Excavation of a prehistoric site in France dated 110,000 years ago showed deer as being the third most commonly eaten large mammalian food (after horse, most often eaten, and the aurochs, ancestors of modern cattle). Deer are browsers of twigs and leaves as much as grazers, and they are totally unsuited to feedlot management. Thus, modern farmed deer meat is very similar to the meat our ancestors ate. As a general rule, deer meat contains very little fat.

Horse

The horse evolved in North America millions of years ago. Various species crossed into Europe and Asia during the Pleistocene glacial periods when sea levels dropped so far that North America and Europe were connected. By about 75,000 years ago, various species and subspecies were well established in the grasslands of Eurasia. This animal and its Asian relative was a major food source for European and Central Asian human ancestors at this time. In fact, at one stage it was the predominant large animal eaten.

In Upper Paleolithic Europe the horse was the animal most frequently featured on cave paintings, followed by the bison. The paintings are considered to be pictures of animals that the ancestors of the Europeans ate. Ironically, the horse in North America became extinct, possibly through hunting by Clovis people around 11,000 years ago. A skeleton of Equs conversidens, a small North American horse species, has been found in Alberta, Canada with cut marks on its bones, and a spear point found 500 meters away tested positive for horse protein residues.

Horse muscle tissue has substantial stores of glycogen, an instantly available form of carbohydrate energy. Presumably this is needed to power the horse's flight reaction – it may run at full speed for many miles to escape a predator. The result is that the flesh is both slightly sweetish in taste, and possibly a useful energy source. Apart from it not being as dangerous an animal as other big game, it was possibly easy to kill by panicking it over a cliff, or into a pit trap.

In spite of its leanness and excellent nutritional value, and our long evolutionary history of eating this meat, very few Western people eat this ancestral food animal. In Europe horsemeat is relatively common only in Belgium, and to a lesser extent Sweden and France.

Grass-fed horse meat would most likely have the evolutionary correct fat profiles. The wild horse ate grasses and bulbs, and lived in a fairly marginal environment, so it was probably only seasonally fat. When horse meat is available, it may have had some grain feeding, chiefly oats or similar high-carbohydrate food, but probably was still chiefly grass-fed, except where old or "broken down" racehorses are used – often fed grains and pellets. Exclusively grass-grazed horse meat would have the most natural biochemical composition of fats, but even in France, where horses are still sometimes raised as a meat animal, they may be "fattened" off grass before slaughter. Some of the Belgian and French horsemeat is now imported from horse feedlots in USA and Canada.[14]

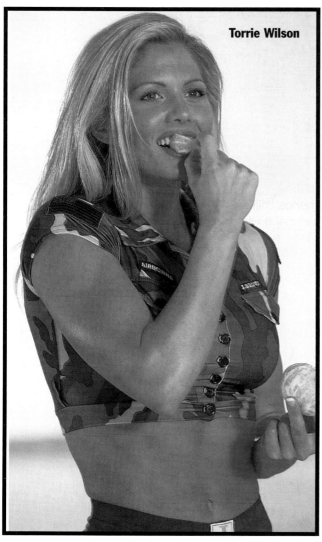

Torrie Wilson

Diet

We now know what nutrients we want to incorporate into our diet, and the best foods to get them from. First remember this: It doesn't matter if everything you eat is perfect, if too much of it is consumed you will get fat. And if your goal is to get lean, that will work against you. Again, if your goal is to build muscle, you had better make sure you are eating enough protein. So how do you go about putting together the game plan? There are a million different diets, just as there are a million different training routines. You've got everything from the high-protein diet to the high-fat diet, and to this day experts in our field still argue as to which is the best.

Human nutrition is part science and part art. Provided you eat a balanced diet that resembles that of our ancestors, heavy in natural fruits, vegetables and meats, and totally lacking in processed foods, then you'll be fine. It may not be politically correct, but it will be evolutionarily correct!

"The majority of them give the impression of being men who have been drafted into the job during a period of martial law and are only waiting for the end of the emergency to get back to a really congenial occupation such as slum demolition or debt collecting."
– Alan Brien, describing waiters.

Getting Started

There are seven basic rules that everyone should follow when setting up their own diet plan:

Rule #1: Eat small but nutritious meals throughout the day. This will help speed up you body's metabolism and help discourage you from storing fat. It will keep your hunger under control, and more realistically reflect the style of eating our ancestors followed.

Rule #2: Keep the protein high. Remember, if you are incorporating a strength-training routine into your program, you need at least 1 full gram of protein per pound of bodyweight. Even if you decide not to use weights, keep in mind that dietary protein taken every three to four hours will prevent you from losing lean muscle tissue, even while doing aerobic training. The last thing you want to have happen is for your body to rob the amino acids from your own muscles!

Rule #3: Keep dietary fats to a minimum. While fat is essential, our ancestors were always limited in the amount of fat they could eat. You have to do the same.

Rule #4: Watch your carbohydrate intake. Carbohydrates are considered protein-sparing, but too much of them in your diet will prevent you from losing unwanted bodyfat. If you are burning the carbohydrates from your diet all day long, it will be virtually impossible for your body to burn stored bodyfat for energy. And that's how the Atkins diet works. By not consuming carbs, you trick the body into thinking that it's starving, and it burns stored bodyfat. Consume carbohydrates, and the body releases insulin to store fat.

Rule #5: Make sure to eat protein right after you train. This is your golden "window of opportunity." Your muscles need that protein to help with repairs right after they have been broken down in the gym.

Rule #6: Include carbohydrates and fat with each of your meals. That will stop any hunger pangs that might lead to late-night refrigerator raids.

Rule #7: Drink lots of water. Protein and exercise has a dehydrating effect on the body and water will help moderate that as well as help transport nutrients.

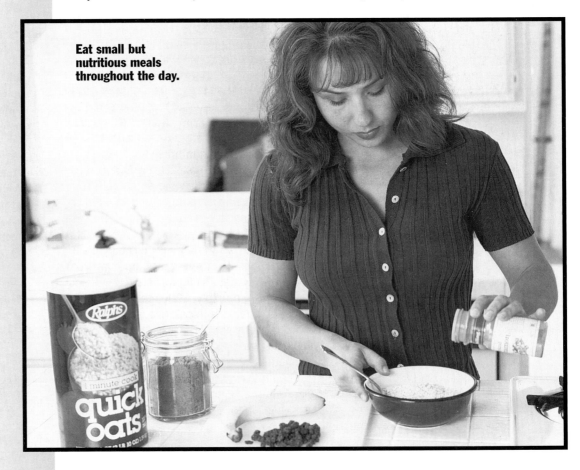

Eat small but nutritious meals throughout the day.

Determining Your Calorie Intake

If you eat and you gain, you're eating too much. If you eat and you lose, you're not eating enough. Sorry, we can't make it any more complicated than that.

Measuring Bodyfat Percentage

The easiest method is the skin-fold test. It uses an instrument called a caliper and calculates your bodyfat by measuring the thickness of skin folds at various sites around your body. The test is painless and can be done pretty quickly. Many gyms and health centers offer free bodyfat testing.

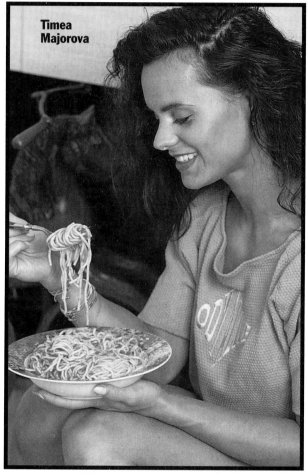

Timea Majorova

> *"If Broadway shows charge preview prices while the cast is in dress rehearsal, why should restaurants charge full price when their dining room and kitchen staffs are still practicing?"*
> *– Marion Burros*

A Formula for Lowering Bodyfat Levels

The starting point is to decide where you want to be, so the first thing we need to do is make some adjustments. Let's start with protein. As we just mentioned, you should be eating at the very least 1 gram of protein per pound of your bodyweight. Since protein and carbohydrates are both 4 calories per gram, subtract the same number of carbohydrates from your diet, and add the protein to keep the caloric total the same. The calories remain the same because we just switched the protein and carbohydrates.

Next take a look at your dietary fat and cut it by about 5 percent. So, if your total calories were 2000 and 20 percent of your diet was from fat, then we know you are eating about 45 grams of fat per day in your diet. To figure this out, we just multiply 2000 calories by .20 and get 400 calories. Now remember that 400 value is in calories, so we have to divide it by 9 (because there is 9 calories in one gram of fat). That leaves us with approximately 45 grams of dietary fat. Since we are going to start out by cutting your fat intake by 5 percent, we need to figure out 15 percent of your diet from fat which would be 300 calories or 33 grams (2000 x .15 = 300 ÷ 9 calories = 33.3 grams of fat). That leaves us with a difference of 12 grams of fat (45 grams of fat minus 33 grams of fat). Now all we have to do is look at your diet and decide where we are going to cut the 12 grams of fat.

"The Americans are a funny lot. They drink whiskey to keep them warm, then they put some ice in it to make it cool; they put some sugar in it to make it sweet, and then put a slice of lemon in it to make it sour. Then they say 'Here's to you' and drink it themselves."
– B.N. Chakravarty

Don't Be Afraid to Make Changes

The first time you change your diet many different things are bound to happen because of the initial shock to the system. If you lose more than a couple of pounds it's okay, your body will just acclimate itself to the changes. But if you are still losing more than a couple pounds after the second week, then you should add some calories. Chances are, though, if you just make a subtle change, you will probably lose only a pound or two. Let's assume everything is going great, you are losing 1 pound a week. Then, after five weeks, all of a sudden you stop losing weight. Time to go in and make another adjustment.

This time you subtract another 5 percent from fat calories, or if you feel your dietary fat is getting too low, subtract some calories from the carbohydrates. The only number that should stay pretty constant throughout the whole diet is your protein intake. However, even this may need to be adjusted higher. There is a definite correlation to getting lean while eating a high-protein diet. Be prepared to lose a little energy. While a high-protein diet is awesome for getting ripped, it is not the best diet for enhancing energy levels. Don't be afraid

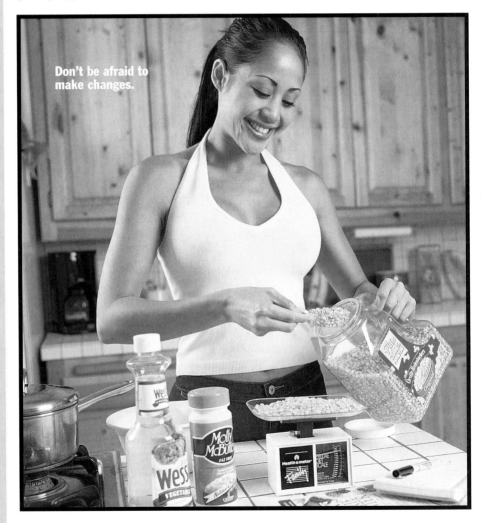

Don't be afraid to make changes.

to go in and change things around. No one, including yourself (unless you've done this before), is going to know exactly how their body will respond.

The Best Foods

Many different foods are good for you – we've listed them throughout this chapter. What must be determined now is, which foods will be best to incorporate into your diet plan to help you attain the best results and achieve your goal. Below is a list from which you can choose foods when structuring your nutritional plan:

Protein
Lean turkey breast (unprocessed)
Lean ground beef or flank steak
Chicken breast
Egg whites
Tuna

Carbohydrates (starchy)
Pasta
Rice
Potatoes
Oatmeal
Cream of rice
Whole-wheat bread

Carbohydrates (fibrous)
Spinach
Green beans
Peas
Broccoli
Cauliflower
Salad

Fats
Flaxseed oil
Safflower oil
Primrose oil

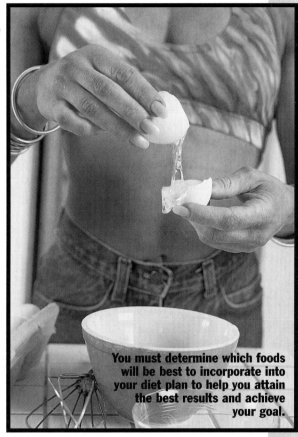

You must determine which foods will be best to incorporate into your diet plan to help you attain the best results and achieve your goal.

You will always find a combination of the macronutrients in all foods. However, most foods derive the majority of their calories from one macronutrient – and that is why they are classified as such. The protein foods above are very good sources for your protein because they all have very little carbohydrates and fat. When choosing your protein sources at the grocery store, make sure to pick the leanest cuts of meat. Remember, there *will* be saturated fat in your protein sources, so we want to minimize that amount as much as possible. It is better to get your fat from the essential fatty acids in unsaturated fat.

In the following chapter on supplements, you will see how easy it is to incorporate them into your diet. After reviewing all the great foods there are from which to obtain nutrients, you may be left wondering why you need to take any type of supplement. The truth is, you really don't. Everything you need to build muscle and lose fat is right there in the perfect diet. The problem most people encounter is, they don't eat the perfect diet. They have the "No" syndrome – no time, no knowledge, no money. Most of us don't have the time to prepare the meals needed to make up the prefect diet and on the rare occasion that we do, many of us fall short on knowledge or money. Enter, supplements …

REFERENCES

1. www.maxmuscle.com/guide/guidemain.htm
2. www.ods.od.nih.gov/whatare/whatare.html
3. www.cc.nih.gov/ccc/supplements/vita.html
4. www.cc.nih.gov/ccc/supplements/vitb6.html
5. www.cc.nih.gov/ccc/supplements/vitb12.html
6. www.cc.nih.gov/ccc/supplements/vitd.html
7. www.cc.nih.gov/ccc/supplements/vite.html
8. www.cc.nih.gov/ccc/supplements/folate.html
9. www.cc.nih.gov/ccc/supplements/magn.html
10. www.cc.nih.gov/ccc/supplements/selen.html
11. www.cc.nih.gov/ccc/supplements/zinc.html
12. www.naturalhub.com/natural_food_guide_grains_beans_seeds.htm
13. www.naturalhub.com/natural_food_guide_meat.htm
14. www.naturalhub.com/natural_food_guide_meat_common.htm
15. www.fantasyfit.com/php/faqdisplay.php3?category_id=4&topic_id=3#question1
16. www.vita-men.com/FAQs/faq-k.htm#Q1
17. www.vita-men.com/FAQs/general.htm#Q3
18. www.hcrc.org/contrib/coleman/fiber.html
19. www.members.nbci.com/nutration/vkfaq.htm
20. www.ma.essortment.com/vitaminsmineral_rwva.htm
21. www.cybervitamins.com/vitamin_k.htm
22. www.bayho.com/MM011.ASP?pageno=335
23. www.who.int/inf-fs/en/fact113.html
24. www.199.97.97.16/contWriter/yhdnutrition/2001/02/12/medic/1408-0187-pat_nytimes.html
25. www.shs.ilstu.edu/hpo/Nutrition_Mission/Nutrition percent 20Web/Nutrition-Carbohydrate.htm
26. www.mendosa.com/gi.htm

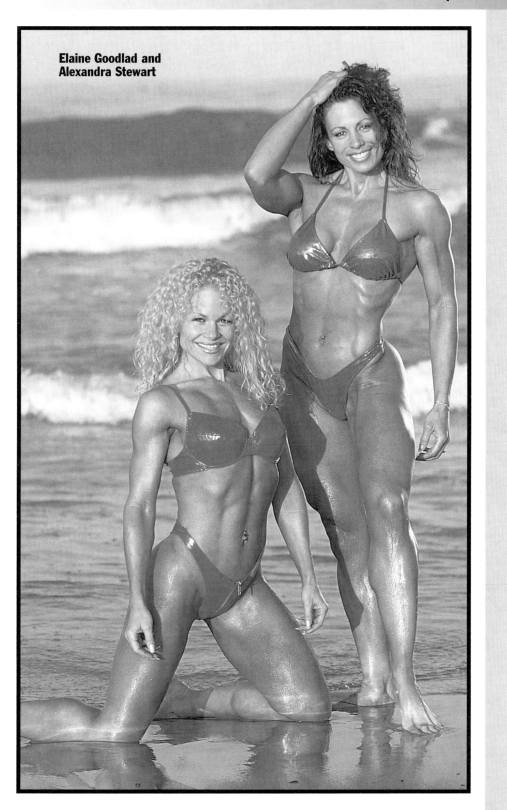

Elaine Goodlad and
Alexandra Stewart

CHAPTER EIGHT

The Intermediate Level

With three to six months of introductory training behind you it's time to progress to the intermediate ranks. At this point the waters get a bit murky regarding what is "right," "best," or whatever. We are not going to try to tell you that after three months you must start following intermediate routines. Most people progress at different speeds. What's best for you may be useless for someone else. However, we hope the suggestions in the next few pages will enable you to keep progressing and perhaps more important, help keep your motivation levels high.

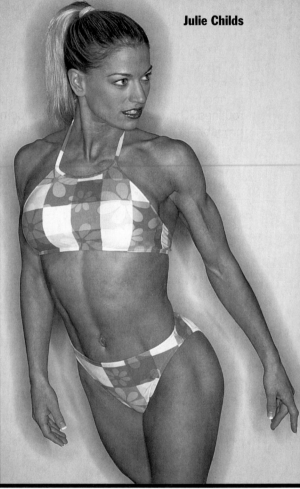

Julie Childs

It's Time to Split!

Perhaps the biggest change you'll make in your training during the intermediate phase is dividing or splitting your training into sections. Up until now you've been training the whole body on nonconsecutive days, performing only one exercise per bodypart. Although such training is productive, and certainly has its advantages, most serious strength trainers eventually switch to a split routine.

By *split routine* we mean training certain muscles on one day and others the next. One of the disadvantages to full-body routines is the diminished intensity factor that creeps in toward the end of the workout. Often you are only going through the motions on the last couple of muscle groups. Splitting, however, allows you to do more for the muscles as you don't have to partition your energy reserves to hit the entire body. In fact this is the primary advantage to split routines; the reduced number of muscles trained in the session allows you to do more for each muscle group. Instead of one exercise for 3 sets, you can do two, three, even four exercises for the same muscle. There are several ways to split up your routine.

Push/Pull
This routine consists of training your pulling muscles (back and biceps) on one day and your pushing muscles the next (chest and triceps). You can then train your legs, shoulders and abdominals in between the other workout days.

Upper Body/Lower Body
This split routine consists of training your upper body one day, your lower body the next. Even though the legs are only one muscle group, they constitute 50 percent of the body's muscle mass.

Random
Random muscle combinations are perhaps the most common split routines. There's really no right way to combine muscle groups. It probably doesn't make sense to combine legs, chest and back on one day, as these are the three largest muscle groups. Instead put legs with a smaller muscle group like arms or shoulders. The bottom line is, try to divide the body up evenly so that you are training about the same amount of muscle mass on each day.

How Often?

Besides deciding which muscle groups to combine, you also need to decide how often to work out. As there are many options here, let's look at the pros and cons of each.

Four Days per Week
This is probably the most popular routine split. You divide the body in two, then train two days in a row followed by a day off. You can go two on/one off indefinitely, or follow the traditional week as follows:

Monday – Day 1
Tuesday – Day 2
Wednesday – Day 3
Thursday – Day 1
Friday – Day 2
Weekends – Off
Monday – Day 3, etc.

The two-on/one-off split has many advantages, the chief of which is, you are only in the gym two days in a row. The day off in between gives the body ample time to recover. For some, even training two days in a row is too taxing on the recovery system and a modified version of the split is called for. In this case

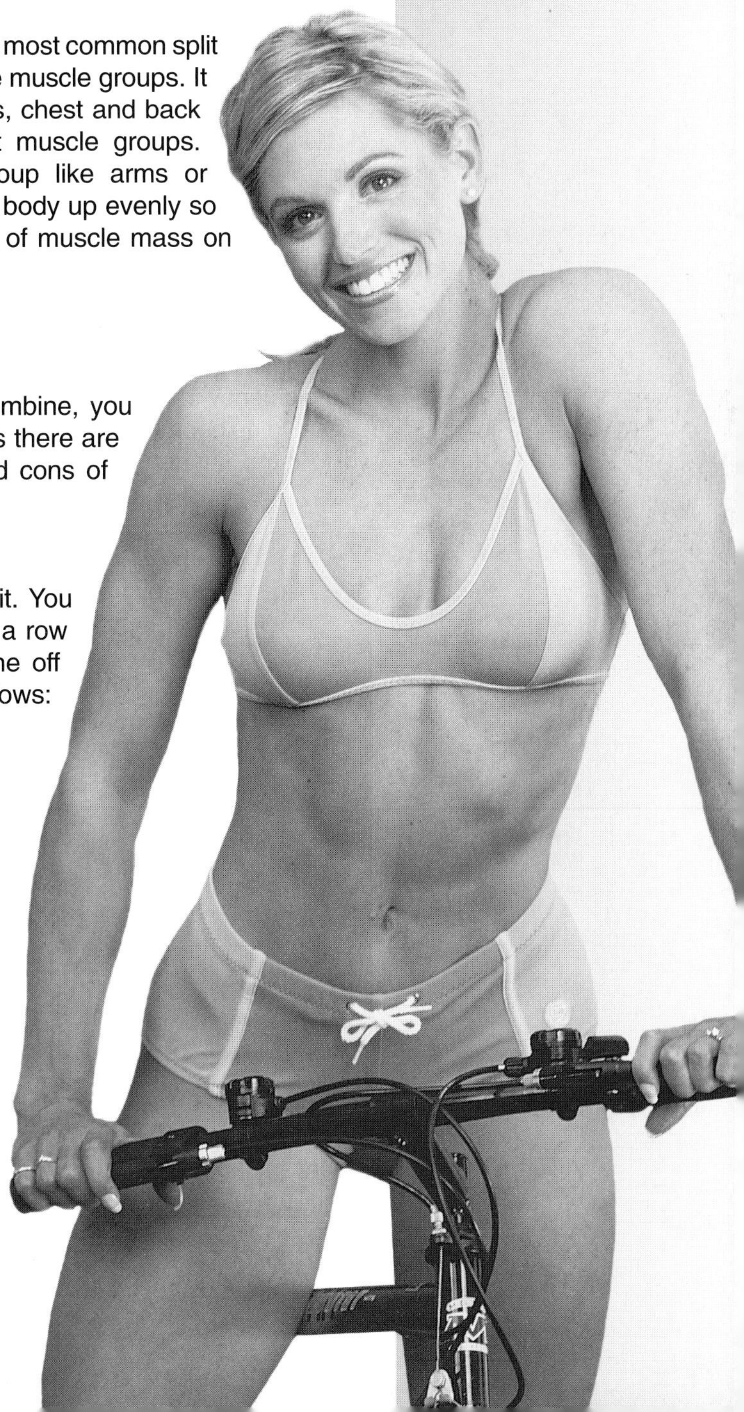

Kim Lyons

you train one day, take a day off, then train the other half of the body on the third day. The one-on/one-off routine gives your bodyparts 48 hours of rest between workouts.

A third variation of the four-day training split is great for those who want to split the body in two halves but can only get to the gym three times per week. In this case the two-week split can be followed:

Week 1   Day 1
            Day 2
            Day 1

Week 2   Day 2
            Day 1
            Day 2

Notice how in the first week the day 1 routine is worked twice, while the day 2 exercise routine is done only once, but during the second week you switch things around. This means during a two-week period you hit the same muscles three times. Such a split is great for those with school, work or family commitments. With an average workout lasting an hour, you can get away with a total time investment of only three hours per week. Even the busiest women can usually scrounge three hours of time to train.

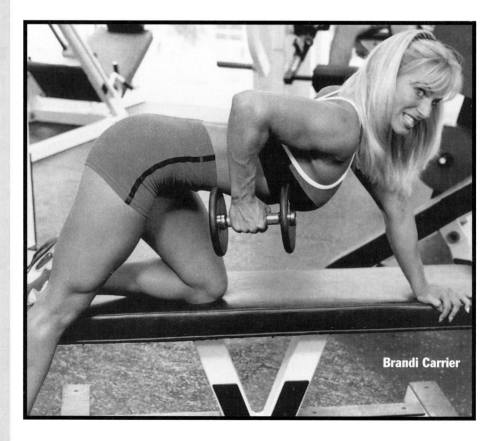

Brandi Carrier

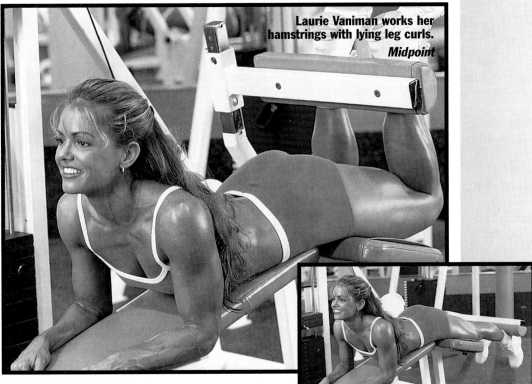

Laurie Vaniman works her hamstrings with lying leg curls.
Midpoint

Start

Sample Routines

Split Routine A:
Day 1

Thighs	Squat	3 sets	8-12 reps
	Leg extension	3 sets	8-12 reps
Hamstrings	Lying leg curl	3 sets	8-12 reps
	Stiff-leg deadlift	3 sets	8-12 reps
Calves	Standing calf raise	3 sets	6-8 (15-20)*
	Seated calf raise	3 sets	6-8 (15-20)*
Biceps	Cable curl	3 sets	8-12 reps
	Incline curl	3 sets	8-12 reps
Triceps	Lying dumbell extension	3 sets	8-12 reps
	Cable pushdown	3 sets	8-12 reps
Abdominals	Lying leg raise	3 sets	15-20 reps
	Crunch	3 sets	15-20 reps

*Note: Alternate low reps (6 to 8) one week and high reps (15 to 20) the next for the calves.

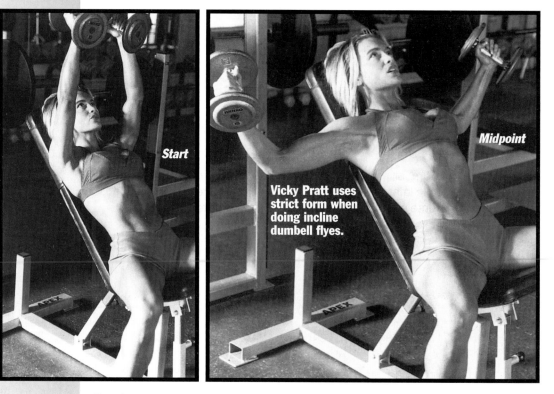

Start

Midpoint

Vicky Pratt uses strict form when doing incline dumbell flyes.

Day 2

Chest	Flat dumbell press	3 sets	8-12 reps
	Incline dumbell flye	3 sets	8-12 reps
Back	Front lat pulldown	3 sets	8-12 reps
	One-arm row	3 sets	8-12 reps
Shoulders	Machine press	3 sets	8-12 reps
	Lateral raise	3 sets	8-12 reps
	Bent-over lateral	3 sets	8-12 reps

Split Routine B:
Day 1

Chest	Flat barbell press	3 sets	8-12 reps
	Incline dumbell press	3 sets	8-12 reps
Back	Chinup	3 sets	8-12 reps
	T-bar row	3 sets	8-12 reps
Biceps	Preacher curl	3 sets	8-12 reps
	Concentration curl	3 sets	8-12 reps
Abdominals	Crunch	3 sets	15-20 reps
	Reverse crunch	3 sets	15-20 reps

Day 2

Thighs	Leg press	3 sets	8-12 reps
	Leg extension	3 sets	8-12 reps
Hamstrings	Seated leg curl	3 sets	8-12 reps
	Lying leg curl	3 sets	8-12 reps
Calves	Toe press	3 sets	6-8 (15-20)
	Seated calf raise	3 sets	6-8 (15-20)
Shoulders	Dumbell press	3 sets	8-12 reps
	Cable lateral raise	3 sets	8-12 reps
	Reverse pec-dek flye	3 sets	8-12 reps
Triceps	Dumbell extension	3 sets	8-12 reps
	Bench dip	3 sets	8-12 reps

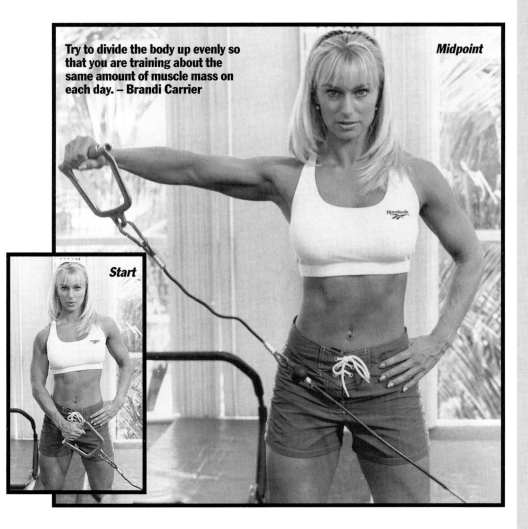

Try to divide the body up evenly so that you are training about the same amount of muscle mass on each day. – Brandi Carrier

Midpoint

Start

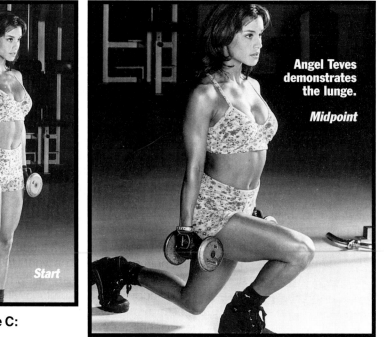

Angel Teves demonstrates the lunge.

Midpoint

Start

Split Routine C:
Day 1

Thighs	Lunge	3 sets	8-12 reps
	Leg press	3 sets	8-12 reps
Chest	Incline dumbell press	3 sets	8-12 reps
	Flat dumbell flye	3 sets	8-12 reps
Shoulders	Front barbell press	3 sets	8-12 reps
	Upright row	3 sets	8-12 reps
	Bent-over lateral	3 sets	8-12 reps
Triceps	Lying barbell extension	3 sets	8-12 reps
	Kickback	3 sets	8-12 reps
Calves	Standing calf raise	3 sets	6-8 (15-20)
	Seated calf raise	3 sets	6-8 (15-20)

Day 2

Back	Front pulldown	3 sets	8-12 reps
	Seated cable row	3 sets	8-12 reps
Hamstrings	Lying leg curl	3 sets	8-12 reps
	Stiff-leg deadlift	3 sets	8-12 reps
Biceps	Standing dumbell curl	3 sets	8-12 reps
	One-arm cable curl	3 sets	8-12 reps
Abdominals	Hanging leg raise	3 sets	15-20 reps
	Crunch	3 sets	15-20 reps

Six-Day Splits

If four-day splits have a disadvantage, it's they require you to train three muscle groups during one workout. Even doing only two exercises per muscle group, there's still a lot of ground to cover. By the time you get to the third group you may be just going through the motions. One solution is to follow the three-day split, where you divide the body into three distinct areas. This means only having to hit two muscles per workout.

Besides the time factor, six-day splits allow you to do three or more exercises for each muscle group. Even though increasing the weight is often enough to keep the muscles responding, sometimes an increase in volume is needed. By having to train only one or two muscle groups per workout you have time for a few more exercises.

There are two primary ways in which to implement a six-day split routine. The most popular is to train three days, and then take a day off (three on/one off). A few individuals prefer training six on and resting on the seventh. Of the two we recommend the former. Training six days straight can leave the body in a state of overtraining. Even the three on/one off may be too taxing as you are essentially working out six days out of eight. Or put another way, in a two-week period you are in the gym 12 days. The top strength athletes in the world usually limit six-splits to a few months of the year, just enough time to shock the body without draining it entirely. Of course you will be the best judge of when you need to reduce your training volume. As soon as you start recognizing the symptoms of overtraining (see Chapter Twelve), either reduce your workload or take a few days off (perhaps weeks).

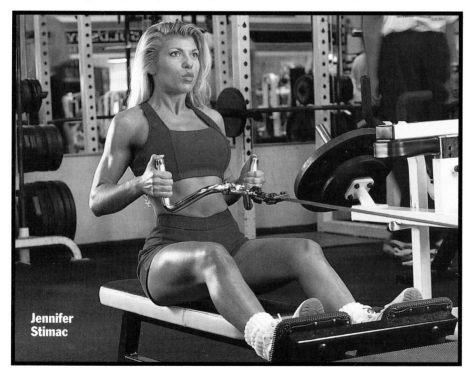

Jennifer
Stimac

Split Routine A:
Day 1 – Chest and Arms

Chest	Flat barbell press	3 sets	8-12 reps
	Incline dumbell press	3 sets	8-12 reps
	Pec-dek flye	3 sets	8-12 reps
Biceps	Standing barbell curl	3 sets	8-12 reps
	Concentration curl	3 sets	8-12 reps
Triceps	Pushdown	3 sets	8-12 reps
	Dumbell extension	3 sets	8-12 reps

Day 2 – Legs and Waist

Legs	Squat	3 sets	8-12 reps
	Leg extension	3 sets	8-12 reps
	Lunge	3 sets	8-12 reps
	Lying leg curl	3 sets	8-12 reps
	Stiff-leg deadlift	3 sets	8-12 reps
	Standing calf raise	3 sets	6-8 (15-20)
	Seated calf raise	3 sets	6-8 (15-20)
Abdominals	Reverse crunch	3 sets	15-20 reps
	Crunch	3 sets	15-20 reps
	Rope crunch	3 sets	15-20 reps

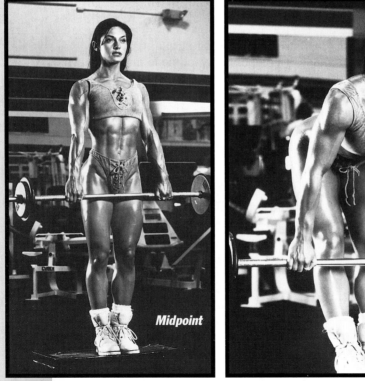

Midpoint

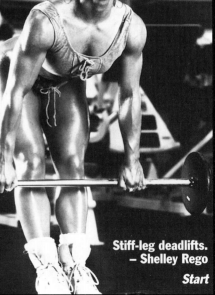

Stiff-leg deadlifts.
– Shelley Rego

Start

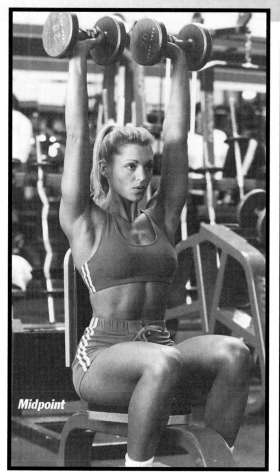

Midpoint

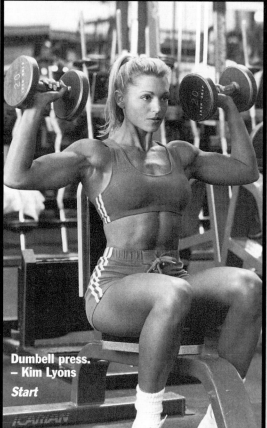

**Dumbell press.
– Kim Lyons**

Start

Day 3 – Back and Shoulders

Back			
	Front pulldown	3 sets	8-12 reps
	Seated cable row	3 sets	8-12 reps
	One-arm row	3 sets	8-12 reps
	Back extension	3 sets	15-20 reps

Shoulders			
	Dumbell press	3 sets	8-12 reps
	Lateral raise	3 sets	8-12 reps
	Reverse pec flye	3 sets	8-12 reps
	Dumbell shrug	3 sets	8-12 reps

Routine B:
Day 1 – Chest and Back

Chest			
	Incline dumbell press	3 sets	8-12 reps
	Flat barbell press	3 sets	8-12 reps
	Flat dumbell flye	3 sets	8-12 reps

Back			
	Chinup	3 sets	8-12 reps
	T-bar row	3 sets	8-12 reps
	One-arm row	3 sets	8-12 reps

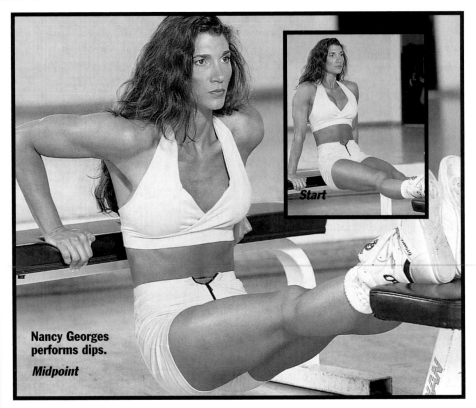

Start

Nancy Georges performs dips.

Midpoint

Day 2 – Legs and Waist

Legs	Leg press	3 sets	8-12 reps
	Hack squat	3 sets	8-12 reps
	Seated leg curl	3 sets	8-12 reps
	Stiff-leg deadlift	3 sets	8-12 reps
	Donkey calf raise	3 sets	6-8 (15-20)
	Seated calf raise	3 sets	6-8 (15-20)
Abdominals	Hanging leg raise	3 sets	15-20 reps
	Crunch	3 sets	5-20 reps
	Rope crunch	3 sets	5-20 reps

Day 3 – Shoulders and Arms

Shoulders	Machine press	3 sets	8-12 reps
	Cable lateral raise	3 sets	8-12 reps
	Reverse pec-dek	3 sets	8-12 reps
	Upright row	3 sets	8-12 reps
Biceps	Barbell curl	3 sets	8-12 reps
	One-arm preacher curl	3 sets	8-12 reps
Triceps	Rope extension	3 sets	8-12 reps
	Bench dip	3 sets	8-12 reps

Split Routine C (machine only):
Day 1 – Legs and Waist

Thighs	Leg press	3 sets	8-12 reps
	Leg extension	3 sets	8-12 reps
Hamstrings	Lying leg curl	3 sets	8-12 reps
	Seated leg curl	3 sets	8-12 reps
Calves	Standing calf raise	3 sets	6-8 (15-20)
	Seated calf raise	3 sets	6-8 (15-20)
Abdominals	Machine crunch	3 sets	15-20 reps

Day 2 – Chest and Back

Chest	Flat machine press	3 sets	8-12 reps
	Incline machine press	3 sets	8-12 reps
	Pec-dek flye	3 sets	8-12 reps
Back	Front pulldown	3 sets	8-12 reps
	Seated cable row	3 sets	8-12 reps
	Pullover machine	3 sets	8-12 reps

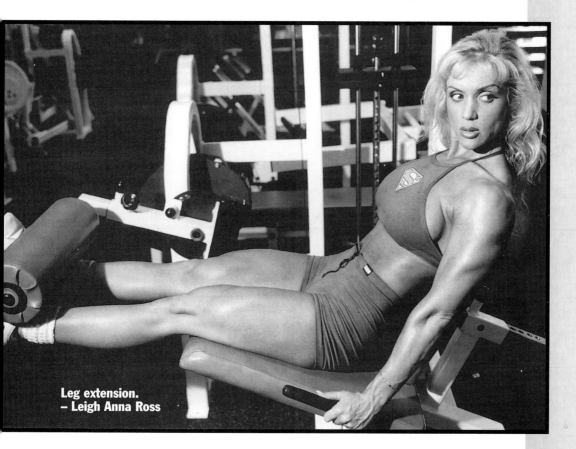

Leg extension.
– Leigh Anna Ross

Day 3 – Shoulders and Arms

Shoulders	Machine press	3 sets	8-12 reps
	Lateral raise machine	3 sets	8-12 reps
	Reverse pec flye	3 sets	8-12 reps
Biceps	Machine preacher curl	3 sets	8-12 reps
	Cable curl	3 sets	8-12 reps
Triceps	Pushdown	3 sets	8-12 reps
	Rope extension	3 sets	8-12 reps

Split Routine D (free weights only):
Day 1 – Legs and Abs

Thighs	Squats	3 sets	8-12 reps
	Lunges	3 sets	8-12 reps
Hamstrings	Stiff-leg deadlift	3 sets	8-12 reps
	Back extension	3 sets	8-12 reps
Calves	Donkey calf raise	3 sets	to failure
	One leg calf raise	3 sets	to failure
Abdominals	Lying leg raise	3 sets	15-20 reps
	Crunch	3 sets	15-20 reps
	Reverse crunch	3 sets	15-20 reps

Day 2 – Chest and Arms

Chest	Flat dumbell press	3 sets	8-12 reps
	Incline dumbell press	3 sets	8-12 reps
	Dumbell pullover	3 sets	8-12 reps
Biceps	Barbell curl	3 sets	8-12 reps
	Incline dumbell curl	3 sets	8-12 reps
Triceps	Dumbell extension	3 sets	8-12 reps
	Bench dip	3 sets	To failure

Day 3 – Back and Shoulders

Back	Chinups	3 sets	8-12 reps
	Barbell row	3 sets	8-12 reps
	One-arm row	3 sets	8-12 reps
Shoulders	Dumbell press	3 sets	8-12 reps
	Lateral raise	3 sets	8-12 reps
	Bent-over lateral	3 sets	8-12 reps

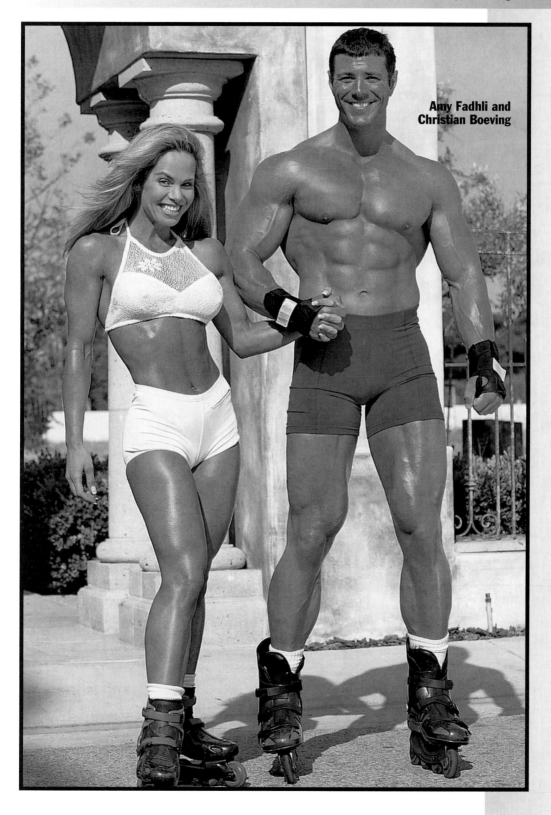

Amy Fadhli and
Christian Boeving

CHAPTER NINE

Exercise Descriptions

ABDOMINALS

CRUNCHES – You will need a flat bench or chair to perform this exercise. Lie down on the floor and rest your calves on the bench. Adjust your distance from the bench so that your thighs are perpendicular with the floor. Now bend forward and try to touch your thighs.

COMMENTS – Most bodybuilders consider crunches one of the best ab-builders. At first you may want to perform the movement with your arms by your sides. As you get stronger, place your hands at the sides of or behind your head. Doing so adds the weight of the arms to your upper body, thus making the exercise more difficult.

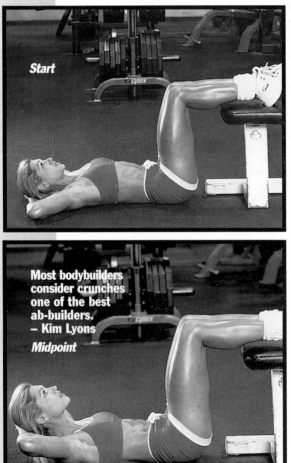

Start

Most bodybuilders consider crunches one of the best ab-builders.
– Kim Lyons

Midpoint

MUSCLES WORKED – Crunches primarily work the upper abs, but there is some lower ab stimulation as well. The exercise also brings the hip abductors into play, although to a much lesser extent than situps.

BENT-LEG RAISES – You can use the chinup bar on the Universal multistation or a freestanding version. Jump up and grab the bar with both hands. With the legs slightly bent, raise them up to the parallel position. Lower slowly until your thighs are once again in line with the upper body.

COMMENTS – Some bodybuilders perform this movement with the legs straight – *not recommended.* Straight-leg raises place unwanted stress on the lower back. While perhaps not noticeable now, this practice may lead to problems down the road. And don't swing the legs up and down – you'll defeat the purpose of the exercise. You want to lift the lower body using abdominal power, not momentum.

MUSCLES WORKED – The bent-leg raise primarily works the lower abdominals, but there is some upper abdominal and hip abductor stimulation.

LYING LEG RAISES – Lie down on the abdominal board, with your hands grabbing the hand-grip behind your head (i.e. your head is toward the hand grip/foot rest, unlike situps where your feet are closest to the hand grip/foot rest). With your legs slightly bent, raise them to the vertical (or just short of the vertical) position. Pause a second and then slowly lower them. Try not to touch the board at the bottom so as to keep the tension on the abdominals throughout the exercise.

COMMENTS – Once again, don't perform the movement with straight legs. Also, resist the urge to use your upper body to pull your legs up. Use only abdominal strength. Finally, start with the abdominal board placed in the lowest position. As you get stronger you can increase the incline to make the exercise more difficult.

MUSCLES WORKED – Lying leg raises primarily work the lower abdominals, but the upper abs and hips also come into play.

ROMAN-CHAIR SITUPS – The Roman chair looks similar to a low incline bench, but it has a pair of foot supports at one end. Anchor your feet under the supports (they are usually round padded rollers) and lean back on the bench to the starting position. Try to use only your abdominals and not your hip flexors.

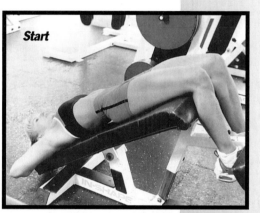

Start

COMMENTS – Roman-chair situps are very effective for working the lower abdominal region. By bending and locking the legs, it's virtually impossible to cheat. If there's a disadvantage to this exercise it's the stress placed on the lower back. Many bodybuilders find arching the back in this manner very painful. Our advice is to give them a try and see how they feel. If there's any back pain, substitute one of the other ab exercises.

MUSCLES WORKED – Roman-chair situps primarily work the lower abdominal region, but the upper abs are also stimulated. Depending on the ratio of your leg/upper body length, you may find the hip flexors take much of the strain. Only you can judge how effective the exercise is for the abdominals. If you feel your abs are doing very little, switch to another exercise.

Try to use only your abdominals and not your hip flexors when doing Roman-chair situps. – Brandi Carrier

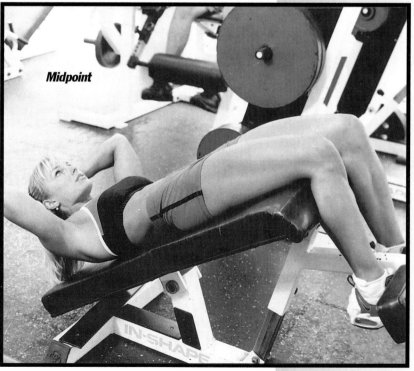

Midpoint

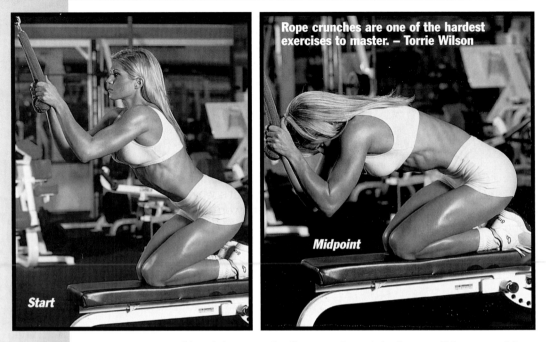

Rope crunches are one of the hardest exercises to master. – Torrie Wilson

Midpoint

Start

ROPE CRUNCHES – Kneel down on the floor or a bench facing a pulldown machine. Grab the attached rope. Bend forward so that the rope is straddling your neck (i.e. one side of the rope touching each ear). With the knees and feet kept firmly on the bench, bend forward until your forehead is within a couple of inches of touching down – and crunch. Return to the starting position by raising the torso about a foot and a half from the bench.

COMMENTS – This is one of the hardest exercises to master as the body tries to cheat by rocking the torso up and down. Even with good technique, some individuals get nothing out of it. Others find they have to tire out the abs first with another exercise before they derive any benefit from rope crunches.

MUSCLES WORKED – Rope crunches work the entire abdominal region. The obliques, hip flexors and serratus also come into play.

LEGS (THIGHS)

SQUATS – Place the barbell on the squat rack, at about shoulder height. Step under the bar and rest it across your traps and shoulders. Step back, away from the rack, and place your feet slightly less than shoulder width apart. Now in a slow and controlled manner bend your knees and descend. Stop when your thighs are approximately parallel with the floor. Pause for a second and then return to the starting upright position.

COMMENTS – Most consider squats to be the king of the thigh-builders. If done properly they will build you a phenomenal set of quadriceps. Done improperly they may put you in traction! For starters, try to use a squat rack with "catchers." These are pins which will stop the weight if you get in trouble. If none are available, make sure you have one or two spotters watching you. (Besides the safety aspect, a spotter can tell if you are not performing the exercise properly.)

It's most likely a good idea to wear a belt when performing squats (see Chapter Two). Belts are seldom worn during exercise demonstrations, however, their use is advised during training. Also don't bounce at the top or bottom of the exercise. Remember you have a loaded barbell on your shoulders, which is putting a lot of stress on your spine. Keep control of the weight throughout the movement. Make sure you rest the bar across your shoulders and traps, not on the bony protrusion at the base of your skull. Do so and you will need regular chiropractic visits!

To put most of the stress on the thighs, try resting your heels on a two-inch block of wood. If you perform squats flat-footed, much of the lifting will be done by your glutes. In addition, keep your stance shoulder width or less. The wider the stance the more glute involvement. (That's why powerlifters use a fairly wide stance. They need the tremendous power of the glutes to help in lifting such huge poundages.)

MUSCLES WORKED – While primarily a thigh-builder, squats will stimulate the whole leg region. Even with a narrow stance the glutes will come into play. Also, the calves and hamstrings are used in stabilizing the legs as you move up and down. Finally, and much less obvious, the spinal erectors (lower back muscles) are needed to keep the body upright. In fact they are often the weak link in the chain. Most injuries obtained while doing squats center around the lower back region. You must concentrate totally when performing this exercise.

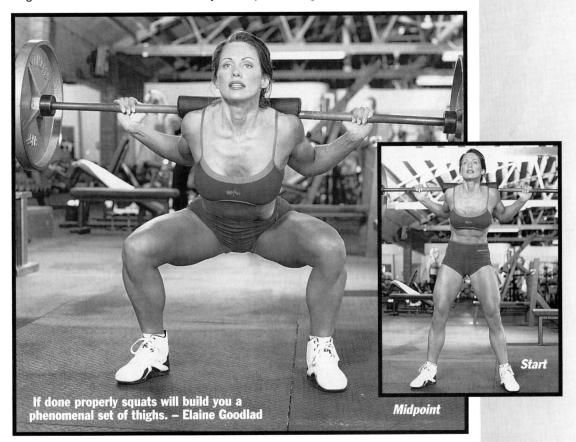

If done properly squats will build you a phenomenal set of thighs. – Elaine Goodlad

Midpoint

Start

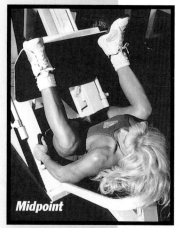

Midpoint

LEG PRESSES – You will need to use the leg-press machine to perform this exercise. Sit in the seat and place your feet on the pressing board. Your stance should be about shoulder width, but this can be varied to work different parts of the thigh. Extend your legs to the locked out position, pause, then bring them down until your knees touch your chest. Perform the movement in a slow, controlled manner.

COMMENTS – Although leg presses don't give the degree of thigh development as squats, they are a close second. And if you have knee or back problems, the leg press will adequately work the thighs without aggravating these areas. As with squats, the wider the stance, the more glute involvement. By making a V with the feet (heels together, toes apart) you can do wonders with the inner thigh region (vastus medialis).

Perhaps the greatest advantage of the leg press is the amount of weight you can use. Unlike squats, where the lower back is a limiting factor, the leg press allows you to pile on hundreds of pounds of plates. It won't be long before you have 6 to 8 (or more) 45-pound plates on each side. Provided you maintain good form, you can really let the ego go wild on this exercise. Lower back involvement is virtually eliminated, and even the knees don't have the same stress placed on them.

A word of caution concerning hyperextending the legs. If you place the feet too low on the pressing board, there is the risk of locking the legs and actually forcing them into a hyperextended position at the knee joint. When performing this exercise, don't forcefully lock out the legs. This may damage the supporting connective tissues of the knee (ligaments, tendons and cartilage).

MUSCLES WORKED – The leg-press machine is designed to place most of the stress on the thighs. There is very little glute involvement, and the spinal erectors are all but eliminated from the exercise. The calves and hamstrings play a small role in stabilizing the legs over the course of the movement.

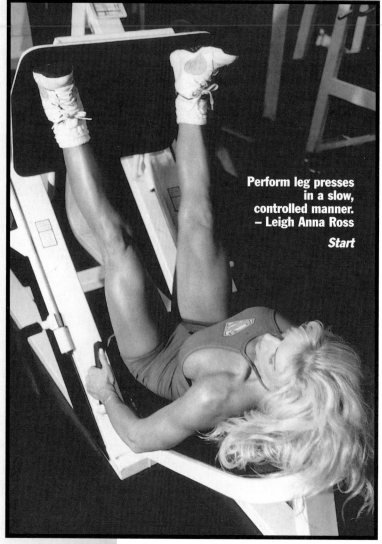

Perform leg presses in a slow, controlled manner.
– Leigh Anna Ross

Start

HACK SQUATS – You need a special machine to do this one. Place your feet about shoulder width apart on the machine's inclined footboard. Rest the pads on your shoulders and slowly squat down until your thighs are parallel with the floor. Using thigh power alone, return to the starting position.

COMMENTS – There are two variations of the hack machine. One version uses shoulder pads for supporting the weight, the other relies on two handles placed low on the machine (the user grabs the handles to lift the weight). Most bodybuilders find the shoulder pad version the most comfortable.

To get the full benefit of the hack squat, make a slight V-shape with your feet (heels together, toes apart). As with any type of squat, don't bounce at the bottom as this places tremendous strain on the knee ligaments.

MUSCLES WORKED – Hack squats will give your outer thighs that nice sweeping look. By bracing yourself against the backboard, the strain often associated with regular squats is greatly reduced.

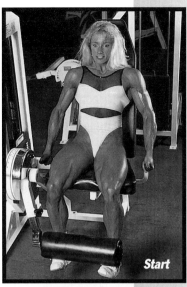

Start

LEG EXTENSIONS – If you've ever had a sports-related knee injury, then this exercise should be familiar. The leg extension is among the most popular of rehabilitation exercises. Sit down on the machine's bench and place your feet under the padded rollers. Raise the legs to a locked position and squeeze your thighs. Lower back to the starting position and repeat.

COMMENTS – Most gyms have a machine that incorporates the leg curl and leg extension. In other words, you perform both exercises on the same machine. The same weight stack is used, but for leg extensions you sit on the end and use the lower rollers, while for leg curls you lie face down and use the upper rollers. Your gym, however, may have these exercises on separate machines. Many bodybuilders lie on their back when doing leg extensions. They can't use as much weight, but this is made up for by working the thighs through a greater range of movement.

Resist the tendency to *drop* the weight to the starting position. As with other exercises, 50 percent of the movement is the negative (lowering) phase. For variety you can perform the exercise one leg at a time.

MUSCLES WORKED – Extensions are great for building the thigh muscles around the knee area. They're also a very effective physiotherapy exercise. Following knee surgery,

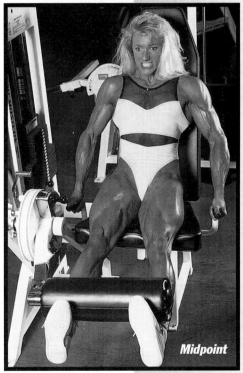

Midpoint

Squeeze the thighs at the top of the movement. – Ericca Kern

most athletes are limited in the amount of direct leg exercise they can perform. Leg extensions are great for strengthening not only the lower thigh, but also the associated tendons and ligaments.

SISSY SQUATS – Depending on your level of strength, you may need to hold a weight plate during this exercise. Place your feet in the V position, and leaning back, squat down until your thighs are at least parallel with the floor. If you have trouble holding your balance, grab a stationary upright for support. If you can do 15 to 20 reps with relative ease, hold a plate against the chest with your free hand.

COMMENTS – You can do this exercise with a dumbell or weight plate held to the chest. Most bodybuilders find the plate most convenient, but it's personal preference. Don't get carried away with the amount of weight. Save the heavy poundages for your regular squats and leg presses.

MUSCLES WORKED – Sissy squats are similar to hack squats in that they will add a great sweep to your outer thighs. Although more isolated than regular squats, sissy squats involve the glutes to some degree.

LEGS (HAMSTRINGS)

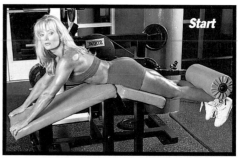

LEG CURLS – Lie down on the leg-curl machine, with your feet placed under the round foot supports (often called rollers). Pretend you are doing biceps curls (which in fact is what the hamstrings are – leg biceps) and curl the legs toward your butt. Pause at the top, and slowly lower the legs back to the starting position.

COMMENTS – Some gyms have three types of leg-curl machine, two of which force you to lie face down on a bench. The bench may be either straight or partly angled. The angled bench forces you to do the exercise more strictly. It keeps you from swinging the legs up. Many gyms have a third leg curl machine that allows you to stand up and work one leg at a time – similar to one-arm concentration curls for the biceps.

Just as you wouldn't do biceps curls in an awkward

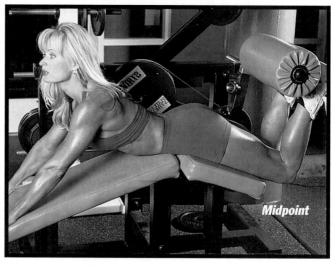

Leg curls must be performed under full control, in a slow, rhythmic style. – Sherry Goggin-Giardina

manner, so too must leg curls be performed in a slow, rhythmic style. No jerking or bouncing the weight, and try to avoid lifting your hips off the bench. If you have to raise your hips, you're probably using too much weight.

MUSCLES WORKED – Leg curls primarily work the hamstrings, although there is some calf involvement. The glutes and thighs only come into play to stabilize the legs during the exercise.

STANDING LEG CURLS – Position yourself in the machine with the knee of the working leg resting on the pad. With the supporting leg locked straight, curl the other leg upward to just short of the butt. Lower back down until the leg is just short of a lockout.

COMMENTS – Standing leg curls can be considered the concentration curls of hamstring exercises. They offer the advantage of devoting full attention to each

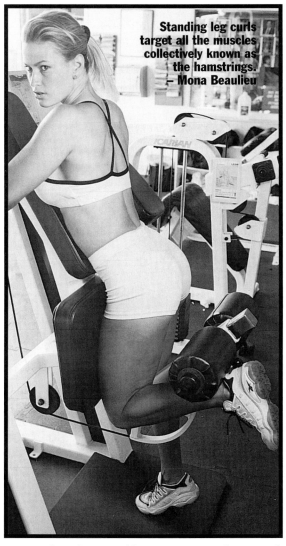

Standing leg curls target all the muscles collectively known as the hamstrings.
– Mona Beaulieu

leg separately. The downside is that you have to support the bodyweight on one leg. For the average body-builder this is no big deal, but for someone with knee or back problems it may be too stressful. The other disadvantage is that many gyms don't have this particular style of leg-curl apparatus.

MUSCLES WORKED – Standing leg curls target all the muscles collectively known as the hamstrings. The glutes and calves play a secondary role.

SEATED LEG CURLS – Once again you'll need a special machine to do this exercise. As each brand is slightly different, we'll describe the version manufactured by Atlantis of Laval, Quebec, Canada. Set the machine so that the roller rests on your heels. Sit down in the chair and push forward on the upper handle. This lowers the roller arm so you can place your feet on top. With the feet positioned on top of the roller, return the adjustment handle to the starting position. Lower the knee pads until they are snug on your thighs. Curl your legs back until they almost touch the main frame underneath. Raise the legs back up to just short of locking out.

COMMENTS – The advantage of the seated leg curl over the lying version is strictness. It's very easy to cheat on the lying leg curl, by throwing the butt up into the air, or pulling with the arms. The seated leg curl, however, forces you to move the weight with just your hamstrings. As a word of caution, many seated leg-curl machines allow the legs to go past the point of lockout, thus hyper-extending at the knee joint. Always keep control of the weight on the way up, and don't let the legs straighten out completely.

MUSCLES WORKED – Seated leg curls primarily work the hamstrings, but the glutes and calves also play a small role.

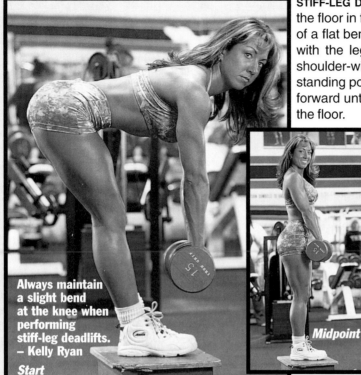

Always maintain a slight bend at the knee when performing stiff-leg deadlifts. – Kelly Ryan

Start

Midpoint

STIFF-LEG DEADLIFTS – Place an Olympic bar on the floor in front of a block of wood, or on the end of a flat bench. Stand on the block or bench and with the legs slightly bent, grab the bar with a shoulder-width grip. Raise the torso up to the standing position, pause for a second, then bend forward until the plates are just short of touching the floor.

COMMENTS – Although the name says "stiff-leg," keeping the legs completely locked can put excessive stress on the lower back. Always maintain a slight bend at the knee. Also never bounce for the same reason. The lower back ligaments receive enough abuse in life without you giving them another reason to act up.

MUSCLES WORKED – Although the lower legs do not bend as in a traditional leg curl, the hamstring muscles do cross the hip joint and are thus stimulated by extension at the hip. The lower spinal erectors and glutes also come into play on this exercise.

CHEST

FLAT BARBELL BENCH PRESSES – Lie on your back and take the barbell from the supports, using a grip that is six to eight inches wider than shoulder width. Lower the bar slowly to the nipple region, then press it back to the locked out position.

COMMENTS – King of the chest exercises, the bench press is performed by virtually every top bodybuilder. A few points to consider. Don't drop the bar and bounce it off your chest. Yes, you can lift more weight that way, but you are robbing the exercise of its effectiveness. You also run the risk of breaking ribs or splitting your sternum. Then there is the pec-delt tie-in to worry about. Drop the bar in a loose fashion and you increase the risk of tearing the area where your chest muscles connect to your shoulder muscles. To avoid the previous nasties, lower the weight in a slow, controlled manner, then push it back to arms' length.

Lock the arms out or not, its your personal preference. Some bodybuilders find stopping just short of a lock keeps the tension on the muscles throughout the movement. Others find locking out feels more comfortable. As the split is about 50-50 on this issue, try both methods and choose one (this applies to virtually all exercises).

Another point to mention, don't arch your back off the bench. Once again you may increase your lift by a few pounds, but at what cost? Arching decreases the amount of pectoral stimulation, and it certainly is of no benefit to your lower back.

If you have trouble keeping your back on the bench, perform the movement with your legs up in the air. You will not be able to use as much weight, but there is no way you can arch your back when in this position.

MUSCLES WORKED – Flat bench presses primarily work the lower chest region, but the whole pectoral-deltoid area is stimulated. You will also find your triceps receiving a great deal of stimulation. Finally, the muscles of the back and forearms are indirectly used for stabilizing the upper body during the exercise.

INCLINE BARBELL PRESSES – If using an adjustable bench, set the bench to an angle of about 25 to 30 degrees. Incline bench presses are performed in the same manner as flat benches, the only difference being instead of lowering the bar to the nipple region, bring it down to the center of the chest, just under your chin.

COMMENTS – Most bodybuilders find angles above 30 degrees place too much stress on the front delts, and not the upper pectorals. Of course your bone structure may dictate the opposite. You may have to play around with the angle of the bench to see what's best for you. If you don't have access to an adjustable bench, make do with the fixed version. In many cases these fixed benches are closer to 45 degrees, which is too steep for working the upper pecs. You may find that slightly arching the back can shift most of the stress from the shoulders to the chest. But be careful – the lower back was not meant to be arched to any degree. Here's a better solution: Raise one end of a flat bench. You can use a couple of pieces of wood, another bench, or a specially constructed wooden block (most gyms have these for performing bent-over rows) to prop up the flat bench.

MUSCLES WORKED – The incline barbell press primarily works the upper chest. It also stresses the front delts and triceps. Most bodybuilders find inclines excellent for the pec-delt tie-ins. Remember, as you increase the angle, the stress shifts from the upper chest to the shoulders.

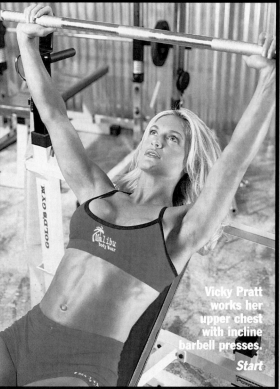

Vicky Pratt works her upper chest with incline barbell presses.

Start

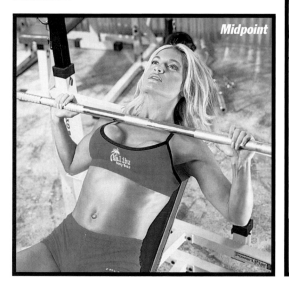

Midpoint

FLAT DUMBELL PRESSES – This exercise is similar to the barbell version, but you use two dumbells instead. Start by sitting on a flat bench, and cleaning (lifting) a pair of dumbells to your knees. Lie back on the bench, and with the dumbells pointing end to end (i.e. they form a straight line across your chest like a barbell), lower them down to your sides. Pause at the bottom, and then press to arms' length.

COMMENTS – The advantage of using dumbells is the greater range of movement at the bottom. A barbell can only be lowered to the rib cage, whereas the dumbells can be dropped below the rib cage, which gives the chest muscles a greater stretch. But be careful – the lower part of the movement is the most dangerous. If you drop the dumbells in an uncontrolled manner, you run the risk of tearing the pec-delt tie-ins. Although there is much personal preference, most bodybuilders find a dumbell spacing of about 6 to 8 inches wider than the shoulders to be the most effective.

MUSCLES WORKED – Dumbell presses are great for developing the pec-delt tie-ins. If you squeeze them together at the top, the inner pecs are also worked. And no matter how much you try to eliminate them, the triceps and shoulders will be involved. That's fine. At the beginning stage you want to work as many muscles in conjunction as possible.

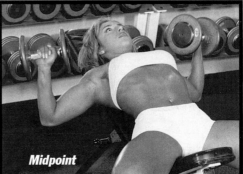

Midpoint

INCLINE DUMBELL PRESS – This is the inclined version of the flat dumbell press. With the exception of the angle, the exercise is performed in the same manner.

COMMENTS – Because you have to hoist the dumbells up higher to get them into starting position, it might be a good idea to recruit the help of a spotter. Most bodybuilders lift one of the dumbells up and have a partner pass the other one. If possible have both dumbells passed to you. Without sounding too repetitious, lower the dumbells slowly, and go for a full but controlled stretch at the bottom.

MUSCLES WORKED – Incline dumbell presses are an excellent exercise for developing the upper chest. Because of the increased angle, they also hit the front deltoids. And like most chest exercises, there is some secondary triceps involvement. If your shoulders are taking too much of the weight, lower the angle of the bench a few degrees.

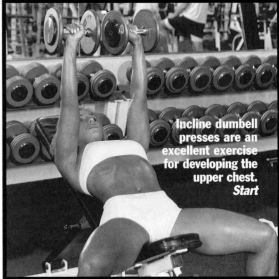

Incline dumbell presses are an excellent exercise for developing the upper chest.
Start

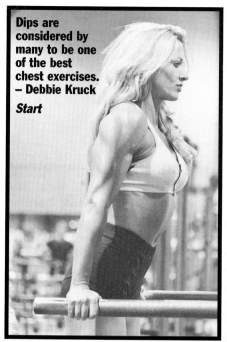

Dips are considered by many to be one of the best chest exercises.
– Debbie Kruck

Start

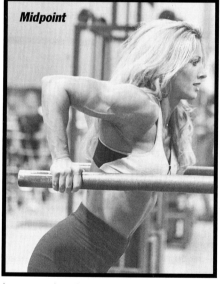

Midpoint

DIPS – One of the simplest but most effective chest exercises. Most gyms have a set of parallel bars for doing dips. If your gym doesn't, you can make do with the Universal shoulder press. Start the exercise with your arms straight, in locked-out position. With chin on chest, lower your body down between the bars, pause, and push yourself back up to arms' length.

COMMENTS – Dips are considered by many to be one of the best (and *the* best by the late Vince Gironda) chest exercises. To keep the stress on the chest, lean forward and flare your elbows out to the sides. If you keep vertical and have your elbows in tight, the exercise is more of a triceps-builder. As with other chest exercises, don't bounce at the bottom. Doing so places too much stress on the pec-delt tie-ins.

MUSCLES WORKED – Dips primarily work the lower, outer chest. They produce that clean line under the pecs. They also stimulate the front delts and triceps, so for this reason, dips are an excellent beginning exercise.

FLAT FLYES – Start this exercise in the same position as the dumbell press. Instead of having the dumbells pointing end to end, rotate your hands until the palms are facing and the dumbells are parallel with your body. With your elbows slightly bent, lower the bells for a full stretch. Pause at the bottom, then squeeze the dumbells up and together over the center of the chest.

COMMENTS – Flyes are more of a stretching exercise than a mass-building movement. Still, with practice you'll eventually be using a considerable weight. Always lower the dumbells in a controlled manner, no matter what the poundage. Drop them too fast and you could rip the pec-delt tie-in. Treatment for such an injury is surgery and many months of rehabilitation.

MUSCLES WORKED – Flyes work the whole chest region. Fully stretching at the bottom works the outer chest region, squeezing together at the top develops the inner chest. This gives your chest that clean line up the middle. As there will be some pec-delt tie-in strain, be careful at the bottom of the movement.

INCLINE FLYES – This is the same exercise as the previous, but this time you use an incline bench. Once again go for a full, slow stretch at the bottom.

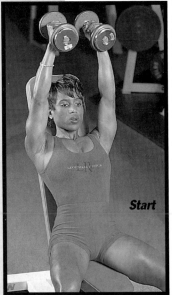

Start

COMMENTS – As with incline dumbell presses, the incline bench dictates lifting the dumbells higher. You may need a partner to hoist the bells into position. In fact it's probably a good idea to have them passed to you, whether you can lift them or not. Jerking heavy dumbells from the floor puts a great deal of stress on the biceps and lower back. Better to be safe than macho.

MUSCLES WORKED – Incline flyes put most of the stress on the upper pectorals. They also strongly affect your chest/shoulder tie-ins. Once again, by squeezing the dumbells together at the top, the inner chest can be worked.

DECLINE BARBELL PRESSES – Position a decline bench (the Roman chair is often used) so that the bar can be brought down to the lower chest. The reps are performed in the same manner as flat and incline bench presses.

COMMENTS – Many gyms have decline benches that have the bar supports welded to the back of the bench. If the angle of the bench is adjustable, vary the angle to get the maximum feel in your pectoral muscles. You can substitute dumbells in place of the barbell.

MUSCLES WORKED – Decline presses are similar to dips in that they work the lower, outer chest region. They are a good substitute if you find your front delts taking most of the strain during flat bench presses.

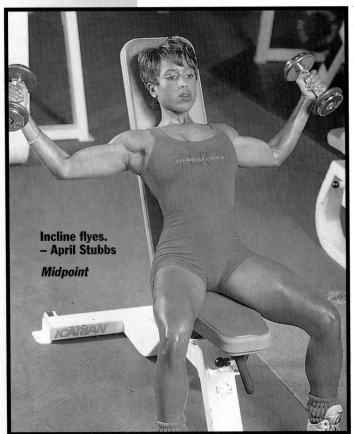

Incline flyes.
– April Stubbs

Midpoint

CABLE CROSSOVERS – Stand between the two cable uprights and grab an overhead pulley handle in each hand. Adopt a runner's stance (one leg forward and bent the other back and bent just slightly). Bring the handles forward and down so that they meet about waist high. Return to the starting position with the arms stretched out to the sides about head high.

COMMENTS – Cable crossovers are another exercise where proper technique is an absolute must. If you let the arms fly back too fast you run the risk of tearing the pec-delt tie-in. Also, to ease the stress on the shoulder joint, keep a slight bend in the elbows.

MUSCLE WORKED – Cable crossovers are great for working the center of the chest. There is some front delt involvement as well.

PEC-DEK FLYES – Sit down on the seat of the machine and grab the handles (Apex style) or place the elbows behind the pads (Nautilus style). Push the arms forward until the handles or pads are just about touching. Return slowly to the starting position with the handles or pads positioned out to the sides or just behind the body.

COMMENTS – Don't let the arms fly back too fast. That's a great way to tear the chest or shoulders. Also try to use as little arm power as possible. Think of the arms as extensions of your chest muscles. If using the Nautilus model open the hands and just push with the arms.

MUSCLES WORKED – Pec-dek flyes are similar to cable crossovers in that they are great for hitting the inner chest. They also work the pec-delt tie-ins.

BACK

CHINUPS – You will need access to an overhead bar to perform this exercise. Most Universal multistations have one attached but a wall-mounted version is just as good. Jump up and grab the bar with a grip that is about twice your shoulder width. Now pull yourself up and try to touch the chest to the bar. Lower back down to the starting position in a controlled manner.

COMMENTS – Chins are considered by most to be the best back exercise. In fact bodybuilders of all levels have made them the mainstay of their back routines.

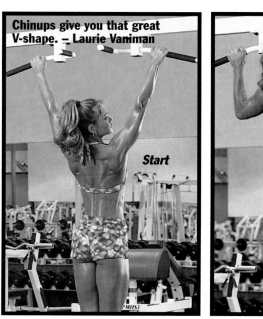
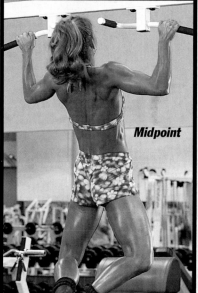

Chinups give you that great V-shape. – Laurie Vaniman

Start

Midpoint

They give you that great V-shape. When doing this movement, try to pull with the large back muscles (latissimus dorsi), not with the biceps and forearms. Don't *drop back* to the starting position in such a manner that you yank your arms out of the shoulder sockets! Do the exercise nice and slow.

At first you will find it easier to do chinups to the front. As you get stronger you can pull up so the bar is behind your head. There is little difference between the two exercises. When you reach a point that you are doing 12 to 15 easy reps, attach a weight around your waist, or hold a dumbell between your legs to increase the resistance and keep the muscles growing.

MUSCLES WORKED – Chins primarily work the large latissimus (lats) muscles. They also stress the smaller back muscles like the teres. Finally, the rear delts and biceps are brought into play. You will find that by pulling to the front, the lower parts of the lats are worked the most. Conversely, pulling behind the head stresses the upper section. Keep in mind that these divisions are not carved in stone, and at the beginning level it is adequate to do either one. If you have the strength, you might alternate the two on the same day or alternate days.

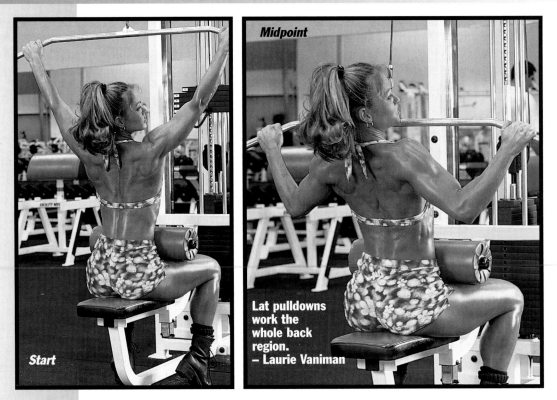

Midpoint

Lat pulldowns work the whole back region.
– Laurie Vaniman

Start

LAT PULLDOWNS – Although not quite as effective as chins, pulldowns enable you to adjust the amount of weight. Chins force you to use your bodyweight, whereas the lat machine allows the trainer to select the desired poundage. Instead of pulling yourself up to an overhead bar, the bar is brought down to you. Take a wide grip (about twice shoulder width) and sit on the attached seat, or kneel down on the floor. Now pull the bar down – either behind your head or to the front and touch your chest. Pause at the bottom and squeeze your shoulder blades together. Return to the outstretched arms position.

COMMENTS – Pull to the front or to the back, it's a personal decision. There is little difference between the two. Either version will add tremendously to back width, giving that much coveted V-shape. Generally speaking, when you pull to the front you hit more of the lower upper back (i.e. the lower insertions of your lats). Pulling behind the head works the upper regions of the lats and the rear delts. There is so much overlap between the two movements, however, that at the beginning level, doing either movement is sufficient. You might want to rotate both, either on the same day or on alternate back days.

Keep your grip fairly wide – narrow-grip pulldowns place much of the stress on the biceps. In fact many bodybuilders often perform narrow-grip chins and pulldowns as a biceps exercise! Finally, because you have to grip the bar, the muscles of the forearms get a good workout. In fact they may be the weak link in the chain.

MUSCLES WORKED – Lat pulldowns work the whole back region, from the large latissimus muscles to the smaller teres, rhomboids and rear deltoids. They also stress the biceps and forearms.

BENT-OVER BARBELL ROWS – Bend over at the waist so that your upper body is just short of parallel with the floor. Grab a standard barbell. Using a wide grip, pull it up to the abdomen. Lower slowly, then repeat. Concentrate on using the upper (lats) back muscles and not your spinal erectors.

COMMENTS – You must be especially careful on this exercise. Any sudden bouncing or jerking will put great stress on your lower back. If you have to "throw your lower back into it" you are using far too much weight. Take off a few plates and do it more strictly. The only part of the body that should move is your arms. Your upper body and legs should remain stationary. To get a full stretch, stand on some sort of low platform. Most gyms have specially constructed boxes for you to stand on to perform bent-over rows. The extra 10 to 12 inches of stretch will add greatly to the effectiveness of this one. Here's a final point: Bend your knees slightly to help reduce the stress on your lower back.

MUSCLES WORKED – The bent-over barbell row is considered by most to be one of the best back-builders. It's particularly effective in producing thickness in the back. Besides the back muscles, this exercise stresses the biceps and forearms. Finally, because of the bent-over position, the hamstrings and spinal erectors are stretched.

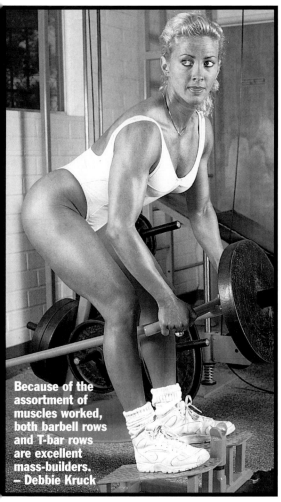

Because of the assortment of muscles worked, both barbell rows and T-bar rows are excellent mass-builders.
– Debbie Kruck

T-BAR ROWS – Many gyms have a long bar that has one end bolted to the floor. By placing plates on the free end, and grabbing the short crossbar, a variation of the barbell row can be performed. Called T-bar rows (because of the shape), they are an effective substitute for the barbell version. Grab the crossbar and pull the plates up to the chest/abdominal region. Squeeze at the top and then lower back to the floor. Don't touch the plates to the floor, but stop a few inches from it.

COMMENTS – Once again don't bounce or jerk the weight up. As with the barbell row, T-bar rows place a great deal of stress on the lower back. Keep your upper body stationary, and lift the plates with your back muscles and arms only. If your gym does not have a specially designed T-bar, you can do the same movement with one end of a regular Olympic bar pinned in a corner. Check with the gym's management first, however. Rotating an Olympic bar on one end may damage the sleeve/ball-bearing mechanism. If you are allowed to do the exercise, try to use an old bar. In fact your gym may have set aside an old bar just for this exact purpose.

MUSCLES WORKED – T-Bar rows work the same muscles as the regular barbell row. The lats, teres, rhomboids, rear delts, biceps, forearms and lower back – all come into play. Because of the assortment of muscles worked, both types of rows are excellent mass-builders.

Note: If you have lower back problems, you might want to avoid these exercises. If you must do them, start off by using light weight. Gradually build up the poundage over time. Don't make the mistake of slapping on 45-pound plates from day one. Your strength will increase with time. Keep in mind that lower back injuries often don't heal. You may have them for life. Therefore the emphasis should be on *prevention.* In a manner of speaking, rows can be a double-edge sword. Done properly they will help strengthen the lower back, thus reducing the chances of future injuries. Done improperly they may be the cause of injury! So pay strict attention to your exercise style. Don't get carried away with the weight, and don't lift with your lower back.

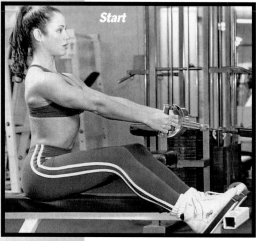
Start

SEATED PULLEY ROWS – You will need a cable machine to do this back exercise. Grab the V-shaped pulley attachment and sit down on the floor or associated board. With the legs slightly bent, pull the hands toward the lower chest/upper abdomen. Pause for a second and squeeze the shoulder blades together. Now bend forward and stretch the arms out fully.

COMMENTS – You can perform this exercise with a number of different pulley attachments. The most frequently used is the V-shaped double-handle bar. Some bodybuilders like to use a straight pulldown bar. Others use two separate handgrips. Our advice is to experiment with the different attachments and select the one that feels the most comfortable. You can also per-form cable rows on the lat pulldown machine. To get the full effect, lean back and pull the hands to the lower chest. The direction of force should be about 90 degrees to the body.

When doing the seated version, keep the legs slightly bent. Performing this exercise with straight legs won't do your lower back any good.

MUSCLES WORKED – Seated pulley rows are another exercise that works the whole back area. They are more of a thickness movement than a width-builder. As with other rowing exercises, seated pulley rows work all the major muscles of the back. They also stimulate the biceps and forearms.

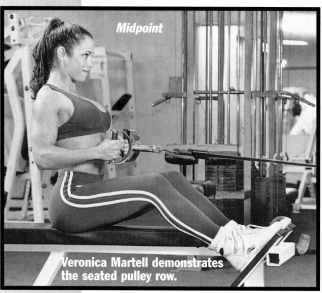
Midpoint

Veronica Martell demonstrates the seated pulley row.

ONE-ARM DUMBELL ROWS – Instead of using a barbell or cable, you can do your rows using a dumbell. Bend over and lean one hand and knee on a bench for support. Place the other leg behind you, in a running-type stance. Grab a dumbell with the free arm and stretch it down and slightly forward. Pull the dumbell up until the arm is fully bent, slowly return to the starting position, pause, and then go on to your next rep. It's like sawing wood.

COMMENTS – One-arm rows are great because they allow you to brace your upper body, essential if you have a lower back injury. Even though your biceps will be involved in the exercise, try to concentrate on using just your back muscles. Once again, no bouncing or jerking the weight. If you have to contort the body to lift the weight, the dumbell is too heavy.

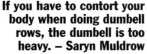

If you have to contort your body when doing dumbell rows, the dumbell is too heavy. – Saryn Muldrow

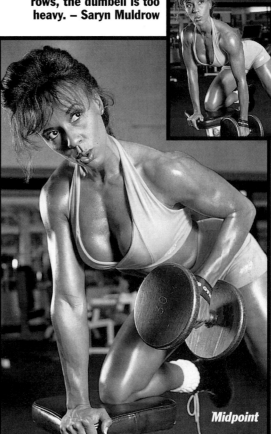

STRAIGHT-ARM PUSHDOWNS – Stand two to three feet out from the front of the lat-pulldown or triceps-pushdown machine. Grab the attached bar with a shoulder-width grip and with the arms kept in a locked out position, push the bar down to the thighs. Raise the bar back up until the moving plates are about an inch from the stationary plates.

COMMENTS – For the taller members out there, you may find the plates touch before you get a good stretch at the top of the exercise. One suggestion is to adopt a wide stance. The wider you spread your legs the lower you'll go to the floor. Those with a gymnastics background will benefit the most from this technique. Because of the virtual elimination of the biceps and forearms, you won't be able to use nearly as much weight as a regular pulldown.

MUSCLES WORKED – This is as pure a back exercise as you'll find. It is especially useful for hitting the upper and outer lats, just under the armpits. Straight-arm pushdowns make an excellent first exercise in a pre-exhaust superset.

DUMBELL PULLOVERS – Grab a dumbell and lie face up *across* a flat bench. With the hips dropped below bench height, and the arms kept nearly straight, lower the dumbell in both hands behind your head to a comfortable stretch. Return to the top position with the dumbell positioned at arms' length above the chest.

COMMENTS – Some people prefer doing this exercise while lying lengthways on the bench. Others prefer doing the movement with an EZ-curl bar. Try all three positions and see which works best for you.

MUSCLES WORKED – Pullovers are one of those exercises that incorporate a large number of muscles. For some it's a great lat exercise; others get a great chest stretch. The serratus and shoulders also play a role.

MACHINE PULLOVERS – Sit on the seat of the machine and (depending on the model) place your elbows behind the pad or grab the overhead bar. Push the arms down in front of the body to the maximum range of motion of the machine. Return to the overhead position.

COMMENTS – At the risk of being hounded out of the bodybuilding hall of fame, this is one of the few machine exercises that are actually better than the free-weight equivalent. With dumbells you only get about 90 degrees of motion before gravity starts to interfere. But most pullover machines keep the tension on the lats for 150 degrees or more.

MUSCLES WORKED – Machine pullovers are another great exercise to hit the back muscles without the biceps playing a major role. The serratus and shoulders play a minor role.

SHOULDERS

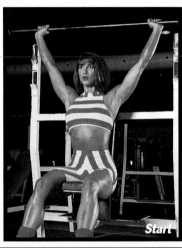

Start

BEHIND-THE-HEAD SHOULDER PRESSES – With a grip that is about six to eight inches wider than shoulder width, take a barbell from the rack. Lower the bar behind your head, stopping just short of your traps. Push the bar up to arms' length, then repeat.

COMMENTS – Don't bounce the bar off your neck. If you strike either of the top vertebrae (atlas and axis) you run the risk of nerve damage. Perform the exercise in a slow and controlled manner. You don't need a rack to position the bar, but cleaning a loaded bar to your shoulders, doing your reps, and then having to lower it back to the floor is very energy-consuming. After a few months it will be impossible. So use the squat rack, or better still, the shoulder-press rack. Most gyms have a special seat with a vertical back support. Two long supports enable the user to position the bar behind the head. All you have to do is reach back and lift the bar from the racks. Once your reps are finished, it's a simple matter of setting the bar down behind your head.

MUSCLES WORKED – Behind-the-head presses work the entire shoulder region, particularly the front and side delts. They also stress (to a lessor degree) the rear delts and traps. Finally, as with most pressing movements, the triceps are also brought into play.

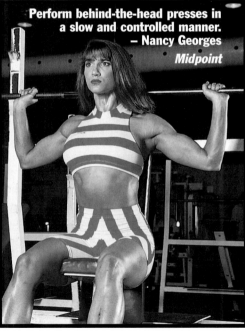

Perform behind-the-head presses in a slow and controlled manner.
– Nancy Georges

Midpoint

FRONT MILITARY PRESSES – This exercise is performed in the same manner as the previous, except instead of lowering the bar behind the head, you lower it to the front. Bring the bar down until it just touches the upper chest. Once again, no bouncing, just smooth controlled reps.

COMMENTS – Most bodybuilders find it more comfortable to lower the bar to the front. It also eliminates the risk of striking the head or neck. There is a tendency to arch when doing the exercise, so be careful. A slight arch to bring the bar to the upper chest is fine, but nothing excessive.

MUSCLES WORKED – Front presses put most of the stress on the front and side delts. The rear delts and traps receive some stimulation, but not to the extent as in rear presses. The upper pectorals are worked if you lean back when doing the exercise.

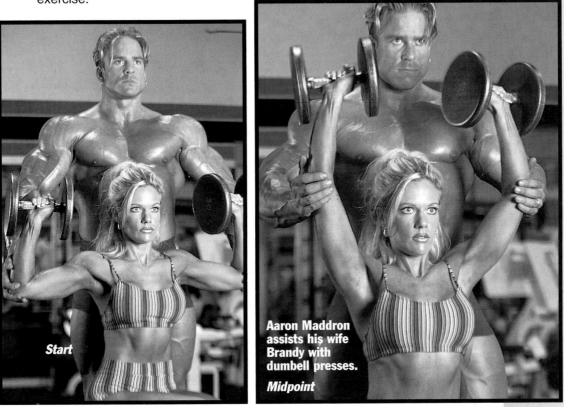

Start

Aaron Maddron assists his wife Brandy with dumbell presses.

Midpoint

DUMBELL PRESSES – Instead of performing your pressing movements with a barbell, grab two dumbells and hoist them to shoulder level. You can stand or sit when pressing the bells, but if standing, be careful not to excessively arch the lower back.

COMMENTS – You can press both dumbells at the same time or in an alternating fashion, it's up to you. As with the barbell version, be careful of the lower back. Try not to arch excessively, and don't drop the dumbells back to the starting position.

MUSCLES WORKED – This exercise stresses the whole deltoid region. Particular emphasis is placed on the front and side deltoids. There is some secondary trap and rear delt involvement.

BARBELL SHRUGS – Grab a barbell using a shoulder-width grip. With your arms locked, raise the bar up trying to touch the shoulders against your ears. Squeeze at the top of the movement, then lower the bar.

COMMENTS – There are a number of variations to this exercise. Instead of raising and lowering the bar in a straight line, you can rotate the bar in a circular motion. Also, you're not limited to using a barbell for the exercise. Many bodybuilders find the Smith machine is more comfortable. Instead of taking the bar from the floor, you can have it set at any desired height, making it easier on your lower back. The Universal bench press can also be used for shrugs. (In fact more serious bodybuilders use the machine for shrugs than for bench presses!) Try to keep the arms, legs and back straight throughout the movement. And watch your lower back!

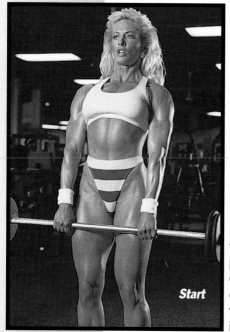

Start

MUSCLES WORKED – Barbell shrugs are by far the best trapezius-builder. Make them a regular part of your training and you will have traps that add to your overall V-taper. Besides the traps, your forearms, hamstrings, lower back and rear delts will be indirectly stimulated.

DUMBELL SHRUGS – This is simply a variation of the barbell version. Hold the dumbells about shoulder width apart and perform the movement as you would the barbell variety.

COMMENTS – You can hold the dumbells parallel or pointed end to end. The choice is yours. If you hold them end to end, watch you don't bang them off your thighs. Try to keep them in front of the body and slide them up the front of the thighs.

MUSCLES WORKED – Dumbell shrugs work the same muscles as the barbell version. Since you will be using less weight (you can generally lift more weight with one barbell than two dumbells), the lower back will not have the same strain placed on it. In fact we strongly recommend using dumbells if you have a pre-existing back problem.

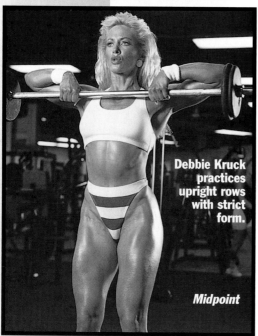

Debbie Kruck practices upright rows with strict form.

Midpoint

UPRIGHT ROWS – Start the exercise by holding a barbell at arms' length. Using a narrow grip (about three to five inches) lift the bar up the front of the body, keeping the elbows flared to the sides. Squeeze the traps together at the top, then lower into the starting position.

COMMENTS – Which muscles are worked depends on the grip used. Generally, any hand spacing of five inches or less puts most of the stress on the traps. Widen the grip and the side deltoids come into play. In the routines presented above we are suggesting the exercise as a trap-builder, but it can easily substitute for one of the delt exercises. Just remember to keep the grip wide when doing so.

If you have weak or injured wrists, you might want to think twice about attempting this exercise. Upright rows place tremendous stress on the forearms and wrists. If you experience minor pain when doing the exercise, try wrapping the wrists with support bandages. This should enable you to complete your sets in comfort. Of course you're the only one who can determine if the "pain" is just a nuisance or representative of something more serious. If in doubt, skip the exercise.

As with barbell curls, upright rows give you the option of adding a few cheat reps at the end of the set. Limit such cheat reps to one or two. Don't make the mistake of cheating from rep one.

MUSCLES WORKED – With a narrow grip, upright rows primarily work the traps, with some secondary deltoid stimulation. A wide grip (six inches or more) will shift the strain to the side delts, with the traps now playing a secondary role. The forearms are worked no matter what grip you use.

LATERAL RAISES – You can perform this exercise seated or standing. Grab two dumbells and, with the elbows slightly bent, raise them out to the sides of the body. As you raise the dumbells, gradually rotate the wrists so that the little fingers point up. Many bodybuilding authorities, including Robert Kennedy, liken the wrist action that of to pouring a jug of water.

COMMENTS – You can do this exercise with the arms completely locked, but most bodybuilders find it more effective to bend the arms slightly and use more weight. Lateral raises can be done to the front, side or rear (explained in full detail later). Instead of using dumbells, a cable may be substituted. Either version may be performed with one or two arms at a time.

MUSCLES WORKED – You can use lateral raises to work any head of the deltoid muscle. Most intermediate bodybuilders use them for the side delts, as the front delts receive ample stimulation from various pressing movements. Lateral raises to the side will give your delts that half-melon look. There's not much you can do to widen the clavicles, but you can increase your shoulder width by adding inches to the side delts.

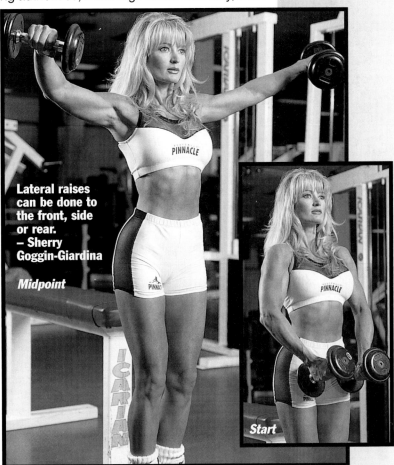

Lateral raises can be done to the front, side or rear.
– Sherry Goggin-Giardina

Midpoint

Start

BENT-OVER LATERALS – This is the bent-over version of regular lateral raises. By bending over, the stress is shifted from the side to the rear delts. You can do this exercise free standing, seated, or with your head braced on a high bench. The latter is for those with lower back problems or individuals who have a tendency to swing the weight up.

COMMENTS – Concentrate on lifting the dumbells with your rear delts, not your traps and lats. For variation try using a set of cables. You will have to grab the cable handles with your opposite hands, so the cables form an X in front of you. This exercise is popular with bodybuilders in the months leading up to a contest.

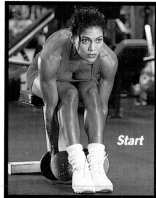
Start

MUSCLES WORKED – When performed properly, bent-over laterals primarily work the rear deltoids. There is, however, secondary triceps, trap and lat stimulation. If you're not sure what a fully developed rear deltoid looks like, check out a recent picture of Paul Dillett. His rear delts contain as much muscle mass as most bodybuilders' whole deltoid region!

SMITH-MACHINE SHRUGS – With a shoulder-width grip, lift the bar from the support catches. Keeping your arms straight, lower the bar as far as the traps will allow. Shrug your shoulders as high as you can, trying to touch your deltoids to your ears. Pause, then lower to the starting position.

COMMENTS – Smith-machine shrugs are great for those with lower back problems. Unlike using a standard barbell, which has to be lifted from the floor, the Smith machine allows you to start and finish the exercise at waist height.

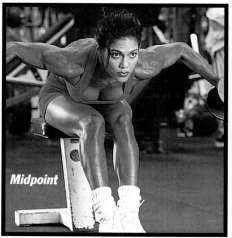
Midpoint

Bent-over laterals are popular with bodybuilders in the months leading up to a contest. – Kristie Alvarado

MUSCLES WORKED – As with barbell and dumbell shrugs, this exercise primarily works the trapezius muscles. Smith-machine shrugs also place secondary stress on the delts and forearms.

REVERSE PEC FLYES – Sit down in the pec-dek machine, facing the backrest. Depending on the model, either grab the handles or place your forearms in front of the pads. Bring the arms back to a comfortable stretch, which for most people means with the elbows slightly behind the body, or arms straight out to the sides (depending on the model). Return to the starting position.

COMMENTS – The advantage of this exercise over bent-over dumbell laterals is that it puts little or no stress on the lower back. The machine also makes it a bit more difficult to swing and bounce the weight up with body momentum, something many people do on bent-over laterals.

MUSCLES WORKED – Reverse pec flyes primarily hit the rear delts, but the teres, rhomboids and traps also come into play.

TRICEPS

TRICEP PUSHDOWNS – You will need to use the lat pulldown machine for this exercise. Grab the bar with a narrow grip, anywhere from two to eight inches. With your elbows tight to your sides, press the bar down to a locked out position. Pause and flex the triceps at the bottom, then return the bar to about chest high.

COMMENTS – Take a false (thumbs above the bar) grip when performing triceps pushdowns, and resist the urge to flare the elbows out to the sides. If you have to swing to push the bar down, you're probably using too much weight.

MUSCLES WORKED – Triceps pushdowns work the entire triceps region, especially the outer heads.

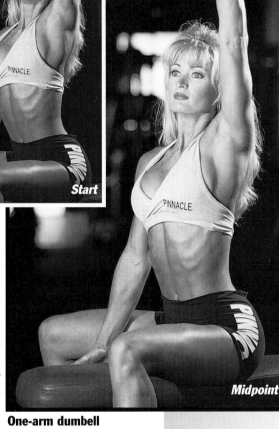

Start

Midpoint

ONE-ARM DUMBELL EXTENSIONS – Grasp a dumbell and press it above your head. Keeping the upper arm stationary, lower the dumbell behind the head to the starting position. Then press back up to the extended position using triceps power only. Try to perform this movement in a slow rhythmic manner.

COMMENTS – It's possible to work up to 75-plus-pound bells, but keep this in mind: The elbow joint and associated tissues (ligaments, cartilage, tendons) were not designed to support huge poundages. Never bounce the dumbell at the bottom (arm bent) of the exercise. Try to emphasize good form rather than weight.

MUSCLES WORKED – Although it works the whole triceps region, this exercise is great for the lower triceps.

One-arm dumbell extensions are great for the lower triceps. – Sherry Goggin-Giardina

LYING TRICEPS EXTENSIONS – Place an EZ-curl bar across the end of a bench. Lie down on the bench so that the bar is above your head. Reach back, grab the bar, and hoist it to arms' length. Keeping your elbows by your sides, lower the bar to your forehead. Now extend the bar to arms' length and slowly back down.

COMMENTS – If you are wary about lowering the bar to your head, lower it behind your head and lightly touch the bench. Don't bounce the bar off the bench, but merely pause before going on. Try to keep the elbows tight against your sides.

MUSCLES WORKED – This is one of the main triceps mass-builders. It stresses the whole triceps, particularly the long rear head of the muscle. Lowering the bar behind your head brings the lower lats and upper chest into play. This exercise also works the intercostals, located just below the rib cage.

UPRIGHT DIPS – For this exercise you use the same apparatus as when performing dips for the chest. With a few minor modifications you can shift the strain from the chest to the triceps. For starters, keep the elbows tight against the body. Flaring them to the sides will work the chest. Also, unlike dips for the chest (where you bend forward) keep your body as vertical as possible. In fact some bodybuilders lean back slightly to get that extra degree of triceps stimulation.

COMMENTS – As with most exercises that rely on lifting your bodyweight, you will eventually reach a point where you can bang out 12 to 15 reps with ease. To increase the resistance, hold a dumbell between your legs or attach a plate to a special dipping chain. Before you know it you will dipping with 50 to 100 pounds!

With regard to safety, be careful at the bottom of the movement. Although dips are an excellent triceps exercise, they also place much stress on the front delts, particular the pec-delt tie-ins. Don't bounce at the bottom. Perform this exercise in a slow and controlled manner. (You might want to write out the phrase *"in a slow and controlled manner,"* in black letters and post it on your bedroom wall. This is perhaps the most important piece of advice we can give, and that's why it's emphasised so often.)

MUSCLES WORKED – Performed in an upright manner, dips place most of the

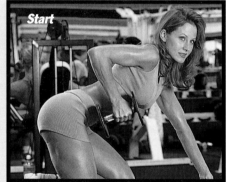

Start

strain on the long rear head of the triceps. Because of the weight used (minimum of your bodyweight), they also work the other two heads quite nicely. And even though you may attempt to eliminate other muscles from the exercise, the front delts and chest will take some of the strain. Once again this is fine at the beginning level where the goal is to add overall muscle mass.

TRICEPS KICKBACKS – With your body braced on a bench, bend over and set your upper arm parallel with the floor. Grab a dumbell and extend the lower arm back until it's in the locked position (i.e. your whole arm is now parallel with the floor). Pause and squeeze at the top, then lower back to the starting position.

COMMENTS – Resist the urge to swing the dumbell up using body momentum. True, you can use more weight that way, but it won't give the same triceps development. Keep the upper arm locked against the side of the body. As with bent-over laterals, if you have trouble keeping stationary, or if you have a weak lower back, place your free hand on a bench or other such support.

MUSCLES WORKED – Triceps kickbacks are great for giving the triceps that horseshoe look. They are especially useful for developing the long rear head of the triceps. They are a favorite exercise of competitive trainers during the precontest months.

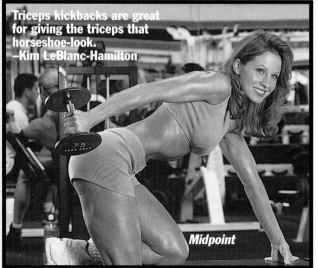

Triceps kickbacks are great for giving the triceps that horseshoe-look.
–Kim LeBlanc-Hamilton

Midpoint

REVERSE PUSHDOWNS – This exercise is performed in the same manner as regular pushdowns. The main difference here is that you grab the bar with your palms facing up. Keep your elbows locked against your sides and extend (push) the bar downward. Flex the triceps at the bottom, then return to the starting position.

COMMENTS – You won't be able to use as much weight in this version of the pushdown, so don't become alarmed if you have to drop your poundage by 20 to 30 pounds. This exercise is great for finishing the triceps off after a basic movement like lying triceps extensions or dips. Concentrate more on the feel rather than the amount of weight used.

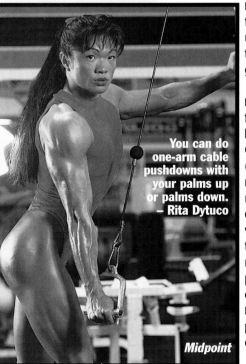

Start

Midpoint

You can do one-arm cable pushdowns with your palms up or palms down.
– Rita Dytuco

MUSCLES WORKED – This is another great movement for the long rear head of the triceps. A couple of sets and you will feel your triceps burning from elbow to armpit!

ONE-ARM CABLE PUSHDOWNS – With your body in the standing upright position, grab one of the upper cable handles. Push the handle down, lock out the arm at the bottom, then return to the starting position.

COMMENTS – You can do this exercise either palms up or palms down. You might want to reach across with your free hand and grab your shoulder on the side being exercised. Besides the bracing effect, you have your free hand in a position to spot yourself on the last couple of reps. As with the previously described reverse push-downs, go more for the burn than for huge poundages.

MUSCLES WORKED – This is another great finishing exercise for the triceps. A palms up grip will place most of the strain on the rear triceps, whereas a palms-down grip will hit more of the side head.

NARROW-GRIP PRESSES – Lie down on a flat bench with an Olympic bar or EZ-curl bar placed on the supports above you. Grab the bar with a narrow grip (shoulder width or less) and lower it to midchest. Push upward as if doing a regular bench press.

COMMENTS – You will need to experiment with different grip widths to find the one that maximizes triceps involvement and minimizes wrist stress. As with flat bench presses, don't bounce the bar off the chest or arch the lower back.

MUSCLES WORKED – Narrow-grip presses primarily work the triceps, but the front delts and pecs also come into play.

BICEPS

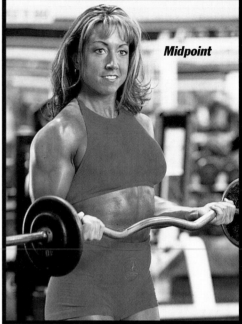

Midpoint

STANDING BARBELL CURLS – Perhaps this is the most used (and abused!) exercise performed by bodybuilders. You can use the standard Olympic bar, a smaller straight bar, or an EZ-curl bar. Grab the bar slightly wider than shoulder width and curl it up until the biceps are fully flexed. Try to keep your elbows close to your sides, and don't swing the weight up with your lower back. Lower the weight back to the starting position in good form. Don't simply let the thing drop! Not only would you be losing half the movement, but you run the risk of tearing your biceps tendons. (You can ask Dorian Yates, Lou Ferrigno or Tom Platz what that feels like.)

COMMENTS – Barbell curls are considered the ultimate biceps exercises. But many bodybuilders seem to forget that the negative (lowering) part of the movement is just as important as the positive (hoisting) portion. Try to lower the bar at about the same speed as you curl it up.

Keep your back straight – and no swinging. If you want to cheat, save it for the last couple of reps. For example, perform 8 to 10 reps in good style, then "cheat" 1 or 2 more. Don't abuse a good thing, however. One or 2 cheat reps are fine, but cheating from the start is counter-productive. At your level of development, you'll get all the stimulation you want from strict reps.

If you have weak forearms or wrists, you might want to give the EZ-curl bar a try. The bent shape of the bar allows you to rotate the forearms slightly,

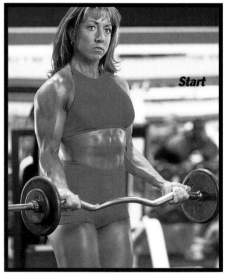

Start

Barbell curls are considered the ultimate biceps exercises. – Kelly Ryan

thus reducing the tension on the wrists and forearms. We should add that most bodybuilders use a straight bar, but you're best to play it by ear. Give both types a try and pick the one that is the most comfortable and produces the greatest biceps stimulation.

MUSCLES WORKED – The standing barbell curl works the entire biceps muscle. Also, because you have to forcibly grip the bar, this exercise will give you a great set of forearms. The front delts and lower back also come into play for stabilizing purposes.

STANDING DUMBELL CURLS – Instead of using a barbell, grab two dumbells. Although it's possible to simultaneously raise both dumbells, most bodybuilders do what are called alternate dumbell curls. As the name implies, you curl the bells one at a time. Start with the dumbells by your sides, the ends pointing to the front and back (i.e. the dumbells are parallel to one another). As you curl, rotate your palms from the "facing in" position to "facing up." This is called supination. Many bodybuilders are not aware that the biceps has two main functions. Besides the better-known curling movement, the biceps also rotate the forearms. You can see this if you hold your arm by your side and rotate the hand back and forth. Notice the biceps flexing as the hand approaches the palm-up position. By using dumbells, you can take advantage of this physiological trait. Now we should add that you would have to use a really heavy dumbell (more than you could curl) to get the full effect of supination. Still, every bit helps, so give it a try.

COMMENTS – Once again, limit any swinging to the last 1 or 2 reps. And even then it's probably not necessary at this stage of your development. Try to put total concentration into each and every rep.

Besides the psychological aspect of curling one dumbell at a time, there may be a physiological basis. Neurologists suggest that when two arms are used simultaneously, the brain has to split the nerve impulses. Whereas by alternating, you get full nerve transmission to each biceps. How much is fact and how much is theory? That's open to debate. And although you have no control over nerve impulses, you do have control over exercise performance. So choose the version that feels most productive. As a final comment, Arnold favored the alternating version. Need we say more?

MUSCLES WORKED – Dumbell curls are great for working the belly of the biceps. They also reduce the stress on the wrist and forearm. In fact many bodybuilders suggest starting your biceps workout (this only applies to intermediate and advanced bodybuilders who are performing more than one exercise for their muscles) with dumbells so as not to overstress the weaker areas.

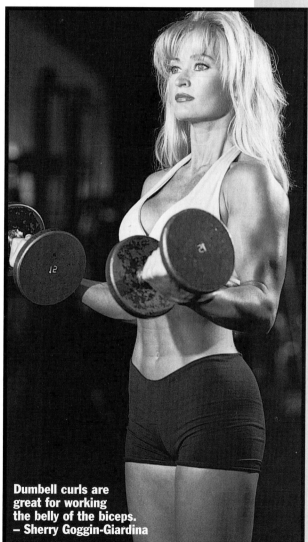

Dumbell curls are great for working the belly of the biceps.
– Sherry Goggin-Giardina

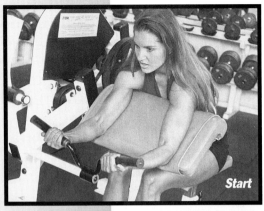

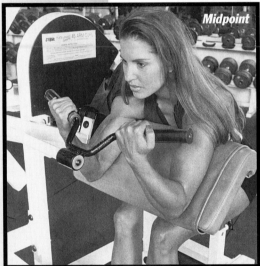

Preacher curls performed by Veronica Martell.

PREACHER CURLS – Also called Scott curls, this exercise is great for working the lower biceps region. Start by sitting on the stool or bench connected to the preacher board. Adjust yourself so that the padded board fits snugly into your armpits. Take the barbell (straight or EZ) from the supports and curl it until the biceps are fully flexed. Lower to the starting position and repeat.

COMMENTS – Although biceps length is genetic, you can create the illusion of length by building the lower regions. Some Scott benches are positioned fairly high and require you to stand up when doing the movement. If your gym has both, give them a try and pick the one that suits you.

Of all the biceps exercises, this one is the most dangerous if not performed in good style. Under no circumstances drop the barbell to the bottom position. You can easily rip the biceps tendon from where it inserts on the forearm bone. The only option open to you then would be surgery and many months of inactivity. With a little attention paid to good style and strict form, you can avoid the aggravation.

MUSCLES WORKED – Although they work the whole biceps muscle, Scott curls are primarily a lower biceps exercise. Because you are braced by the padded board, its virtually impossible to cheat and bring your lower back into the movement. Finally, you will notice a great deal of forearm stimulation. This is fine. You will need a strong grip for many of your other exercises.

INCLINE CURLS – You will need an incline bench to perform this one. Unlike incline presses for your chest, use a bench with an angle of at least 45 degrees. Anything less will place too much strain on your front delts. Grab two dumbells and lie back on the bench. Curl the bells up until the biceps are fully flexed. All the tips suggested for standing dumbell curls apply here as well (rotate the hands from a facing in, to a facing up position, don't swing the weight up, etc.).

COMMENTS – Once again you have the option of curling both dumbells simultaneously or alternating. When you lower the dumbells, be careful not to hit the side of the incline bench. In fact, this is another reason for starting the dumbells in a forward pointed position. If they were in the standard end-to-end position, they would have less clearance with the bench.

The advantage of using the incline bench is that it limits the amount of cheating you can do. Let's face it, you can't swing very much if you have your back braced against a rigid board.

MUSCLES WORKED – Incline curls work the whole biceps region. Many bodybuilders find them great for bringing out the biceps peak. Of course this attribute is more genetic than anything else is. The exercise does provide some forearm stimulation, but not to the same extent as the various barbell curls.

CONCENTRATION CURLS – Sit on the end of a bench and grab a dumbell. With your elbow resting on your inner thigh, curl the bell up, flex, and then lower it again. Do one complete set, then switch arms.

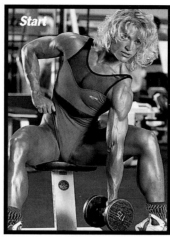

COMMENTS – Most bodybuilders perform concentration curls in the seated position. A few (including Arnold Schwarzenegger) like to do the movement standing bent over. Instead of bracing the elbow against the thigh, it's held down and away from the body. Keep the shoulder on the exercising side lower than the one on the free side. Resist the urge to swing the weight – use only biceps power. As with all dumbell curls, you may want to supinate the hands when performing the exercise.

MUSCLES WORKED – Most bodybuilders consider concentration curls more of a shaping and peaking exercise than a mass-builder. Keep in mind that peak and shape are primarily due to genetics. Unless you have the genetics, you will never develop biceps peaks like Robby Robinson. Still, you'll never know unless you try, and this is where concentration curls come in. This exercise cannot change your genetics, but it can maximize whatever potential you do have.

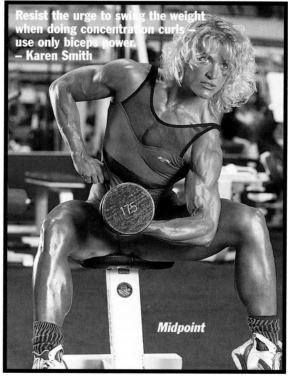

Resist the urge to swing the weight when doing concentration curls – use only biceps power. – Karen Smith

Midpoint

ONE-ARM PREACHER CURLS – Instead of using a barbell, try preacher curls with a single dumbell. Remember to lower slowly and not bounce the weight at the bottom.

COMMENTS – By using a dumbell you can adjust your upper body to take some of the stress off the biceps tendon. Many bodybuilders find preachers hard on the forearms and elbows. Using a dumbell allows you more flexibility than the rigidity of a barbell. A barbell puts the force at 90 degrees to the upper body. A dumbell allows you to vary this angle, thus placing less stress on the forearms and elbows.

MUSCLES WORKED – Dumbell preacher curls place most of the stress on the lower biceps. As discussed above, they treat your forearms and elbows with more kindness than the barbell version!

STANDING CABLE CURLS – For variety try standing biceps curls with a set of cables. Work one arm or both at the same time. It's up to you. If doing them one arm at a time, grab the machine with your free hand for support. It's extremely difficult to stay stationary when exercising one side of the body.

COMMENTS – As with most cable exercises, go for the feel rather than the amount of weight. Cable curls are an excellent way to finish off the biceps after a basic movement such as the standing barbell curl. Of course you can take the opposite approach and use them as a warmup exercise. Many bodybuilders (including Franco Columbu) suggest starting your biceps workout with cables or dumbells. This warms up the area and doesn't put the same stress on the elbows and forearms that barbell curls do.

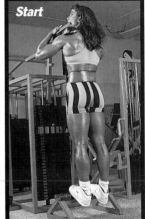

Start

MUSCLES WORKED – Standing cable curls are another so-called peaking and shaping exercise. They work the whole biceps region, and if performed one arm at a time, allow you to really concentrate. For a great pump, try finishing your biceps workout with a couple of high-rep (15 to 20) sets of cable curls.

NARROW REVERSE-GRIP CHINUPS – Grab an overhead chinning bar with a shoulder-width reverse grip. Pull your body up until the bar is touching your midchest. Lower back down until your arms are just short of locking out.

COMMENTS – Despite being a variation of the regular chinup, one of the best back exercises, the narrow reverse-grip chinup puts much of the stress on the biceps. As with regular chins, avoid swinging the body when performing your reps. You may need to experiment with different grip widths to maximize biceps tension.

MUSCLES WORKED – Narrow-grip chins primarily work the biceps and lats, but the forearms, teres and rhomboids also come into play.

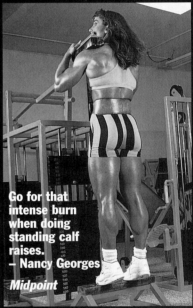

Go for that intense burn when doing standing calf raises.
– Nancy Georges

Midpoint

CALVES

STANDING CALF RAISES – You will need access to the appropriate machine to do this exercise. Rest your toes on the attached block of wood, and rest the pads on your shoulders. Lower your body so that your heels are lower than your toes. From here the exercise is straightforward. With your knees locked, raise yourself up on your toes, stretch all the way down, pause, and flex up on your toes as far as possible. Go for that intense burn!

COMMENTS – Even though this is primarily a stretching exercise, don't be afraid to load the machine with hundreds of pounds of weight. Keep your back and legs straight. The only movement is at the ankle joint. Although calf injuries are very rare (the calf muscle is composed of extremely dense muscle fiber, which makes tearing very difficult), you still shouldn't bounce at the bottom of the movement, as you might strain the Achilles tendon.

MUSCLES WORKED – Standing calf raises work the entire calf muscle, with the primary focus on the upper (gastrocnemius) region.

CALF FLEXES ON LEG-PRESS MACHINE – Here is another example of using a machine for an exercise it was not designed for. Instead of pressing the weight with your thighs, you "flex" the weight platform using only your feet. As with the standing version, go for the maximum amount of stretch at the top and bottom.

COMMENTS – The advantage of this exercise – you don't have the entire weight pushing down on your spine. The disadvantage – it will take a bit of practice to get the foot positioning correct. Still, this exercise is an adequate substitute if you don't have access to a standing calf machine.

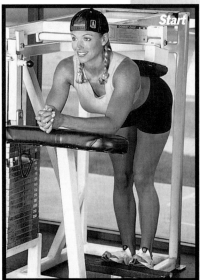

MUSCLES WORKED – Most of the stress is placed on the lower portion, but the upper calves are also worked. If you really want to get that extra burn in the lower calf, use less weight and bend your legs slightly. This will shift all the stress to the lower area. After one set of these your calves will be burning like crazy!

DONKEY CALF RAISES – With your toes resting on a block of wood (at least 4 inches thick is recommended), bend over at the waist and have a training partner sit on your lower back. Flex up and down on your toes, going for the maximum stretch. If you find one rider too light, try to fit a second on your back.

COMMENTS – The bashful and shy might want to avoid this exercise! Also, many upper-class gyms (health spas) advise against doing them. You see, the general public is intimidated by people riding on top of one another, especially if they are moving up and down!

Having said that, donkey calf raises are considered by many to be the best calf exercise. Bodybuilders such as Arnold, Larry Scott, Franco Columbu and Frank Zane made extensive use of donkey raises. The exercise is seen less frequently in gyms today. No doubt the presence of fancy new equipment and increased numbers of general fitness trainers has contributed to the decline. Still, if you check out Gold's or World Gym in California, you will see numerous bodybuilders burning their calves with donkey raises. And one look at their lower legs gives testament to the effectiveness of this exercise.

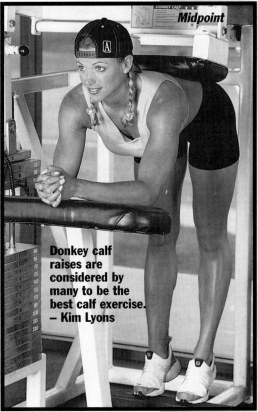

Donkey calf raises are considered by many to be the best calf exercise.
– Kim Lyons

MUSCLES WORKED – Donkey calf raises work the whole calf region. If you keep the legs completely locked, most of the work is done by the upper calf. Bend the knees slightly and the lower calves take most of the strain. For variety you might want to include both versions in your training. Remember, when doing the bent-leg variety, you will need to use less weight as the lower calf cannot handle as much weight as the upper calf.

SEATED CALF RAISES – You will need a special machine to do this exercise. Sit down on the seat and place the padded knee rests on your legs. With your toes on the block of wood, stretch up and down as far as you can.

COMMENTS – Because it works the lower calf, you will need to use less weight. Go for at least 20 reps and try to feel every one of them. No bouncing the weight on your legs. Even though the supports are padded, improper style can injure your knees.

MUSCLES WORKED – Since the legs are bent, most of the stress is placed on the lower calf (soleus), but there is some secondary upper-calf involvement.

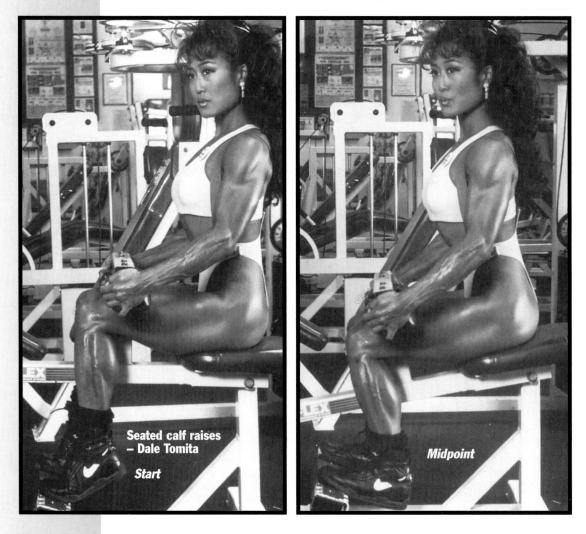

Seated calf raises
– Dale Tomita

Start

Midpoint

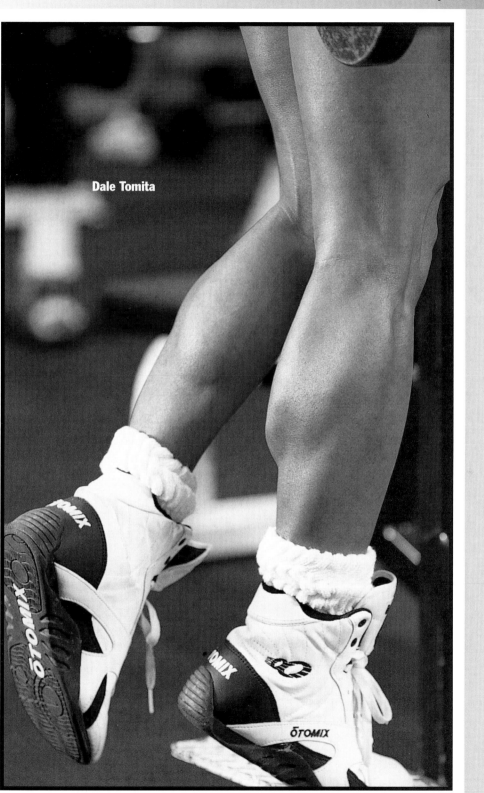

Dale Tomita

Injuries

Your technique may be perfect, your warmup straight from the textbook, but sooner or later you will incur an injury. We know this sounds blunt but it is the reality of the situation. Just think about what you are asking the muscles to do. One set of 10 reps on the leg press with 200 pounds means you've moved one ton of weight in less than a minute. Do the math for an entire workout and see exactly how much weight you've lifted. Even though the benefits far outweigh the risks, we'll be the first to admit that weightlifting is inherently dangerous.

Chapter Ten is not meant to be a self-diagnostic tool. If you think you've sustained an injury, go see your physician. He or she has anywhere from five to ten years of medical training to offer you – far more than the few paragraphs we are about to present. If you have access to a sports physician better still, as he or she will have treated literally thousands of similar injuries. Our goal is to highlight some of the common causes of weight training injuries, and then look at the most frequent injuries seen in gyms.

Causes

Poor Technique

Without doubt the number one cause of weight training injuries is poor technique. For men poor technique stems from those large but frail male egos that are constantly put to the test every time they hit the gym. If John lifted 225 pounds on the bench press, then Mark has to try 230 pounds. Now there's nothing wrong with that kind of competitiveness. In fact such mini-competitions do wonders to maintain one's intensity and enthusiasm, so don't be afraid to put a few extra pounds on the bar, or go for that extra rep – but *never* at the expense of good technique.

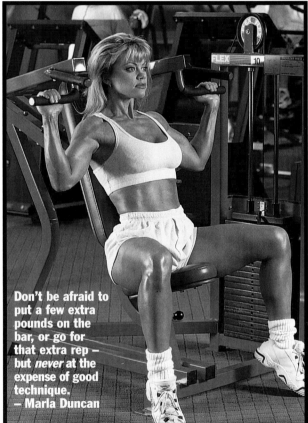

Don't be afraid to put a few extra pounds on the bar, or go for that extra rep – but *never* at the expense of good technique.
– Marla Duncan

Unfortunately many individuals try to lift a heavier weight sooner than their muscles are capable. To compensate they start letting other muscles come into the exercise, and perhaps more important (at least from an injury point of view), their technique goes straight out the window. They may get away with it for a period of time, but sooner or later something gives. In the case of pressing movements it's usually the shoulder muscles, particularly the small underlying rotator complex. The next time you're in the gym listen to how many guys you hear complaining about their shoulders. For every one person who developed the problem through no fault of their own, we bet there are ten others whose problem was self-inflicted through bad technique.

Perhaps the best example to illustrate the relationship between technique and injury is squats. Few other exercises have developed the horrendous reputation of squats. They've been called everything from knee-wreckers to lower back destroyers. The fact is squats are the best leg exercise around. From a kinesiology point of view they are safer than leg extensions – the movement most commonly prescribed for knee rehab. The reason squats seem to cause so many lower back and knee injuries is, you guessed it, *poor technique.* Take a glance toward the squat rack the next time you go for a workout. Watch how many people bounce at the bottom, or lean way too far forward. The knees should not be used as elastic bands to help you "bounce" the weight back up. Is it any wonder so many people develop ligament problems? As for leaning forward, the problem should be obvious. Try bending forward at the waist to about a 45-degree angle. Feel that extra pressure on the lower back. Now imagine how it would feel with a couple of hundred pounds on your back. The human spinal column is a marvel of engineering, but like any work of architecture, it can bear only so much weight.

If you get nothing else from this book, take this advice: Always perform your exercises in good style. Your muscles, joints, and other soft tissues will thank you.

Overtraining

As later in the book we'll be devoting an entire chapter to this topic, we'll only touch on it here. *Overtraining* is the term used to describe any amount of training that places more stress on the body than it can handle. In other words the training volume is so high that the body is unable to recover sufficiently between workouts.

As we saw in the chapter on biology, exercising causes damage to the muscles at the microscopic level. Over a short period of time (usually 48 to 96 hours) the muscle tissue rebuilds, but at a slightly thicker level. Despite popular belief it's not the actual workout that causes improvement but the time period between training sessions. If the body is not given adequate time to make repairs, not only will the muscle tissue not rebuild, but the risk of injury goes way up.

Two classic signs of overtraining are an increase in the number of injuries and the presence of nagging injuries that simply don't want to heal. If you start experiencing either of these, stop your training and take a few days or weeks off. In the case of a major injury see a physician.

Mia Finnegan

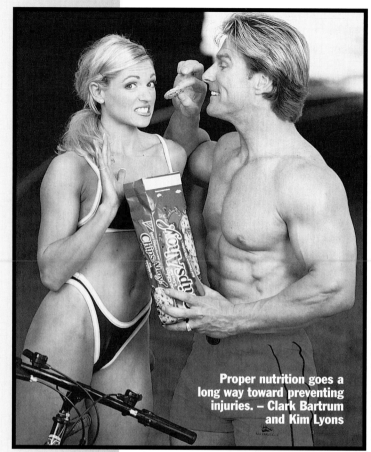

Proper nutrition goes a long way toward preventing injuries. – Clark Bartrum and Kim Lyons

Poor Nutrition

Although not a direct cause, poor eating habits can lead to injuries. Despite the proclamations of a few holdouts, regular exercise places increased nutrient demands on the body. A bricklayer needs a certain number of bricks to complete a wall. Likewise the body needs a certain amount of nutrients to meet its metabolic activities. Insufficient protein can slow down muscle tissue repair. Not enough carbohydrate and your energy levels will suffer. And yes, even the much-maligned fat is needed in certain amounts.

If you are one of those individuals who skip breakfast, eat a small lunch, and then have a huge cooked supper, we suggest reevaluating your eating habits. Try eating smaller but more frequent meals throughout the day. Not only will this ensure better nutrient utilization, but it also increases the body's recovery ability. This will go a long way toward preventing injuries.

Poor Exercise Choice

The purchase of this book is one of the best steps toward eliminating this common cause of injury. There are literally hundreds of exercises you can do in a gym. Most are safe and productive. Some are productive but questionable in safety. And then there are those that are neither productive nor safe.

One of the most popular warmup exercises you'll witness in the gym is broom twists. Basically the individual will place a broomstick or similar straight bar behind his or her head and commence to twist the torso in a corkscrew fashion. We're not sure where this one originated but we are sure it's not doing your spinal column any good. One of the prevailing myths in exercise is that you can spot-reduce. Many people think that by vigorously twisting the torso they can somehow shrink the obliques. Sorry, but, it's not that simple. All this exercise does is place undue stress on the lower back ligaments and vertebrae.

Another popular exercise is good mornings. Once again the familiar broomstick is used, but instead of twisting, you bend forward at the waist until the torso is parallel with the floor. Ouch! Twists are bad, but this one is worse. You'll even see misguided individuals doing this exercise with a weighted barbell. We'll let the mathematicians calculate the forces involved. Suffice to say, as soon as you bend forward with the legs kept straight, there is literally hundreds of pounds of pressure placed on the lower back.

We could go on, but we hope you get the message. The exercises recommended here have been chosen because of their effectiveness and safety. If you are in doubt as to the merits and risks of an exercise after reading this book, ask a qualified strength-training instructor.

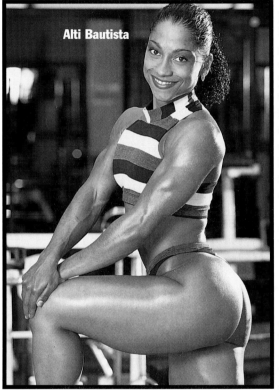

Alti Bautista

Poor Equipment

Unless you work out in an old gym (or one equipped with old machines) you won't have to worry about this cause of injury. All of the new lines of strength-training equipment have been designed by kinesiologists and biomechanical engineers. This means they come very close to duplicating the natural movements of the body. The same, however, cannot be said for some of the older apparatus still in use.

Even though their modern lines are state of the art and take a back seat to no one, a couple of pieces of the long-standing Universal line of equipment are questionable, in particular the Universal leg press.

Universal was one of the first companies to get into the manufacturing of gym equipment. Most high schools and colleges still have the familiar Universal multistation front and center in their gyms. The fact that so many of these large units are still working perfectly despite being 20 or 30 years old is testament to Universal's workmanship. Having said that you may want to give the leg-press station on the unit a pass. Numerous individuals have injured their knees while performing this exercise. Unlike the newer leg presses which come with a large pressing platform that allows you to change your stance, the foot rests on the old Universal leg press are very small, to the point of being pedals. If your bone structure happens to suit this arrangement, then no problem. But let's face it, most people have different bone lengths, tendon attachments, and muscle proportions. The small pedals on the Universal leg press lock your feet, and hence your stance, in one position. For many this stance is biomechanically incorrect and the knees (and occasionally the lower back) may suffer because of it.

Commercially manufactured strength machines may cause problems, but the homemade jobs may mess you up for good. With the typical piece of strength-training equipment costing $2500 to $3000, it's not surprising that some gym owners go the garage route. Iron can be bought fairly cheap, and most people know someone who's handy with a welding torch. For a couple of hundred dollars you can assemble a strength-training machine that would rival any commercial product. The problem of course is that most welders know little or nothing about the way the human body works. Ask them how to ratio gases for a good burn, and you'll get lost in the vocabulary. But request a simple explanation of how the thigh muscles move the legs and most are left scratching their heads. It has nothing to do with intelligence, just background and training.

It takes more to build an effective and safe strength-training machine than just slapping together a few pieces of iron. You need to know the proper biomechanics of the muscles. It takes computer simulations and skilled professionals to design safe and effective strength-training machines.

Before you start condemning every piece of equipment you come across, we should add that some of the safest and most effective lines of equipment were built by "handymen." The most famous was Joe Gold, the founder of the Gold's Gym chain. Arnold Schwarzenegger and other top bodybuilders flocked to his gym in California in the late 1960s – and one of the reasons was Joe's expertise in designing equipment.

However, we warn you – Joe Gold was an exception and not the norm. If your gym has a large inventory of homemade machines, proceed with caution. If there seems to be an unusually high number of injuries associated with using a certain piece of equipment – avoid it like the plague. If a certain piece of equipment doesn't get used, except by novices, it's probably because the long-time regulars discovered a few dangerous quirks. Again, skip that machine.

We are by no means suggesting you read the design specs of every piece of apparatus you use, but we do advise you to always be on guard for machines that "don't seem right."

Categories of Injuries

There's an old saying in the legal profession that states that anyone who represents themself in court has a fool for a client. The same theory holds true for diagnosing injuries. Let the professionals determine whether or not you have an injury and to what extent.

Sprains
The joints of your body are supported by ligaments – strong bands of connective tissue that join one bone to another. A sprain is a simple stretch or tear of the ligaments. The areas of your body most vulnerable to sprains are your ankles, knees and wrists. A sprained ankle can occur when your foot turns inward. This can put extreme stress on the ligaments of your outer ankle and could cause a sprain. A sprained knee can be the

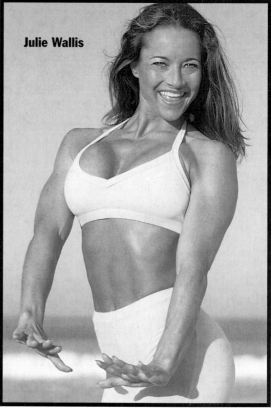

Julie Wallis

result of a sudden twist. Few injuries have ended as many athletic careers as the dreaded ACL (anterior cruciate ligament) tear. Wrist sprains most often occur when you fall on an outstretched hand.

What Are the Signs of a Sprain?

While the intensity varies, pain, bruising and inflammation is common to all three categories of sprains – mild, moderate and severe. The individual will usually feel a tear or pop in the joint. A severe sprain produces excruciating pain at the moment of injury, as ligaments tear completely or separate from the bone. This loosening makes the joint nonfunctional. A moderate sprain partially tears the ligament, producing joint instability, and some swelling. A ligament is stretched in a mild sprain, but there is no joint loosening.

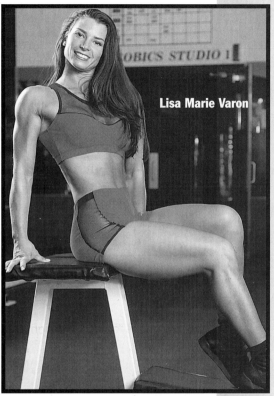

Lisa Marie Varon

The recommended treatment for a sprain is *RICE* – rest, ice, compression and elevation. In simple terms, stop training, apply ice to reduce swelling, wrap the area if need be, and elevate the area if possible.

Strains

Your bones are supported by a combination of muscles and tendons. Tendons connect muscles to bones. A strain is the result of an injury to either a muscle or a tendon, usually in your foot or leg. The strain may be a simple stretch in your muscle or tendon, or it may be a partial or complete tear in the muscle-and-tendon combination.

What Are the Signs of a Strain?

Typical indications include pain, muscle spasm, muscle weakness, swelling, inflammation and cramping. In severe strains, the muscle and/or tendon is partially or completely ruptured, often incapacitating the individual. Some muscle function will be lost with a moderate strain where the muscle/tendon is overstretched and slightly torn. With a mild strain the muscle/tendon is stretched or pulled slightly. Some common strains are:

• Back strain. When the muscles that support the spine are twisted, pulled or torn, the result is a back strain. Athletes who engage in excessive jumping (during basketball, volleyball, etc.) are vulnerable to this injury.

• Hamstring muscle strain. A hamstring muscle strain is a tear or stretch of a major muscle in the back of the thigh. The injury can sideline a person for up to six months. The likely cause is muscle strength imbalance between the hamstrings and the muscles in the front of the thigh, the quadriceps. Kicking a football, running or leaping to make a basket can pull a hamstring. Hamstring injuries tend to recur.

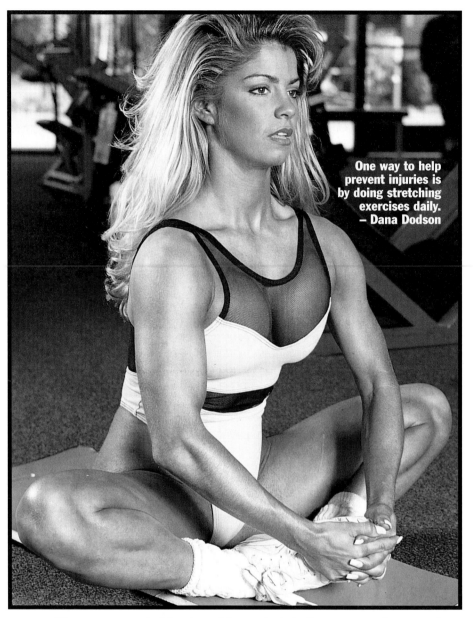

One way to help prevent injuries is by doing stretching exercises daily.
– Dana Dodson

The recommended treatment for a strain is the same as for a sprain – rest, ice, compression and elevation – followed by simple exercises to relieve pain and restore mobility. For a serious tear, see your physician. You may need surgical repair.

Contusions

A contusion is a bruise caused by a blow to your muscle, tendon or ligament. The bruise is caused when blood pools around the injury and discolors your skin. The most frequent causes of contusions in gyms are the ends of barbells and machine handles.

Most contusions are mild and respond well when you rest, apply ice and compression, and elevate the injured area. If symptoms persist, medical care should be sought to prevent permanent damage to the soft tissues.

Tendonitis

Inflammation is a healing response to injury, and is usually accompanied by swelling, heat, redness and pain. An inflammation in a tendon or in the tendon covering is called *tendonitis.* What usually causes tendonitis is not just a single injury but a series of small stresses that repeatedly aggravate the tendon.

Professional baseball players, swimmers, tennis players and golfers are susceptible to tendonitis in their shoulders and arms. Soccer and basketball players, runners and aerobic dancers are prone to tendon inflammation in their legs and feet. And we hate to admit it but weight training could cause tendonitis in all areas.

Tendonitis may be treated by rest to eliminate stress, anti-inflammatory medication, steroid injections, splinting, and exercises to correct muscle imbalance and improve flexibility. Persistent inflammation may cause damage to the tendon, which may necessitate surgical correction.

Bursitis

A bursa is a sac filled with fluid. It is located between a bone and a tendon or muscle, and it allows the tendon to slide smoothly over the bone. Repeated small stresses and overuse can cause the bursa in your shoulder, elbow, hip, knee or ankle to swell. This swelling and irritation is called bursitis, and many people experience it in association with tendonitis. Bursitis can usually be relieved by rest and possibly with anti-inflammatory medication. Some orthopedic surgeons also inject the bursa with additional medication to reduce the inflammation.

Stress Fractures

When one of your bones is stressed by overuse, tiny breaks in the bone can occur. The injury is termed a *stress fracture.* Early symptoms may be pain and swelling in the region of the stress fracture. The bones of your lower leg and foot are particularly prone to stress fractures. The fracture may not be seen on initial routine ex-rays, requiring a bone scan to obtain the diagnosis. We should add that stress fractures are very rare in strength training. In most cases the surrounding soft tissue will give way first. Not that this is any comfort to sufferers, but just to let you know that the odds are good to excellent that you'll never experience a stress fracture from regular strength training.

Prevention Tips

No one is immune from injury, but here are six tips developed by the American Academy of Orthopedic Surgeons to help reduce the risk:
• Participate in a conditioning program to build muscle strength.
• Do stretching exercises daily.
• Always wear shoes that fit properly.
• Nourish your muscles by eating a well-balanced diet.
• Warm up before any sports activity, including practice.
• Use or wear protective equipment appropriate for that physical activity.

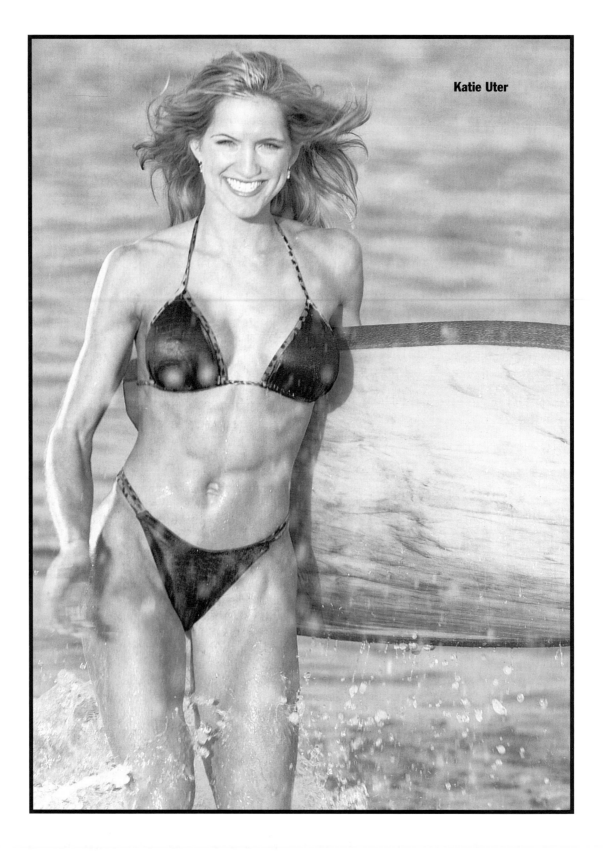

Katie Uter

Book 2

CHAPTER ELEVEN

Advanced Training Techniques and Principles

It would be great if we could tell you when you'll know you've reached the advanced stage of training, but we can't. Everyone progresses at different rates. One individual may be ready for advanced training in three months, while another may take three years. Of course these are the extreme ends of the spectrum. Most people fall somewhere in between. Generally speaking the average person can start incorporating advanced techniques into her routine after six to 12 months of consistent training.

The Case for Advanced Training

The old saying "All roads lead to Rome" is certainly true for most beginners. It seems no matter what type of training program beginners follow, they make great gains on it. After years if not decades of inactivity their muscles and cardio system are begging to be used, and just about any form of stimulation will bring the desired results. A point, however, will be reached when the results start to plateau. Great gains drop to slow gains, which in turn lead to stagnation. When this happens you essentially have three options. You can get frustrated with the whole training thing and give it up, you can keep slugging away following the same old tired routine, or you can start using advanced training techniques to kick-start your system. We don't need to go into detail on the folly of the first option, right? Giving up training will lead to a whole host of problems down the road. You've come this far, don't quite now. Option two may yield results. Sometimes the body will start responding again, even with the same stimulation, month after month. But in all honesty that probably won't happen. Often months lead to years and you're no further ahead. Despite their best efforts, most people get frustrated and fall back on option one and quit.

The best way to keep the body responding is to follow option three and employ variety in your training. You have to keep the body guessing. If it "knows" that at 5:30 on Tuesday it's going to be doing 3 sets of incline dumbell presses, you must come in and do something entirely different. You have to catch it off guard

Mona Beaulieu

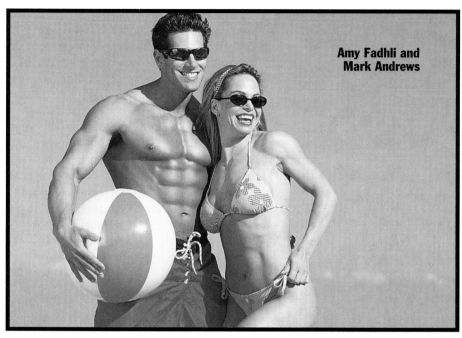

**Amy Fadhli and
Mark Andrews**

so to speak. All of the following techniques and strategies fall into the category of advanced training. In this section we are going to describe how each works. Then later in the book we'll show you how to incorporate the techniques into your training.

Time of the Day

Earlier we discussed how there is no "best time" of the day to train. For the most part this is true, but only to a certain degree. Eventually the body reaches a point where it becomes accustomed to doing the same thing at the same time every day. One of the easiest ways to catch the body off guard is to change your workout time. If you normally train at 5:00 p.m. try 7:00 in the morning. Likewise if you are a morning person try a late evening workout. We realize many readers train at the most convenient time of the day, and school or work may prevent you from changing your workout time. But for those readers who have some flexibility in their daily schedule, try switching things around once in a while.

Order of Exercises

If changing your workout time is not an option, try switching the order of your exercises. Most people become complacent and follow the same exercise sequence day after day. For example a common chest routine is the flat barbell press, incline dumbell press, and flat dumbell flye. This is a great workout, but why always start with flat presses? Why not do the inclines first? True, you won't lift the same weight on the flats, but then you'll lift slightly more on the inclines. And if you're like most people, odds are your upper chest needs more work than the lower chest anyway.

Order of Muscles

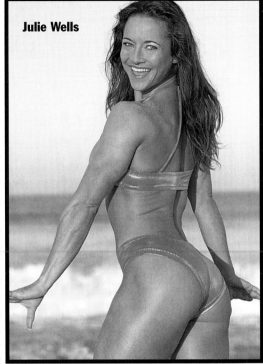

Julie Wells

Closely related to the previous is the issue of muscle order. Using the same example, most people start with chest, then hit back, and finish off with a small muscle group like biceps or triceps. Once again the question arises, Why start with chest? For most people the answer is "Outta sight, outta mind." Because the chest muscles are out front and very visible they tend to get a lot more attention than the back muscles, which are sort of hidden. Go to any bodybuilding contest and you'll see that great chests are a dime a dozen, but outstanding back development is a rarity. In fact the competitors with the best backs tend to get the greatest reaction from the audience. Now we realize competitive body-building is not in the future of most readers, but what if we told you there was a health issue involved?

Bet we have your attention now. Over time most individuals become slope-shouldered because the muscles of the upper back and lower shoulders become weak. As soon as the shoulder girdle starts sagging forward, the body's center of gravity changes, with the lower back having to take up the extra strain. By keeping the back muscles strong, however, you help offset the slope-shoulder effect brought on by time. So if you are one of those individuals who tend to train the most visible muscles first, please reconsider.

Before leaving the topic we should add a few precautionary points. Even though switching around the order in which you work the larger muscles makes perfect sense, the same does not hold true for the smaller muscles like biceps, triceps, abs and lower back. These smaller muscles play a major role in most exercises for the larger muscles. If you train them first and tire them out, you will diminish the intensity with which you can hit the larger muscles. For example the biceps are heavily involved in back-training. Likewise the triceps come into play on most chest and shoulder exercises. The abs and spinal erectors are major stabilizers for just about every exercise. In the case of squats they play a vital role. If the abs and spinal erectors are fatigued before commencing squats, you run the risk of severely injuring the lower back.

Muscle Combinations

Besides playing around with exercise order you can also group muscles on different days. The muscle combinations are almost endless and later in the book we'll discuss different combinations you can use to add variety to your workouts. Suffice to say, generally speaking, try to split things up so you are training roughly the same amount of muscle mass on each day. For example it wouldn't make sense to train legs, chest and back on the same day – these are the three largest muscle groups in the body. It would make more sense to put a small muscle group like arms with legs, and then train the medium-sized muscles on a separate day. In any case don't become a slave to the same muscle combinations. You need variety – change it up!

Types of Exercises

It would be brave and bold on our part to claim this book contained a description of every exercise out there. We are, however, confident there is enough variety within these pages to add spice to your workouts. On average you should change your routine every four to six weeks. Now keep in mind this is a general time period. Some individuals need to make changes every workout, while others go literally years on the same program and still make progress. The old saying "If it ain't broke, don't fix it" applies to strength training just as well as anything else in life.

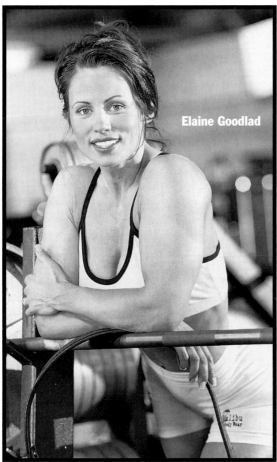

Elaine Goodlad

The bottom line? As soon as you feel the muscles becoming stale, or perhaps more important, when you begin to get bored with it all, start mixing it up. As soon as you do you'll notice the muscles are much more sore for the next few days. This is good evidence that the muscles had adapted to the routine you were following.

Reps and Sets

Where is it written that you must do 3 sets of 10? Yet go into any gym and that's what you'll observe the vast majority of members doing. There are a number of reasons why people do this, of course, and we'll start the blame with ourselves. Most writers list "3 sets of 10 reps" on workout programs for convenience. This does not mean, however, that you have to become a slave to these numbers. Another factor is that most people learn by observation, and as we just stated, the most common routine in any gym is based on the old 10 reps x 3 sets scheme. A third reason could be attributed to memory, or more precisely lack thereof. It's far easier to remember to perform 3 sets of 10 for every exercise than to employ a whole host of rep and set schemes.

Despite these somewhat valid reasons, we urge you to vary your sets and reps on a regular basis. Instead of 3 sets of 10, try 4 sets of 15, or 2 sets of 6. The combinations are endless. As we said earlier, muscles are composed of different fiber types that respond better to different rep ranges. Sticking with the same number of reps often neglects parts of the muscles.

Cheat Reps

Despite the negative connotation, cheating does have a role to play in strength training. At its basic level, cheating means to utilize other muscles to help lift the weight during an exercise. Cheating is probably the first advanced technique people lean in the gym; it's also probably the most abused. From day one you'll see individuals swinging their whole body in the sole attempt to lift more weight. The barbell curl is the best example. Everything from the lower back and legs to the shoulders and abs can be brought into play. Oh, and did we tell you, you can also work the biceps with this exercise!

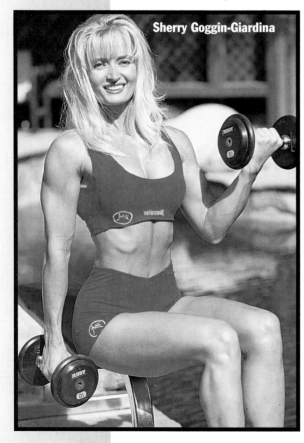

Sherry Goggin-Giardina

Unless otherwise stated you should perform all exercises in this book in good style. There are a few instances, however, where a couple of cheat reps at the end of a set may be productive. Let's use that great source of abuse once again, the barbell curl. Select a weight that causes you to fail at about 2 reps short of the desired number. Instead of stopping the set, use just a little body momentum to help you keep the bar moving. Try as hard as possible to let the biceps do most of the lifting. They are after all the muscles you are trying to work with this exercise.

The biggest advantage to cheat reps is also their disadvantage; they can be performed on just about any exercise at any time. Cheat reps should only be used to complete an additional couple of reps, not for the entire set.

Negatives

It's only logical to follow the topic of cheat reps with negatives as the two complement one another. Let's use that barbell curl once again. On the last couple of reps when you cheat the bar into the top position, don't let it simply drop back down again. In fact don't even lower it at the normal speed. Lower it as slow as possible, periodically trying to stop the bar and reverse direction. Negatives are based on the principle that a muscle is capable of lowering a much heavier weight in good style than it can lift in proper style. You may be able to lift only 100 pounds on the bench press in an upward direction, but you could probably lower 150 to 175 pounds slowly. The latest research suggests that not only are negative reps just as productive as positive reps, but they may be even more productive when it comes to pure strength gains.

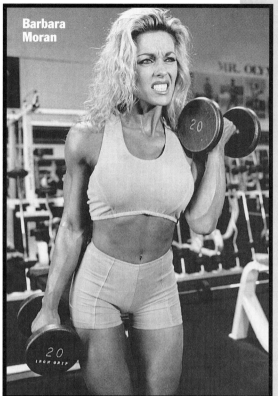

Barbara Moran

Many exercises set themselves up perfectly for negatives. Besides the barbell curl, you can perform negatives on just about any biceps exercise. It's also relatively easy to perform negatives on many shoulder exercises such as lateral raises to the front and side.

You can also take advantage of negatives on many other exercises, but the presence of a spotter is almost mandatory. Trying to lower a heavy weight on a bench press is not the issue, but getting it back to the starting position is. You will need a spotter to stand behind you and help lift the bar back to the arms locked out position. The same holds true for most shoulder-pressing movements. You may be able to sway up 10- or 20-pound dumbells on a lateral raise exercise, but most people can move considerably more weight on pressing movements, especially barbell exercises.

Before leaving the topic we should warn you that there are a few exercises where you might want to give negatives a pass. The squat is perhaps the best example. Most people will be using 100 pounds or more. It's one thing to go to failure with a set of 10-pound dumbells in your hands, but it's something else entirely to do the same thing with 100 pounds or more on your back. Granted a good spotter should able to help you get back up from a deep squat position, but even then there is considerable risk involved. If you want to perform negatives for thighs, stick with the leg-extension or leg-press machine.

Partial Reps or Burns

As with cheat reps, you should perform most of your exercises in strict style for a full range of motion. Nevertheless there are a few instances when partial reps, also called "burns," play a role. As the name suggests, with partial reps you don't complete a full range of motion. You'll see it all the time in the gym on the leg press. Guys will put 1000 pounds or more on the machine, lower the platform

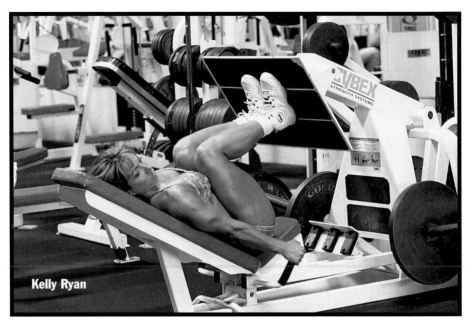

Kelly Ryan

by 10 to 12 inches, and then push it back up. Such training (and we use the word loosely) may do wonders for the ego, but very little for the thighs.

As with cheat reps, partial reps should only be employed after you get 6 or more good reps in good style. Then at the end of your set you could lower the weight partway down and back up again. Even though you are not stimulating the entire muscle for a full range of motion, you are still working it in a productive manner.

No doubt many readers can see where the potential for abuse creeps in. Performing an exercise for a limited range of motion doesn't "hurt" as much, and you can easily lift more weight. We should add that partials are not just for the egotistical types, either. The body will always try to take the easy way out when exercising. Many well-intentioned trainers will unconsciously start doing half-reps without even realizing it. Everyone succumbs to the temptation at some point in their lives. Always be on guard for such "cheating." Sure, throw in a couple of partial reps at the end to really fatigue the muscle, but don't make the common mistake of doing partial reps on most of your exercises.

21s

Just as negatives logically follow cheat reps, so too do partial reps lead perfectly into 21s. To perform a set of 21s select a weight that is about 50 percent of what you could normally handle for 8 to 12 reps. Start by moving the weight from the start position *halfway* to the top. Then return to the starting position. Continue for 7 such partial reps. At the seventh rep raise the weight to the full top position and lower back down halfway. Again complete 7 partial reps. Now comes the hard part. Without stopping, try to finish off the set by completing 7 full reps. Congratulations, you've just completed a set of 21s. It will take you a couple of such sets to fine-tune your poundage. Try to pick a weight that causes you to fail at 5 to 7 on the full-range reps. As soon as you reach the point where 8 or more are possible, increase the weight.

Even though you can do 21s on just about any exercise, they seem to work best with pulling movements like back, biceps and hamstrings exercises. It's very difficult to control the weight with pushing muscles such as chest, shoulders and triceps.

We confess, we are not sure where the name "21s" came from. Why not 18s (3 x 6) or 24s (3 x 8)? Who knows? In fact who cares! Give them a try in your workouts to shock the muscles.

Rest-Pause

Rest-pause is one of those principles that have been around for years and is one of the most intense forms of training. It was formally known as the California set, and was used primarily for strength-building. Because of the training philosophies of the time, rest-pause was not overly popular with many bodybuilders and practically nonexistent for the general population. It made a comeback, however, in the mid-'70s, thanks primarily to the works of one bodybuilder, the late Mike Mentzer. Even though Mike was considered a non-conformist by many, his "heavy-duty" principles have changed the training philosophy of countless individuals wanting to achieve muscular conditioning.

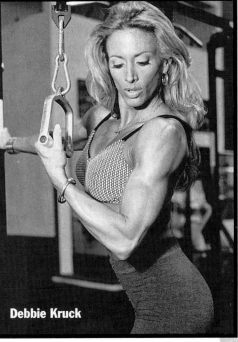

Debbie Kruck

The key element to rest-pause is oxygen. When muscles fatigue the body is no longer able to provide the working muscle with the oxygen necessary to continue a set. But under the rest-pause system, the body is allowed time to replenish the working muscles with oxygen, thus enabling the set to be completed. This is done by simply putting the weight back on the rack for a brief period of time (usually 10 seconds) once failure has been reached. The set is then continued with the recharged muscles being able to perform more reps.

We should warn you that rest-pause is such an intense form of training that you can easily slip into a state of overtraining if you employ it too frequently in your workouts. A good rule of thumb is to do only one rest-pause set per exercise – just enough to stimulate the muscles without overtaxing the body's recovery system

10 x 10

Sometimes the best solution to a problem is the simplest one. In recent years there has been a movement by many trainers and writers to get back to basics.

Their view is that modern training techniques are getting too confusing and starting to stray away from the fundamentals. One of the "basics" that is getting good promotion these days is what's called 10 x 10. There's certainly nothing fancy here. Pick an exercise and do 10 sets of 10 reps. It may sound simple, but trust us, your attitude will change after you give it a try. The goal is to select a weight that allows you to complete a comfortable 10 reps for the first set. Each successive set then becomes harder. You will really have to work to get 10 reps on your last couple of sets.

Probably the greatest advantage to 10 x 10 is thoroughness. Let's face it, on many days the first exercise for a given muscle only serves as a warmup. In fact it's often only after you complete 2 or 3 sets of your second exercise that the muscle starts to fatigue. But with 10 x 10 there's no "wastage" of the first couple of sets as you are doing another 7 or 8 of the same movement.

Besides the quality of 10 x 10, there also a practical advantage. Unless you go into a gym at a down time, chances are you will have to fight for access to most machines. Even getting a bench to do some barbell or dumbell exercises can be a chore. But 10 x 10 means you only have to access one piece of equipment – be it machine, bench, or set of dumbells or barbell. Once you have it there's no need to wait on other members.

We should add that most gyms don't want members to monopolize the one piece of equipment for extended periods of time. Even though they probably won't limit you to a certain number of sets, members are expected to cooperate with one another – and that means you must share. Always keep an eye out for someone waiting to jump in.

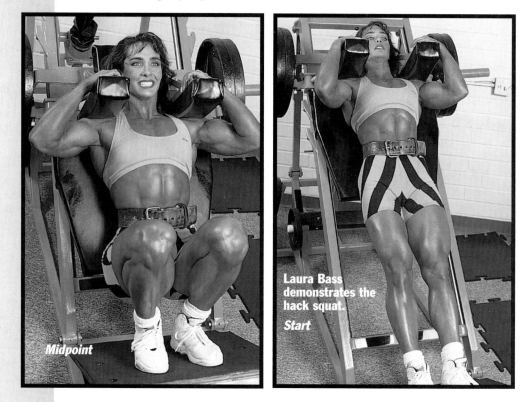

Laura Bass demonstrates the hack squat.

Start

Midpoint

Supersets

For those who work out in a crowded gym or just want to add variety to their training, supersets are ideal. Supersetting involves performing two exercises back to back with little or no rest in between. Supersets can be done for the same muscle group or two different muscle groups – usually opposing muscles, i.e. biceps and triceps, chest and back, etc.

The nice thing about supersets is that they are fast and very efficient. By performing two exercises back to back you can work twice as much muscle mass in a given period of time. And if you are supersetting for the same muscle group, you can hit the muscle from many different angles in a short period of time. Finally ... supersetting is fun! Performing endless sets and reps of the same exercises gets boring after a while, but add a couple of supersets to your routine and your enthusiasm will go through the roof. Here are a few superset combinations you can try.

Supersets for the Same Muscles

Legs:
Leg press – leg extension
Leg extension – squat
Leg curl – stiff-leg deadlift
Standing calf raise – seated calf raise

Chest:
Flat dumbell press – incline dumbell press
Incline dumbell press – flat dumbell flye
Pec-dek – incline machine press

Back:
Wide-grip pulldown – narrow-grip pulldown
Seated row – T-bar row
Chinup – T-bar row

Shoulders:
Front dumbell raise – side dumbell raise
Side dumbell raise – upright row
Bent-over lateral raise – dumbell press

Biceps:
Preacher curl – narrow reverse-grip chinup
Dumbell curl – hammer curl

Triceps:
Lying EZ-bar extension – narrow-grip press
Two-arm dumbell extension – bench dip
Rope extension – pushdown

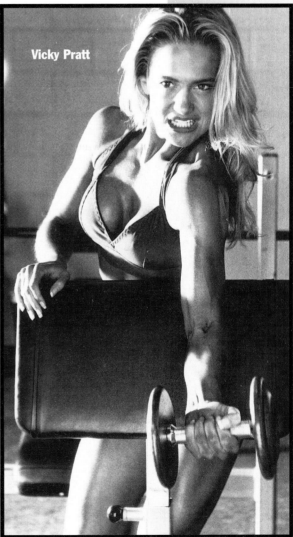

Vicky Pratt

Abdominals:
Crunch – reverse crunch
Leg raise – crunch
Hanging leg raise – reverse crunch

Supersets for Opposing Muscles

Thighs and hamstrings:
Leg press – lying leg curl
Lying leg curl – leg extension
Squat – stiff-leg deadlift

Chest and back:
Flat bench press – chinup
Flat dumbell press – lat pulldown
T-bar row – incline dumbell press

Biceps and triceps
Lying EZ-bar extension – standing barbell curl
Seated dumbell curl – two-arm dumbell extension
Preacher curl – bench dip

Front and rear shoulders:
Front dumbell raise – bent-over lateral raise
Dumbell press – reverse pec-dek flye

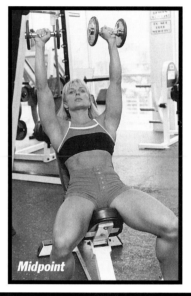

Incline dumbell presses.
– Brandi Carrier

Midpoint

You'll notice we listed shoulders by themselves. In many respects the shoulders are a physiological oddity, as they don't really have an opposing muscle group. There are all sorts of theories as to why the body didn't evolve a large muscle group to work in the opposite direction of the shoulders. The simplest reason is the body didn't need to! Think about it, the primary function of the shoulders is to lift things up and away from the direction of gravity. Over the few million years of human evolution, any time an individual wanted to put something down, he or she let gravity do most of the work. There wasn't a need for a large muscle group to "push" downward. Now we realize this is a very simplistic explanation, and the anatomists among you are probably laughing, but essentially that's what happened. In evolutionary biology terms "Use it or lose it." or in this case "don't evolve it."

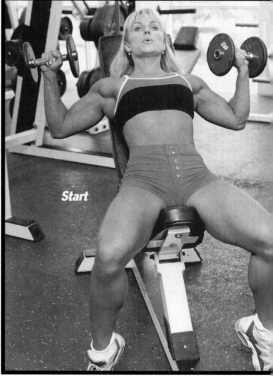

Start

As with many advanced training techniques there are practical considerations. Putting two dumbell exercises back to back shouldn't be too difficult even at the most crowded of times. But trying to alternate two separate pieces of strength machines at suppertime is practically impossible. You no sooner leave one piece of machinery than someone else hops on. In fact there is the possibility you could lose both machines in the transition time between one and the other. Our suggestion is to limit supersets to dumbell exercises at busy times, and save machine supersets for slow times.

Trisets

The next step up from supersets is trisets. Instead of performing two exercises back to back, you do three. You could perform one exercise for three different muscles but the most common practice is to do three exercises for the same muscle group. As with supersets, trisets are a great way to apply maximum stimulation to a muscle in as short a period of time as possible. In addition, by choosing three different exercises you can hit the muscle from different angles, thus ensuring that every muscle fiber is being stimulated.

The downside to trisets mirrors that of supersets – trying to do them at peak times in the gym. If it's difficult to obtain two pieces of equipment for a superset, it's virtually impossible to hold on to three for a triset. Once again, choose your exercises based on the time of the day you work out – free weights for peak times and machines for slower time periods.

Triset Combinations

Thighs:
Squat – leg press – leg extension
Lunge – leg extension – leg press
Leg extension – hack squat – lunge

Hamstrings:
Leg curl – stiff-leg deadlift – back extension

Chest:
Flat barbell press – incline dumbell press – pec-dek flye
Incline barbell press – flat dumbell press – dumbell pullover
Flat dumbell press – incline dumbell press – flat dumbell flye

Back:
Chinup – front pulldown – T-bar row
Front pulldown – seated cable row – dumbell pullover
T-bar row – straight-arm pushdown – reverse pulldown

Shoulders:
Dumbell press – side raise – reverse pec-dek
Machine press – cable side raise – bent-over lateral
Upright row – dumbell press – dumbell shrug

Biceps:
Seated dumbell curl – barbell curl – narrow reverse-grip chinup
Preacher curl – incline curl – standing barbell curl

Triceps:
Lying EZ-bar extension – narrow-grip press – bench dip
Pushdown – rope extension – two-arm dumbell extension

Abdominals:
Hanging leg raise – crunch – reverse crunch
Lying leg raise – reverse crunch – crunch

Giant Sets

Some readers may ask, if it's possible to put two or three exercises back to back, what about four or more? The answer is, by all means. Performing four or more exercises back to back is called giant setting – the most intense form of combination training. Again the option exists to train two or more muscles within the one set, but most people stick to one muscle group.

Giant sets are the most difficult of the three to perform. By the time you reach the fourth or fifth exercise, both your muscles and cardiovascular system are begging for mercy. But then that's one of the primary benefits of giant sets – you can bring maximum stimulation to a muscle and give the cardiovascular system a workout as well.

As you might expect there's no way you'll be able to handle the same weight on your exercises in a giant set as you could for a straight set. This is especially true for those exercises placed third and beyond in the set.

Given the level of intensity, we suggest performing only one or two giant sets for large muscle groups. If you do two giant sets of four or five exercises each, that's a total of 8 to 10 mini-sets for the muscle. For smaller muscles like biceps and triceps we suggest you do only one giant set. These small muscles are easily overtrained and receive a good deal of stimulation from training the larger torso muscles.

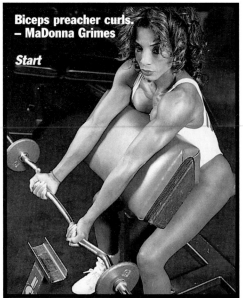

Biceps preacher curls.
– MaDonna Grimes

Start

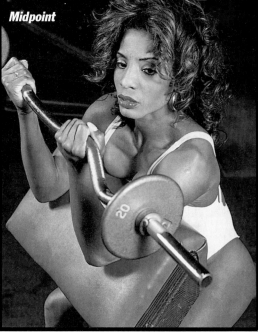

Midpoint

Giant Set Combinations

Thighs:
Leg extension – squat – leg press –
lunge – hack squat

Chest:
Flat barbell press – incline dumbell press –
flat dumbell flye – pec-dek –
dumbell pullover

Back:
Chinup – T-bar row – front pulldown –
seated pulley row – dumbell pullover

Shoulders:
Dumbell press – dumbell side raise –
reverse pec-dek – upright row –
dumbell shrug

Biceps:
Barbell curl – seated dumbell curl –
cable curl – preacher curl

Triceps:
Lying barbell extension – narrow press –
pushdown – bench dip

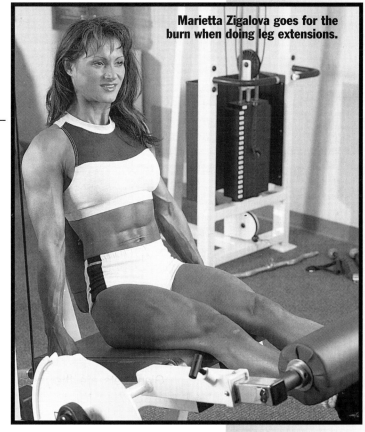

Marietta Zigalova goes for the burn when doing leg extensions.

Pre-Exhaustion

In a manner of speaking, pre-exhaustion is a form of supersetting. But instead of picking exercises at random, there is a logical sequence. After a few weeks you'll discover that on many exercises the smaller muscles give out before the larger primary muscles being targeted. For example the front shoulders and triceps often fatigue before the chest muscles on various pressing exercises. Likewise the biceps are usually tired long before the larger back muscles give out. Thanks to the writings of *MuscleMag's* own, Robert Kennedy in the late 1960s, there is a well-known technique to get around this "weakest link" phenomenon.

Pre-exhaustion: the selection and performance of an isolated movement directly stressing the larger target muscle with limited involvement of the smaller muscles that will be acting to assist this target muscle. In effect you "pre-exhaust" the larger muscle so that it becomes the weak link in the chain. Still with us? Here is an example:

Suppose it is chest day. You have performed your usual warmups and are ready to begin your chest-training. To incorporate pre-exhaustion into this workout, grab a pair of dumbells and start with a few moderate to intense sets of flat flyes for chest, taking care to keep the elbows slightly bent and stationary through the entire range of motion. Performed properly this movement exhausts the pecs with little effect on the anterior delts and triceps muscles. Then move directly to a basic compound movement for chest, like the bench press. Since the pecs are somewhat exhausted from the isolation set, they should fail first, before the front delts and triceps muscles, thus providing greater stimulation to the pecs.

Want another example? Start your back-training with an isolation exercise like straight-arm pushdowns or machine pullovers. Both exercises fatigue the lats while placing little stress on the biceps. Then when you move to a compound exercise like pulldowns or T-bar rows, the biceps will still be fresh and won't give out before the lats.

Other Pre-Exhaustion Combinations

Thighs:
Leg extension – leg press or squat

Chest:
Flat dumbell flye – flat barbell press
Pec-dek flye – flat dumbell press

Back:
Straight-arm pushdown – front pulldown
Machine pullover – T-bar row

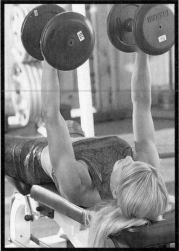

Shoulders:
Side dumbell raise – front machine or dumbell press
Side cable raise – front barbell press

Staggered Sets

Sooner or later you'll discover that no matter how much attention you pay to developing symmetry, one or more muscles will start lagging behind. For larger muscles you'll need to be creative, but for smaller muscles there is a simple solution – staggered sets.

Let's say your calves are being a tad stubborn. Although training these muscles can be downright painful, given their small size, it doesn't take a lot of energy to train

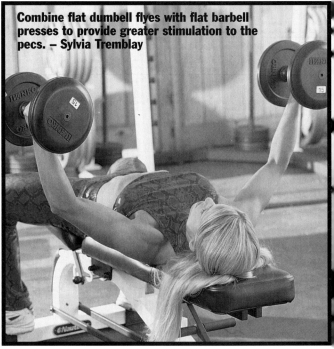

Combine flat dumbell flyes with flat barbell presses to provide greater stimulation to the pecs. – Sylvia Tremblay

them. This means you can fit in extra sets for calves between sets for larger muscles. For example, while waiting to do another set of bench presses, you could run over to the standing calf machine and do a set. Likewise, use your one to two minutes of rest between sets of shoulder presses to perform a set of seated calf raises.

Here's another example. For some people, training is limited by a weak grip, the result of less than adequate forearm strength. The forearm muscles like the calves are painful to train but require little energy. You could easily fit in a couple of sets of wrist curls between sets of squats or leg press (or any other leg exercise for that matter).

You'll notice we recommended calf exercises be done with upper-body muscles, and forearms with legs. It wouldn't make sense to train forearms with upper-body movements as you need a strong grip to execute these exercises. Likewise the calves play a stabilizing role on most leg exercises.

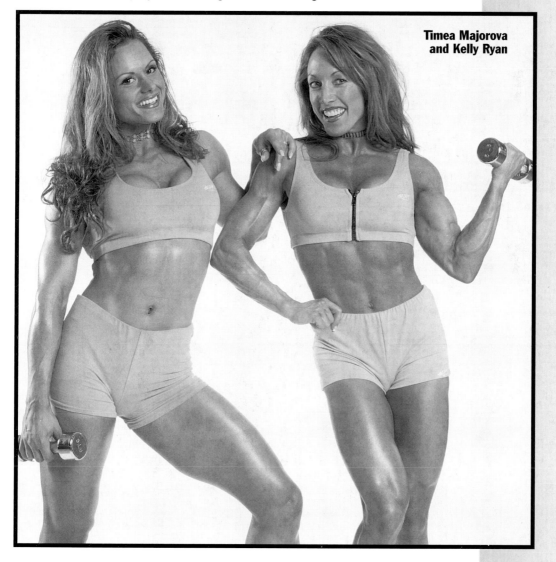

Timea Majorova and Kelly Ryan

CHAPTER TWELVE

Overtraining

It is no secret, especially among athletes, that in order to improve performance you've got to work hard. Hard training, however, breaks down muscle tissue and in some respects makes you weaker. Rest is what makes you stronger. Physiologic improvement in sports only occurs during the rest period following hard training. This adaptation is in response to maximal loading of the cardiovascular and muscular systems and is accomplished by improving efficiency of the heart, increasing capillaries in the muscles, and increasing glycogen stores and enzyme systems within the muscle cells. During recovery periods these systems build to greater levels to compensate for the stress that you have applied. The result is that you reach a higher level of performance.

But if sufficient rest is not included in a training program, regeneration cannot occur and improvements will reach a plateau. Further, if this imbalance between excessive training and inadequate rest persists, level of performance will actually decline. Overtraining can best be defined as the state where the athlete has been repeatedly stressed by training to the point where normal rest periods are no longer adequate to allow for recovery. The "overtraining syndrome" is a new term coined to describe the collection of emotional, behavioral and physical symptoms due to an excess that has persisted for weeks to months. Athletes and coaches also know it as "burnout" or "staleness." This is different from the day to day variation in performance and post exercise tiredness that is common in conditioned athletes. Everybody has slow periods, but when a few weeks turn into a few months or more, you can bet that overtraining is high on the list of suspects.

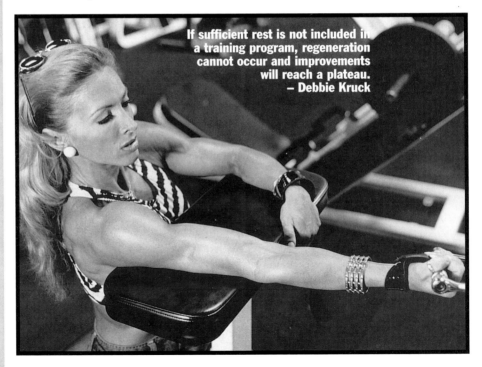

If sufficient rest is not included in a training program, regeneration cannot occur and improvements will reach a plateau.
— Debbie Kruck

Even though symptoms vary from person to person, the most common sign of overtraining is usually chronic fatigue. This tiredness may limit workouts and may be present at rest. The individual could also become moody, easily irritated, have altered sleep patterns, become depressed, or lose the competitive desire and enthusiasm for the sport. Some will report decreased appetite and weight loss. Physical symptoms of overtraining include persistent muscle soreness, increased frequency of viral illnesses, and increased incidence of injuries.

Several clinical studies have been done on athletes with the overtraining syndrome. Exercise physiologic, psychological and biochemical laboratory testing have been done. Findings in these studies have shown decreased performance in exercise testing, decreased mood state, and, in some, increased cortisol levels – the body's "stress" hormone. In men there will also be a decrease in testosterone. For both sexes there will be altered immune status, and an increase in muscle breakdown products will be observed.

Medically the overtraining syndrome is classified as a neuroendocrine disorder. The normal fine balance in the interaction between the autonomic nervous system and the hormonal system is disturbed and "athletic jet lag" results. The body now has a decreased ability to repair itself during rest. Heaping more workouts onto this unbalanced system only worsens the situation. Additional stress in the form of difficulties at work or personal life also contributes. We often get caught up in a chicken and egg situation where increased life stressors decrease the body's recovery abilities, which of course increases the degree of overtraining. This in turn makes the individual less able to deal with life's daily stressors. A snowball effect occurs that requires a great deal of time and effort to break out of.

Generally speaking there are two forms of the syndrome. The sympathetic form is more common in sprint sports and weight training, and the parasympathetic form is more common in endurance sports. Results from various measurements taken during exercise physiologic testing differ between the two forms, but decreased overall performance and increased perceived fatigue are similar. In the parasympathetic form there may be a lower heart rate for a given

Never underestimate the importance of rest. – Cathy Miller

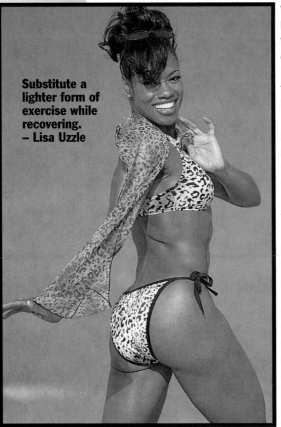

Substitute a lighter form of exercise while recovering.
– Lisa Uzzle

workload. Athletes training with a heart rate monitor may notice that they cannot sustain the workout at their normal level. Fatigue takes over and they have to terminate the workout. Regulation of glucose can become altered and the athlete may experience symptoms of hypoglycemia during exercise.

We won't comment on all of the differences between the two forms of the overtraining syndrome, but one example is resting heart rate. In the sympathetic form the resting heart rate is elevated. In the parasympathetic form, however, the resting heart rate is decreased. If this sounds confusing, you are not alone. There is very little agreement in the literature about abnormal laboratory findings. Additionally, it is possible to have the overtraining syndrome but show completely normal physical findings and biochemical tests. At this point there is no single test that will confirm whether or not an individual is in a state of overtraining. The overtraining syndrome should be considered in any person who manifests symptoms of prolonged fatigue, and performance that has leveled off or decreased. Make sure to exclude the possibility of any underlying illness that may be responsible for the fatigue.

I Have It, Now What Do I Do?

The treatment for overtraining is simple – rest, and lots of it. The longer the overtraining has occurred, the more rest is required. Therefore, early detection is very important. If the overtraining has occurred for only a short period of time (e.g., three to four weeks) then interrupting training for three to five days is usually sufficient rest. After that workouts can be resumed on alternate days. The intensity of the training can be maintained but the total volume must be lower. The factors that led to overtraining must be identified and corrected. Otherwise, the overtraining syndrome is likely to recur. The alternate-day recovery period is continued for a few weeks and then an increase in volume is permitted. In more severe cases the training program may have to be interrupted for weeks, and it may take months to recover. An alternate form of exercise can be substituted to help prevent the exercise withdrawal syndrome.

We should add that most of the medical studies and advice on overtraining have involved single-sport athletes. For triathletes and other multisport athletes the recovery process may be different depending on the circumstances. If you discern that the overtraining has occurred in only one discipline, then rest from activity along with significant decreases in the other sports can bring about full recovery. The following is vitally important: Do not suddenly substitute more workouts in one sport in an attempt to compensate for rest in another. Athletes who do this will not heal the overtraining, but will drive themselves deeper into a hole. Overtraining affects both peripheral and central mechanisms in the body. Resting from overtraining on the bicycle by swimming more will help a pair of fatigued quadriceps, but to the heart, pituitary and adrenals, stress is stress.

Prevention

As with almost everything else health related, prevention is the key. Well-balanced gradual increases in training are recommended. A training schedule design called periodization varies the training load in cycles with built-in mandatory rest phases. During the high workload phase, you alternate between high-intensity exercise and low-intensity exercise. This approach is used by a number of elite athletes in many sports.

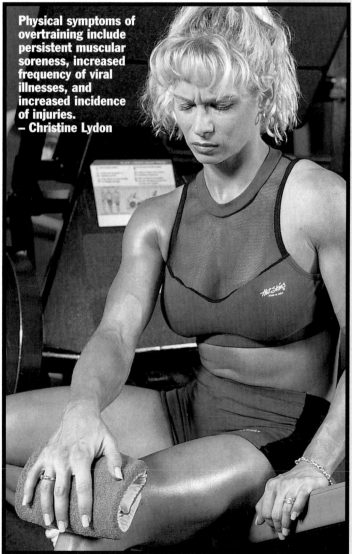

> Physical symptoms of overtraining include persistent muscular soreness, increased frequency of viral illnesses, and increased incidence of injuries.
> – Christine Lydon

Another suggestion is to use a training diary. In addition to keeping track of training volume and intensity, you can record your resting morning heart rate, weight, general health, how the workout felt, and levels of muscular soreness and fatigue. Significant progressive changes in any of these parameters may signal overtraining. Avoiding monotonous training and maintaining adequate nutrition are other recommendations for prevention. Vigorous exercise during the incubation period of a viral illness may increase the duration and severity of that illness. Athletes who feel they are developing a cold should rest or reduce the training schedule for a few days. In fact if you seem to be getting another cold every month or so, or you just can't seem to shake one, that in itself may be a sign of overtraining.

In conclusion, the prevailing wisdom is that it is better to be undertrained than overtrained. A small amount of training will produce some improvement, but too much may set you back. Rest is a vital part of any woman's training, no matter what her level. A well-planned training program involves as much art as science, and should allow for flexibility. Early warning signs of overtraining should be heeded and schedule adjustments made accordingly. Smart training is the path to faster times and good health.

Common Warning Signs of Overtraining
- Mild but prolonged soreness
- Pain in muscles and joints
- Washed-out feeling, tired, drained, lack of energy
- Sudden drop in exercise performance
- Insomnia
- Headaches
- Inability to relax, twitchy, fidgety
- Insatiable thirst, dehydration
- Lowered resistance to common illnesses; colds, sore throat, etc.

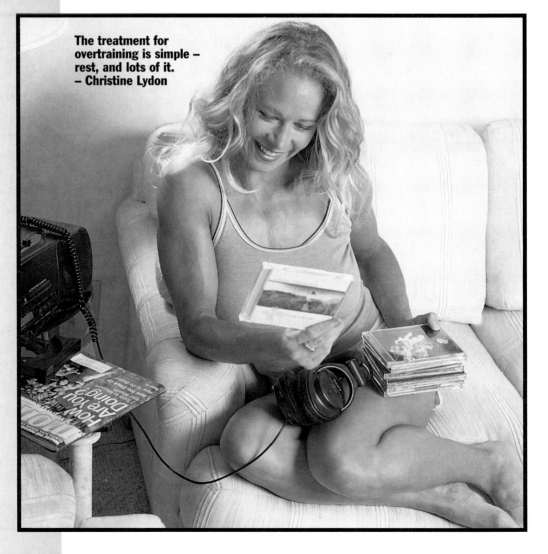

The treatment for overtraining is simple – rest, and lots of it.
– Christine Lydon

What If I Have Some of These Warning Signs?

If you're suffering from several of these warning signs, see your physician so that any potentially serious problem can be ruled out. Otherwise just stop and rest. Take a few days off. Drink plenty of fluids. Check and alter your diet if necessary. Maybe plan an alternative training routine so that you're not constantly working just the same muscle groups. If you don't receive consistent massage work, this would be a good time to get one or two sessions to help flush metabolic wastes out of your system and loosen up.

To prevent further overtraining injuries, check out some of the more common overuse factors associated. You may need to modify all or part of what you're doing.

How to Avoid Overtraining

If you've recently "pumped up" your workout regimen, there are some steps you can take to avoid overtraining.
• Get enough rest. In addition to taking adequate time to recover between workouts, make an extra effort to get a full night's sleep.
• Increase your load slowly. Make incremental changes in the duration and intensity of your exercise sessions. Many experts recommend 10 percent as a weekly target.

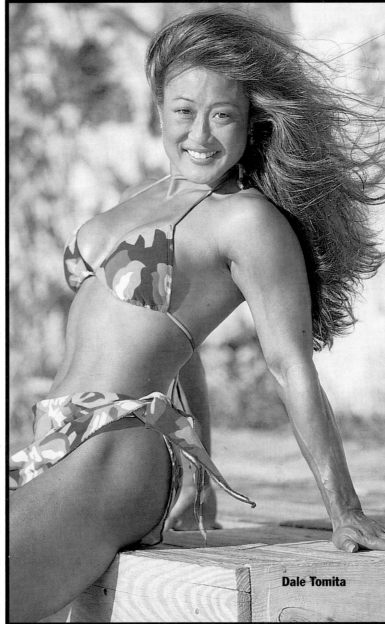

Dale Tomita

• Keep a training diary. By noting factors such as the type of workout (running, swimming, cycling, dancing, etc.), its length and intensity, what you ate that day, how you felt while exercising and so forth, you may reveal important patterns to aid in your recovery.
• Eat a balanced diet that is low in fat and high in complex carbohydrates.
• Alternate intense workouts with lighter exercise sessions and perform a variety of exercise activities.

CHAPTER THIRTEEN

Cardiovascular Training

It's one thing to look like you're in great shape, but something else entirely to be in great shape. Despite our bias toward strength training, the authors are the first to admit that this is only half the battle to developing a fit body. Many readers no doubt have heard their boyfriends or husbands say out loud, "I wonder what he's got under the hood?" while looking at a sports car. In essence your other half is wondering what size engine is powering the car. On the outside there may be chrome and quality galore, but what really counts is the engine powering the vehicle. The human body is much the same. If you limit yourself to weight training you can build a great-looking physique, but what good is it if you can't climb a flight of stairs without gasping for breath? The muscles are only as functional as the engine powering them, which in this case is the cardiovascular system. In fact the better developed your muscles the more nutrient and waste removal demands are placed on the cardiovascular system.

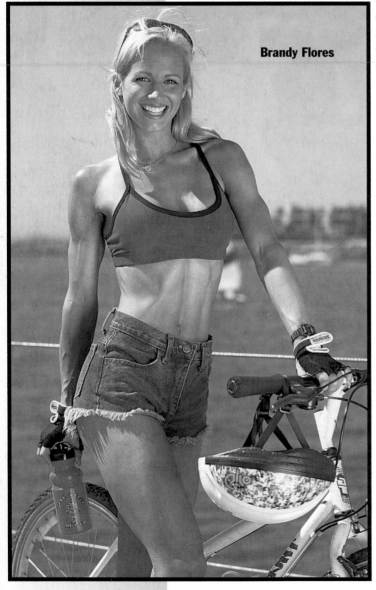

Brandy Flores

For maximum effectiveness and safety, cardiovascular exercise has specific instructions on the *frequency, duration* and *intensity*. These are the three important components of cardiovascular exercise you need to recognize, understand and implement in your program. In addition, your cardiovascular program should include a warmup, a cooldown, and stretching of the primary muscles used in the exercise.

Warm Up Before Stretching

You must not stretch until after your muscles are warm (after blood has circulated through them) – never stretch a cold muscle. First warm up. A warmup should be done for at least five to ten minutes at low intensity. Usually the warmup is done by performing the same activity as the cardiovascular workout but at an intensity of 50 to 60 percent of maximum heart rate (max HR). After you've warmed up sufficiently at a relatively low intensity, your muscles will be ready. To prevent injury and to improve your performance, you should stretch the primary muscles used in the warmup before proceeding to the cardiovascular exercise.

Don't Forget to Cool Down

The cooldown is similar to the warmup in that it should last five to ten minutes and be done at a low intensity (50 to 60 percent of max HR). After you have completed your cardiovascular exercise and cooled down properly, it is now important that you stretch the primary muscles being used. Warming up, stretching and cooling down are very important to every exercise session. These three steps not only help your performance levels and produce better results, but also drastically decrease your risk of injury.

Frequency of Cardio Training

The first component of cardiovascular training is frequency of exercise, which refers to the number of exercise sessions per week. To improve both cardiovascular fitness and to decrease bodyfat or maintain bodyfat at optimum levels, you should exercise at least three days a week. The American College of Sports Medicine recommends three to five days a week for most cardiovascular programs. Those of you who are very out of shape and/or who are overweight and doing weight-bearing cardiovascular exercise such as an aerobics class or jogging, might want to have at least 36 to 48 hours of rest between workouts to prevent an injury and to promote adequate recovery from bone and joint stress.

Duration of Exercise

The second component of cardiovascular exercise is duration, which refers to the length of time spent exercising. Not including the warmup and cooldown, the cardiovascular session should vary from 20 to 60 minutes to gain significant cardiorespiratory and fat-burning benefits. Each time you do your cardiovascular exercise, try for at least 20 minutes or more. Of course, the longer you go the more calories and fat you'll burn and the better you'll condition your cardiovascular

Nicole Rollolazo

system. All beginners, especially those who are out of shape, should take a very conservative approach and train at relatively low intensities (50 to 70 percent max HR) for 10 to 25 minutes. As you get in better shape, you can gradually increase the duration of your sessions.

It is important that you gradually increase the duration before you increase the intensity. That is, when beginning a walking program, for example, be more concerned with increasing the number of minutes per exercise session before you increase the intensity by increasing your speed or walking hilly terrain.

In simple terms remember this: Cardiovascular exercise should be done a minimum of three times a week, 20 minutes per session. Once your muscles are warmed up, and after the cardiovascular exercise and cooldown, you should stretch the muscles you used. For example, after bicycling stretch your quadriceps, hamstrings, calves, hips and lower back. After doing the rowing machine, stretch your legs, back, biceps and shoulders.

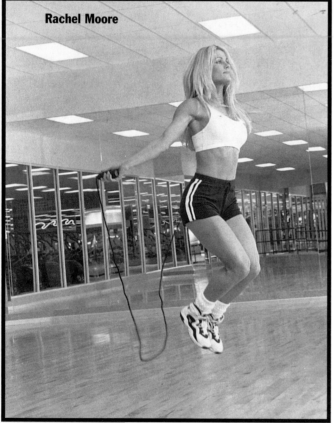

Rachel Moore

Heart Rate

There are two ways in which to check your heart rate during exercise. The most accurate method is to strap a heart-rate monitor around your chest. It will give you feedback on a digital watch that tells you exactly what your heart rate is at a specific time in the exercise session. The other way to obtain your heart rate is by palpating (feeling) either the carotid artery, the temporal artery or the radial artery. The easiest site is usually the carotid or the radial artery. The carotid artery may be felt by gently placing your index finger on your neck, between the middle of your collarbone and jaw line. Palpating the radial artery is done by placing your index and middle fingers on the under side and thumb side of your wrist.

You measure your heart rate in beats per minute (counting the number of beats for 60 seconds). For convenience, many people take their pulse for 6 seconds and multiply that number by 10, or simply add a zero behind the number just obtained. So, if in 6 seconds you count 12 beats, that means your heart rate is 120 beats per minute (bpm). Although counting for 6 seconds is most convenient, keep in mind that the longer the time interval used, the more accurate the results will be. For example, counting your heart rate for 30 seconds and then multiplying that number by 2 will give a slightly more accurate reading than counting your heart rate for 15 seconds and multiplying by 4, or 10 seconds and multiplying by 6. Whatever time interval you use, be consistent.

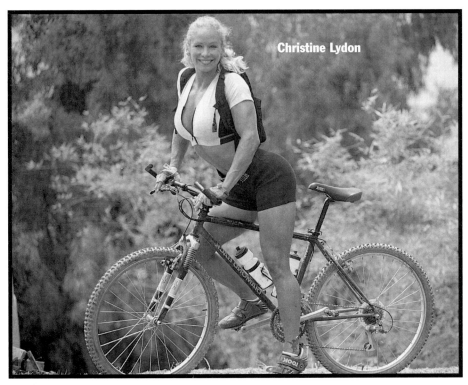

Christine Lydon

Heart Zone Training

How do you know if you are training too intensely or not intensely enough for what you want to achieve? This is where Target Heart Zone training comes in. To use this method you must first determine your maximum heart rate (max HR).

You can determine your max HR in one of two ways. One method is to use the age-predicted max HR formula whereby you subtract your age from 220. If you are 40 years old, your predicted max HR would be 180 bpm. The other method, which is much more accurate and more individualized, is actually to have a medical or fitness professional administer a max HR test for you, which is usually taken on a stationary bicycle or treadmill for several minutes and requires very hard work. Thus, only those cleared by a physician should do this test. No need to explain how to administer this test because only trained professionals should be involved. Please refer to the Global Health and Fitness Personal Training Directory for professionals in your area who are trained in administering a max HR test.

Healthy Heart Zone
The first zone is called the Healthy Heart Zone – 50 to 60 percent of your max HR. This is the easiest and most comfortable zone within which to train and is the one that is best for people who are just starting an exercise program or have low functional capacity. Those of you who are walkers most likely train in this zone. Although this zone has been criticized for not burning enough total calories, and for not being intense enough to get great cardiorespiratory benefits,

it has been shown to help decrease bodyfat, blood pressure and cholesterol. It also decreases the risk of degenerative diseases and has a low risk of injury. In this zone 70 percent of carbohydrates burned (used as energy) come from carbohydrates, 5 percent from protein and 25 percent from fat.

Fitness Zone

Next is the Fitness Zone, which is 60 to 70 percent of your max HR. Once again, 85 percent of your calories burned in this zone are fats, 5 percent protein and 10 percent carbohydrates. Studies have shown that in this zone you can condition your fat mobilization (getting fat out of your cells) while conditioning your fat transportation (getting fat to muscles). Thus, in this zone you are training your fat cells to increase the rate of fat release and training your muscles to burn fat. Therefore, the benefits of this zone are not only the same as the Healthy Heart Zone training at 50 to 60 percent – you are now slightly increasing the total number of calories burned and providing a little more cardiorespiratory benefits. You burn more total calories in this zone simply because it is more intense.

Aerobic Zone

The third zone, the Aerobic Zone, requires that you train at 70 to 80 percent of your max HR. This is the preferred rate if you are training for an endurance event. In this zone your functional capacity will greatly improve and you can expect to increase the number and size of blood vessels, increase your vital capacity and respiratory rate, and achieve increases in pulmonary ventilation, as well as increases in arterial venous oxygen. Moreover, your stroke volume (amount of blood pumped per heartbeat) will increase, and your resting heart rate will decrease.

What does all this mean? It means your cardiovascular and respiratory system will improve and you will increase the size and strength of your heart. In this zone 50 percent of calories burned are from carbohydrates, 50 percent are from fat, and less than 1 percent from protein. And because of the increase in intensity, there is also an increase in the total number of calories burned.

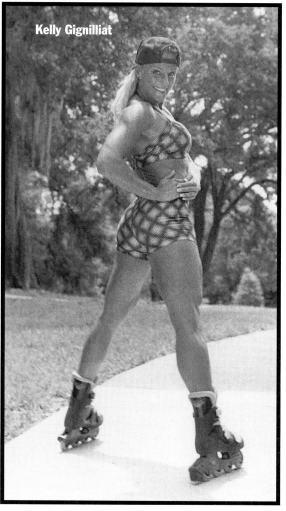

Kelly Gignilliat

Anaerobic Zone

The next training zone is called the Threshold or Anaerobic Zone, which is 80 to 90 percent of your max HR. Benefits include an improved VO2 maximum (the highest amount of oxygen one can consume during exercise), and thus an improved cardiorespiratory system and a higher lactate tolerance ability. Your endurance will improve and you'll be able to fight fatigue better. Since the intensity is high, more calories will be burned in the Anaerobic Zone than within the previous three zones. Although more calories are burned in this zone, 85 percent of the calories burned are from carbohydrates, 15 percent from fat, and less than 1 percent from protein.

Red-Line Zone

The last training zone is called the Redline Zone, which is 90 to 100 percent of your max HR. Remember, training at 100 percent is your maximum heart rate (maximum HR), your heart rate will not get any higher. This zone burns the highest total number of calories and the lowest percentage of fat calories. Ninety percent of the calories burned here are carbohydrates, but only 10 percent are fats and again less than 1 percent is protein. This zone is so intense that very few people can actually endure for the minimum 20 minutes – or even five minutes. (Only those who are in very good shape and have been cleared by a physician should train in this zone). This zone is usually targeted for interval training. For example, one might do three minutes in the Aerobic Zone, one minute in this Redline Zone, then back to the Aerobic Zone. This is called interval training.

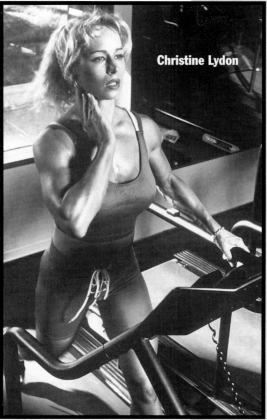

Christine Lydon

Cardiovascular Training: Which Apparatus Do I Use?

The best type of cardio machine is the one that you use regularly! If you find that you especially like one machine, then you are likely to spend more time on it and exercise at a higher intensity. Conversely, if you particularly dislike a machine, you will probably not want to exercise as long or hard on it. Having said that, if your main exercise goal is improved fitness (rather than increased performance in a particular sport) it is beneficial to use a variety of cardiovascular machines in your workout, as long as your heart rate remains in the targeted training zone during the exercise. Add variety to your workout to help prevent overuse injuries that could arise from repetitive joint motion. In addition, each cardiovascular machine places unique stresses and demands on the muscles of your body. Vary the type of stress and the muscles used and you will enjoy the benefits of more balanced muscle development.

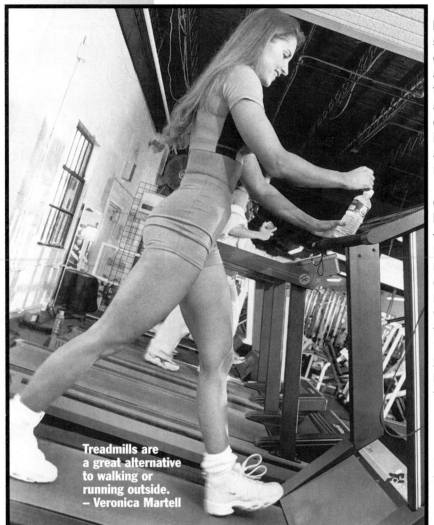

Treadmills are a great alternative to walking or running outside.
– Veronica Martell

That's right, no one should be doing his or her cardio the same way or on the same piece of equipment every week. Just as you need to regularly change the way you perform your resistance exercises, so should you change up your cardio routine, including aerobic classes if they are part of your cardiovascular regimen.

Your gym or workout center should offer at least three basic types of cardio equipment – treadmill, stationary bike and recumbent bike. The three machines work the bodyparts differently. We hope you have many more choices. In selecting which piece you are going to use there are two basic aspects: 1. the degree of difficulty, and 2. the biomechanics, which bodyparts it will exhaust the fastest.

Treadmills

Most novices seem to select the treadmill as their first adventure in cardio training. The treadmill is a great alternative to walking or running outside, especially when it's hot and humid and the last thing you want to do is pass out from heatstroke. The only real problem with the treadmill is finding a gym that's open on a Monday night after work, right? So, how effective are treadmills? Do you get the same benefits as you would from walking or running outside? Here are the answers.

The Good ...

The good news is, walking on the treadmill burns about the same number of calories as walking outside, provided you're walking at the same intensity. Of course, outside you have things like hills and valleys that may boost your calorie expenditure, but you can do the same on the treadmill by simply using those incline buttons.

In some ways a treadmill is better than walking outside. The belt you're walking on is usually a bit more forgiving than the cold hard concrete of the sidewalk, so your legs may thank you. You might want to adjust your incline to about 1 or 2 percent since you don't have any wind resistance to slow you down like outside. You don't want to end up walking faster on the treadmill and a slight incline will help compensate for that.

Another plus of using a treadmill is the fact that you can keep track of your distance and speed much better than you can outside. With the belt moving at a constant pace, you either stay with it or you fall off. Outside it's easy to find yourself strolling rather than briskly walking. Plus, you know exactly how far you've gone on a treadmill and you can at least estimate how many calories you've burned.

Another benefit of the treadmill is you have a place to put your water bottle and Walkman. It's a small matter, but try carrying a bottle of water in your hand while walking outside and you'll see what we mean. Most fitness clubs also provide a bookstand so you can read your way through your 45-minute walk without breaking stride.

According to some studies walking the treadmill burns the most calories and puts the most aerobic demand on the heart and lungs for the same amount of perceived effort on the part of the exerciser. That doesn't mean you can't work as hard on another machine. Remember, it's not necessarily what you're doing, it's how hard you're doing it!

The last reason to hit the treadmill? That's easy! After all, what's more natural than walking? No matter what your fitness level, almost anyone can hop on a treadmill and go for a walk. Some other gym machines are not that forgiving.

The Bad ...

You know why the treadmill is so darn great, but what are the disadvantages? Number one is the sweat factor. When you're on a treadmill indoors, there's no wind resistance. That means you're going to get hotter faster and you're probably going to sweat like a pig. A fan is a must, so beg your gym to place a few fans strategically around the club.

Another bad thing about treadmills is the solitude factor. Unless you can drag a friend with you to talk you through the hard parts of your workout, you're pretty much on your own with nothing to think about except how long this workout is taking. We've seen lots of people throw their towel over the control panel so they don't have to see how long they've been walking. Note: this doesn't work! Each minute will still feel like a lifetime unless you find something to occupy your mind.

And The Ugly ...

What's the worst thing about walking on a treadmill? Boredom wins, hands down. You can only look at your neighbor's rear for so long before you start sinking into a coma. Most clubs have televisions and you can tune in there, which helps. Reading a magazine is also a pleasant way to pass the time, but if you're running on the treadmill, it's almost impossible to follow tiny lines of print with jiggling eyes. A minute can drag on forever on a treadmill, but that just doesn't happen when you're outside. Outside you've got plenty to distract you (the man who just drove by and whistled at you, the pile of dog poop you must try to avoid, etc.) and you're actually going somewhere. Time doesn't stop like it does when you're going nowhere.

Get the Most out of Your Treadmill Workout

Change your intensity. I cannot stress this enough, ladies! Don't just get on there and walk for 30 minutes at 3.0 mph every single day. Those incline buttons were put there for a reason, so start using them! You can mimic going up a hill by increasing your incline 1 percent every 15 or 30 seconds. You can go for a hike by cranking the incline up to 8 or 9 percent. Not only will this variety increase your endurance, it will also decrease your boredom. You always want to monitor your heart rate. Are you in your Target Heart Zone? If not, either you're working too hard (you poor thing ... slow down!) or you're not working hard enough (you mean you're not even sweating?).

Elipticals or Cross-Trainers

Another favorite apparatus is the new "elliptical-style" cardio equipment. These are the new machines that have the steps moving in a circular motion. Many

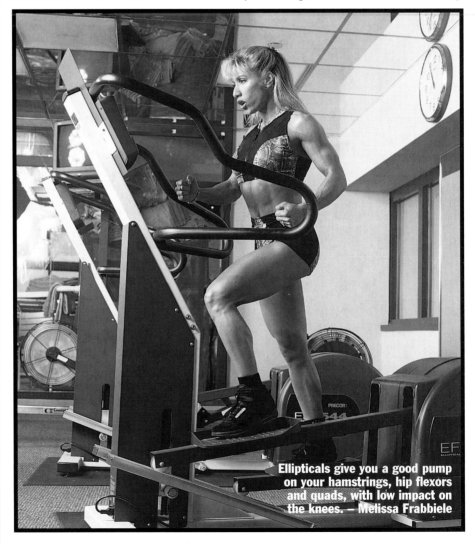

Ellipticals give you a good pump on your hamstrings, hip flexors and quads, with low impact on the knees. — Melissa Frabbiele

different companies are capturing this new craze and for a reason. They give you a good pump on your hamstrings, hip flexors and quads, with low impact on the knees. You can give your heart a good workout while tightening your butt and pumping up your legs. Some companies have added arm movements to the machine which allows you to work the upper body muscles as well. We should add that working the arms probably doesn't add much in the way of extra

cardiovascular stimulation. The legs are such a large muscle group that once they get moving they'll quickly bring your heart rate up to your target zone. Moving the arms doesn't add that much more to the exercise. The one advantage, however, is comfort. Many people find that they must move their arms when exercising the lower body. But then others find it more convenient to grab a stationary handle. Most gyms have both versions, so simply try them out and pick the one you prefer.

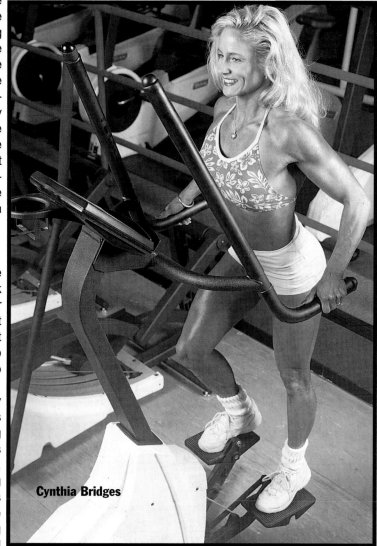

Cynthia Bridges

StairMaster

StairMasters were the rage in the 1980s but have since taken a back seat to the elipticals. StairMaster is actually a trade name and most gyms call them "steppers," but any cardio machine you step up and down on is often referred to as a StairMaster.

The problem for many trainers with these machines is that the up and down stepping motion places tremendous stress on the ankles and knees. After all, the entire bodyweight is pivoting on these two joints. On the plus side the stepper is a very effective piece of equipment for burning bodyfat, improving stamina and endurance, and conditioning the lower body. But it's also probably one of the most poorly executed indoor movements. Most people take short choppy steps while moving and they hold on for dear life. To improve the workout effectiveness take full steps, as if you were climbing real stairs, and pump your arms. But if you find the knees start to take the brunt of the exercise, switch to another type of cardio machine.

Ergometers

The common name for ergometers is "rowers" and a quick glance will tell you why. These are perhaps the simplest cardio machines in terms of size and complexity. Most consist of a long frame on which a sliding seat is mounted. You simply sit in the chair, strap your feet to a set of footrests, and grab a short straight bar connected to a chain and chord wrapped around a circular column. Then, with visions of the great Harvard/Oxford rowing rivalry, you push your body backwards while at the same time pulling the handle into the lower rib cage. Ergometers are to rowing what stationary bikes are to ten-speed cycles; they allow you to mimic an outdoor activity while indoors.

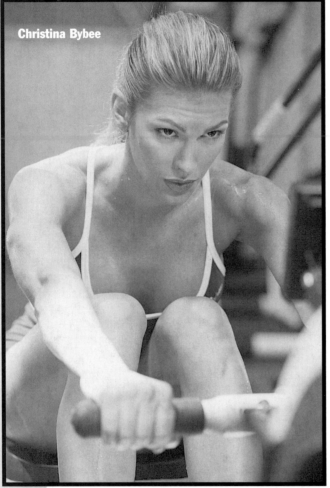

Christina Bybee

Despite their simplicity, rowers are a great way to stimulate the cardiovascular system. The sliding seat also puts less stress on the lower back than a fixed-seat version. The key with rowers is to keep the torso upright at all times. You don't pull with the lower back. Use the thighs, arms and back muscles to do the pulling and sliding.

As a bit of trivia, rowers are among the oldest of cardio machines, and even the fabled *Titanic* had a rowing machine in its gymnasium.

Stationary Cycles

They're simple, they're usually plentiful, and they're probably the oldest of cardio machines. A trip back in time would see stationary cycles as the only piece of cardio equipment found in gyms. In fact most gyms still have a couple of old Monarch bikes kicking around. They are durable and easy to use. No bells or whistles, just a simple tension lever for increasing the resistance on the wheels.

Cycling has numerous benefits, chief of which is its simplicity. Virtually anyone can hop on a bike and start pedaling. For someone carrying a few excess pounds, bikes are great as they support most of your weight. With the exception of the knees and ankles, there is little stress on the body's joints.

For those with pre-existing back and knee problems, most of the major manufacturers now offer recumbent bikes. Instead of the standard upright position, the seat is lower with regard to the pedals. This means you are sitting back with the legs more in front of you than underneath.

Besides manually operated cycles, most gyms have the more elaborate electronic versions. Besides being much larger, electronic bikes have a programmable console that allows you to select different courses with varying degrees of difficulty. Most work by measuring your actual heart rate and comparing it to your theoretical heart rate. The bike then adjusts the tension in the pedals to increase or decrease your heart rate depending on how it compares to your target heart rate. Most programmable cycles also allow you to set a constant tension in the pedals. (For perhaps the ultimate in indoor cycling see Spinning in Chapter Twenty-Four.)

Variety

Most indoor machines offer a variety of program options, so try to avoid the habit of always punching in the same level of intensity and duration. By mixing up your workout routine, you'll stimulate your body differently and train all levels of energy systems. You should also do other activities throughout the week. This will help you develop a more toned physique overall and reduce your risk of repetitive-stress injuries. Plus, watch out for boredom! Most exercisers have no difficulty going for a two-hour bike ride outside, but after 10 minutes on a stationary bike or treadmill you can go stir-crazy. The more fun you make it the more consistent you'll be.

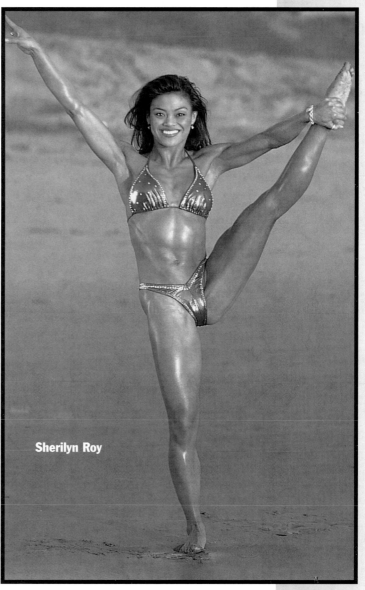

Sherilyn Roy

CHAPTER FOURTEEN

Staying Motivated

I no longer have the time. My job takes all my energy. It's not in my budget. Am I really getting anywhere? Any of these excuses sound familiar? It is usually easy to acknowledge a barrier, but the best solution is always the simplest. So instead of visualizing the barrier, look for a way through it. You don't have the time? Why? How much time do you spend watching TV? Do you sleep in on weekends? Could you squeeze in a workout early in the morning before work?

I don't have the money for a gym membership. Seriously? Most gyms are going to cost you around $2 or $3 a day. If you brown bag it to work, you'll have the money. If not, buy some gym equipment, alone or with a friend, and work out at home. Ask the gym owner if you can work off your membership. And it doesn't cost anything to go walking.

With the exception of those with serious health problems or living in the depths of poverty, there is nothing to stop most of you from getting off your backside and lifting some weights or going for a walk. Those buns aren't going to tighten up all by themselves. There is a look you want to achieve, a level of fitness you desire. That's why you're reading this book.

"Most people are more deeply influenced by one clear, vivid, personal example than by an abundance of statistical data."
– Eliot Aronson, social psychologist.

"I want it all, and I want it covered in chocolate."
– bumper sticker.

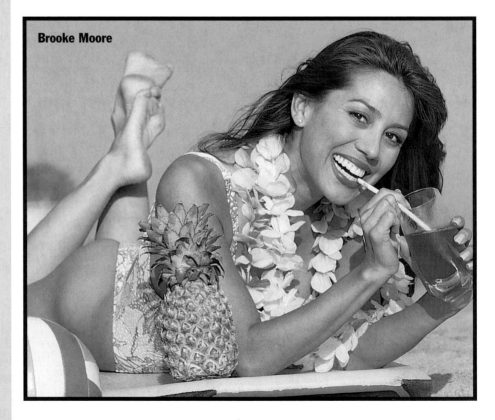

Brooke Moore

The other chapters cover diet and training. Chapter Fourteen examines how to overcome the mental challenges faced by a person who is out of shape and wants to change. Motivating yourself is based on the following concepts:

1. Training is the catalyst for change.
2. What you don't know, training will teach you.
3. Each exercise is measured in single reps.
4. Focus on where you are going, not on where you have been.
5. Failure is not a crime. Failing to learn from failure is a crime.
6. It's not the difficulties in life, but how you deal with them.
7. Aim high.

"I've had a wonderful time, but this wasn't it."
– Groucho Marx (1895-1977)

Training is the Catalyst for Change

Training changes your life. Once you start exercising, your body experiences physical changes. So does your personality. It's subtle at first. Your body resists. Muscles that haven't been used for a long time will quickly let you know they are not amused! Everyone feels sore at first, but after a couple of weeks you begin to feel refreshed. You sleep better.

Your priorities change. Once you decide your body has value, you find you start making other lifestyle changes. Smokers quit smoking. Late nights and booze just don't jive with early morning workouts. Junk food doesn't satisfy you the way healthful foods do. Best of all, your old clothes no longer fit! And you make friends with people who understand the importance of good physical health. This peer group becomes a new social network you can turn to for guidance and friendship. There is a very simple litmus test for a "healthy gym." It should meet the following three conditions:

Torrie Wilson

1. The atmosphere is informal, comfortable and relaxed. No one wants to work out in a gym full of prima donnas who are out to show how they're better than everyone else, or anyone who expects that the moment they arrive they own the equipment you're using. Everyone should be equal, or it's not going to work.
2. There is a lot of discussion in which everyone participates. Socializing is the best part of going to the gym! Joking around, gossiping, talking politics and business ... It's all part of the rich atmosphere that turns the gym into a mini-vacation.

3. The goal of fitness is well understood and accepted. It's a gym, not a meat market. There are places for that sort of thing. If you find yourself attracted to someone, start up a casual conversation and mention where you're going later. If the other person is interested, you'll find out. But otherwise, focus on improving your body, not using it.

What You Don't Know, Training Will Teach You

How long should I jog? What should I lift? How many stretches should I do? This book provides guidelines, but every person is different. Your body will teach you about what it can and cannot do. As you train, you will also learn to observe those around you. Exercise is both science and art, and the ability to do something is not as important as how you do it. Being able to do 50 situps is not a great achievement if you do them wrong – or worse, if you injure your back in the process!

> *"I have not failed. I've just found 10,000 ways that won't work."*
> – *Thomas Alva Edison (1847-1931)*

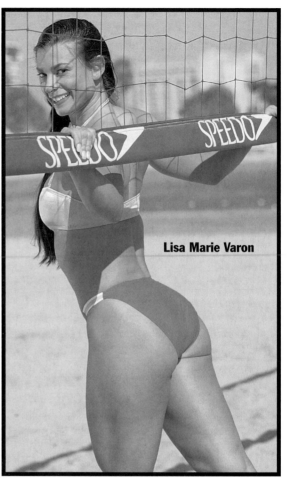

Lisa Marie Varon

Each Exercise is Measured in Single Reps

Training is a commitment. You just don't join a gym and two weeks later go from XL to a size small. Getting in shape is a gradual, long-term process. To put it in perspective, no one goes to university with the expectation of walking out after two weeks with a degree. It takes a minimum of three years of study to achieve that goal. Training is no different. You will not become a fitness goddess overnight. You must struggle through the early days, being satisfied with very small achievements. But even if you do just one single rep, that accomplishment is still more than if you had not tried. Gradually, as your body adapts, your movements will become more fluid and you will break through these early plateaus.

Don't wallow in the past. It's too easy to think about all the times you cheated on a diet, or gave up on working out. Think about what you want to look like, and what you want to be doing with that new body. By focusing on what will be, you keep a positive attitude where you never give up.

To maintain that focus, keep a daily journal. Record what you ate, what you lifted, how far you ran, how fast, what you weighed. You will see concrete evidence of your progress. The changes may be very small, but over time they become impressive. Remember to focus on the performance and not on personal qualities. The idea is to dwell on how you can improve your body. Personal traits make us individuals. How much we can change, and whether we should, is more a matter of how you fit in with society. If you can change for the better, great! If you can at least not get any worse, then join the club!

Failure is Not a Crime ... Failing to Learn From Failure is a Crime

If it doesn't work, stop! Doing an exercise because that hot trainer "Gunther" said you should do it that way (and you hate it) is stupid! You won't hurt Gunther's feelings. Don't do it if it doesn't feel comfortable. The idea is to keep training. If you don't like what you're doing, pretty soon you will find all kinds of excuses to avoid going to the gym.

"The artist is nothing without the gift, but the gift is nothing without work."
– Emile Zola (1840-1902)

"Success usually comes to those who are too busy to be looking for it."
– Henry David Thoreau (1817-1862)

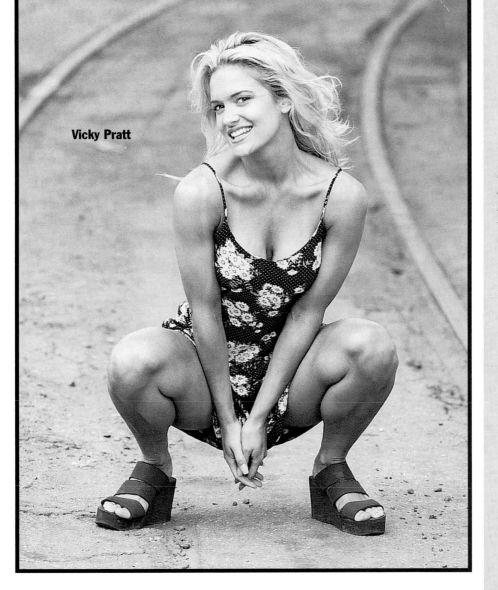

Vicky Pratt

It's Not the Difficulties in Life, But How You Deal With Them

If it can go wrong, it will. That doesn't mean you have to give up on yourself. People get the flu but they recover. So you're out of the gym for two weeks – get back into it gradually. You won't be able to start from where you left off, but you'll catch up pretty fast. Remember that people used to die from the flu. Thanks to medicine and good nutrition, we survive, but it still exhausts the immune system. Give your body time to recover.

Relationships and jobs will hit rocky points – they may even end. The best you can do is part ways with dignity. As we age, we change our expectations and priorities. Sometimes those changes result in a relationship or job that no longer fits. The one constant throughout these difficult periods will be your body. And good physical health has been shown to prevent, or at least alleviate, mental health issues. Emotional turmoil will send adrenaline hurtling through your body. By working out, you allow your body to deal with the chemical results, and prevent stress from harming your body. In the long term, both your mind and your body will be stronger.

> *"If you are going through hell, keep going."*
> – Sir Winston Churchill
> (1874-1965)

> *"Fill what's empty, empty what's full, and scratch where it itches."*
> – The Duchess of Windsor, when asked what is the secret of a long and happy life.

Aim High

Always have incredible goals. You may never climb Mt. Everest, and so what? The idea is to train like you are planning to. Visualize yourself achieving incredible feats. Ever thought about jogging the entire length of the Great Wall of China? How about swimming the St. Lawrence Seaway?

Without a goal you have no direction. But that lofty dream shapes your short-term goals. I'm going to have shapely buns in nine months. I'm going to have a smaller waistline in a year. I'm going to be able to jog two miles by next year. Slowly, even if it takes a lifetime, you will get closer to that incredible goal. And if you can dedicate the rest of your life to regular training, that in itself will be a worthwhile achievement.

Laura Mak

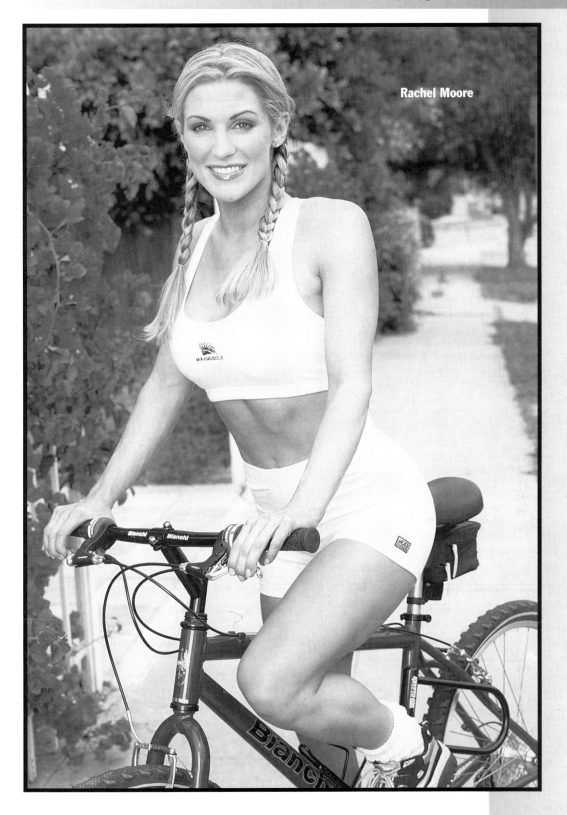

Rachel Moore

CHAPTER FIFTEEN

Getting "Back" At It!

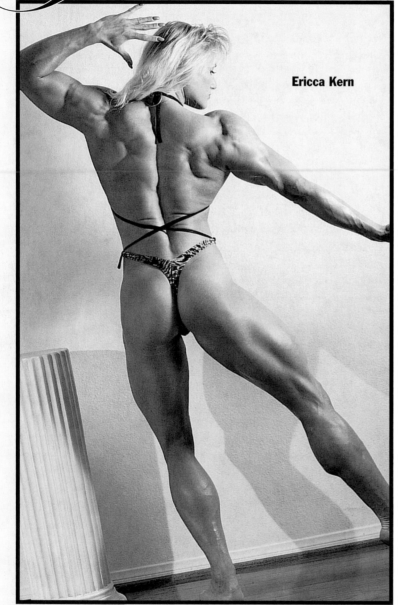

Ericca Kern

Anatomy and Function

For bodybuilders the back can be the decisive muscle group that wins the contest. For women a good back can help create the illusion of a smaller waist. Unfortunately, despite its importance, this muscle group is often neglected. The back is really a collection of muscles that cover the entire dorsal region of the torso. The largest muscles are the triangle-shaped latissimus dorsi – the lats. The lats give the back its characteristic V-shape and run from the armpits to the center of the spine, to the lumbar or lower back region. The primary function of the lats is to draw the arms toward the body and downward from an overhead position.

Assisting the lats are various smaller muscles including the teres (major and minor) and the rhomboids. Both these muscles attach to the lats around the shoulder blade (scapula) region. Besides helping the lats move the arms, they also help move and stabilize the shoulder blades.

Located at the very top of the back are the trapezius – the traps. Even though the traps are anatomically part of the back musculature, most people train them with shoulders (most traps exercises seem to stimulate more shoulder muscles than back muscles). The traps are triangle-shaped and run from the base of the neck to the midspine. Their main function is to elevate and rotate the shoulder-girdle complex.

Finally we have the two long chord-like spinal erector muscles located at the base and center of the torso. Even though the lats and traps are the larger, more impressive muscles, it's the spinal erectors that play the biggest role in a healthy life. A profound statement to be sure, but the lower back probably causes more grief than all the other areas combined. It seems half the population has "back problems." In this chapter we are going to show you how to keep yours healthy.

Training

With the exception of the spinal erectors, back-training can be divided into two primary types of exercises, widening and thickening. Widening exercises hit more of the outer edges of the lats and do the most to highlight the much sought after V-shape. The best exercises for width are different variations of chinups and pulldowns.

Thickening exercises are those that hit the center parts of the lats, as well as the teres, rhomboids, and to a lesser extent the traps. The best thickening exercises are rowing movements such as seated rows, one-arm dumbell rows and barbell rows.

We should add that all widening movements hit the center back muscles, and all rowing exercises activate the outer lats. Total isolation is impossible, but it is possible to stimulate different regions of the back by varying your training.

Back-Training With the Stars

Brandy Maddron

Brandy Maddron's story is one of the most inspiring in female fitness. At one time she was a frightening 71 pounds – the result of a teenage bout with anorexia. At 5'3" she was about 45 pounds short of her ideal weight. With low self-esteem problems to begin with, it took a lot of courage, determination and fortitude for Brandy to walk into a gym. In three months she gained over 70 pounds, but unfortunately much of it wasn't in the form of muscle. The same people who expressed negativity about her previous body form were now telling her she still looked unhealthy at the new weight.

Brandy Maddron

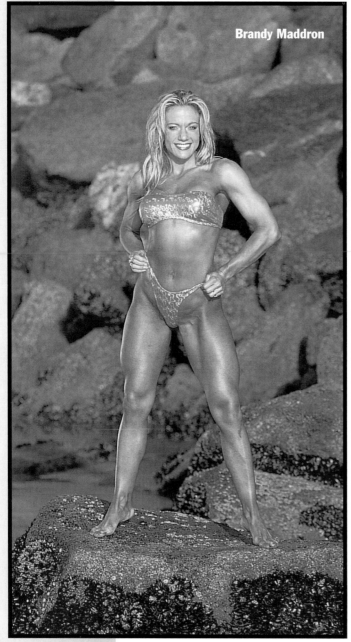

Brandy Maddron

At this point many people would succumb to the yo-yo effect and fall back into the clutches of anorexia, but Brandy was made of tougher stuff. For the next two years she engaged in an aerobics-only program, being careful not to become too obsessive or extreme about her training. One of the best things that could have happened to her was meeting Aaron Maddron. Not only was she convinced to start weight training, but Brandy also found her future husband in the process!

After just six months of training Brandy entered her first bodybuilding contest. When she looks back now she realizes she looked pretty skinny, but compared to the 70 pounds she weighed when suffering from anorexia, she was the picture of health. Realizing she didn't have the potential to gain the muscle mass necessary for bodybuilding, Brandy switched to competitive fitness – where she won her first two contests.

Brandy's back is one of her best bodyparts. That's not surprising given her approach to training. Where many women rely on cables and pulleys, Brandy relies on basic exercises using heavy weights. A typical back workout will see her choose four exercises to address width, shape, depth and detail.

Brandy usually starts with that king of back exercises, pullups. Like most women she has trouble lifting her bodyweight, but she still manages to do 3 sets of 6 to 8 reps. If she can't complete the set she'll have a training partner give her a few forced reps.

Brandy's second back exercise is standing cable rows. Rather than perform the standard seated cable row, she prefers to stand up and use a rope. To minimize back stress Brandy always keeps her back slightly curved and not rounded. Sometimes she pulls the rope ends to the sides of her body; other workouts she pulls to the center of her body.

To make sure both sides of her back are receiving equal stimulation, Brandy performs one-arm dumbell rows as her third exercise. Again she does 3 sets of 6 to 8 reps, making sure to keep her back slightly arched.

To finish off her back, Brandy does 3 sets of either stiff-leg deadlifts or good mornings. In either case she keeps a slight bend at the knees to reduce lower back stress. Brandy feels the lower back is one of the keys to overall physical health, as most exercises rely on the lower back muscles to a greater or lesser degree.

Brandy's Back Workout
1. Pullups – 3 sets x 6 to 8 reps
2. Standing rope cable rows – 3 sets x 6 to 8 reps
3. One-arm dumbell rows – 3 sets x 6 to 8 reps
4. Stiff-leg deadlifts – 3 sets x 6 to 8 reps

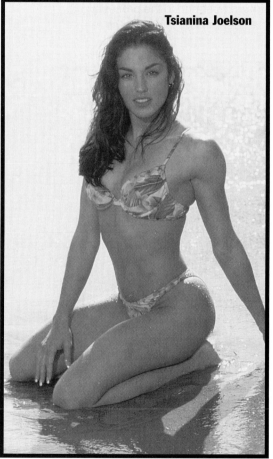

Tsianina Joelson

Tsianina Joelson's Fitness American Back

It started with baton twirling at age 9; progressed to volleyball and cheerleading by high school. Within a few years the relatively unknown Tsianina Joelson had captured the prestigious Fitness America Pageant over 120 other talented hopefuls in 1997. Tsianina almost purposely missed the America Fitness Pageant when she observed the size and muscularity of the competitors in another contest a few weeks before. But her husband convinced her that she had a good routine and was in great shape, and she reconsidered. The outcome is now in the history books.

Since winning the Fitness America Tsianina's career has exploded – from photo shoots and magazine coverage to public appearances and guest posing. The biggest change in her life has been the launching of her own fitness show – *Daily Burn*. With her vast knowledge of fitness and outstanding physique, Tsianina serves as an inspiration to millions of women everywhere.

During her competitive days Tsianina was known for her wide back. In fact it reached the point where she had to cut back on training to keep it in proportion with other muscle groups.

Tsianina is not a slave to rigid programming, and to use her own words, "I like to feel my way through workouts." She's a great believer in instinctive training. Sometimes she'll perform straight sets and reps, other days she may mix things up with a few supersets.

Over the course of many years, Tsianina has evaluated just about every conceivable back exercise and what areas they hit. Early in her training she was trying to add size and shape to the whole back region so she blended a mix of widening and thickening exercises. Nowadays she feels her back needs additional width so she opts for more pulldowns and pullups.

Tsianina usually starts her back-training with pulldowns. For variety she alternates wide and narrow grips, and on occasion adds in a reverse grip. She does 4 sets of 12 to 20 reps but as competition draws near she increases the reps and picks up the pace.

With her back fully warmed up Tsianina moves on to pullups. She admits she has never found this exercise easy and must work at trying to perfect the movement. Tsianina considers pullups a great overall upper-body movement as the abs, shoulders and lower back all come into play. Unlike pulldowns, Tsianina maintains a wide grip on all 4 sets of pullups. She does 8 reps on the first 2 sets and tries to get 6 on the last 2 sets.

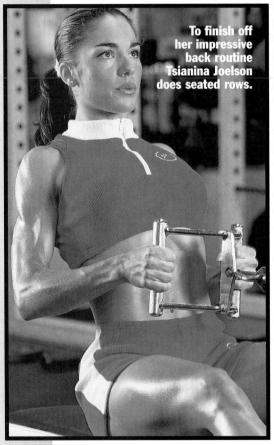

To finish off her impressive back routine Tsianina Joelson does seated rows.

For her third exercise Tsianina performs one-arm dumbell rows. Of all the back exercises, one-arm rows are her favorite. She finds she can isolate the lats best with this one. She also likes the fact that you can isolate the lats one side at a time, which helps give her feedback on whether one side is weaker than the other (something almost impossible to do with two-arm back exercises). Tsianina performs one-arm rows in a slow and controlled manner and does 4 sets of 15 to 20 reps.

To finish off her impressive back Tsianina does seated rows. As the previous three exercises hit more of the outer lats, she does seated rows with a narrow grip to hit the inner portion of the back. Tsianina stresses that, to get the most out of this exercise, you must squeeze the shoulder blades together and arch the chest as you pull the handle toward the lower rib cage. She also recommends developing a good muscle-mind link as the arms try to dominate this movement. Even though it's her last exercise she still does 4 sets of 15 to 20 reps.

Tsianina Joelson's Back Routine
1. Pulldowns – 4 sets x 12 to 20 reps
2. Pullups – 4 sets x 6 to 8 reps
3. One-arm rows – 4 sets x 15 to 20 reps
4. Seated rows – 4 sets x 15 to 20 reps

Debbie Kruck

Along with Marla Duncan and Mia Finnegan, Debbie Kruck is one of the founding members of fitness. There were fitness shows back in the 1980s, but it was the 1990s that saw the explosion we now recognize as modern fitness championships. Debbie started training when she was only 12, and her early start paid big dividends in 1989 and 1990 when she won the coveted Fitness USA and the Fitness America Championships.

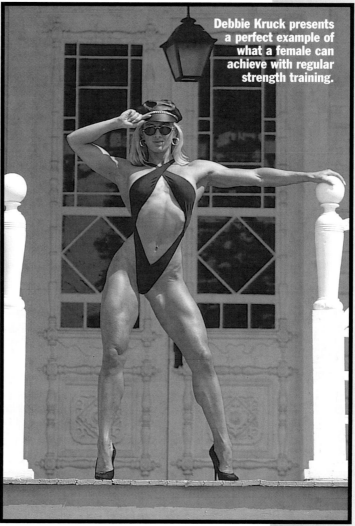

Debbie Kruck presents a perfect example of what a female can achieve with regular strength training.

Watch Debbie onstage and you'll easily see why many of today's fitness stars have been influenced by her physique. From her wide shoulders and stunning back, down to her miniscule waist, Debbie presents a perfect example of what a female can achieve with regular strength training.

Debbie is famous for her back. She attributes much of its size and shape to many years of doing little more than chins and pulldowns. She also varied the grips from wide and narrow to reverse, and used special attachments. Those two basic exercises evolved into six to eight variations.

Debbie trained her back once or twice per week. She usually selected four or five exercises and did 4 sets of each. This high-volume approach is frowned upon by some, but she found it did wonders for her back. Let's take a look at a typical Debbie Kruck workout to see just what it takes to build a championship back.

Debbie usually started her back workout with chinups. For most of her career she did them on an overhead chinning bar using the previously mentioned wide, narrow and reverse grips. Later she adopted a more unorthodox approach to chinning. She'd go over to the pulldown machine and put significantly more plates on the stack than she weighed. She'd then do chins while holding on to the pulldown bar. Debbie is the first to admit that this form of chins is only suited to advanced trainers. A typical workout would see Debbie perform 4 or 5 sets of chins, but there were times when she'd keep going until she was only getting 4 or 5 reps per set. That's a total of 8 to 10 sets of chins!

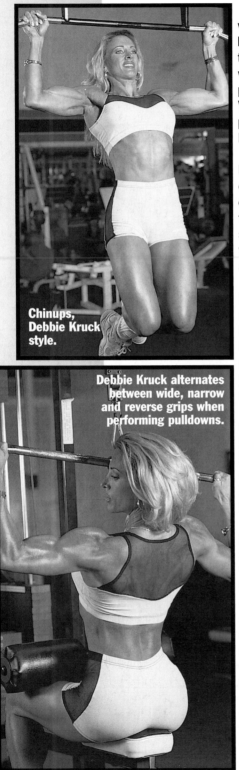

Chinups, Debbie Kruck style.

Debbie Kruck alternates between wide, narrow and reverse grips when performing pulldowns.

After chinups Debbie moved on to another favorite widening exercise, pulldowns. Again the grips alternated between wide, narrow and reverse. Debbie was exceptionally strong on this exercise and 4 sets with 140 pounds was normal. On occasion she even went up to 200 pounds for a couple of reps just to check her strength. When you realize that most men can't do a 200-pound pulldown, you get an indication of how strong Debbie Kruck really was.

With two basic width movements out of the way, Debbie next moved on to her thickening exercises. She often started with T-bar rows, and as with pulldowns and chins, alternated between a wide and narrow grip. She typically did 4 sets of 12 reps, using as much weight as she could handle. Debbie adds that rows are exercises where the arms want to take over. You need great focus and concentration to isolate the lats.

For her second width exercise (fourth overall) Debbie did upright seated rows. The exercise is performed on a special machine that enables you to rest your chest against an upright pad and hold on to two vertical handles. Unlike regular seated cable rows this machine takes the stress off the lower back. Pull the handles toward you until your elbows are slightly behind the torso. Debbie usually did 4 sets of 12 reps.

To finish off her back, Debbie performed one-arm dumbell rows. Leaning over with one knee and hand braced on a bench, she'd pull the dumbell up until it was in line with her chest. The weight was then lowered until her arm was just short of a lockout. Debbie usually did one heavy set of 8 to 10 reps and 3 sets with a lighter weight for 10 to 15 reps.

Mia Finnegan

Mia Finnegan has a knockout physique from every viewpoint – but her symmetry and muscle tone was not built in a day. She had to spend thousands of hours in the gym balancing out weak bodyparts. Like most former competitive gymnasts (from the age of 6 all the way up to college) Mia was left with a world class set of legs, but a small (albeit muscular) upper body. When she decided to venture into the highly critical worlds of bodybuilding and fitness, Mia knew she had to bring up her upper body. One area that needed special attention was her back. Through trial and error Mia discovered that the high-volume style of physique training worked best for her. Heavy weights and few sets may do it for some, but in her case only many sets using moderate weight did the trick.

Another Finnegan discovery was, to complement her fitness routine, she had to have functional muscle – not just "all show and no go." In terms of training this meant primarily doing compound power movements as opposed to isolation exercises.

A typical Finnegan back workout began with an extensive warmup – so extensive that many people would call it a workout in itself. She first did 4 sets of lower-back extensions for 12 to 15 reps, then an equal number of hanging pelvic tilts to loosen the lower part of her back even further. Then, as if this were not enough, she threw in 3 sets of chinups on an assisted chinup machine (i.e. Gravitron). She used the offset resistance to prevent total fatiguing of her back but at the same time make the muscle work slightly. Only after she felt her back was fully warmed up and filled with blood would Mia start her primary back-training.

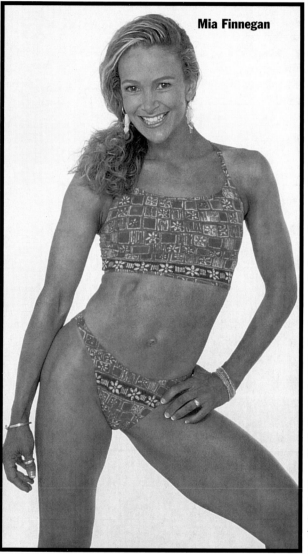

Mia Finnegan

For her first back exercise Mia did wide-grip chinups to failure. On a typical day she could do 16 or 17 reps on the first set, then lose a couple of reps with each set until she was just managing to complete 12 on the third set.

With her back reaching the point where it could no longer do chinups, Mia switched over to wide-grip pulldowns. She always pulled the bar to the front. She considers the behind-the-head version too hard on the rotator cuff. Mia would do 4 sets of pulldowns, adding weight with each set, going from 80 to 100 pounds.

With these two basic widening exercises out of the way, Mia moved on to her first center-back exercise, seated pulley rows. Mia found this movement great for the rhomboids and lower lats. Pulling the weight to the lower rib cage, she concentrated on squeezing her shoulder blades together. She would use about 70 pounds on her first set, then add 10 pounds per set until she reached 90 pounds for 2 sets of 8 to 12 reps.

On those days when she had the extra time and energy, Mia would add in 4 sets of standing cable rows. Again she emphasized keeping her back straight and not bouncing at the bottom of the movement.

"Most women think that if they start working out they will become muscular like a professional body-builder. What they don't realize is that it takes a lot of hard work to put on even a small amount of quality muscle."
– *top fitness competitor and regular* Oxygen *contributor Mia Finnegan, reassuring women that they won't gain huge amounts of muscle from a regular weight-training program.*

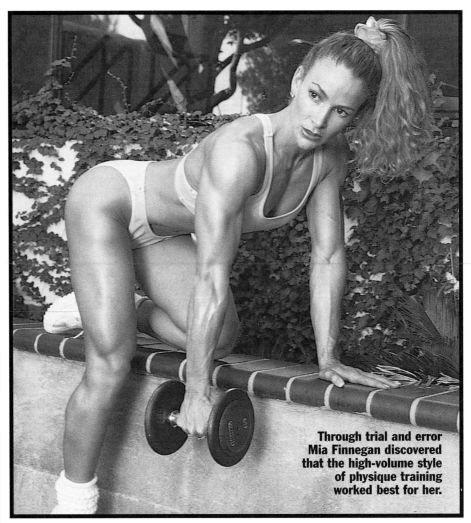

Through trial and error Mia Finnegan discovered that the high-volume style of physique training worked best for her.

To finish off her back, Mia performed one-arm dumbell rows. With one knee and hand braced on a flat bench, Mia would lower the dumbell down and forward slightly for a good stretch, then pull upward until her upper arm was parallel with the floor. She usually performed 3 sets of 12 to 15 reps.

Mia Finnegan's Back Routine
Warmup sets:
1. Back extensions – 4 sets x 12 to 15 reps
2. Hanging pelvic tilts – 4 sets x 12 to 15 reps
3. Chinups on Gravitron – 3 sets x 12 to 15 reps
Working sets:
1. Wide-grip chinups – 3-4 sets x 12 to 17 reps
2. Wide-grip pulldowns – 4 sets x 8 to 12 reps
3. Seated cable rows – 4 sets x 8 to 12 reps
4. Standing cable rows (optional) – 4 sets x 8 to 12 reps
5. One-arm dumbell rows – 3 sets x 12 to 15 reps

Kelly Ryan

In a way we're not surprised Kelly Ryan has achieved so much so fast. At one time she was a top gymnastic prospect training under the tutelage of famed coach Bela Karoyli. For those you who don't recognize the name, Bela is the Romanian coach who helped Nadia Comaneci score perfects 10s at the 1976 Olympic Games in Montreal. From the age of 5 until 13, Kelly tumbled her way toward Olympic destiny, but gave up the sport when she realized just how much pressure was involved. Instead she turned her athletic prowess to other disciplines including cheerleading, volleyball and track and field. When fitness gained recognition as a legitimate sport in the 1990s, Kelly knew her vast athletic talents would propel her to the top. And you know something? She was right. Within a couple of years she had won the 2000 Arnold Classic, Ms. Fitness International, and runner-up in the 1999 Ms. Olympia – her first IFBB show!

Nowadays Kelly's back is one of her outstanding bodyparts but it wasn't always that way. Like many former gymnasts, Kelly's lower body had far outstripped her upper body in terms of size and strength. As soon as she knew fitness was to be a big part of her future, Kelly set to work to improve her upper body.

With regard to her back, Kelly found that her inner back responded quicker than her outer back. As the V-taper is one of the most important parts of any great physique, Kelly modified her routine to stress her outer lats. She also changes her routine on a frequent basis to keep the muscles guessing. Finally Kelly always starts her workout with back-training. That way she can put most of her energy into the area.

A typical Kelly Ryan back workout starts with perhaps the best widening exercise there is, pullups. Kelly includes both wide- and narrow-grip pullups in her training. She primarily uses the exercise as a warmup, but on many occasions will throw in a few sets at the end of her back workout, usually 3 to 4 sets of 12 reps.

Kelly's second back exercise is seldom seen – reverse cable flyes. Kelly stands between a cable crossover machine and grasps a handle in each hand. She then pulls her elbows behind her torso. Unlike conventional pulldowns, which bring a lot of biceps into play, Kelly finds this exercise can be done with little biceps involvement. Kelly typically does 3 or 4 sets of 12 reps.

Kelly's third back exercise is two-arm dumbell rows. She prefers the two-arm version to the traditional one-arm version, although she's the first to admit it – you have to pay extra attention to form as there's no lower-back support. Kelly leans forward until her torso is about 45 degrees from horizontal, and keeps her knees slightly bent. She then pulls both dumbells up until they're in line with her hips. Again she does 3 or 4 sets of 12 reps.

Kelly's fourth back exercise is low cable rows using the rope attachment. Again you must watch the lower back as you pull the rope to the lower rib cage.

"I prioritize my lats first in almost any routine because that V-taper is what's so desirable to judges. I also watch my form to make sure I'm pulling with just my lats and not with my biceps."
– top fitness competitor Kelly Ryan, commenting on the importance of form and order when it comes to training her lats.

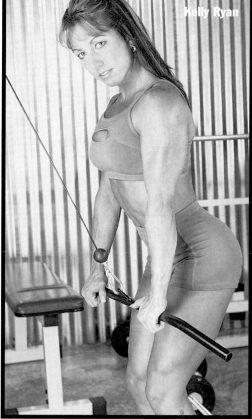
Kelly Ryan

Kelly prefers the rope because it allows her to pull through a slightly greater range of motion. This adds a few extra degrees of contraction to the lats. You guessed it. She does 3 or 4 sets of 12 reps.

To finish off her back routine, Kelly does straight-arm pushdowns (sometimes referred to as cable pullovers). Standing about two feet from the weight stack she grabs a straight bar connected to an overhead pulley. With her arms locked straight out, she pushes the weight down until the bar is an inch or two from her thighs. She then raises the bar upward as high as possible (which in most cases is limited by the height of the weight column). Kelly finds this exercise great for working the lats up high in the armpit region, as well as bringing out her serratus. As with all her back exercises, she does 3 or 4 sets, 12 reps per set.

Kelly Ryan's Back Workout
1. Pullups – 3 or 4 sets x 12 reps
2. Reverse cable flyes – 3 or 4 sets x 12 reps
3. Two-arm dumbell rows – 3 or 4 sets x 12 reps
4. Standing cable rows – 3 or 4 sets x 12 reps
5. Pullovers – 3 or 4 sets x 12 reps

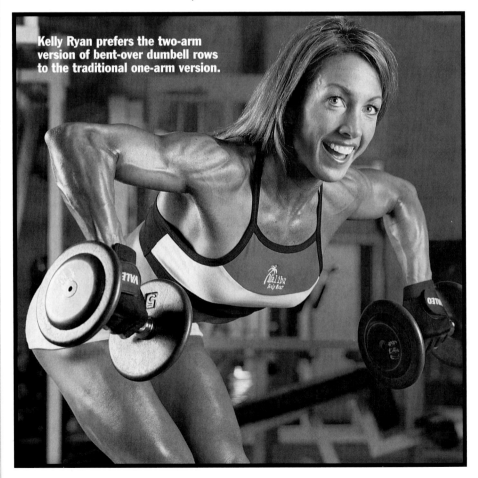

Kelly Ryan prefers the two-arm version of bent-over dumbell rows to the traditional one-arm version.

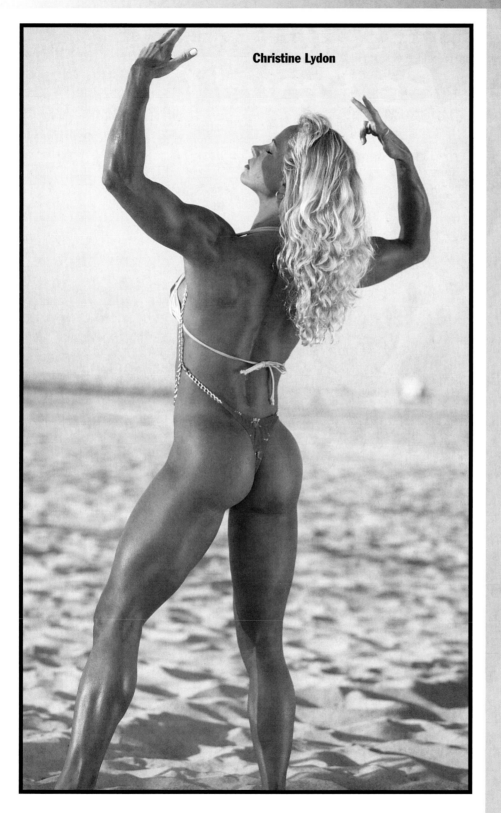

Christine Lydon

CHAPTER SIXTEEN

A Chest to Be Proud Of

Anatomy and Function

With the possible exception of the biceps, the chest is probably the most trained muscle in gyms, particularly among the male segment of the population. And women are not immune to chest favoritism, as a well-developed pectoral base helps to uplift and highlight the breasts.

There are numerous reasons why the chest receives so much attention. For one thing you can't miss it. It's right up there in front of you for all to see, whether you're trying to impress the guys or girls. The back, on the other hand, is sometimes "out of sight, out of mind."

Another reason for focusing on the chest is its importance in sports. Just about every form of athletic endeavor requires a good strong set of pectorals.

Finally, the chest is the primary muscle used in that most famous of exercises – the barbell bench press. Somehow "how much you can bench" is a right of passage, especially for guys. The fact that other chest exercises are probably just as effective seems to get overlooked. Hoisting a couple of hundred pounds off the supine body is part of the gym experience.

The chest is composed of two muscles (or four, depending on your point of view). The larger outer pectoralis major are by far the main part of the chest and appear as two fans starting from the collarbone and extending about a third of the way down the front torso. The smaller underlying pectoralis minor serve more to assist the larger pectorals major than take a leading role. In any case the primary function of both pectorals major and minor is to draw the arms forward and together. They are the primary pressing muscles of the upper body.

Training

Chest exercises can generally be divided into upper and lower movements. As time goes on and weaknesses develop, you can add exercises to your program to hit the inner, outer and pec-delt tie-in. Hitting the lower or upper chest is not so much a case of doing different exercises as modifying the angle of the bench you are using. Exercises performed on a flat bench

Gabrielle Resnick

(horizontal with the floor) primarily target the lower pecs. Increase the angle toward vertical and you will start bringing in the upper chest. Although it depends on the individual, generally speaking most people find an angle between 20 and 45 degrees best. Anything higher than 45 degrees seems to stimulate too much deltoids.

Besides playing with the angle, you can also vary the type of equipment you use. Barbells and dumbells are best for building a good foundation, while cables and machines make great finishing movements. A good chest routine should incorporate exercises from all categories of equipment.

Dr. Christine Lydon

Since she retired from competitive bodybuilding and started putting her talents to writing, Christine Lydon has modified her chest-training considerably. When she first started training Dr. Lydon lifted about nine months of the year, hitting chest twice a week. Typically she would do 4 sets each of 3 different exercises for a total of 12 heavy sets (not counting warmup sets). On most days she started with flat barbell presses, proceeded to incline barbell presses, then finished off with dumbell flyes or a machine exercise. No slouch in the strength department, Dr. Lydon could bench press 160 pounds for reps. Despite her best intentions, she realized her chest muscles had reached a plateau.

While chatting with some guys backstage at a bodybuilding contest she received an important piece of advice. They told her she was overtraining her chest muscles and that they had become accustomed to doing the same exercises week after week. Dr. Lydon took the advice to heart and cut back her chest-training from twice to once per week. She also dropped most of the barbell work in favor of dumbells. After a few weeks not only had her chest muscles responded, but she could then bench press 175 pounds for reps.

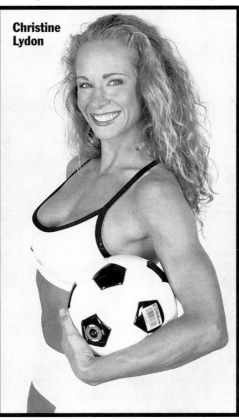

Christine Lydon

Dr. Lydon is convinced that, while it is a great exercise for beginners, the flat barbell bench press does have its limitations. The natural full range of the chest is to bring your arm all the way across in front of your body to the opposite shoulder. With the typical medium to wide grip used on the barbell press, this vital across-the-body movement is eliminated.

These days Dr. Lydon starts her chest routine with either flat or incline dumbell presses. She brings the dumbells all the way together at

"In this age of silicon enhancement, many women are probably wondering if chest-training is necessary for a proportioned physique. While chest-training cannot increase breast tissue, it will optimize both natural and surgically enhanced chests by building the muscle that lies beneath."

– former bodybuilder and regular Oxygen *contributor Dr. Chris Lydon, commenting on the importance of chest-training for women.*

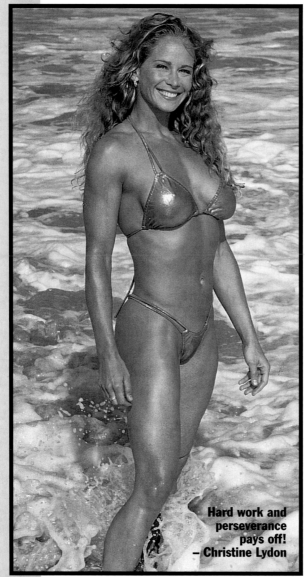

**Hard work and perseverance pays off!
– Christine Lydon**

the top, pauses, then lowers until her elbows are just below her torso and the dumbells are at chest height. Dr. Lydon finds pyramiding works best for her, and she'll start with a weight that allows 15 to 20 reps and work up to a weight that limits her to 6 to 10 reps. In all she does 4 sets.

Even though she seldom if ever does flat barbell presses any more, she occasionally chooses incline barbell presses as her second exercise. Even though there is more shoulder involvement than with flat presses, she finds the incline version less stressful on the shoulder joint. She uses a wide grip and lowers the bar to the top of her chest. As with dumbell presses she prefers to use an ascending pyramid scheme of weights, starting light for high reps and finishing heavy for lower reps.

With two free-weight exercises completed, Dr. Lydon next moves on to a couple of machine exercises. Her first (or third in the sequence) is the Hammer press machine. She finds this machine forces her to execute the movement in perfect form. She'll typically do one light set of 15 to 20 reps, then 3 working sets of 10 to 15 reps.

For her fourth and final exercise Dr. Lydon will do either pec-dek flyes or cable crossovers. She finds both great for the inner pecs which, she adds, go along way toward emphasizing cleavage. She typically does 4 sets of either exercise, preferring to go lighter for higher rep ranges than for any of the other chest exercises.

Dr. Chris Lydon's Chest Routine
1. Dumbell bench presses – 4 sets x 6 to 20 reps
2. Incline barbell presses – 4 sets x 6 to 20 reps
3. Hammer press machine – 3 sets x 10 to 15 reps
4. Pec-dek flyes – 4 sets x 12 to 18 reps
or: cable crossovers – 4 sets x 12 to 18 reps

Jenny Worth

If they gave an award for perseverance, Florida's Jenny Worth would win hands down. Take a look at the following competitive record:

1999 IFBB Fitness Olympia – 9th place
1998 IFBB Fitness Olympia – 10th place
1998 IFBB Midwest Pro Fitness – 2nd place
1998 IFBB Jan Tana Pro Fitness – 6th place
1998 NPC USA Fitness Championships – Overall Short Class
(IFBB professional qualifier)
1998 NPC Florida State Fitness Championships – Overall
1997 3rd Annual NPC Debbie Kruck Fitness Classic – Overall
1997 NPC Team Universe Fitness Championships – 5th place
1997 NPC Women's National Fitness Championships – 14th place
1996 NPC Southern USA Fitness Championships – Overall
1996 NPC Tallahassee Fitness Championships – Overall
1996 NPC Junior National Fitness Championships – 2nd place
1996 2nd Annual NPC Debbie Kruck Fitness Classic – 3rd place
1996 NPC Women's National Fitness Championships – 14th place

A typical day for Jenny Worth starts at 4:00 a.m. when she does her first cardio session. Following a quick meal she then bikes 12 miles to the center of Miami for her first personal training client. Depending on whether or not she has another client booked, Jenny may hop on a treadmill for yet another cardio session. Throughout the day she alternates training clients, eating and preparing for her next fitness show. Then just before bed she jams in another cardio session. A quick shower and it's off to sleep, only to rise and begin all over again the next morning.

It's easy to see how Jenny has developed a reputation as one of the most dedicated fitness competitors in the world, but surprising when you realize that she's not even 25 years old. When you find out that Jenny's training partner is a 300-pound guy named Dodd Romero, you get some idea of how hard she

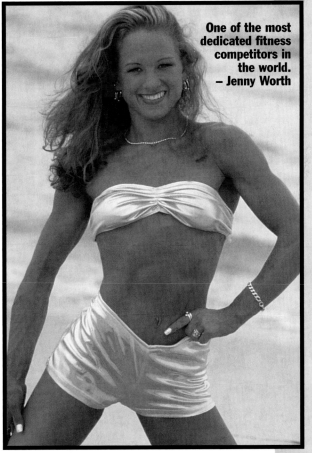

One of the most dedicated fitness competitors in the world. – Jenny Worth

trains. Dodd gave Jenny a job at Gables Personal Fitness in Miami, and after witnessing her workouts realized that, despite her diminutive size (5'1" and 112 pounds), she would make a great training partner.

Jenny and Dodd usually start their chest workout with what they consider the king of upper-body movements, the bench press. For variety they'll alternate barbell presses with Smith-machine presses and dumbell presses. They do a warmup set of about 15 reps and then start adding weight. In Jenny's case this means working from the 20-pounders up to the 70s. Yes, you read correct. Jenny can do 4 reps with 70-pound dumbells. On the Smith machine she has worked up to 205 pounds for 4 reps.

For their second exercise, Jenny and Dodd do incline dumbell presses. When she started training Jenny's upper chest lagged far behind her lower chest so Dodd had her doing nothing but inclines for a whole year. Depending on the day, Jenny will do either 2 straight sets of 15 reps, or 3 drop sets.

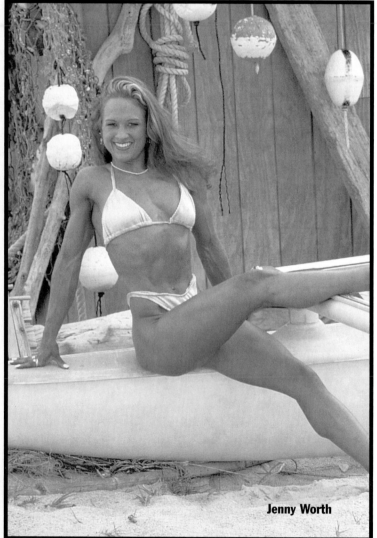

Jenny Worth

To bring out the detail in her chest, Jenny does cable crossovers, but with her own unique variation. She does 21 reps straight, changing her body position three times. She does 7 reps where her hands meet in front of her eyes, 7 reps to her waist, and then 7 reps where she kneels on the ground. In some respects it almost like the popular 21s routine many people do for their biceps. Jenny usually subjects her chest to 2 sets of such madness.

Jenny's final weight exercise is dumbell or machine pullovers. Even though this exercise is a great lat-builder, it also brings the chest into play. Jenny says all the great body-builders like Arnold, Haney and Yates did pullovers in their routines, so why not her? Jenny typically does 2 sets of 21 reps of pullovers.

Although that finishes her strength exercises, Jenny has one more move-ment in store for her chest. At the end of her workout she drops to the floor and does a set of pushups to failure. Sometimes she'll get 50 reps, other times it's up to 75 or more. It all depends on how she feels that day and what kind of chest workout she just had.

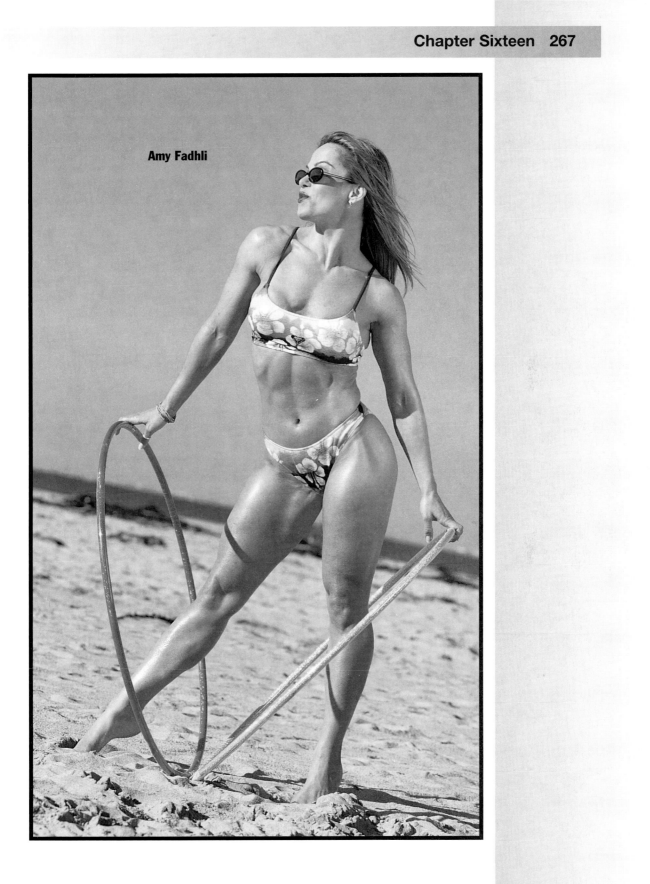

Amy Fadhli

Shoulder-Training

For those readers who plan on competing, great shoulder development is an absolute necessity. A weak chest or back can sometimes be hidden with creative posing, but the shoulders are visible in every pose. For the majority of readers, those who no doubt never plan to compete, good shoulder development will not only add symmetry to the physique but will actually reduce lower-back problems down the road. With time the muscles in the upper back and rear shoulders tend to become proportionally weaker than the muscle located in the front of the torso. The result is the sloped-shoulder look, which changes the body's center of gravity and places additional stress on the spinal erectors (as if they needed more). The decline of posture is one of the primary theories as to why so many people develop "a bad back" later in life. The bottom line here is, you need to incorporate an adequate shoulder program into your training.

"One thing is certain. Because I compete in a sport where overall fullness and size of the delts is becoming more and more important, I make sure I get in at least one heavy workout each week."
– 1998 Fitness Olympia winner Monica Brant, commenting on her shoulder-training.

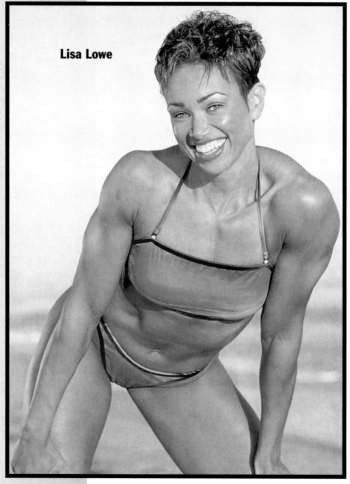

Lisa Lowe

Anatomy

The shoulders are actually made up of four distinct regions – the larger, outer deltoids consist of the front (anterior), side (lateral) and rear (posterior) heads. The smaller muscles located on the scapula (shoulder blade) are collectively called the rotator complex or rotator cuff. Although the larger deltoids get most of the attention in both the gym and physique contests, it is the underlying rotators that cause so many problems down the road. Usually what happens is, the delts gain strength so rapidly that the smaller rotators can no longer keep up. It doesn't help matters either when they've been subjected to years of heavy pressing movements.

Besides the delts and rotators, the trapezius or traps can be considered part of the shoulder group. As noted earlier, the traps are anatomically considered part of the back, but the vast majority of people prefer to include them in their shoulder workouts.

Training

Deltoid-training can be divided into pressing movements (barbells, dumbells or machines) and dumbell raises (front, side and rear). To hit the rotators, both internal and external, a number of dumbell or cable-rotation movements should be performed. The traps can also be stimulated with various types of shrugs and upright rows.

Monica Brant

Since winning the 1998 Fitness Olympia, Monica Brant has had little time to sit back and enjoy the spoils of her victory. From posing exhibitions and seminars to endorsements – and yes, more competitions – Monica's appointment book is full.

Monica is a firm believer that most people overtrain their muscles. That's why she prefers to alternate a heavy workout with a lighter one for each muscle. Monica is also a great believer in instinctive training. This Fitness Olympia winner is definitely not a slave to conformity.

The first thing Monica does when starting her shoulder workout is a simple check for any soreness. The shoulders are involved in just about every upper-body exercise and are very susceptible to injury. Monica usually spends a couple of minutes stretching the shoulders from as many angles as possible. This test gives her the feedback she needs to customize her shoulder routine for that day. Excessive soreness usually means lighter weights for higher reps, but if everything feels good she'll use heavier weights.

In regard to the exercises, if one word could summarize Monica's approach it's *variety*. She likes to hit her shoulders from as many different angles as possible. She also modifies her training to suit the time of the year. During the off-season she'll use more basic barbell and dumbell movements; close to a competition she'll incorporate more functional exercises. For example pressing a barbell onstage is not a necessity, but doing a handstand is. So in the months leading up to a show she'll perform handstand pushups in place of pressing movements.

A final Brant generalization is to incorporate as many isolation exercises as possible. During most workouts you'll observe her doing various dumbell and cable lateral movements. She's particularly fond of one-arm laterals as by lifting with one arm you can put total focus into that area. Here's a typical Monica Brant shoulder workout.

Monica Brant

Seated dumbell presses – Monica does seated dumbell presses when her strength levels are high and muscle soreness is low. For variety Monica alternates the bench angle from a high incline (75 to 80 degrees) to vertical. She also alternates from the standard palms-forward grip to an underhand grip. Finally she may play around with rep speed and do both fast- and slow-rep sets – it all depends on how she feels. Typical weights and reps for Monica are 25- to 30-pound dumbells for 3 or 4 sets of 6 to 8 reps.

Upright rows – Through trial and error, Monica has found that using dumbells stimulates her shoulders and traps more effectively than using a barbell. The problem she finds with a barbell is that it locks you in one plane of motion. Dumbells, however, allow you to move your arms and shoulders in such a manner that you can apply maximum stimulation to the muscles. Monica usually does 3 sets of 8 to 10 reps.

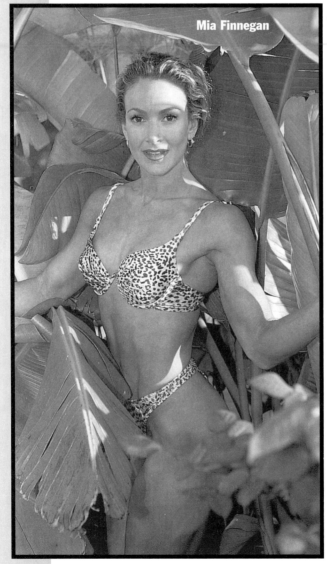

Mia Finnegan

One-arm cable lateral raise – To finish off her delts, particularly her side delts, Monica heads to a cable crossover machine and does 3 sets of one-arm cable lateral raises. For variety Monica alternates both the angle she raises the cable and the height to which she brings the handle. On some days it's just short of shoulder height; on others she raises her hand above her shoulder. As this is an isolation finishing exercise, Monica prefers to use lighter weight and execute the movement in ultrastrict style.

Mia Finnegan

You'd never know it by looking at her, and it's not a conclusion easily drawn from her competitive record, but, Mia Finnegan was not blessed with the greatest shoulder width in the world. It took years of hard work to widen her genetically narrow shoulders. Even though she was blessed with narrow hips, she knew the judges favored a big hip-to-shoulder differential. To achieve this Mia embarked on an extensive shoulder program employing high reps to failure.

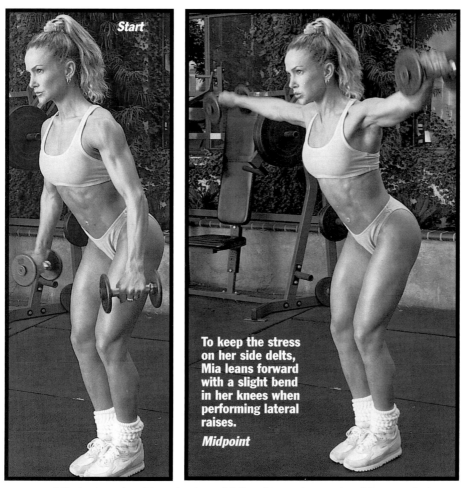

Start

To keep the stress on her side delts, Mia leans forward with a slight bend in her knees when performing lateral raises.

Midpoint

Mia trains shoulders in the middle of her chest, shoulders and triceps routine. Even though she finds her shoulders are good and warm after her chest exercises, she still likes to add in a few light direct shoulder sets to complete the preparation. One of her favorite warmup exercises is lateral raises using three-pound dumbells for 25 reps. Mia doesn't care if people laugh. Her goal is not to impress them at this point (that comes later onstage), but to get as much blood into her shoulders as possible. Even though she's aware that some people start heavy and go lighter, she prefers to start light and gradually work up to the heavier weight.

Mia has two distinct training styles when it comes to shoulders. If she's on the road, or stuck for time, she selects three exercises and performs 3 trisets. A typical triset would start with side raises, progress to dumbell presses, then finish with dumbell rows. Yes, you read the last exercise correctly. Even though most people perform dumbell rows as a back exercise, by having her shoulders pre-exhausted, Mia finds most of the stress is shifted to her rear delts when she does one-arm rows. Averaging 30 seconds between sets, Mia can complete 3 such trisets in 30 minutes. In and out of the gym in half an hour and on to other things.

When not stuck for time Mia incorporates four exercises into her delt-training. She carefully selects the exercises to hit the front, side and rear heads of her deltoids. The first exercise after her warmup is usually dumbell laterals. To keep the stress on her side delts, Mia leans forward with a slight bend in her knees. To keep the exercise honest, she concentrates on leading with her elbows as she raises to shoulder height. Mia is not a slave to reps and she may do 12 or she may do 20. It all depends on how she feels that day.

To shift the stress from her lower to upper side delt, Mia performs one-arm lateral raises. Holding a light dumbell in one hand she grabs a stationary upright with her free hand and leans away from the support. Mia then raises the dumbell to shoulder height. To keep tension on her side delts, she starts the exercise 6 to 8 inches away from her body. The key to this exercise, says Mia, is to keep the working shoulder lower than the other shoulder. A typical workout will see her do 3 sets of 12 to 20 reps.

For her third exercise Mia moves to the seated dumbell row. As we said earlier, Mia finds this exercise excellent for hitting the rear delts. Instead of the traditional one-arm version, Mia prefers to stand up and work both sides at the same time. She starts with her knees slightly bent, arms hanging by her sides, and pulls up until her upper arm is parallel with the floor. To keep most of the stress on her rear delts and not her lats, she doesn't squeeze her shoulder blades together. Again she does 3 sets of 12 to 20 reps.

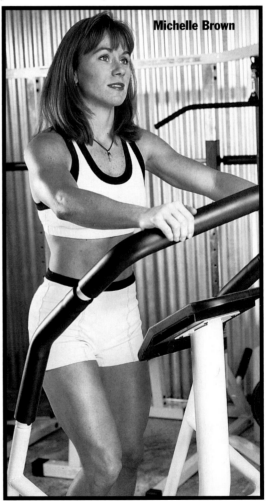

Michelle Brown

To finish off her shoulders, Mia performs a unique version of the press. Instead of dumbells or a barbell, she places a flat bench between a cable crossover machine and grabs a set of handles hooked to the low pulleys. From here she presses upward as if doing a dumbell press. Mia finds the cable version of this exercise keeps her delts under constant tension. Once again she goes to fatigue for 3 sets.

Michelle Brown

Although she never managed to win a major fitness competition, Texas native Michelle Brown was one of the regulars during the industry's growing days in the mid-1990s. With a fourth in the '96 Texas Fitness Championships, and a very respectable tenth at the 1997 Ms. Fitness USA contest, Michelle has far surpassed her dream of merely making the top 15.

Michelle received her introduction to weight training in college to both improve her cheerleading and avoid the dreaded "freshman ten" (the gaining of ten pounds from living on fast food during the first year of college). From 1991 to 1996 Michelle also taught aerobics, and it was an advertisement in a copy of *Ms. Fitness* magazine that got her inspired to enter the Texas Championships.

Perhaps Michelle's biggest source of guidance came from her boyfriend, whom she met in the gym. Not only did he introduce her to the full spectrum of exercises, but he also pushed her to the limit during each and every workout. In fact they had such great workouts together that Michelle now finds it difficult to train with other women. Her boyfriend's greater strength forced her to try to keep up. And even though she had to use lighter weight, she did an equal number of sets and reps.

Michelle thinks a training partner is a necessity during shoulder-training. The shoulders are very susceptible to injuries and a good training partner knows when and how to offer a helping hand.

Michelle usually starts her shoulder routine with that old standby, the military press. She sits in the special chair/rack combination that supports the bar and provides back support. She alternates front and behind-the-head presses – typically 3 sets to the front and 3 sets behind the head. For both variety and to give her shoulder joint a rest, she alternates heavy days of 8 to 10 reps and light days of 15 to 20 reps.

Michelle's second exercise is usually front dumbell raises. Given the smaller amount of muscle mass worked, and the reduced amount of weight as compared to barbell presses, Michelle takes less rest between sets. To minimize stress on her lower back she keeps a slight bend in her knees. She typically does 3 sets of 12 to 15 reps.

Exercise number three is seldom seen, the reverse-grip dumbell press. Michelle finds this exercise great for hitting both the front delts and the pec-delt tie-ins (the area where the front shoulders meet the upper chest). She does 3 sets of 10 to 15 reps.

With her front delts bombarded into submission, Michelle moves on to side delts. Michelle likes to do drop sets on this exercise and will start with 15-pound dumbells for 10 reps. Without resting she drops to 12s for another 10 reps. Michelle adds that you should experiment with different start and finish positions to see which version works best for you. Some individuals find starting at the sides most effective, others prefer to have the dumbells meet in front of the body. The same holds true for height. Most people stop once the dumbells are parallel with the floor, but a few individuals need to raise the dumbells higher.

For most trainers the shoulders would be finished by now, but Michelle has one more exercise up her sleeve. She grabs an EZ-curl bar and commences to do upright rows. She finds this exercise great for finishing off the side shoulders as well as bringing in the rear delts and traps. For variety she alternates between an EZ-curl and a straight bar. Since this is her finishing exercise, she keeps the weight light and does 3 sets of 12 reps.

"It sort of just took on a life of its own once I saw the benefits it provided. I found myself signing up for P.E. classes in college so I could stay active even beyond my cheerleading."
– former Ms. Fitness USA contestant and long-time fitness advocate Michelle Brown, commenting on how the training bug grabbed a hold of her.

Ericca Kern

In many respects the modern fitness movement owes its popularity to the unpopularity of female bodybuilding. In the late 1980s and early 1990s female bodybuilding started mirroring that of male bodybuilding – primary emphasis on size and muscularity. Toned but feminine physiques were pushed aside in favor of women whose bodies would not look out of place in a male contest. Even though the sport kept its die-hard fans, the vast majority of the public and competitors started looking for an alternative. Female fitness, a sport that lingered in relative obscurity, was all of a sudden thrust into the limelight … all of which brings us to Ericca Kern.

Despite the size of some of the competitors surrounding her, Ericca Kern has managed to combine the best of both worlds. She carries enough muscle mass and muscularity to please bodybuilding fans, while at the same time she maintains the grace and femininity that drives hot-blooded males wild.

"Female bodybuilders have for a long time struggled with the marriage of muscle and grace. Only a few female physiques in our sport have attained this level of aesthetic harmony. Blonde bombshell Ericca Kern fits naturally into this mold."
– MuscleMag International contributor Ron Harris, commenting on the muscular yet feminine appearance of 1995 North American champion Ericca Kern.

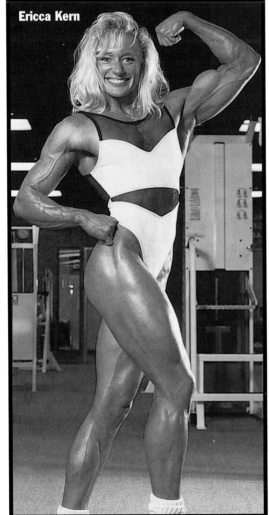

Ericca Kern

Ericca first started lifting weights in college. At the time she was 105 pounds and battling anorexia. She ran 15 miles every day to keep her weight down and in her own words "to try to feel in control of my life." A friend suggested she take a weightlifting course and in quick time she discovered she could control her body without having to ravish it with unhealthy practices. Ericca responded to the weights with amazing speed and within two years turned professional.

Although picking out a "best feature" on Ericca's physique is difficult, her deltoids are two of the best on the pro circuit. They don't have the mass of some of the larger competitors, but then that's not her goal. Instead she trains her delts for shape, proportion and detail.

Ericca usually begins her shoulder workout with lateral raises. Ericca admits she has always had wide shoulders, the result of a genetically wide shoulder girdle. Still she feels extra width is a bonus as it plays a major role in bringing out that much desired X-frame. Ericca

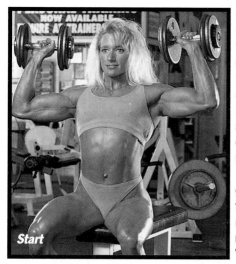

Start

Midpoint

Ericca Kern works
her shoulders with
dumbell presses.

does 1 set with a pair of 10-pound dumbells for 15 to 20 reps, then a set with 15s for another 15 reps. Then comes her first workout set with the 20-pounders for 8 to 12 reps, and the last 3 sets with the 30-pounders for 8 to 12 reps. We should add that, even though she primarily uses dumbells, Ericca will occasionally substitute cables or a machine for lateral raises.

With her side delts given a good going over, Ericca switches to presses to blast her front delts. Once again she relies mainly on dumbells, but will add machine and barbell presses for variety. With her shoulders already warmed up from laterals, Ericca jumps right into the presses using the 50- or 60-pound dumbells for 4 sets of 8 to 12 reps.

For her third and fourth exercises she does a superset of front dumbell raises and upright rows. For the front raises Ericca uses 20- or 25-pound dumbells for 4 sets of 8 to 12 reps. For the upright rows she will use an EZ-curl bar with 60 to 80 pounds on it and do 4 sets.

To finish off her shoulders, Ericca does either lying lateral raises or rear-delt flyes. She prefers doing bent-over laterals face down on a low-incline bench as it allows her to go as heavy as she wants without having to worry about her lower back. She keeps her elbows slightly bent and raises the dumbells until they are parallel with the floor. She typically does 4 sets of 8 to 12 reps using 15- or 20-pound dumbells.

Ericca Kern's Shoulder Routine
1. Dumbell lateral raises – 4 sets x 8 to 12 reps
2. Dumbell presses – 4 sets x 8 to 12 reps
3. Upright rows/front raises – 4 supersets x 8 to 12 reps
4. Lying lateral raises – 4 sets x 8 to 12 reps

CHAPTER EIGHTEEN

Thighs and Glutes

Ask any engineer what's the most important part of a building and he or she will answer – the foundation. The same holds true in weight training. Nothing looks as stupid as a great upper body teetering about on two pencil-stick legs.

"Great legs" are one of the most attractive features on the entire female body. They are one of the main pieces of artillery any woman can use to reduce most hot-blooded males to drooling idiots (drooling optional). Sexy legs can make you look good in just about any piece of clothing whether it's a dress, a skirt or shorts.

Finally, if you play sports, great leg strength is an absolute must. Just about every sport requires leg strength and coordination. From tennis and golf to basketball and hockey, the legs make or break the game.

The glutes rank right up there with the thighs when it comes to practical function and appearance. The glutes are the strongest muscles in the body and in conjunction with the thighs, enable you to lift hundreds of pounds. From an aesthetics point of view the glutes form what has over the years become known as "a great ass." Most things look better coming toward you than going away, but not the glutes. For most men, a great ass ranks right up there with the breasts as one of the first things they notice about a woman's body. And if the surveys are right, a tight butt is one of the most attractive things women find about men. So no matter what side of the fence you're on, the glutes go a long way in getting you noticed by the opposite sex.

Anatomy and Training

The thighs or quadriceps are composed of four large heads (rectus femoris, vastus internus, vastus lateralis and vastus intermedius). All four of these muscles function to straighten the leg from a fully bent position. And each of the four quadriceps muscles works harder at certain points along the full range of motion of leg extension. Collectively the quadriceps muscles are often called the "thigh extensors."

The glutes are located on your backside and act as a hinge between your torso and legs. Any time you straighten up, as when you stand up out of a chair or pick something up off the ground, the gluteus is one of the prime mover muscles that drives the motion. The glutes, as they are commonly called, work in conjunction with the spinal erector

Amy Fadhli

muscles or the lower back and the hamstrings on the back of the thighs. These three muscle groups are commonly referred to as the "posterior chain."

Training the thighs and glutes is as simple as it is painful (particularly the thighs). One of the reasons why leg-training gets neglected is that it requires a great deal of energy. You're training half the body's muscle mass, after all. Another reason is that the thigh muscles hurt like few others when being exercised. The old saying "go for the burn" is redundant here. You don't need to go for it, it will find you!

The glutes are less painful to train than the thighs. All those years of sitting on our ass has reduced the nerve sensitivity in the region. Most thigh exercises also involve the glutes, so the two muscles complement each other in training.

The best exercises to hit both the thighs and glutes are squats, lunges, leg presses and hack squats. To isolate the thighs the leg extension works best. Likewise, to shift most of the stress to the glutes, backward leg sweeps do the job.

Butt-Building the Czechoslovakian Way With Timea Majorova

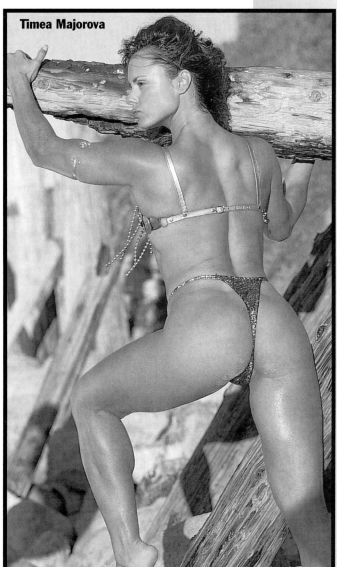

Timea Majorova

Timea Majorova is quick to credit her brothers with getting her involved in athletics. Like many girls with brothers, she became a tomboy and spent many years romping and wrestling. Besides the physical conditioning, that may account for her quest for independence at such a young age. At 14 she struck out on her own for Bratislava to go to secondary medical school. As luck would have it there was a small gym located close to her dormitory. A combination of weight training and aerobics (not to mention skating, skiing and swimming) led to a physique that was good enough to place second at a local fitness competition. From there it was on to the Slovakian Championships, where she placed first. She then followed this up by winning both the European and World Championships.

"I work on my butt very hard. It's such a problem area for most women, so I must stay on top of the game by doing specific exercises for it."
– Timea Majorova

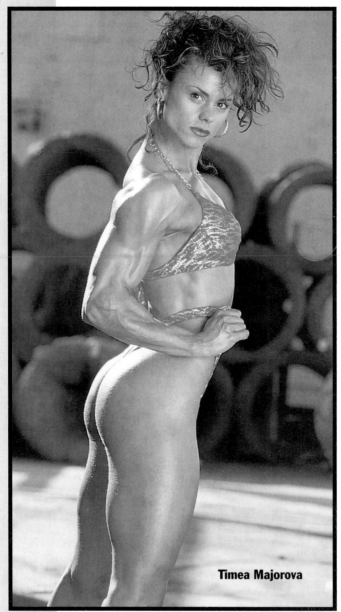

Timea Majorova

Since coming to America Timea has focused all her energy on filling in her five-foot-nine frame, and has been rewarded with top-ten finishes in both the Fitness Olympia and Arnold Fitness International.

It's not surprising that Timea trains hard, and hits the gym five or six times per week. She also runs or cycles daily and is constantly practicing her moves to look better onstage. As her legs and butt are two of her best features, it only made sense to find out what she does for such a "great ending."

Even though she has access to just about every type of equipment since coming to America, she still relies on basic exercises like leg presses, squats and hack squats for her glutes. Timea starts her glute-training with squats. She performs standard squats, sinking down until her thighs are parallel with the floor. As she starts rising back up, she squeezes her glutes and exaggerates the issue by sticking her butt out. To keep most of the stress on the glutes she uses a wide stance and points her toes outward. She does 3 sets of squats, keeping the reps in the range of 12 to 15.

Timea's second glute exercise is the leg press. If she did leg presses earlier in the week to hit her legs, she will use a lighter weight and do higher reps. She also keeps her feet higher on the pressing platform so her butt does most of the work, as opposed to a lower stance which brings in more of the quads. Typically she does 3 or 4 sets of 15 to 20 reps.

For her third exercise Timea opts for hack squats. Again she varies the exercise from the position she would normally use for thighs. Instead of leaning back on the support, she faces the machine. As with regular barbell presses she flexes her glutes on the way up and down. To keep the tension on the glutes at all times, she doesn't lock out at the top. She does 3 sets of 15 reps.

Next up it's barbell lunges. Timea adds that, since lunges are also a primary thigh exercise, you must focus total concentration on the glutes. To minimize knee stress she cautions that the knees must never move out past the toes. Sometimes she does stationary lunges, other times she "lunges across the gym." She usually does 4 sets of 20 reps.

To finish off her glutes Timea does stiff-leg deadlifts. To both minimize lower-back stress and maximize glute involvement, she keeps the knees slightly bent and lower back slightly arched. She also sticks her butt out as far as possible when performing the exercise. On a typical day she will do 3 sets of 15 reps. Timea finishes off with a series of stretching exercises.

Timea's Glute Workout
1. Squats – 3 sets x 12 to 15 reps
2. Leg presses – 3 to 4 sets x 15 to 20 reps
3. Reverse hack squats – 3 sets x 15 reps
4. Lunges – 4 sets x 20 reps
5. Stiff-leg deadlifts – 3 sets x 15 reps
6. Stretches

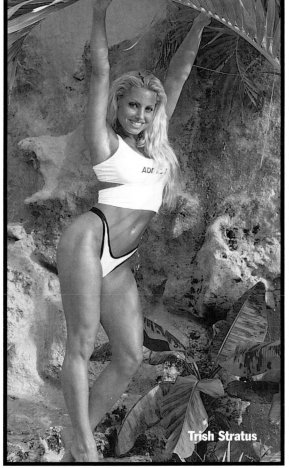

Trish Stratus

Trish Stratus

Even though she knows she inherited great genetics, Trish Stratus had to work hard to turn her good body into a great one. And as one of the most photographed fitness models in the industry, Trish knows she must maintain near-perfect condition year-round.

Trish was first spotted by top Canadian trainer Scott Abel, while she was working out at his gym in Ontario. He convinced her that she had both the body and facial looks to make it as a fitness model. In fact he was so convinced that he took her to meet *MuscleMag* founder Robert Kennedy. If there's one thing Bob has developed over the years it's his uncanny ability to spot new talent. A test shoot was followed by her first cover and her career was launched almost overnight. It's reached the point now that Trish has dozens of covers to her credit, numerous magazine articles, and travels the world with the WWE, World Wrestling Entertainment.

Early in her training Trish focused almost entirely on her legs. The result was a "bottom-heavy" physique that would never have won awards for symmetry. Under Scott's tutelage, however, Trish started to focus on her upper body – and the result is one of the most balanced female physiques around. Unlike many women, Trish isn't afraid she'll turn into Arnold by hitting the weights hard. Even though she considers herself a fitness athlete, she trains as a bodybuilder. That is, she uses heavy weights to build quality muscle.

With her demanding schedule, Trish has had to develop a training program based on flexibility. One week she may be in a large city with numerous gyms to choose from. The next it's some small town with nothing more than a few barbells and dumbells at her disposal. To keep in great shape while on the road Trish utilizes supersets, trisets, giant sets and drop sets.

A typical leg and glute day will see Trish start with barbell squats. Trish doesn't believe in half-assed squats either (no pun intended!). She squats down

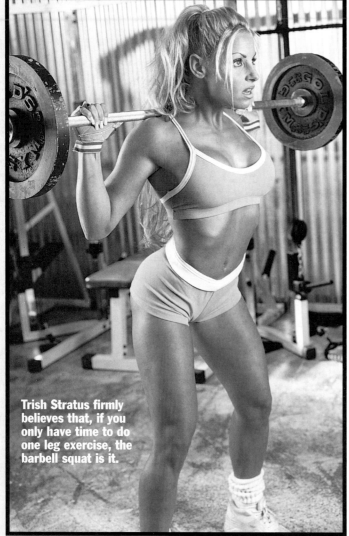

Trish Stratus firmly believes that, if you only have time to do one leg exercise, the barbell squat is it.

to below parallel to hit not only the thighs but the glutes and lower back as well. Trish firmly believes that, if you only have time to do one leg exercise, this is it. Trish always wears a belt to give her lower back support and wraps her knees for the last couple of heavy sets. The latter precaution is important as her knees suffered numerous injuries from years of playing competitive soccer. Trish always uses strict form on squats – slowly lowering to the full squat position, then exploding back up to just short of locking out.

Trish normally does 7 sets, pyramiding the weight up for 5 sets and then dropping the weight for the last 2. She usually gets 20 reps per set.

After squats come leg presses on a 45-degree machine. She does one warmup set, then puts about 225 pounds on the machine and pumps out 3 sets of 25 reps. As with squats, the reps are slow and strict. No bouncing at the bottom or locking out at the top.

Her third leg exercise is leg extensions. She finds this movement great for adding separation between her quad heads. She pyramids the weight each set for 4 sets of 12 to 15 reps.

With her thighs and glutes burning like crazy, Trish switches over and starts her hamstrings training. She does 2 sets of 15 reps, then adds more weight and goes for an additional 2 sets of 12 reps.

Trish's second hamstrings exercise is good mornings. She places the bar low on the traps and not on the neck, and is careful to maintain a slight arch in her lower back. She also keeps the legs slightly bent to minimize lower back strain. Trish adds that this is one exercise that must be done slow and controlled with no sudden jerky movements.

The previous is Trish's primary leg and glute program, but if she feels her glutes need extra work she'll utilize a specialty program. One of her favorite butt exercises is one-leg cable kickbacks. She does these by attaching one ankle to a low pulley and adopting a runner-type stance (unattached leg in front). From there Trish kicks or lifts the attached leg back behind her as far as possible. She pauses midway at the top and squeezes her butt muscles, then returns her leg to the starting position. Trish does 3 sets for each leg, averaging 25 reps per set.

Another Stratus favorite is what she calls "tush pushes." Trish lies on the floor on her back and bends her knees so that her glutes come off the floor. She keeps her upper body flat on the floor and extends her arms and hands along the sides for support. She then arches or pushes her pelvis as high as she can toward the ceiling, squeezing hard for a count of five, then lowering her lower body back down. Trish does 25 reps per set but has gone up to 50 or more on occasion.

A third butt specializer is an old favorite of Rachel McLish's (the first Ms. Olympia) – kneeling one-leg raises. Trish kneels on the floor on all fours and supports her body on her palms. She releases one leg from the floor, tucks it up against her chest, then extends it back behind her as far and as high as possible. The higher you lift the leg the harder the glute contraction. She does 3 sets per leg for 50 reps.

Mia Finnegan

As one of the first superstars of the fitness industry, Mia Finnegan set the standard for what the ideal fitness physique should look like. It's no exaggeration to say literally millions of women have been influenced by her physique and knowledge.

Mia got her first introduction to weights back when she was 16 and a competitive gymnast. She continued using weight-training exercises to help her gymnastics right up until college. At 23 the competitive bug bit and she began entering in bodybuilding contests.

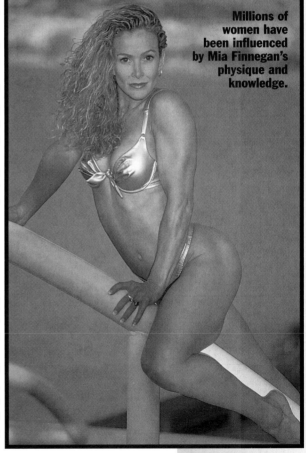

Millions of women have been influenced by Mia Finnegan's physique and knowledge.

When she switched over to fitness competitions, Mia re-evaluated her physique and realized that the muscle she had built for gymnastics and body-building had to go. She also decided her hamstrings and glutes needed more work than her thighs. This is not surprising as most women store more fat on their glutes and hamstrings than on their thighs.

Currently Mia has nine exercises in her leg routine and she picks four or five per workout, mixing them up for variety. She always does leg extensions, lunges and hyperextensions, but she frequently rotates the others. A typical Mia Finnegan leg workout is as follows.

1. Leg extensions – 3 sets x 15 to 20 reps
2. Lunges – 3 sets x 15 to 20 reps
3. Machine kickbacks – 3 sets x 15 to 20 reps
4. Hyperextensions – 3 sets x 15 to 20 reps

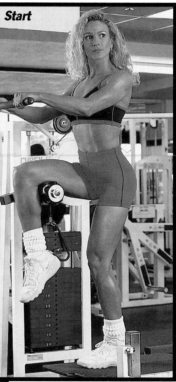

Start

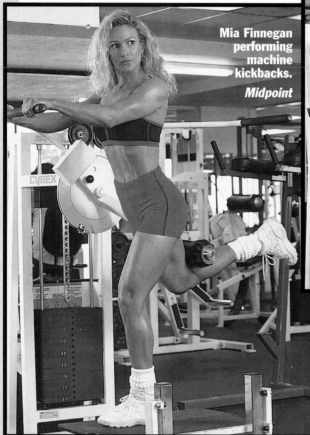

Mia Finnegan performing machine kickbacks.

Midpoint

Monica Brant

Monica Brant is one of the true superstars in the field of fitness. She is originally from Texas, born in Ft. Hood and raised on a 20-acre ranch in a small town outside San Antonio called Castroville. It's not surprising that someone born on a ranch in Texas would fall in love with horses. Monica has been riding and showing ponies and horses since the age of 5. Her mom had a professional horse training business and she started learning how to help around the stables.

By the time she was 14, Monica was giving riding lessons and training horses on her own with occasional advice from her mom. Along with volleyball and track in high school, Monica competed in many events: Western pleasure, barrels and pole-bending, English pleasure, dressage, and personal favorite – hunter/jumper.

Monica first started lifting weights in 1991, after witnessing Marla Duncan win a national competition. Monica found Marla's beauty and physique so impressive that she wanted to try doing the same – fitness competitions.

Up until 1995 Monica only competed for fun, not as a money-making career. But all that changed in 1994 when she was honored with a *Muscle & Fitness* magazine cover. This accomplishment helped her realize she had potential to earn some real money in the fitness industry. She kept competing, and in April of '95 moved to the Los Angeles area. Upon her arrival she dove into her career and competed in the IFBB organization two or three times per year. Finally, after four tries, Monica was awarded with the 1998 Ms. Olympia title.

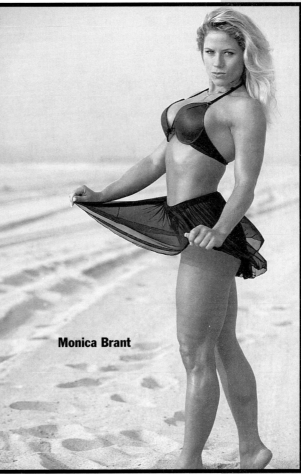

Monica Brant

Monica is another fitness athlete who found her legs responded faster than her upper body. So much so that she took two full years off leg-training and relied on sprints to keep them conditioned and toned. In 1996 she noticed her upper body had caught up, so once again she started strength training for her legs.

Today Monica works her legs with high repetitions. She rarely uses weight, and keeps the reps in the 20-to-50-range. Monica is a big believer in supersets and often combines two leg exercises back to back, resting only 30 seconds between sets. Monica is also a great believer in the principle of instinctive training. She doesn't have a set pattern of exercises when she trains legs, preferring to take each day as it comes, depending on how she is feeling. The one thing that does remain constant is the amount of time she takes to train her legs. "I'll typically do legs for 20 to 30 minutes – no more than that. The reason I can get it done in that time is, I don't take a normal amount of rest between sets."

Prior to any leg work with weights, Monica starts out by getting on the treadmill for five minutes. She finds this is the right amount of time to warm up her legs without interfering with her leg-training.

After some light stretching, Monica starts her routine with some sort of leg press. She may only use a 45-pound plate on one side, or one on each side. If she's doing a lying leg press she'll go very light and bang out 30 to 45 repetitions. No matter what leg press she uses, Monica alternates her foot positioning. She starts with a medium-width stance for the first set, then switches to a wide stance for the next set. Finally she uses a narrow set for the last set. Monica adds that those who have knee problems may want to avoid the latter position – the narrow stance does stress the knees more than the other two.

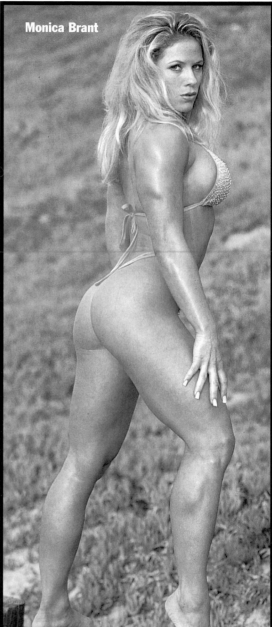

Monica Brant

After leg presses Monica moves on to leg extensions. While the leg press is great for increasing the size of the thighs, Monica feels the leg extension has done the most to add the separation between her quad heads. Monica will do as many as 6 sets of leg extensions. As with leg presses she varies her foot position to hit the entire surface of her quads. She alternates between toes pointing in and toes pointing out for 2 sets each. She keeps the weight fairly light on this exercise, preferring instead to go for higher reps in the 25 to 40 range.

With leg extensions out of the way, Monica moves on to lunges. Again variety is the order of the day on lunges. Some days Monica will rest the back leg on a bench. She finds this not only hits the thighs but also brings more hamstring into play. The key here, says Monica, is to never let the knee lunge out past the toes.

Another Brant favorite is the walking lunge. Monica finds a long stride works best for her, but you will have to experiment to see what feels best for you. Here's another tip: Keep the upper body erect and avoid looking down. As soon as you start looking down, the back and torso will follow. Pretty soon everything is pointed downward – a dangerous position to be in when performing lunges. The safety aspect is one of the reasons Monica prefers to use dumbells rather than resting a barbell on her shoulders. Not only do they provide a bit more stability, but also if something goes wrong it's just a matter of letting them drop.

To finish off her quads, Monica does freestanding squats. Unlike regular barbell squats, freestanding squats are done holding a dumbell in each hand. She prepares for this exercise by placing two 10-pound plates on the floor on which to rest her heels. Monica finds this exercise great for bringing out the "teardrop" of the thighs. She goes to failure on this exercise, in all doing 4 to 6 sets.

Lisa Lowe

Glutes

With her background in jazz dance and bodybuilding it's not surprising that Lisa Lowe has two of the best legs and glutes on the pro fitness circuit. They're symmetrical, toned, and built to boot (no pun intended!).

Glute kickbacks – Lisa usually selects this as her first exercise because it utilizes just the "natural" weight of each leg, involves a stretch without that addi-

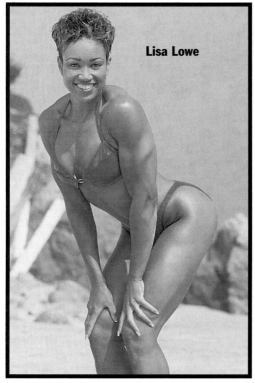

Lisa Lowe

tional resistance, and utilizes the highest number of repetitions per set. Lisa suggests "about 20" for each of 3 sets. "Your glutes really start to burn at that point."

You begin with the working leg extended and the foot cocked to a point that places it in line with the head. You then raise it to about a 45-degree angle with the foot elevated above the head. "The entire idea is to keep tension on the glutes throughout the exercise," emphasizes Lisa.

One-leg machine presses – "This exercise ties in your glutes, some of your quadriceps on the front of your thigh, and the hamstring along the rear of the leg," notes Lowe.

To begin the exercise, you simply place your back firmly against the angled support, keeping your rear tucked well back and firmly against the seat. After warming up with no weight, begin by loading the appropriate weight resistance and extend your leg until it almost locks out. (Some people use both legs to extend the weight to begin the exercise and then remove the non-working leg.) Allow your leg to come back until your upper and lower leg forms a 90-degree angle. Then push the weight back until it is again almost locked out. Lisa does 3 sets of 10 to 12 repetitions.

Walking lunges – "This an excellent exercise to both work the glutes and develop a better sense of working balance," observes Lowe, who uses light dumbells for 4 sets of 8 reps. She suggests that beginners start without weights and do just 2 sets.

Lisa begins by lunging forward until her lower leg forms a slightly sharper than 90-degree angle with the floor. She then continues to drop the following leg until it almost touches the floor. (Note that the following leg beneath the knee is parallel with the floor.) To finish the exercise, pull the following leg forward as you begin to stand.

Stiff-leg deadlifts – "This exercise has always been a miracle worker for me," notes Lisa. "Before I performed it regularly I always had a problem getting and feeling a tie-in from the glutes to the hamstrings. This really concentrates on that area. The key to this exercise," says Lisa, "is really concentrating on keeping your back absolutely straight throughout the movement." Note that the weight goes directly down, rather than being thrust forward as Lisa lowers and raises it. The weight is never allowed to touch down. Lisa performs 3 sets of 8 to 10 repetitions.

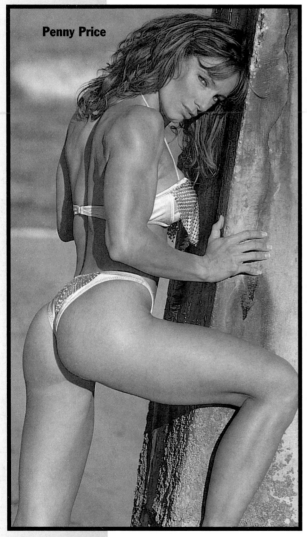

Penny Price

Penny Price

Unless you knew otherwise, from reading Penny Price's biography you'd think more than one individual was involved. She started with professional bodybuilding, progressed to women's fitness, switched over to triathlon, and in her "spare time" picked up a degree in nutrition. Oh, and did we mention she gave birth to two children as well?

Penny Price is the consummate over-achiever. Most women would be content with one of the previous accomplishments, but Penny constantly challenges herself and raises the bar another notch higher.

For Penny to achieve success in any of the previous disciplines, a strong pair of legs was an absolute necessity. As a top personal trainer she also recognizes that the legs are a problem area for most women. Her advice to those women with large legs is to use lighter weight and do high reps. She also recommends doing a lot of aerobic activity that includes climbing stairs, biking and running. In this case your goal is to thin the legs out while preserving good muscle tone. Of course too much aerobics can make the legs look stringy, but that's where weight training comes in.

For those with lean legs the goal is to increase size. The best way to do this is to use heavier weights for lower repetitions, and take longer periods of rest between sets. With regard to aerobics Penny suggests avoiding running. She believes it will interfere with gaining weight. Riding the stationary cycle would be a much better option.

Penny's current leg routine consists of five basic exercises – two for thighs and three for hamstrings. We'll discuss her hamstring exercises in the next chapter. Penny's two primary thigh exercises are squats and lunges. Let's take a closer look.

Squats – Penny places a bar across her shoulders and stands with her feet about shoulder width apart. To reduce the stress on her lower back, Penny keeps her shoulder blades contracted and chest up. This helps prevent her from leaning too far forward, probably the biggest cause of squat-induced lower-back problems.

Penny says to start the exercise you should lead with the tailbone, and squat down as if sitting in a chair. She executes this movement in a slow and controlled manner and so must you. If leaning forward is the primary cause of lower-back problems, then bouncing at the bottom is the primary cause of knee problems on this exercise. Penny typically does 3 sets of 10 to 15 reps. These are working sets of course. She usually does a few high-rep sets of squats at the beginning to warm up her thighs.

Penny's second thigh exercise is the lunge. For those new to weightlifting, Penny recommends starting out by practicing this exercise with no weight. Lunges require a great deal of balance, perhaps even more so than squats. The objective is to lunge as far forward as possible without having the knee move out past the toes. As with squats the torso must be held high and straight to prevent leaning forward.

To keep her thighs and glutes guessing, Penny alternates different versions of the lunge. On some days she'll do walking lunges. On others she'll elevate the front leg on a box. The key is to never let the muscles adapt to one movement. Penny usually does 3 sets of 10 to 12 reps.

Stacey Lynn

Stacey Lynn is one of the world's most popular fitness models. Whether she's at a trade show behind the counter at a MuscleMag booth, or seductively sprawled on a beach doing a photo shoot, Stacy is the envy of millions. Stacey trains twice daily, six days a week, working her legs and glutes Monday, chest Tuesday, back Wednesday, and her glutes again on Thursday. Fridays and Saturdays are then spent on shoulders and arms.

As with most muscle groups, Stacey likes to vary her leg exercises and the order she performs them to keep her body guessing. A typical workout, however, often starts with lunges off a bench. She finds by having the back leg elevated on a bench requires more balance and control. The end result she feels is better muscle development. Elevating the rear leg also places more weight on the front leg, which means she doesn't have to hold on to huge poundages. As with any lunge exercise the key is to never let the knee move out past the toes. Stacey typically does 3 sets of 20 to 25 reps.

"I devote a lot of time to leg-training. I usually do two or three exercises per muscle group with 20 to 25 reps per set. My leg regimen lasts one and a half hours."
– MuscleMag *cover girl and top fitness model Stacey Lynn, commenting on what it takes to build world-caliber legs.*

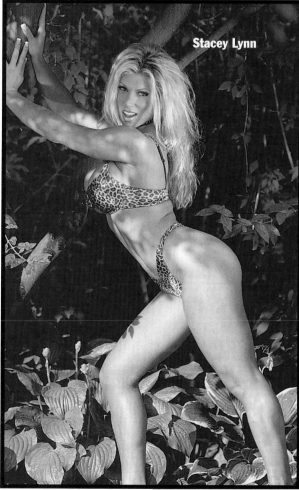
Stacey Lynn

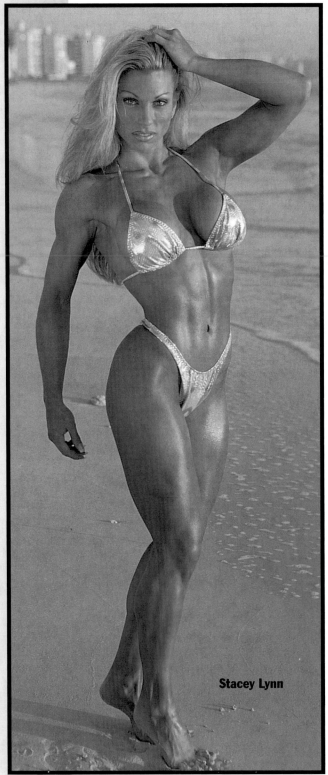

Stacey Lynn

To isolate her quads Stacey relies on that great old standby, leg extensions. This is one of Stacey's favorite leg exercises as it allows her to see the muscles working with each rep. The movement also allows her to concentrate, pause the weight in the contracted position, and give her quads a welcome squeeze. She does 3 sets of 20 to 25 reps.

At this point Stacey performs a hamstring exercise like standing leg curls. As we'll be going into her hamstring-training in greater detail in the next chapter, we'll skip ahead to her next exercise for thighs, the reverse lunge.

The finish position of the reverse lunge is identical to that of the standard lunges but getting there is somewhat different. Stacey stands with her arms at her sides holding two dumbells. Then, instead of stepping forward, she extends one leg backward and bends the knee until it's at 90 degrees. She holds this position for two seconds, then slowly rises to the starting position. As with her other thigh exercises, Stacey does 3 sets of 20 to 25 reps.

For her fourth attack on quads and glutes Stacey switches to barbell squats. To reduce knee stress and place more emphasis on the inner thighs and glutes, Stacey adopts a fairly wide stance. She then squats down until her thighs are parallel to the floor. As she rises back up she squeezes her glutes. A typical leg workout will see Stacey perform 3 sets of 20 to 25 reps of barbell squats.

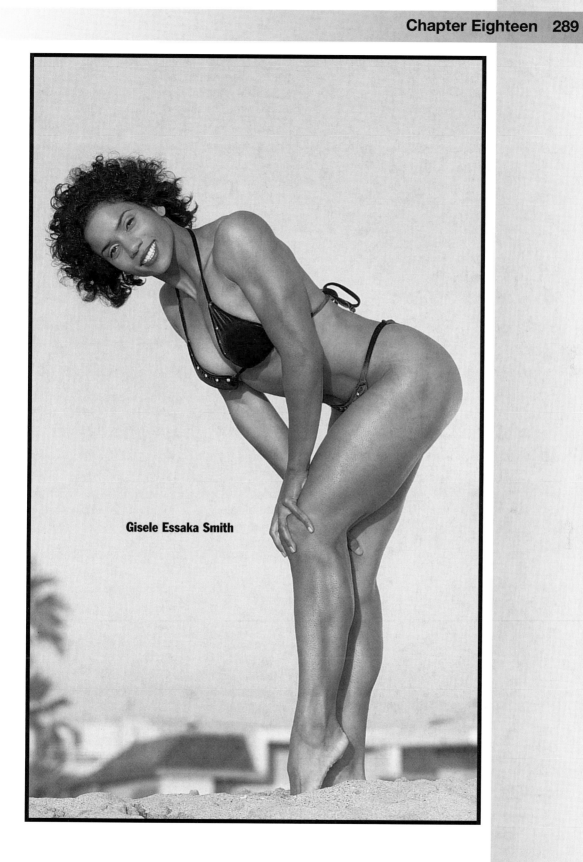

Gisele Essaka Smith

CHAPTER NINETEEN

Hamstrings

Even though the hamstrings are anatomically analogous to the biceps, they get treated like the triceps. Guys will spend thousands of hours training the biceps, while only go through the motions of training the larger triceps. The same holds true for the legs, the thighs get all the attention while the hamstrings get treated as second-class citizens. Even superstar athletes fall victim to this neglect. How many pulled quadriceps do you hear about? Very few, but pulled hamstrings are a dime a dozen.

Anatomy

The three hamstring muscles are the biceps femoris, which has two heads, and the semimembranosus and semi-tendinosus. These muscles are so named because if their tendons are cut behind the knee, the knee cannot be flexed to allow a step to be taken and a person is therefore powerless and is "hamstrung." The primary function of the hamstrings is to flex or curl the lower leg at the knee joint.

Training

Most thigh and glute exercises such squats, lunges and leg presses bring in the hamstrings to a greater or lesser extent. To isolate the hamstrings various leg-curl machines can be used. The stiff-leg deadlift, primarily being a spinal-erector movement, also works the hamstrings as the muscle attaches above the knee joint.

Mia Finnegan

After retiring from competitive gymnastics, Mia Finnegan won her first fitness title in 1992 when she was named Ms. Natural Universe. She has since won Ms. Olympia Fitness '96 (World Champion), Ms. Galaxy Fitness '95, Fitness America National Champion '94 and many others. Mia is currently co-hosting *Fitting It In* and *Fit Cuisine* on the Health Network.

Like most former competitive gymnasts, Mia built a set of legs that overshadowed her upper body. She was left in the enviable position of actually having to *reduce* the size of her legs. Oh, the burdens some people have to endure!

Lisa Uzzle

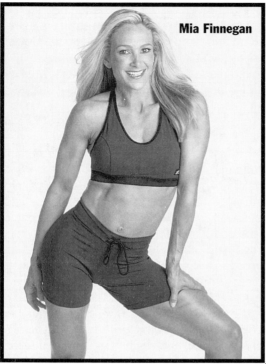

Mia Finnegan

With her focus these days on maintenance, Mia's hamstring routine consists of two versions of the leg curl, (lying, seated or standing), back extensions and stiff-leg deadlifts. As she's reached the point where she doesn't need additional hamstring mass, she keeps the weights light, averaging 3 sets of 15 to 20 reps per exercise.

Mia Finnegan's Hamstring Routine
1. Seated leg curls –
   3 sets x 15 to 20 reps
2. Lying leg curls –
   3 sets x 15 to 20 reps
3. Stiff-leg deadlifts –
   3 sets x 15 to 20 reps
4. Back extensions –
   3 sets x 15 to 20 reps

Penny Price

In the previous chapter we looked at Penny Price's thigh workout. Penny's hamstring routine is a bit more extensive. All the heavy training she did during her bodybuilding days left her with oversized thighs and subpar hamstrings. Many people would shrug this off and proceed full speed ahead, but Penny had loftier goals in minds. She fully understood that proportion was the name of the game, and underdeveloped hamstrings just wouldn't cut it on the competitive stage. So she revamped her leg workouts to bring her hamstrings up to the same standard as her thighs.

Penny usually starts her hamstring training with some form of leg curl. For variety she alternates lying with standing leg curls. She also supersets leg curls with either stiff-leg deadlifts or hyperextensions. Penny found building her hamstrings as difficult as some people find building their calves. This is why she utilizes such a high-intensity approach.

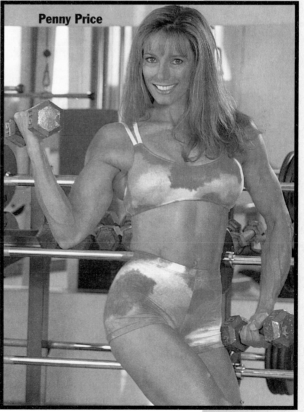

Penny Price

Penny offers a few tips. When doing leg curls try to press the pelvis into the pad to isolate the hamstrings. Letting the butt bounce up and down (or in and out) reduces the stimulation of the hamstring and brings in the glutes and lower back.

Another suggestion is to perform drop sets. Penny usually starts with a weight that just allows her 10 reps. She then reduces the poundage so that she can barely manage an additional 10 reps. Finally a third drop produces another 10 reps. Penny feels the hamstrings are a very stubborn muscle group and need this kind of stimulation.

Penny is the first to admit that stiff-leg deadlifts require a good deal of flexibility to execute properly. She stands on an elevated bench or block and fixates her eyes on a spot on the wall where it meets the ceiling. She keeps her chest out and lower back slightly curved as she bends forward. She also trys to "keep her butt stuck out" for balance and to reduce the stress on her lower back. She says, if there is one exercise that must be performed in immaculate style, it is stiff-leg deadlifts. She typically does 3 sets of 10 to 15 reps.

If she doesn't do stiff-legs as her second exercise in a superset, she'll do hyperextensions. The name is really misleading. As Penny stresses, you should never "hyperextend." Only raise the torso until it is line with the legs. Arching up past the parallel point puts extra stress on the lower-back ligaments. After doing a set of one of the leg-curl exercises, Penny will do a set of 12 to 15 reps of hyperextensions. She'll then repeat for 3 such supersets.

Stacey Lynn

Stacey Lynn realized early on that, given the competitiveness within the fitness industry, she would need to work doubly hard to hold her own against such other stars as Monica Brant, Vicky Pratt and Amy Fadhli. A perfect physique was an absolute necessity. For Stacey this means getting up at 6:00 every morning and doing 45 minutes of cardio. Stacey is also a stickler for details and that's why she designs her workouts to keep all muscle groups in proportion.

In the previous chapter we were introduced to Stacey's quad and glute workout. Unlike many people who either train hamstrings after quads or schedule them on an entirely separate day, Stacey prefers to train hamstrings at the same time as her glutes and thighs. That is, she does a couple of thigh exercises and then switches to a hamstring movement. Then it's back to thighs, and once again back to hamstrings. Stacey is convinced the leg muscles were designed to work together not separately.

Stacey's first hamstring exercise is usually standing leg curls. This is perhaps her favorite hamstring exercise as it's almost impossible to cheat. Stacey advises you to never let the leg lock completely out at the bottom. Stacey does 4 sets of this exercise, alternating legs. One trick Stacey has learned over the years is to contract the hamstrings at the top of the movement and hold for a count of five seconds.

After standing leg curls, Stacey does two more thigh and glute exercises, then performs seated leg curls. Stacey finds this exercise great for working the hamstring/glute tie-in area. As with standing curls, seated curls force you to perform the exercise in strict style. Stacey does 3 sets of 20 to 25 reps.

"I think it's important for everyone to have a goal so they always have a reason to improve. It's not that being in good shape isn't a good enough reason, it is, but I find a goal really helps me visualize the way I want to look all the time."
– former professional bodybuilder, fitness contestant and triathlon champion Penny Price, commenting on the importance of setting goals.

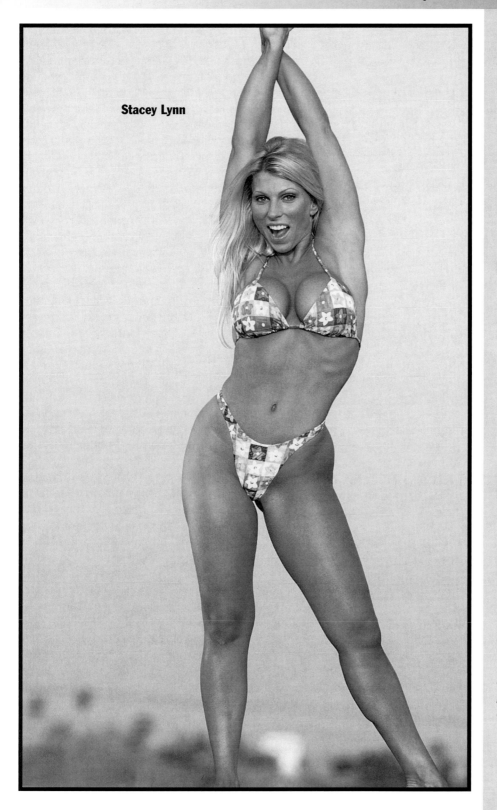

Stacey Lynn

"Simple, I just double up on everything. My normal rep range of 20 to 25 reps becomes 40 to 50, and once-daily cardio becomes two 45-minute sessions, one in the morning and one in the evening. It's exhausting but it works."

– top fitness model Stacey Lynn, in response to an interviewer's question about preparing for photo shoots and guest appearances.

CHAPTER TWENTY

Calves

Bodybuilders call them diamonds, both for their appearance and for what they're worth onstage. The calves fall into the same category as the abs and shoulders – it's next to impossible to hide them when competing. Go to any contest and you'll see that great chests and arms are a dime a dozen. But watch the reaction of the crowd when someone with great calves turns around and starts flexing them. Most audience members are also fitness or bodybuilders at heart. They know how hard it is to build great calves.

Although genetics plays a role in calf development, most people fail to build great-looking calves because of laziness. Even the one and only Arnold Schwarzenegger put calf-training off for years in favor of his chest and arms. Only after seeing South African great Reg Park did Arnold decide to get serious about his calf-training. The rest is, as they say, history. Arnold went on to develop two of the greatest calves in bodybuilding history.

As most women often wear skirts, dresses or shorts, the calves are their most visible muscle group. Well-developed calves not only complement the entire physique, but also give the illusion of leaner-looking thighs – a welcome benefit we are sure.

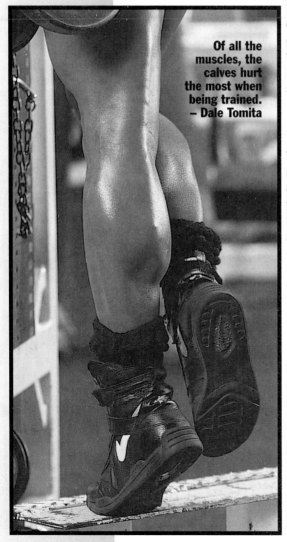

Of all the muscles, the calves hurt the most when being trained.
– Dale Tomita

Anatomy

The calves are made up of many smaller muscles, but two major "show" muscles. The upper gastrocnemius, a two-headed muscle, is responsible for the shape of well-developed calves. The soleus is located beneath the gastrocnemius, and makes up a great deal of lower legs mass. Both muscle groups are prime movers during straight-leg calf raises. You can isolate the soleus from the gastrocnemius by doing calf exercises with the knees bent.

Training

Of all the muscles, the calves hurt the most when being trained, and for many they are the most boring. Sure, everyone wants the end results, but few are willing to make the necessary sacrifices.

Calf-training is as simple as it gets. You will need to do exercises with the legs locked straight to hit the upper gastrocnemius, and exercises with the knees bent to hit the lower soleus. Although kinesiologists say otherwise, most people find that by shifting the foot stance from toes pointed in to toes pointed out, you shift the stress from inner to outer calves, and vice versa. A good calf program should include both standing and seated calf raises, as well as inward and outward toe positions.

Dale Tomita

As the winner of the 1995 NPC Women's Fitness Nationals, Dale Tomita developed a reputation for muscular development, particularly in her calves. In fact Dale's calves rival those of many of the female bodybuilders currently competing. Dale reached the point where she had to back off calf-training to keep them in proportion with the rest of her physique. Most people have to sweat and toil for years to add even an inch to their calves.

Besides great genetics, Dale attributes much of her calf development to her many years of gymnastics. All those years of tumbling, running, and other gymnastics-related activities resulted in a foundation that was perfect for fitness competition.

Dale usually does two exercises per calf workout, one of which is always seated calf raises. She believes this one exercise will do more to bring out the shape of the calves, particularly the lower calves, than any other. Dale's first set is 20 reps. Then she adds weight for an additional 4 sets, going down as low as 12 reps per set. Between sets Dale stands on a ledge and stretches her calves. She firmly believes that regular stretching is the key to calf flexibility and development.

With her calves warmed up from seated raises, Dale moves on to standing calf raises. Unlike some people who go as heavy as possible and do only partial reps, Dales uses relatively light weights and executes the exercise through the full range of motion. For variety Dale alternates her foot stance from toes pointing in to pointing straight ahead, to pointing out. Dale does 4 sets of 15 to 20 reps.

On day two Dale will again start with seated calf raises, but instead of doing standing machine raises she substitutes single-leg dumbell raises. With one hand holding on to a dumbell and the other grasping a stationary upright for support, Dale stands on a heavy wooden block. To keep the free leg from interfering, she bends it back behind her. From there the exercise is performed in a similar manner to the standing machine raise – all the way up on the toes, and down as far as the heels will drop. Again she does 4 sets of 15 to 20 reps.

Dale Tomita

"I've always had the legs I have now for as long as I can remember – not just calves, but entire leg development. Of course they were tinier when I was little, but they were still developed because I was such an active kid."
– 1995 Women's Fitness Nationals champion Dale Tomita, commenting on her leg development.

FREECLIMBER

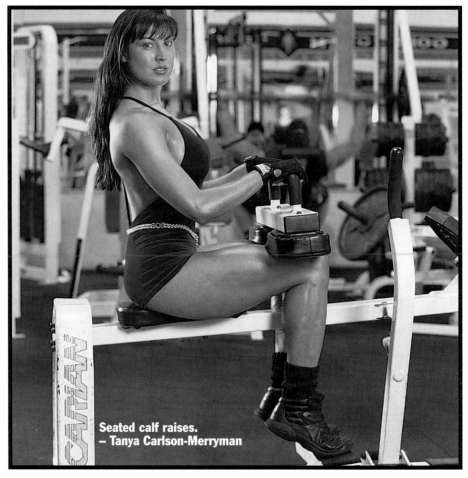

Seated calf raises.
– Tanya Carlson-Merryman

Tanya Carlson-Merryman

Tanya Carlson-Merryman is another of those "unfortunates" who have always had a muscular lower body. Even though Tanya inherited great genes from her parents, she spent up to three hours a day doing ballet and jazz dance. Of course she also busted her butt in the gym doing thousands of calf raises. She's a firm believer that genetics is no substitute for hard work.

One of Tanya's suggestions for those who are having trouble building great calves is *plyometrics*. This means anything that subjects the calves to releasing sudden bursts of power, like jumping rope or aerobics.

Another tidbit Tanya passes on is to never sacrifice form for weight. Every rep must be slow, deliberate, and perhaps most important, taken through the full range of motion. Tanya is convinced that calf-training is as much about stretching as it is about lifting weight. For those who have poor flexibility in the calf region she suggests stretching between sets. You may even need to put in extra time stretching the calves to get the full range of motion.

Tanya Carlson-Merryman trains her calves three times per week after doing some aerobics or plyometrics.

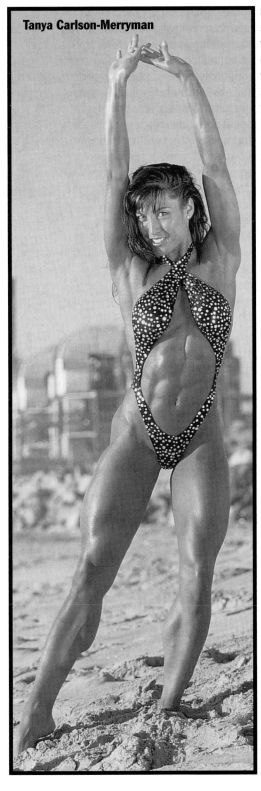

Tanya Carlson-Merryman

Seated calf raises – Tanya usually starts with seated calf raises. She feels the soleus is the real key to great-looking calves. Located on the lower part of the leg, the soleus is the part of the calf that will give the appearance of length. No matter how big you make the gastrocnemius, it won't change how long your calves look. But increase the size of the soleus and people can't but help notice.

Tanya starts with a light warmup set, then does 3 heavier sets of 15 reps. She has found over the years that her calves recover quickly so she rests only about 15 seconds between sets.

Standing calf raises – With the soleus begging for mercy, Tanya next moves on to standing calf raises to hit the gastrocnemius. Tanya does 3 drop sets of this exercise, varying her foot position from toes in, to toes forward, to toes out. Each "subset" consists of 10 reps done 3 times for 30 reps total.

Toe presses – For her third calf exercise Tanya sits in one of the leg-press machines and does toe presses, again 3 subsets of 10 reps for 30 reps total, alternating her toe position (in, out and forward).

Free-standing calf raises – To finish off her calves and to improve her flexibility, Tanya stands on a block of wood, or the foot bar on a regular standing calf machine, and does one-leg calf raises, holding a dumbell in one hand. Tanya does 3 regular sets (as opposed to drop sets) of standing calf raises for each leg.

"First and foremost I have good calf development, and it is genetic. I have always had these legs, and it is mainly because I have been a dancer, an ice skater, and a gymnast. My parents also have beautiful legs."
– 1998 Fitness America Champion Tanya Carlson-Merryman, commenting on the role genetics played in great calf development.

CHAPTER TWENTY-ONE

Biceps

When *Terminator 2* was released, besides the outstanding special effects, one of the features was Linda Hamilton's biceps. Surprising given that her co-star, Arnold Schwarzenegger, sported two of the greatest arms in movie history. But that's how far things have come on the big screen. The days of a Vivian Leigh standing around in a dress and saying "fiddle de de" are over. Today's actress is just as likely to pile up a body count as Arnold, Stallone or Jean-Claude Van Damme. If Clark Gable told one of today's female leads he "didn't give a damn," there is a good chance he'd end up singing soprano in an Austrian choir!

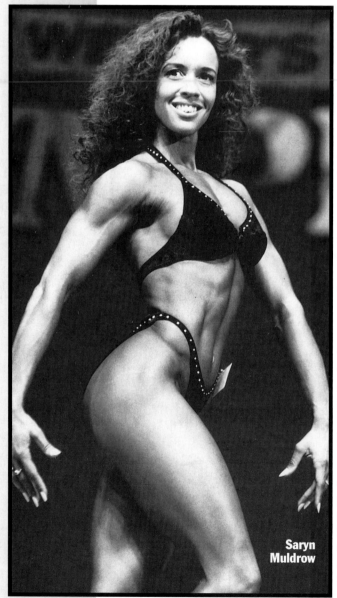

Saryn
Muldrow

Anatomy and Training

The biceps are named as such because they are a two-headed ("bi" and "ceps") muscle that runs from above the shoulder joint to below the elbow joint.

Go into any gym and chances are most patrons will be doing biceps-training, particularly the male side of the spectrum. The biceps are considered the most glamorous muscle because they are easy to see and easy to flex. And as well as being one of the easiest muscles to train, just about every type of exercise equipment (barbell, dumbells, machines, cables) can be used to stimulate the biceps.

Saryn Muldrow

The phrase "overnight sensation" gets tossed around pretty loosely these days, but this is essentially what happened to Denmark native Saryn Muldrow. She came virtually out of nowhere to win the coveted 1996 Ms. Fitness Olympia title.

Muldrow has what most fitness women would kill for, good muscle size, great shape and symmetry, and outstanding separation and detail. Her biceps are among her best bodyparts and she attributes their development to over seven years of training. She recognized early on that while most women have a genetic disposition for gaining size below the waist – whether muscle or fat – the same is not true for the upper body. Saryn was no different and she had to wait a couple of years for her upper body to catch up with her legs before she could compete.

Another important lesson Saryn learned early on was that the biceps cannot take the same degree of punishment as the larger muscles. The arms are easy to overtrain as they are involved in just about all upper-body exercises. This knowledge is one of the secrets to Muldrow's biceps-training. She never subjects her biceps to a workout with too much volume and too little rest. If she does decide to overdo it on biceps-training, she'll make a cor-responding increase in her rest period. But this is the exception rather than the norm. She usually hits the biceps twice a week.

To begin her biceps-training, Saryn typically chooses a power movement. Since fitness athletes need both pure strength and power (strength over time), Saryn always includes such training to help with her gymnastics and strength moves onstage. Although the order may vary, generally Saryn prefers to do EZ-bar curls as her first biceps exercise. First she warms up her biceps with a few light sets of alternate dumbell curls, then does 4 or 5 sets of standing EZ-bar curls. She finds the cambered bar not only gives her better biceps stimulation, but it places less stress on her wrists than a straight barbell. On most days she does 8 to 12 reps per set.

For her sec-ond exercise Saryn moves on to hammer curls using the triceps pushdown rope. She finds this a great exercise to tie in the forearms with her biceps, particularly the brachialus. She completes 3 sets of 10 to 12 reps using as much weight as she can handle to limit her to this rep range.

To finish off her Ms. Fitness Olympia biceps, Saryn does high-pulley cable curls. This exercise is performed on a cable crossover machine with the palms facing inward. Executing the exercise is similar to hitting a double-biceps pose. Both forearms are curled toward the upper body so that the biceps are fully flexed. For maximum effectiveness the upper arms must be kept parallel to the floor. Saryn does 4 sets of this exercise going to failure on each set, which in most cases is approximately 12 to 15 reps.

Kelly Ryan

Dale Tomita

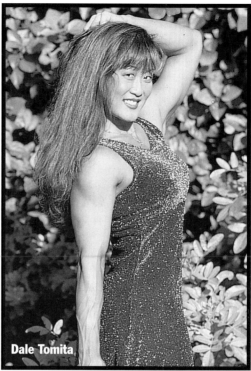

Dale Tomita

Although she had laid a good foundation from many years of gymnastics training, Dale Tomita still needed to work hard to bring her arms in line with her lower body. These days she focuses primarily on shape and explosive movements to help her onstage routine. Dale prefers high-rep sets with as little rest as possible. No wonder she's also a big fan of supersets.

A typical biceps program starts with 3 sets of straight-bar curls and hammer curls. When doing the barbell curls she prefers to keep her elbows further back than most people do. She does 10 reps of barbell curls and moves on to hammers with no break. With hammers Dale has her own unique style. Instead of standard hammer curls she does them in a concentration curl format. After 12 to 15 reps she pauses just long enough to catch her breath, then it's back to barbell curls.

To finish her biceps Dale attaches an EZ-shaped bar to a low pulley and does standing cable curls. To ease the strain on her back she keeps a slight bend in her knees, and to use her own words, "almost sits into the movement." This is one of the few exercises on which Dale likes to perform lower reps, which average 10 per set.

> *"It's my contention that people need to look at their body objectively and work on symmetry. Symmetry is the context of everything that is form. Being balanced in appearance is most important."*
> – top fitness competitor Dale Tomita, commenting on the importance of symmetry.

Lisa Lowe

Lisa Lowe is a perfect example of how fitness women can reap the benefits of a bodybuilder's approach to training. Lean and defined, Lisa is proof that bodybuilding techniques do not necessarily result in bulk and size.

Not long after she started weight training to help with an old dancing injury, Lisa entered her first bodybuilding contest. Lisa placed second at the 1990 Seaside Bodybuilding Classic. But as she said later, the diet was so strict that she didn't do anything for six years!

Despite dropping out of competitive bodybuilding, Lisa kept training to improve her physique, and in 1996 once again took the plunge at a show in Sacramento, California. Despite placing third, she was very pleased with her performance. She realized one thing, though. She had taken her genetics as far as they could naturally go. Lisa had no intention of venturing into the drug culture that had taken over women's professional bodybuilding, so she started looking into the fitness side of the industry. At first she was turned off by the "evening gown" format of some contests, but then she witnessed an NPC contest that had no "fashion" element. In 1997 she entered her first show in California – and won. Lisa Lowe, fitness contestant, had arrived.

Since her debut in 1997, Lisa has managed to place in the top ten in a number of big shows. Lisa has not let her lack of a gymnastics background stand in her way. A combination of perseverance plus some old dance moves has allowed her to remain on equal footing with those women who have a formal gymnastics background.

Among her greatest assets are her beautifully proportioned biceps. Lisa trains biceps and triceps separately, finding that as soon as one side of the arm is fully pumped, it's difficult to do justice to the other side. Even though she changes her workouts all the time, the following is a representative biceps routine she performs on a regular basis.

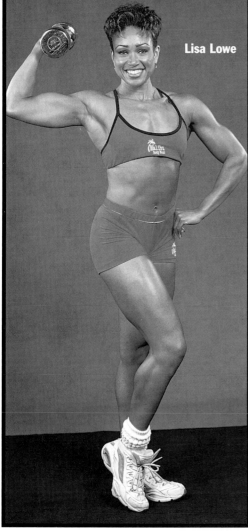

Lisa Lowe

Standing barbell curls – Lisa starts this exercise by making sure her feet are placed firmly on the floor, about shoulder-width apart. She's not a stickler for having her elbows locked by her sides like most people, but even so they come forward only a couple of inches as she curls the bar upward. Lisa starts with one set of 12 reps, then pyramids up in weight and down in reps for the next 3 sets.

Incline dumbell curls – Through trial and error Lisa has found a 45-degree angle works best for her on this exercise. She lets her arms hang by her sides, then curls upward until her forearms are at about a 45-degree angle to horizontal. She does 4 sets of 8 to 10 repetitions, once again pyramiding up in weight.

Machine preacher curls – Even though she occasionally does barbell preacher curls, Lisa finds the machine version much easier to control. She also finds the machine provides stimulation to her biceps through a greater range of motion. She typically does 3 sets of 8 to 10 reps.

Concentration curls – To finish off her biceps Lisa sits down on the end of a bench and does one-arm dumbell concentration curls. She prefers the supported version with her elbow resting on the inside of her thigh. Once again it's 4 sets of 8 to 10 reps.

"When I got into weight training I stuck myself in with the big guys and did whatever they did. I started off as a ballet dancer and did some jazz; however, I injured my back jazz dancing. My therapist said I needed to try lifting some weights to help stabilize my lower-back muscles. And that's when I got into weight training."
– top fitness competitor Lisa Lowe, revealing her introduction to weight training.

Debi Massey

Debi Massey is a perfect example of how fitness can change a person's life. Her initial career was teaching phys-ed, but she gave it all up to pursue her dream of fitness. In short order she went from 11th place at the 1998 USA championships to an impressive 2nd at the NPC Nationals a few months later. To complement her new lifestyle, Debi became a massage therapist and personal trainer along the way.

During the off-season Debi's primary aim is to increase her muscle size and strength. She feels the latter is important as it allows her to incorporate more challenging stunts into her fitness routine. To accomplish this goal, Debi added some basic powerlifting exercises to her training.

Debi is noted for her great biceps development. Her workout usually consists of three movements, utilizing all three basic pieces of equipment – barbells, dumbells and cables. She starts with barbell curls as she feels they are the single best exercise for biceps development. She places her feet shoulder width apart, knees slightly bent. To keep the tension on her biceps, she stops the bar about four inches from her shoulders. At the top she pauses and squeezes her biceps for a second, then lowers to just short of the lockout position at the bottom. In all she does 3 sets of 8 to 10 reps.

Debi's second exercise is dumbell concentration curls. She chooses the conventional style, sitting on the end of a bench and resting the working arm on the inside of the thigh. She tries to maintain a neutral wrist position throughout the full range of motion in order to reduce forearm involvement. As with barbell curls she stops the dumbell about four inches from her shoulder and squeezes her biceps. For those who have trouble holding their elbow against their thigh, Debi recommends a preacher bench. She typically does 3 sets of 8 to 10 reps.

To finish off her biceps (and begin her triceps-training, which we'll cover in the next chapter), Debi supersets high cable curls with one-arm cable kickbacks. For cable curls she attaches a handle to each high pulley of the cable-crossover machine. She then curls the handles toward her as if doing a double-biceps pose. She stops the handles about four inches from her head and gives the biceps a squeeze.

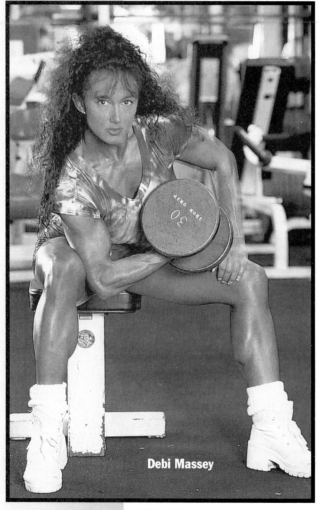

Debi Massey

With little rest she then does a set of cable kickbacks. In all Debi does 3 sets of 12 reps of cable curls as part of her biceps/triceps superset.

Kelly Ryan

Kelly Ryan's climb to the top of women's professional fitness was not an overnight surprise but a carefully constructed plan coupled with a do-or-die attitude on the gym floor. The winner of the 2000 Arnold Classic, Ms. Fitness International, and runner-up in the 1999 Olympia – her first IFBB show – Ryan combines an amazingly muscular body with showgirl charisma and an All-American cheerleader smile (a product of her days as head cheerleader at the University of South Carolina).

Sets and Reps
Kelly doesn't want to put on any more muscular mass, so she keeps her reps for each set at 15 to 20, and does three sets of each exercise.

Barbell curls – Kelly begins with the classic biceps-builder, known to every novice and advanced student of progressive-resistance exercise. The barbell curl works the entire biceps area, with good emphasis on inner biceps thickness to produce an appealing round balance.

Standing dumbell curls – Another classic, this variation of the curl ensures that both biceps are developed equally. While many experts like to markedly turn the hand in toward the body as it nears the top position – Kelly prefers to keep the dumbells relatively steady in their orientation, although she sometimes varies that.

Cable curls – Used as a finishing exercise and to produce pronounced peaks, cable curls can be done in a variety of standing positions. Note that Kelly keeps her free arm stationary and uninvolved in the exercise so that the biceps are truly isolated and does all the work. Her body remains equally stationary throughout, to make sure she does not cheat and bring other muscles into play.

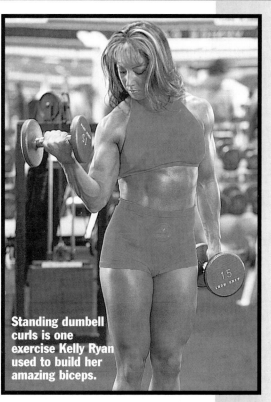

Standing dumbell curls is one exercise Kelly Ryan used to build her amazing biceps.

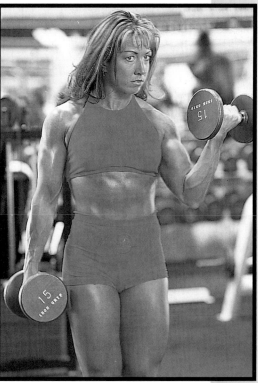

CHAPTER TWENTY-TWO

Triceps

Next to the thighs and hips, the triceps are probably the greatest trouble spot for most women. It's a region the body finds convenient for storing bodyfat and a combination of fat and poor muscle tone will leave the triceps looking like two hammocks. Despite the popularity of the biceps, it is the triceps that provide most of the arm's power, particularly when it comes to pushing.

Anatomy and Training

Like the biceps and quadriceps, the triceps are named because the muscle is subdivided into three heads ("tri" and "ceps"). The triceps are analogous to the thighs in that they are the primary extensor muscles of the upper arms. That is they extend the arms straight out at the elbow joint.

As the triceps affect only a single joint (the elbow), isolation of the three heads is difficult. But by varying your exercises and angles it is possible to shift the stress slightly to each head separately. Even though there are literally dozens of triceps exercises, most fall into two categories – pushdowns and extensions. As will the biceps, all types of equipment can be used (and should be used) to train the triceps.

Dale Tomita

Although she stands just 5'1", Dale Tomita is a virtual powerhouse onstage or off. Packed on her muscular frame are two of the most powerful legs in the women's fitness scene. In fact her legs are so muscularly developed that she's had to work extra hard to bring her upper body into proportion.

Dale got her introduction to competitive sports from 11 years of gymnastics. Only a knee injury at 17 years of age prevented her from the dream of competing in the Olympics. Of course what was the Olympics' loss was the fitness industry's gain, and today Dale is the envy of millions with her outstanding physique.

Dale's triceps are especially eye-catching. She usually trains biceps and triceps together and has a unique method of combining the two muscle groups. After finishing most of her biceps exercises, she supersets the last biceps exercise with her first triceps exercise. On most days she will choose standing cable curls for biceps and one-arm cable kickbacks for triceps. She finds this pair a great superset as you can do both on the same machine,

Danielle Edwards

using the low pulley for biceps and upper pulley for triceps. As we discussed her biceps exercises in the previous chapter, we'll limit ourselves to triceps here.

Dale says the key to performing cable kickbacks is to keep the upper arm completely immobile. Only the forearm and hand must move the weight. Dale keeps her knees slightly bent and the nonworking arm placed on her hips. She then extends the arm down and back until it's completely locked out at the bottom. Dale completes 3 sets (as part of the biceps/triceps superset) of one-arm cable kickbacks.

For her second and third triceps exercises, Dale supersets rope pushdowns and dumbell kickbacks. Again Dale stresses the importance of keeping the elbows "glued to the sides." On the rope pushdowns she recommends experimenting with different elbow positionings to see which works best for you. After one set of rope pushdowns Dale puts her knee on a flat bench and executes a set of dumbell kickbacks. Proper form for Dale on this exercise is to

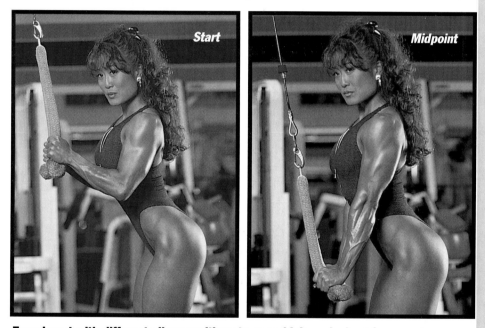

Experiment with different elbow positions to see which works best for you when performing rope pushdowns. – Dale Tomita

lock the elbow against the side so her upper arm is parallel with the floor. She then extends her forearm back until it's locked completely straight out behind. Dale uses a 10- or 15-pound dumbell and completes a set of 10 reps before moving back to rope pushdowns. She does 3 supersets of both exercises.

Dale is also a big believer in stretching, especially between sets. In the short term this will speed up the removal of lactic acid, and in the long term will increase the muscle's range of motion.

A final Tomita tidbit is variety. The previous routine is but one example of Dale's triceps-training. She frequently changes exercises to keep the muscles guessing. It's also much more fun, and that's what getting in shape should be all about.

Lisa Lowe

For IFBB fitness pro Lisa Lowe, balance is everything. That's pretty much what you'd expect from a former ballet dancer who began by studying with the San Francisco ballet, was admitted to the prestigious Juilliard dance department, and performed with the famed Alvin Alley dance troupe in New York City. Lisa is one of the fitness industry's most dedicated professionals. She earned her pro card at the 1998 Team Universe contest, and recently took first place at the 2000 Rimini Pro Fitness Classic in Rimini, Italy.

Lisa usually trains triceps on Mondays after her chest routine. She's found over the years that her triceps respond best to a high-volume approach. Even though she realizes the triceps receive a great deal of stimulation from her chest- and shoulder-training, she still needs to do 12 to 14 sets of direct work to keep them improving.

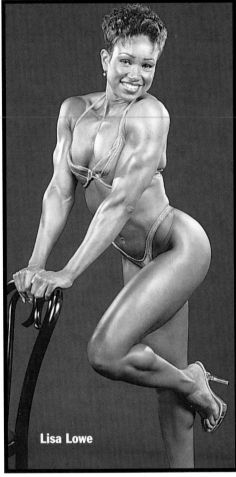

Lisa Lowe

Lisa usually starts her triceps-training with a basic power movement like dips. She tried conventional parallel-bar dips, but found that her chest and shoulders did too much of the work. Instead she places two flat benches together and performs bench dips between them. This exercise allows her to lean back and shift most of the stress from the chest to the triceps. Lisa usually does 4 sets of 12 to 20 reps (20, 15, 12 and 12).

With her triceps now fully warmed up, Lisa moves on to lying EZ-bar extensions. She admits this is a difficult movement to execute properly and advises beginners to go light until they master the technique. Over the years Lisa has tried lowering the bar to different points (chin, nose, top of the head), but found that lowering the bar to her forehead produced the best feel in her triceps. She recommends everyone experiment to see which position is best for them. Lisa typically does 4 sets of 8 to 10 reps.

For her third exercise Lisa moves on to one of her favorites, dumbell kickbacks. The key to this exercise, says Lisa, is to make sure you have your body braced on a flat bench, and your upper arm locked by your side and parallel to the floor. She does 3 sets of 8 to 10 reps.

For her fourth and final set Lisa chooses two-arm dumbell extensions. Again she's tried different versions over the years (one dumbell/one hand, two hands/two dumbells) but the two-hands/one-dumbell version works best for her. She lowers the dumbell down to a comfortable stretch, then returns to the arms-locked-out position. She usually does 3 sets of 8 to 12 reps.

Debi Massey

Given the number of pushing and pressing movements in a typical fitness routine, it's not surprising that Debi Massey takes triceps-training very seriously. The ability to do handstands and pushups relies heavily on triceps' strength, so Debi makes sure hers are up to the job.

Debi's triceps routine consists of four movements, all chosen to increase both strength and development. As we saw earlier, Debi begins training her triceps as she is finishing off her biceps. That is she supersets the last biceps exercise with her first triceps movement. As soon as she completes one set of high-cable curls, she immediately grabs one handle of the cable-crossover machine and does a set of cable kickbacks (also called one-arm cable pushdowns). As with her biceps exercises, Debi holds the contracted position (in this case the arm fully extended at the bottom) for a second and squeezes the muscle. She does one set of 12 reps, then switches back to the overhead cable curl. She does 3 such supersets of 12 reps each.

Debi's second triceps exercise is rope pushdowns. Debi has tried various attachments over the years but found the rope gave her the best feeling in her triceps. Besides placing less stress on the wrists, Debi realized that, by separating her hands at the bottom, she could get a better contraction in triceps. This slight variation is unique to the rope. Bar attachments lock your hands in one position. Debi starts with a heavy weight for the first set of 8 reps, then decreases the weight for 2 additional sets of 10 and 12 reps respectively.

Next up are one-arm dumbell extensions. Debi finds this exercise great for stretching the triceps. For variety she occasionally does the two-hand version, but finds the one-arm version allows for a deeper stretch at the bottom. She does 2 sets of 8 to 10 reps, alternating arms.

To finish off her by now fatigued triceps, Debi does dumbell kickbacks. She places one knee and hand on a bench for support and always keeps her lower back flat, not rounded. To add a few extra degrees of contraction Debi rotates her palm from inward to upward when her arm is fully extended. She typically does 3 sets of 10 reps for each arm, with as little rest as possible between sets.

Kelly Ryan

Triceps pushdowns – The current favorite in triceps-training develops excellent mass over the entire triceps via a full extension and long motion. Note that Kelly uses a straight bar, in contrast to many of the V-bars often seen, and that she begins the pushdowns – also called pressdowns – from a position well above horizontal. She's wedded to neither, and will switch off to a horizontal start or use a cambered V-bar, or both, as she sees fit. The triceps thrive on variation.

"When I'm putting together my stage routine and practicing all the time, my triceps are fried from all the pushups and pressing movements, so I don't train them in the gym at all."
– 2nd place Nationals winner Debi Massey, commenting on her approach to triceps training.

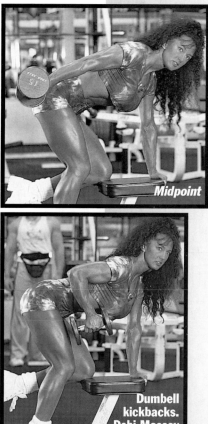

Midpoint

Dumbell kickbacks. – Debi Massey
Start

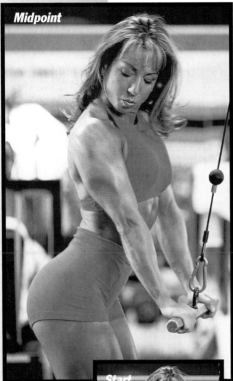

Midpoint

The triceps
thrive on
variation.
– Kelly Ryan

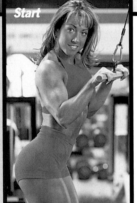

Start

Standing overhead rope extensions – Unlike rope pressdowns, which are usually accompanied by a flare to the outside at the conclusion of the extension, you'll more often see standing overhead rope extensions performed without the flare. They can be flared to provide a variation, but done this way they provide a nice elongating development over the entire length of the triceps. Kelly makes sure her upper arm remains stationary throughout the movement, with movement at a stable elbow, which acts as a fixed pivot to prevent adjacent large muscle groups from taking over the load.

Dumbell kickbacks – Include at least one free weight exercise into your triceps routine to ensure that stabilizing muscles are draw into play and provide a less isolated and more complete look. Although triceps kickbacks, like most triceps exercises, work the entire area, they tend to work the upper and inner head of the triceps a little more aggressively. Kelly keeps the upper arm stationary. As with all her triceps work, Kelly extends her arm to just short of a lockout, keeping constant tension on the triceps, as opposed to letting them rest as the elbow takes the load.

Brandi Carrier

Unlike most other fitness athletes, Brandi Carrier rarely trains arms on a regular basis. This may come as a shock to most readers given the routines of some of the other fitness stars. Brandi has found that her preparations for the obstacle-course round of fitness contests is usually sufficient to keep her arms firm and trim. Brandi admits, however, that if a big photo shoot is on her agenda, she may need to do some serious arm specializing. Even then Brandi has to be careful not to ruin her proportions. Blessed with long muscle attachments she finds her arms respond quickly and tend to overpower the rest of her torso.

Unlike most bodybuilders, Brandi's primary focus when she trains triceps is function. Sure appearance is important, but she knows that winning a tough fitness competition like the Ms. Galaxy requires muscles that are capable of performing.

Brandi's first triceps exercise is usually rope pushdowns. Even though most people consider this an isolation exercise, Brandi considers it one of her primary power movements. She prefers the rope attachment as it allows for more flexion at the lower part of the movement. You can spread your hands apart as you approach lockout at the bottom. Brandi pyramids her weight, going from 10 reps down to just 4. She also pays close attention to exercise tempo. She'll take approximately one second to push the weight down and five seconds to raise it back to the starting position.

For her second exercise Brandi does one-arm dumbell kickbacks. She places one knee and hand on a flat bench for support, and bends forward until her torso is just short of parallel with the floor. She strongly advises you to keep a slight arch in the lower back and not let it round. The upper arm and elbow is then locked tight to the side and the forearm extended or "kicked back" to the lockout position. Brandi prefers an ascending pyramid on this exercise, going from heavy weight that allows just 6 reps, to a very light weight that lets her do 25 reps.

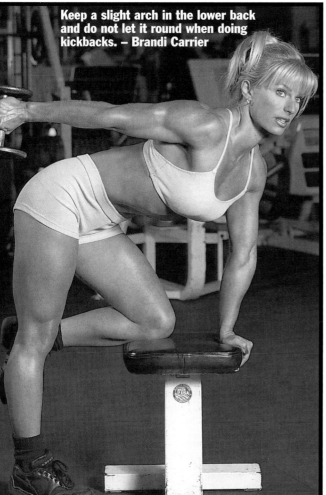

Keep a slight arch in the lower back and do not let it round when doing kickbacks. – Brandi Carrier

Brandi's third exercise is the one-arm cable pushdown. With her free hand placed on her hip, Brandi grasps the overhead pulley and extends her arm down and slightly back to the lockout position. As with any pushdown or kickback, the elbow and upper arm should always be kept stationary against the side. As with rope pushdowns, Brandi considers this a power movement and uses heavy weight that allows for just 3 sets of 4 to 6 reps.

Exercise number four is the one-arm dumbell extension. Brandi sits on a bench with a vertical back support and holds a dumbell straight up in the air. With her free hand placed on her shoulder for support, Brandi lowers the dumbell behind her head until it touches her shoulder blade. She then extends it back to the starting position. The key to this exercise is to keep the elbow pointing at the ceiling at all times. Again Brandi treats this as a power exercise and does 3 sets of 4 to 6 reps.

To finish off her triceps Brand places her feet on a flat bench and her hands on the floor. Then she does 3 sets of pushups to failure, which in her case usually gives a 12, 10 and 8 rep scheme.

Brandi Carrier's Triceps Routine
1. Rope pushdowns – 4 sets x 4 to 10 reps
2. One-arm kickbacks – 3 sets x 6 to 25 reps
3. One-arm cable pushdowns – 3 sets x 4 to 6 reps
4. One-arm dumbell extensions – 3 sets x 4 to 6 reps

"I don't find I need as much weight training for my arms as I do for other bodyparts, mainly because my focus on obstacle-course training provides me with a strenuous workout."
– 1996 Ms. Galaxy winner, Brandi Carrier, commenting on her arm-training.

CHAPTER TWENTY-THREE

Abdominals

Probably more fitness-related books have been devoted to the abdominals than any other bodypart. Everyone wants a trimmer, tighter midsection. Ironically the key to a smaller waist is more cardio and nutrition than direct ab-training. Everyone has abdominals, from the fitness stars onstage sporting "six-paks" to the 400 pounds of obesity sitting in the bleachers. But the fitness stars have their abs exposed, whereas the bleacher-creatures have a considerable covering obscuring theirs.

Anatomy and Training

"I have found that my lean and muscular look sets me apart from the super-skinny models and actresses."
– Galaxy Fitness winner and up-and-coming actress Torrie Wilson, commenting on how she compares to many of today's models and actresses.

The abdominals are a long sheath of muscle that runs from the sternum to the pelvis. Although there are no upper and lower abs (the muscle fibers run north-south not east-west) for practical purposes it is possible to put more emphasis on one area than the other.

The lower abdominal region is very problematic for women. The menstrual cycle causes significant water retention each month, which causes the body to react by stretching the muscle outward. The effects of childbearing can be even more dramatic. As the lower abdominal region is much thinner than the upper, the muscles can only provide limited resistance and eventually the lower abs become softer and more pliable, ultimately causing a bulge in the region.

Training the abs consists of either moving the upper body and keeping the legs stationary, or keeping the upper body stationary and elevating the legs. A good ab routine should include exercises from both categories.

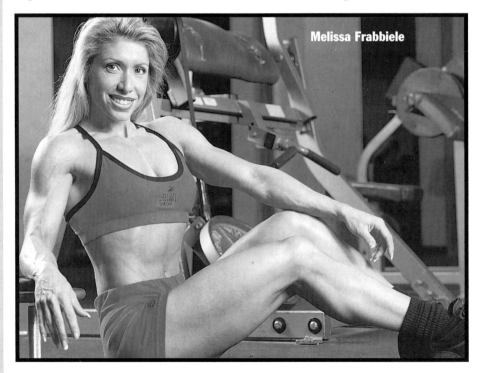

Melissa Frabbiele

Torrie Wison

In September of 1998, McCall, Idaho native Torrie Wilson arrived in Los Angeles in pursuit of a career in acting. Despite the trend at the time for actresses to look like strung-out heroin addicts with their anorexic looks, Torrie vowed to remain true to the ideals of health and fitness. She soon graced the cover of both *Oxygen* and *MuscleMag International* magazines, then proved she was no "show girl" by winning the prestigious Galaxy Fitness crown.

Since arriving in Hollywood Torrie has appeared on *Baywatch* and *Inside Edition,* and regularly appears on WCW wrestling as David Flare's girlfriend.

Torrie feels that Hollywood is moving away from the superskinny look and she regularly gets positive comments on her toned and proportioned physique. Speaking of proportions, Torrie's abs are the envy of millions. Her midsection has that perfect combination of flatness and definition. She trains her abdominals every second day, including both weighted and bodyweight-only exercises. Torrie is convinced that to build impressive abdominals, resistance in the form of weight is necessary.

Besides giving her the results she wants, Torrie has another reason for using weighted abdominal exercises. Since moving to Los Angeles, time has become a premium for Torrie. By adding weights she gets the desired abdominal burn in a shorter period of time. She averages 20 to 50 reps per set on those exercises involving weights, and 75 to 150 reps on bodyweight exercises. Since Torrie alternates the exercises on a regular basis it's difficult to nail down an exact routine, but here are some of her favorite exercises.

Crunches – Torrie always includes some form of crunch in her ab workout. Standard crunches are a great way for beginners to master proper technique. She adds, though, that it is possible to do crunches without utilizing the abs at all. You must learn to concentrate on feeling the abs on every rep. She also adds that many people swing the elbows back and forth. Not only does this form of cheating bring momentum into the exercise and make it less effective, but it also places extra stress on the neck. The elbows must be kept pointed outward at all times. Torrie does 2 or 3 sets of about 75 reps per workout.

Torrie Wilson

Incline crunches – To increase the level of difficulty, Torrie sometimes executes crunches on an incline board. With the angle the abdominal burn kicks in faster, so she doesn't need to do as many reps. She usually crunches 2 sets of about 50 reps.

Hanging leg raise – Torrie's favorite exercise to hit the lower abs is the hanging leg raise. She grabs hold of an overhead chinning bar and slowly raises her legs upward until her thighs are just past the halfway point. This is one exercise where her grip strength is the limiting factor and she gets about 20 reps before having to let go. She usually does 3 or 4 sets of this one, lifting both to the front and to each side.

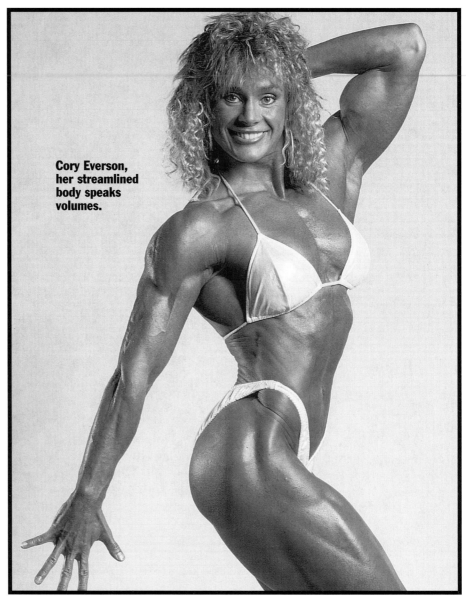

Cory Everson, her streamlined body speaks volumes.

Rope crunches – To really bring on that abdominal burn, Torrie goes over to a triceps pushdown machine and connects a rope to the overhead pulley. From there she kneels on a bench, rests the rope handles behind her head, and crunches forward. She averages 2 sets of 150 reps on this exercise.

Standing cable crunches – To bring in the serratus, Torrie stands next to a cable machine, reaches above her head, and grabs the pulley handle with the opposite hand. She crunches away from the machine, pausing at the bottom to give the abdominals and serratus a good contraction, then returns to the upright position. Torrie likes to use a heavy weight on this exercise and does 2 sets of 25 reps per side.

Cory Everson

It's safe to say Cory Everson was the Arnold Schwarzenegger of female body-building. Her name became synonymous with fitness, and not only does her stream-lined body speak volumes, but she's also been a trusted voice of experience for both men and women. Even though other women came before her, it was Cory who introduced millions of women to the benefits of weight training.

Her top-selling books *Fat Free & Fit* and *Cory Everson's Workout,* along with her complete multi-video series, have served as motivational tools for thousands of people trying to better themselves. In addition she starred in her own TV show, *Gotta Sweat.* Cory has appeared on over 100 magazine covers worldwide, and won the Ms. Olympia competition six consecutive times, from 1984 to '89.

During her Ms. Olympia days in the mid to late 1980s Cory's physique had few if any flaws. Her abdominals were particularly impressive and she always spent 15 to 20 minutes a day training them. The following is but one routine Cory used to make her midsection the envy of millions. Some days she did the exercises as straight sets, on others she performed 3 giant sets.

Six-time
Ms. Olympia
Cory Everson

1. Crunches – 3 sets x 50 reps
2. Rope crunches – 3 sets x 50 reps
3. Decline situps – 3 sets x 50 reps
4. Side crunches – 3 sets x 50 reps

CHAPTER TWENTY-FOUR

Getting In Shape Doesn't Have to Be Boring

One of the prevailing myths about getting in shape is "the process is boring." Nothing could be further from the truth. There are endless ways to lose weight and tone up that body of yours. The following suggestions will help put a little pizzazz back into your training.

Walking – As Effective As it is Simple

You've just met a deadline imposed upon you at the last minute by the boss. Your mind is exhausted and the lower back is starting to serenade you for all those hours sitting at the computer terminal. You could wait until after work and hit the gym as usual – lots of fancy and expensive machines to work out on. And after all, there is a correlation between the quality of a workout and how much money is spent, right? Wrong!

Sometimes the best forms of exercise are the simplest, and perhaps more important, the cheapest. Let's go back to the previous example. Rather than wait untill after work to hit the gym, why not skip most of your lunch break and go for a walk. Assuming a standard 45 to 60 minute break, use 15 minutes to grab a bite to eat, then invest the other 30 to 45 minutes in your mental and physical well-being. Leave the office and go for a brisk walk in the fresh air. We can almost guarantee that within five minutes all thoughts of work will be far behind you, those feeling of anxiety and tension replaced by a healthy dose of the better things in life. Your aching lower back will start feeling its old self again. All of this for the investment of half an hour of your time.

Most people are shocked to learn that brisk walking offers almost the same degree of benefits as jogging or running, and without the same degree of stress on the joints. For example running places three to four times the weight of your body on each step, whereas walking produces one to one and a half times the weight of your body on each step.

For those who think walking offers little in the way of cardiovascular conditioning and calorie-burning, take a look at these numbers. At a pace of 4 mph (15 minutes to do a mile) the average person burns 4 to 6 calories per minute.

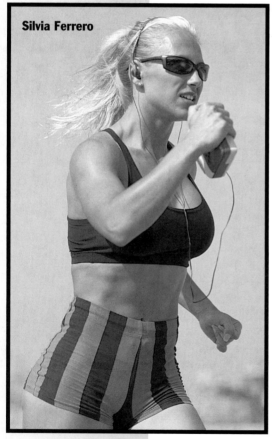

Silvia Ferrero

That works out to 240 to 360 calories per hour. At a slightly faster pace (5 mph, 12 minutes to do a mile) the energy expenditure is 450 to 600 calories per hour, meaning every six walking sessions burns off one pound.

The Way of the Walk

It may seem simple enough, after all most of us have been doing it since we were one or two years old, but walking does have some do's and don'ts with regard to proper form, especially at a faster than normal pace. Your posture should be erect with your abdominals tightened for good back support. Your feet should hit the ground squarely, heels first and toes lifted high. Also, to move faster don't increase your stride. Instead increase the number of steps per minute. To walk a mile in 12 minutes you will need to take approximately 160 steps. For a 15-minute mile you will need to make 135 steps a minute. Keep in mind speed burns calories. As with sprinting your arms should be bent at 90 degrees and your elbows tucked into your waist. A controlled arm swing does not allow your fingertips to cross the midline of your body or reach above your chest. You can close your fingers but don't clench them too tight.

For legs, try to step from the hips. And it's a good idea to do some light stretching before and after your walk to increase flexibility and blood supply to the muscles.

Get in the Habit

Psychologists tell us it takes about three weeks to form a habit, so don't let the first week throw you off. Make a commitment to walking three to five times a week for the next three weeks. Just three times per week is enough to maintain cardiovascular conditioning. For those relying on walking to improve their cardiovascular health, five or six times per week is recommended.

It's easy, it's fun, and it can be done just about anywhere at any time. Give walking a try the next time you want to leave the office behind.

Timea Majorova

Jumping Rope

Looking for a cheap and fun way to add variety to your conditioning? Try regressing to your childhood. Remember how you couldn't wait for recess to get outside and jump rope with your friends? Well, you were doing more than just having fun – you were engaging in one of the simplest yet most effective forms of physical activity.

Jumping rope is practiced by everyone from playground kids to world-class boxers. If you want to see poetry in motion take a look at some of Muhammad Ali's old tapes. The nice thing about jumping rope is the cost. An investment of about $10, plus a good pair of shoes, is about all a person needs to get started. Fitness experts say regular skipping sessions can improve heart rate, breathing, endurance, upper and lower body strength, and coordination. Keep that in mind when you hear someone start bragging about the latest $5000 piece of equipment at her gym!

Learning the Basics

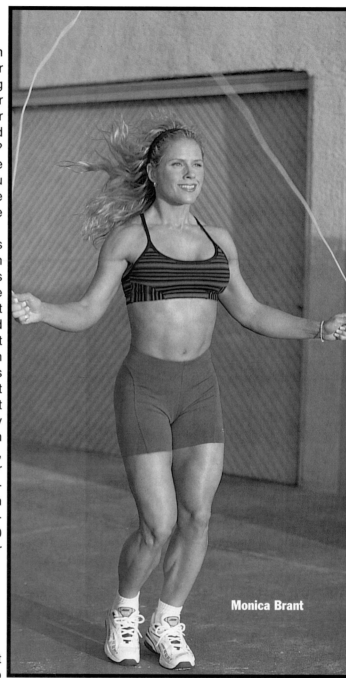

Monica Brant

There are many different lengths of skipping rope. To choose the right length for you, step on the middle of the rope with one foot and bring both hands up to the chest. Your handles should reach just below chest high. Two of the most popular are the colorful beaded ropes and fast-speed leather ropes. Either one will do. When starting to jump, be sure to have enough room around you, including ceiling space as well. Make sure to stay clear of hanging lights and fans!

Jumping Do's and Don'ts

• Wear aerobic shoes or cross-trainers at all times. Don't jump barefoot.
• Stay on the toes and balls of your feet when jumping. Your heels should barely touch, if at all. A wooden or matted floor is easier and preferred rather than carpet.
• Stand tall with abdominals tight, not hunched, your knees slightly bent when landing. Use your calves as shock-absorbers.
• Keep shoulders relaxed with elbows close to your sides.
• Always turn the rope from your wrists without using your full arm.
• Don't try to jump too high. Keep the impact lower for your knees and ankles. Great jumpers need only about an inch off the ground.
• Don't look at your feet! Look straight ahead and concentrate on an even rhythm in your breathing.

Practice Makes Progress!

If it's been a while since you jumped rope, don't worry. You will be the one who sees the most progress the quickest. There are two skills that just keep getting better and better when jumping rope: cardiovascular endurance and coordination. You may be starting at the very beginning with both or maybe you already feel inept at one. A great program to help you see results in both skills is to keep a journal and record your progress.

Endurance – Whether you are naturally trained for anaerobic or aerobic conditioning, jumping rope will help your heart pump more efficiently regardless. It doesn't matter how much time you have. Just start jumping. Put a clock in front of you with a second hand on it. Start with 10 seconds at a time with a 10-second rest. Then move to 20 seconds with a 20 second rest ... and so on! You'll be jumping rope for minutes sooner than you think!

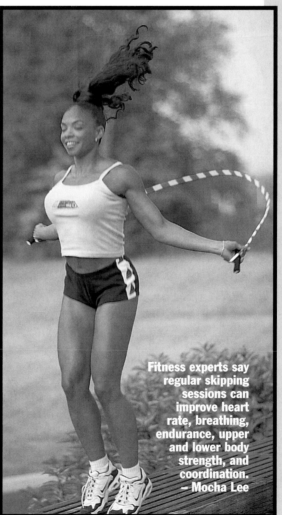

Fitness experts say regular skipping sessions can improve heart rate, breathing, endurance, upper and lower body strength, and coordination.
– Mocha Lee

Coordination – Once you have mastered jumping for approximately 20 seconds at a time landing on both feet, it's time to go on to more challenging moves. The reason is twofold: you want to keep challenging yourself physically with coordination tests and challenging yourself mentally to overcome the great boredom factor. Try this:

- Two-footed landing with double hop between jumps
- Two-footed landing with single hop between jumps
- Single-footed landing: 8 each side, 4 each side, 2 each side, single each side
- Jog, knees up high
- Jog with hamstrings curl
- Scissor legs on landing (front and back with switch)
- Jumping Jack legs on landing (out and in)
- Jumping backwards
- Double-jump (two spins of the rope with one hop)
- Crossovers (cross arms and jump, uncross over head)
- Swing rope side to side and jump in between
- Boxer's shuffle, fast and slow

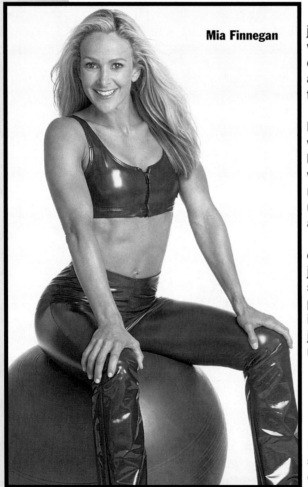

Mia Finnegan

You could incorporate a rope-jumping workout routine in with your weightlifting or other cardiovascular exercises. Jumping to the beat of music and slowly speeding it up is a great way to challenge yourself even more.

Skipping is simple, easy and fun. Keep your jump rope by your bed, where you'll be sure to trip over it or at least look at it every morning when you wake up or every night before you retire. That may remind you to pick it up, even for as little as five minutes at a time.

Hey, we understand. It's the 21st century. Gone are the days of the 9 to 5 job with dinner on the table at 6:00; now some of us don't get home until 7 or 8 p.m. and dinner is bought and eaten just in time to watch the 11 o'clock news and jump into bed to be ready for work the next day.

On the Ball with the Swiss

Every week a quick scan of the home shopping network reveals some new gizmo that supposedly is the greatest invention since sliced bread. You know the commercials, "… just ten minutes three times a week for the midsection you've always dreamed about." Most of these crazy contraptions end up as nothing more than fancy clothes hangers. (One lady told the authors she put a blanket over hers and made an indoor doghouse!) Every now and then, however, one of these inventions actually stands the test of time. Case in point is the stability ball – or Swiss ball.

Swiss balls are large, inflated, rubber and vinyl balls used by physical therapists to enhance the neurodevelopment of their patients. More recently the Swiss ball has been introduced as a strength-training aid to athletes. Training in an unstable environment is said to strengthen stabilizer muscles, reduce chance of injury due to repetitive stress, and improve nervous-system function that leads to functional strength gains. The shape of the ball also facilitates multi-angle training and allows greater range of motion on some exercises – both potentially important factors in properly training certain muscle groups. Exercise-ball workouts increase flexibility, stamina and strength without jarring your body with hard impacts.

We recommend the use of Swiss balls with an anti-burst system to guarantee the safety that is vital for exercising or sitting. These products have the highest quality and safety standards in the world. Due to new technology these balls have extremely high weight limitations. Most importantly, they will not explode if punctured. If a sharp object were to penetrate the skin of the ball, the air would escape slowly, eliminating the risk of injuries.

Although you can use just about any size ball, the following chart provides recommendations based on height. Choosing a ball that fits your body dimensions will make the exercises more effective.

How to determine the correct ball size:

Body Height	Size of Ball	Maximum Inflation
up to 4'10" (up to 145 cm)	small	18" (45 cm)
4'10" to 5'5" (145-165 cm)	medium	22" (55 cm)
5'5" to 6'0" (165-185 cm)	large	26" (65 cm)
6'0" to 6'5" (185-195cm)	X-large	30" (75 cm)
over 6'5" (over 195 cm)	XX-large	33" (85 cm)

One of the biggest advantages of Swiss balls over some of those other crazy TV contraptions is price. An average Swiss ball costs $50 to $75, compared to "four easy payments of $99" for one of those useless home contraptions. There's also versatility to consider. For less than $100 you are getting a piece of equipment that can be used to train just about the entire body. Even the $3000 jobs in commercial gyms can't make that claim.

Another advantage to Swiss balls is their convenience. You can store them just about anywhere (although we'll admit storing the larger-sized balls will take some creative planning).

Finally, and laugh as you may, a Swiss ball makes a great conversation piece. Just think of all the creative and humorous comments friends and relatives will make when they first lay eyes on your "big blue ball." Censors prevent us from repeating them here but we think you get the picture.

The Exercises

The following exercises for most of the major muscles in the body will get you started. As time goes on you can learn and add others. In fact there are videos available (often free with the ball) to take you through dozens of movements.

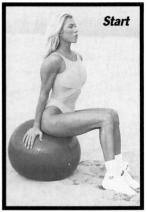

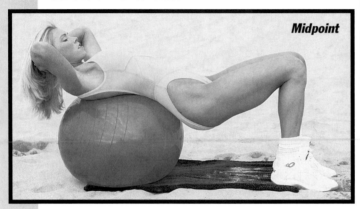

Jennifer Goodwin works her abs on the Swiss ball with abdominal curls.

Wall squats – Stand with your back to a wall or vertical support. Press the ball between your lower back and the wall. Walk your feet one or two steps in front of your body and position them shoulder width apart. Slowly lower your body to a squat position as the ball rolls up your back. Pause when your thighs are parallel with the ground. Return to the starting position.
Muscles worked – quadriceps, hamstrings and glutes.

Hamstring curls – Lie on your back with your legs and feet on top of the ball. The closer the feet are together, the harder the exercise will be. Lift your hips off the ground and roll the ball in toward your glutes. Roll the ball back to the starting position and lower your hips.
Muscles worked – hamstrings and glutes.

Side-lying abduction – Kneel on the floor or ground and place the ball at your side. Lean into the ball and extend your top leg to the side for balance. Keep your bottom leg bent for support. Firmly press your hip into the ball and maintain neutral posture. Try not to let your top hip roll forward or backward. Place your hands on the front of the ball for support. Slowly abduct (raise) the top leg until it is approximately parallel to the floor. Pause at the top of the movement before lowering your leg to the starting position.
Muscle worked – hip abductors.

Knee grips – Lie face up with your arms at your sides. Keeping your feet on the ground, place the ball between your knees. Gently press your knees together to grip the ball. Now squeeze the ball between your knees. Hold the contraction for ten seconds before returning to the starting position.
Muscle worked – hip adductors.

Heel raises – Stand with the ball pressed between your chest and a wall or vertical support. Walk your feet back one or two steps and lean into the ball. Place your hands by your side. Keeping your weight balanced across the balls of your feet, lift your heels as high as possible. Lower to a starting position.
Muscles worked – gastocnemius and soleus.

Abdominal curls – Sit on top of the ball. Keeping your feet about shoulder width apart, walk your feet away from the ball as it rolls up your back. Continue until your lower and middle back are fully supported by the ball. Place your fists at your temples. (If your neck fatigues, place one or both behind your head for support.) Slowly curl your trunk, lifting your shoulders and upper back off the ball. Return to the starting position.
Muscles worked – rectus abdominus, internal and external obliques.

Trunk flexion – Kneel on the floor with the ball in front of you. Place your hands on the ball and lower your body over the ball until your trunk is supported. Keeping your feet and knees on the floor, your head in line with your spine, and your hands to the sides of the ball, use the muscles in your lower back to lift your chest slightly off the ball. Return to the starting position.
Muscles worked – erector spinae.

Pushups – Kneel with the ball in front of your thighs. Place your hands on each side of the ball and lower your torso until it's supported by the ball. Walk your hands forward on the floor as the ball rolls down your body. Stop when the ball is centered under your hips. Rest your toes on the floor, or to add intensity lift your feet off the floor. Place your wrists under your shoulders. Maintain neutral posture and lower your chest to the floor. Pause at the bottom of the movement and return to the starting position.
Muscles worked – pectorals, anterior deltoid, triceps and serratus anterior.

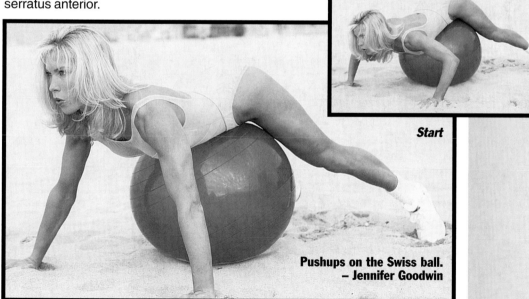

Midpoint

Start

**Pushups on the Swiss ball.
– Jennifer Goodwin**

Seated triceps dips – Sit on top of the ball. Place your hands slightly behind and to the sides of your hips, fingers pointing down. Walk your feet two steps forward and allow your hips to rest on the edge of the ball. Press your hands into the ball. At the same time, bend your elbows and lower your hips into the ball. Return to the starting position by extending the elbows.

Muscles worked – triceps, anterior deltoids, pectorals and lower trapezius.

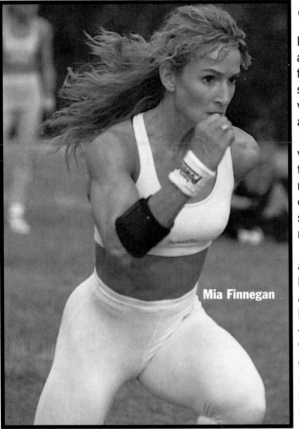

Mia Finnegan

Sprinting

Ironically, while weightlifting tends to treat the muscles as distinct entities, they did in fact evolve to work together. Take the legs for example. The quads, hamstrings and calves all come together to produce a variety of actions from walking and jogging to running and climbing.

Sprinting is one of those activities that tend to be viewed as elitist. It's fine for Olympic athletes and college track stars but "common" people just don't do it. But why not? We have the same muscles, and while the records of Michael Johnson and the late Flo-Jo are probably safe from us mere mortals, nevertheless there's nothing to prevent us from launching into a quick dash.

The only drawbacks to sprint training are that you are dependent on the weather and you have to really know what you're doing. For those who view sprinting as a faster-paced form of jogging, think again. That's like comparing a Dodge K-Car to a Lamborghini Diablo – two entirely different beasts altogether. The next time you watch a big track meet or international athletic competition, take a close look at the 100- and 200-meter sprinters. They are the ones with the incredible physiques. Some of the men would not look out of place at a bodybuilding contest, and many of the women would not look out of place in a fitness lineup.

Although sprinters occasionally pull a hamstring, long distance runners and joggers suffer far more injures. The primary reasons are: length of duration of the activities (seconds as compared to hours), and the direction of body momentum (up and down for long distance runners and forward for sprinters). Among the benefits of sprinting are:

1. Naturally reduces size where you are too big
2. Increases size where you are too thin
3. Balances out leg symmetry
4. Increases cardiovascular fitness
5. Involves just about every muscle in the body
6. Can be done just about anywhere
7. No special equipment needed
8. … and it's fun!

Sprinting can be enjoyed by everyone, young and old alike. As with any form of new physical activity, you might want to touch base with your physician before starting a sprinting program.

Warming Up and Stretching

Start your warmup by shaking out your limbs and bouncing up and down on your toes for three to five minutes. As soon as you feel loose and comfortable, go through a full-body stretching routine. (See Chapter Four.)

The Drills

As with most forms of athletics, sprinting is safer and more effective with proper technique. The following drills are the first half of your workout. You must perform a specified number of sets for each drill at an allocated distance. These drills, recommended by *Oxygen* contributor Wayne Caparas, have stood the test of time and are followed by many top sprinters and football stars (some of the fastest in the world).

Arm swings – This drill teaches proper upper-body movement. Although every muscle is employed, few are under great stress. Stand erect on the balls of your feet. Your head and neck should maintain a relaxed, centered status over your torso. At no time should your facial muscles tighten up or strain. This is perhaps the toughest technique to master since most of use let loose with the facial distortions in the gym.

Other than the secondary use of the pectorals and back muscles, the only major muscles in your upper body that are fully employed while sprinting are your shoulders. Your arms should maintain a 90-degree angle at the elbow. Your arms should swing solely through your shoulders with your forward hand reaching up to eye level and your back hand positioned no further than your butt. Although the arms maintain a fixed angle at the elbow, they should be kept as relaxed and as loose as possible. As you swing your arms back and forth, you should try to find a fluid groove in which to travel.

Now for the feet. As your right arm swings forward you will tip up on your left toe and vice versa. Remember to breathe rhythmically and keep your heels off the ground. Start with a single set of arm swings, reaching forward at least 20 times with each arm (call it 20 reps if you like).

Ankle flips – Combine this drill with arm swings. While maintaining a slight bend in both knees, employ those powerful foot and calf muscles to alternately propel yourself upward as if your legs were like two pogo sticks. Once you establish a hop from foot to foot and have established proper arm swing, gently lean forward. Angling your torso should be all it takes to tell your feet to move you forward. If you are performing this drill correctly, your feet should be less than shoulder width apart, and the lead foot should never reach so far forward that its heel passes the toe of the trailing foot. Sounds complicated, but like all of these drills it's a cinch once you do it. Perform 4 sets of these, 10 meters per set.

High knees – Add this drill in when you have your arm swings and ankle flips down pat. Begin by running in place (never hit your heels), gradually raising your knees in a piston-like motion to their highest point before your torso is forced to lean back. Once you have developed a quick rhythmic pattern of movement, gently lean forward just as you did during the ankle flips. Gravity alone should pull you into a forward path of movement. Do not stride forward and do not allow your heels to strike the ground. Keep your arms swinging and relax. Perform 4 sets of high knees, 10 meters per set.

Overstrides – You will need a little more space for these next two drills. Lightly run for about 10 meters with a proper arm swing and no heel impact. After the 10 meters accelerate your pace, maximizing stride length by reaching with each leg. Move with optimal speed, gliding across your path with grace. Check your form. Your head should not bob up and down. Height is not the goal in this drill, maximum stride length is. Perform 4 sets of overstrides, 20 meters per set (after the 10-meter start up).

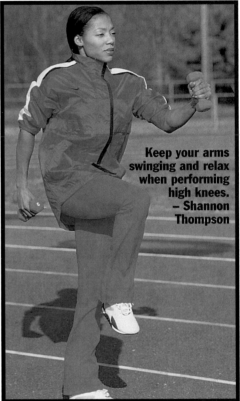

Keep your arms swinging and relax when performing high knees.
– Shannon Thompson

Bounding – Start with the same techniques used for overstrides, but instead of maximizing stride length, bound to maximize stride height or airtime. This move is a cross between overstrides and high knees. Your goal is to bound like a gazelle. You should almost feel as if you are freeze-framing, or profiling, in midair between each stride. Move with speed, but remember, height is your goal here. For some this may be the most difficult drill. Dancers could have an advantage here since they have spent a lot of time learning to leap. If you have weak knees or are presently recovering from a lower-body joint injury, you may want to pass on bounding for now. Perform 4 sets, 20 meters per set.

Cooling Down

Next to the warmup, the cooldown is the most important part of the whole drill sequence. A proper cool down can alleviate injuries, soreness, slow healing and sluggish results. It also increases blood flow to the exercised muscles, speeding waste removal and increasing the supply of nutrients.

Starts

Most sprint races are not won (or lost) at the finish line, but at the very beginning. Nothing is more detrimental to a coach's ears than to hear an announcer say his protégé was "slow off of the blocks."

Starting a sprint is perhaps the most critical part to competitive running. And even if you are sprinting for fun and fitness, you will need to learn proper starts to reach your full physical potential.

In competitive athletics, starting blocks are available to push off from. As most readers probably don't have access to such specialized equipment, we are going to describe the "football player start." Adopt a runner's stance and place one hand on the ground. The idea is to raise your hips so the majority of your bodyweight is resting on your hand. This prepares your legs to propel your body forward, not upward. You are basically jumping out of the start position at about a 30-degree angle to the ground. Using this start technique maximizes your initial speed, establishes proper forward lean, and ensures you don't lose valuable tenths of a second spinning your wheels. Keep your head and eyes down for the first few strides, then shift into overdrive utilizing all the technical skills learned earlier.

Sprinting Sets

No matter what shape you are in, your first few sprints are going to be beneficial. No matter how much weight you can squat, we are almost sure you will experience soreness the next day like you've never felt before. The actual sprints are the easy part – it's honing your skills that takes the time and practice. Given the number of sprint distances (40, 50, 100, 200 and 400 meters being the most common), the combinations are almost endless. As a beginner the most comfortable is 100 meters. It also happens to be the most prestigious in big track meets and the winner of the 100 is often referred to as the world's fastest man or woman.

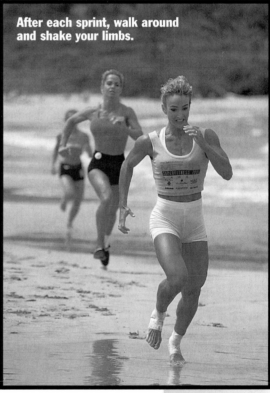

After each sprint, walk around and shake your limbs.

Even though recording your time is not essential, it does allow you to push yourself (the same as knowing how much weight you lift is not that important but we record it anyhow). For a woman 13.5 seconds for 100 meters is considered fast, while 12 seconds is above average for a man.

Once you are comfortable running 100 meters, start to experiment with other distances. Mix things up for variety. By the time you get to 200 and 400 meters your heart and lungs will be saying, "Why didn't we do this before?" For those lucky enough to have the opportunity, a 400-meter sprint on a sandy beach with a gentle breeze on your back is probably as close to utopia as it gets. Here's a sample sprint workout:

12 sprinting sets x 40 meters
8 sprinting sets x 100 meters
4 sprinting sets x 200 meters

After each sprint, walk around and shake your limbs. Do not lie down or sit. You want to keep the blood circulating in your legs.

Snowboarding

It's not surprising that it was a Canadian who first brought international exposure to snowboarding. Canadians are used to wintry arctic conditions for much of the year, and it wasn't long before someone combined the thrill of surfing with the excitement of downhill skiing. The ironic twist to the whole escapade was that it wasn't Ross Rebagliati's winning the gold medal at the Nagano Olympics that garnered all the attention. No, it was his positive drug test for marijuana that made the world media take a closer look at this, until then, obscure sport.

Memories of Woodstock aside, snowboarding is a fun and effective way to strengthen and tone all the muscles of the legs. It's also a great way to alleviate the boredom that sometimes comes with training year round in an indoor gym.

If snowboarding has a downside, it's the start-up cost. An average board will set you back $300 to $600. Add in the $200 to $400 for boots, $100 to $300 for goggles, and $500 to $1000 for quality pants, and you are looking at $2000 to $3000. For most this is a considerable investment. But then again the average golfer or skier will pay about the same. Also keep in mind that these prices are based on new items. As with most sports there is a huge assortment of used equipment on the market from which to choose.

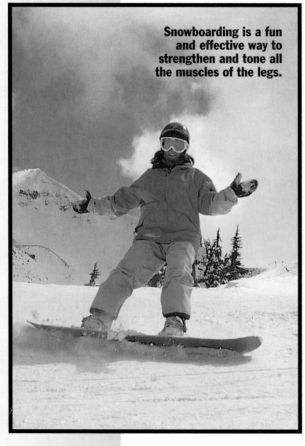

Snowboarding is a fun and effective way to strengthen and tone all the muscles of the legs.

The following drills are presented by Samantha Stenning, a highly sought after snowboarding instructor at Blackcomb Resort in Whistler, British Columbia, Canada.

Rocking But Not Rolling

According to Samantha, maintaining a balanced stance is the most important aspect of your snowboarding career, whether simple side-slipping or hanging big air. Your focus on day one is to learn how to balance your weight on a fast-moving object. Samantha suggests standing on the board on flat ground and rocking from toe to heel. The weight shift will illustrate how to keep your body centered on the board. Lean too far forward and you fall on your knees. Lean too far back and your butt kisses the ground. Try to keep your body aligned with the length of the board.

Heel-Side Stop

Once you've mastered the rocking technique it's time to hit the slopes. Stand with your torso facing downhill and the tip of the board at a slight downward angle. With even pressure kept on both feet, start moving down the hill with the slope on your heel edge. When you want to stop, increase the pressure on your heel.

Heel-Side Go

Samantha uses a car analogy to illustrate the physics of moving and stopping a snowboard. She compares the upper body to the car's steering wheel and the lower body to the gas peddle. By looking and pointing in a given direction you will automatically go in that direction. By the same argument the amount of pressure you apply to the corresponding foot controls your momentum. Try this drill. Position the board at a slight downward angle. Look toward your right and point your right hand in the same direction. Slowly apply pressure to you right heel and you will glide toward the right on your heel edge. To stop, apply pressure on both heels simultaneously. Repeat the drill with your left hand and head facing left. Put pressure on your left heel and ride to your left.

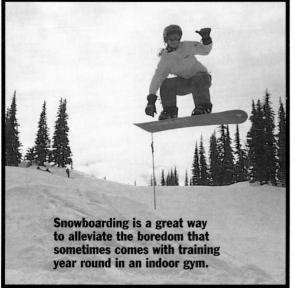

Snowboarding is a great way to alleviate the boredom that sometimes comes with training year round in an indoor gym.

Toe-Side Stop

Start by standing on the board with your body facing up the mountain. Keeping even pressure on both feet, lift your heel edge and side-slip down the slope on your toes. It might be scary to slide backward down the mountain, but don't panic. Take your time and resist the temptation to bend forward at the waist. That would only send you to your knees. Apply pressure to both toes when you are ready to stop.

Toe-Side Go

Start with your torso facing up a gradual incline. Now turn your head to face the right and point your right hand toward the right end of the board. Slowly apply pressure to your right toe, and glide toward the right on your toe edge. Stop by increasing the pressure on both toes simultaneously. Repeat with your left hand and head pointing to the left end of the board. Apply pressure to your left toe and ride to your left on your left toe edge.

Turning

According to Samantha the key to an effective turn is to push on your front foot. This is what actually propels the turn. If you lean back on your heel, the nose of the board will come up and you will almost certainly lose control.

Before you can start practicing turns you need to determine your lead foot. For most people it's the one they'd kick a soccer ball with. It's also the one that usually moves forward first to stop you from falling when pushed from behind.

With your dominant foot identified, it's time to start turning. Most beginners find it easier to turn from their toe side to their heels. Begin with a toe-side go. If you are regular footed, point your arms toward the left, increasing pressure over your left toes as you glide in that direction. Now for the fun part.

While still in motion, gradually decrease the pressure over your toes as you shift your hips. Simultaneously point your arms toward the right as you shift your weight to your heel edge. Let the board turn itself as you complete the transition. Once you've started, commit to the turn. If you don't follow through you may find yourself careening out of control down the mountain. The goal at this point is to ride across it.

Isolated Turn – Heel to Toe

As with the toe-to-heel transition, a heel-to-toe turn calls for a gradual shift in weight from one edge to the other. Once again the adjustment should originate in your hips. Relax and keep your knees bent and your body aligned with the board. Don't flap your arms or double over.

Linking your Turns

Once you can perform each type of turn in isolation (and comfort!), it's no leap of faith to start linking them together. Well done and congratulations, you're a snowboarder! Samantha adds one final word of caution: "Increased speed will come naturally with improvement. But there are tons of speed freaks out there whose style is as sloppy as they are fast. Take your time and you'll live to be a good rider."

Trail Running

"One day I was out hiking and I saw a trail and asked myself why I wasn't running it. I was tired of running through city streets, dealing with traffic, crowds and dogs, and running on the asphalt. Running is an emotional escape for me, a release from society, and it's a perfect escape for me up in the mountains."
– Amber Borowski, self-described trail-running junkie from Salt Lake City, Utah.

With the role concrete and pavement plays in our lives we sometimes forget that humans are animals were living in the woods millions of years before the first brick was fired. Yet we pay hundreds of dollars in gym membership fees and then use equipment that generally costs well over $5000. Add in the reconditioned air and you see just how artificial we've all become. Are you ready for a change? Do you want to get back to nature and get a great workout at the same time? Then give trail running a try.

Trail running is growing by leaps and bounds and is fast becoming a viable alternative to running on pavement or pounding away on a treadmill. It's a fantastic way to take in the beauty of Mother Nature, grab some fresh air, and get a great cardiovascular workout, all in one shot.

The Equipment

After discovering the start-up costs of snowboarding, you'll be happy to hear the only piece of equipment required for trail running is a good pair of shoes. You can start out with any pair of runners, but if you find yourself becoming hooked on the activity, you might want to invest in a quality pair of shoes for trail running.

Shoes designed for trail running are more stable. They have rugged construction and better traction than regular running shoes. They also have better heel and ankle support built in. A word of caution: Beware of imposters. For many manufacturers appearance is everything and you'll see people wearing what look like trail runners but are in fact cheap knock-offs – at least cheap in construction. The price may be just as high as the real thing.

Good trail-running shoes are also water-resistant. There's nothing like trail running early in the morning and overnight dew can play havoc with regular footwear.

Getting Started

Trail running is a great workout but it can be challenging for beginners. The first thing to be concerned about is uneven terrain. For those accustomed to running treadmills and streets, running on a trail will be a whole new experience. Of course the varying terrain is also one of the biggest drawing cards of the activity. Every step is different from the last. You have to negotiate rocks, hills, holes, bumps, fallen trees, streams, and just about everything else Mother Nature throws at you. Hooked yet? Read on.

Besides the physical activity itself you have to keep safety in mind. If you're new to the area, you run the risk of getting lost. Getting lost in the city is one thing, but getting lost in the woods can be life-threatening. We recommend running with a friend, especially if you are not familiar with the trail. Running in pairs also comes in handy if one of you turns an ankle.

Besides the wilderness you have the inhabitants to consider. While the birds, rabbits and other small animals are a welcome sight, the larger forest-dwellers might not be friendly. That idiot grunting and groaning at the squat rack is nothing compared to a grizzly bear or mountain lion (cougar). Most animals avoid humans like the plague and you'll probably never even know they are there. But occasionally, because of wind direction or bad luck, you'll stumble into the path of one of these beasts. We won't go into detail on how to handle the situation. In fact even experts often disagree as to how to react. Most agree that large predatory animals react when an animal starts running away from them. So your best bet is to hold your ground. But if you have the misfortune to stumble on a bear and her cubs, the animal will probably charge no matter what you do. In that case get out of there – it may be your only option. If it's a grizzly bear, climbing a tree is a good start. Black bears, however, are good tree-climbers, so if you are close and running away is not an option, hit the ground and play dead – that might work. Animals rarely

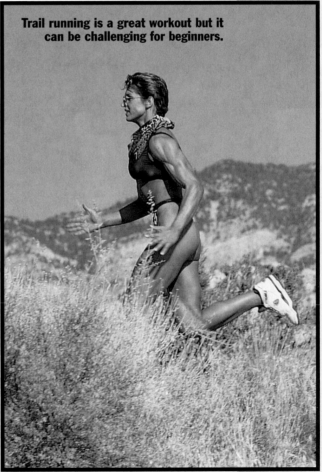

Trail running is a great workout but it can be challenging for beginners.

eat humans unless sick or hungry. If you are running in areas that are frequented by large predatory animals, you might want to contact a wildlife officer for some advice.

In addition to the four-legged variety, two-legged animals can also threaten your safety. It's a sad fact of life – males occasionally attack female runners. These degenerates usually prey on single runners so it's a good idea to link up with a friend or a running club. Hope we haven't frightened you away from trail running. Statistically you are far more likely to be attacked or injured in the city than in the wilderness.

The Trails

As with cardio equipment there is much variety when it comes to running trails. The easiest trails are what are called fire trails (also called jeep or 4 x 4 roads) which are broad and fairly well maintained. The surface might be dirt or gravel and the grades are pretty gradual. Next up we find doubletrack trails, which are just wide enough for two people to pass at once. Finally the single track are only wide enough for one person.

For the ultimate challenge you can go straight into the woods and run old logging paths. You can even leave the path and run randomly through the wilderness. Keep in mind this carries the risk of stepping on some unforeseen object. Proper running trails are usually well maintained and checked for debris. They are like train tracks. You are on your own, however, running through the woods.

A final comment is left by Nancy Hobbs, executive of the All-American Trail Running Association. "The biggest thing is not to measure where you are going by distance but base it on time. Three miles on the trail can be real eye-opening, and you could be out there for an hour. Run for time, not distance."

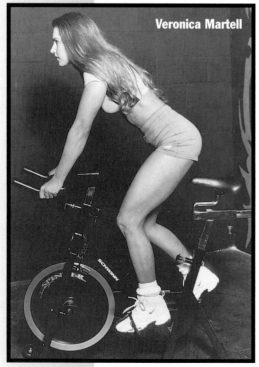

Veronica Martell

Spinning

Spinning is a perfect example of a trendy new form of fitness that seems to have staying power. The name Spinning is actually a trademark of the Schwinn Corporation, but can also refer to any group cycling class on stationary bikes. Just as most people refer to all forms of acetasalicylic acid (ASA) as Aspirin (the trademark name held by the Bayer Corporation of Germany), so too are most group cycling classes called spinning classes.

What makes spinning so popular is that it offers numerous fitness-related benefits, as well as being gender neutral. Despite the advances made in the last couple of decades, weight training is still seen as masculine, and cardio as feminine. But spinning is for everyone, and most classes have an even mixture of men and women.

In terms of conditioning, spinning is a great way to stimulate the cardio-vascular system as well as strengthen and tone up the muscles, particularly the leg muscles.

A lesser-known reason for the popularity of spinning over other forms of fitness is that it is very motivational. A combination of small class size, a dynamic instructor, and tailor-made music all contribute to keep participants interested and determined to finish the class. In a large aerobics class it's easy to slack off and just go through the motions, but in a spinning class there is no room for stragglers. Everyone is motivated to keep up.

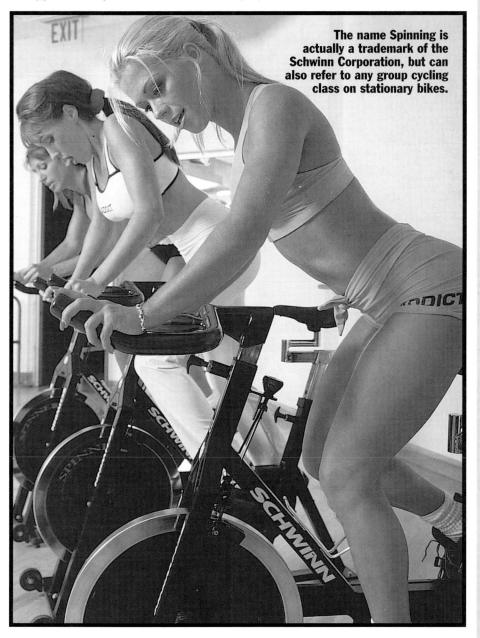

The name Spinning is actually a trademark of the Schwinn Corporation, but can also refer to any group cycling class on stationary bikes.

A typical spinning class consists of one instructor and 10 participants. Instructors have different cycle arrangements but most use a semicircle pattern. As *Oxygen* consultant Lori Grannis put it, "It reminded me of the warm fuzzy feelings I experienced during story time in first grade."

Other than the cycle, the only equipment required is a water bottle and maybe a towel. The cycle itself bears little resemblance to those $5000 cardio cycles that inhabit gyms these days. You won't find any bells or whistles either. In fact no electronics of any kind. This is cycling at its purist. The cycle will have a lever located just beneath the handlebars that allows you to increase the tension on the pedals. Push the lever all the way down and it acts as a brake. Keep this in mind as the large front flywheel weighs 40 or 50 pounds and once it gets going you can't automatically stop it by just locking the legs. You either gradually slow down and stop or push the brake lever down.

If spinning cycles have one big disadvantage over regular cardio cycles it's comfort, or the lack thereof. The seat on a typical cardio cycle is rather small and not blessed with the greatest amount of padding. After 10 or 15 minutes sitting on it your hindquarters are going to start to talk to you in unpleasant terms. Of course, during a spinning class you'll be alternating sitting with standing and sprinting, so you won't be sitting on the seat for long stretches.

The workout itself is like most forms of physical activity and can be divided into three phases – warmup, middle and cooldown. The warmup consists of various stretches that start while standing on the floor, then progress to the cycle. Most instructors start off with slow to moderately paced pedaling, then progress to the faster-paced pedaling and sprinting, either seated or standing. During a typical class you'll alternate various speeds with different tensions on the wheels.

One aspect we almost forgot to mention is ambiance. Along with the instructor yelling at you, and being surrounded by other "victims," spinning classes are conducted with music. Most gyms locate the stereo system controls next to the instructor's cycle so he or she can alternate the tempo throughout the session. Typically slow music is used for the warmup and cooldown, and faster-paced tunes for the heart of the class. Some instructors use rock music, others go for upbeat dance style.

The average spinning class lasts 45 to 60 minutes, and is as good as it gets when it comes to cardiovascular conditioning. Where spinning has an advantage over many others forms of aerobics is in its strengthening effects on the muscles. Most forms of cardio use only the weight of the body as resistance. For the first couple of weeks this may provide some strengthening benefits, but the leg muscles quickly adapt. With spinning the tension lever allows you to increase the resistance on demand. Many weight trainers report their legs get as pumped from a spinning class as a regular squat workout.

Most gyms don't charge extra for spinning. Others require you to pay a small fee. One suggestion is to check out different instructors. They all should have the same qualifications but personality often plays a role. One instructor may motivate you to the point where you could go for two hours, another may make you want to give up after 15 minutes. Of course another member may find just the opposite. It may even come down to music selection. The bottom line is – choose the class and instructor that motivates you to keep coming back.

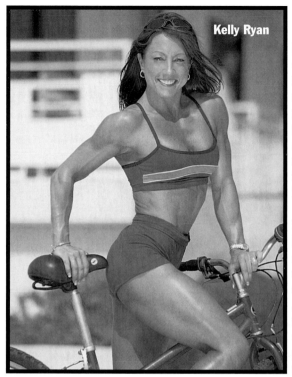

Kelly Ryan

Mountain Biking

For those who want the ultimate outdoor cycling experience, give mountain biking a try. First conceived in California 20 years ago, mountain biking is one of the fastest-growing sports, with 2 to 3 million new riders hitting the slopes each year. For the manufacturers this means 5 billion dollars a year in new bike sales.

The sport of mountain biking has grown so fast that the International Olympic Commission (IOC) has come to recognize the activity (the first bike race was held at the 1996 Olympic games in Atlanta). There are now competitions held worldwide and what was once considered a male sport, now boasts some of the finest women athletes in the world.

Mountain biking has numerous advantages over other forms of physical conditioning. For starters it's classified as low-impact. It doesn't put the stress on the joints to the same degree as other aerobic activities including running and jogging. Mountain biking is also a productive form of aerobic exercise, burning between 500 and 700 calories per hour. This amount compares to the same time weight training or running.

Cycling on dirt, gravel and sand is also a great way to strengthen your legs. Due to the way the legs have to work to pedal the bike and keep the body balanced, the entire leg region (thighs, hamstrings and calves) is stimulated. Don't worry about building huge legs either. Only those competitive bikers who train their legs for the size necessary to climb vertical hills will build tree-trunk-size thighs.

Although considered a lower-body exercise, mountain biking is also a great way to strengthen and tone the upper-body muscles. Steering and balancing a bike over rough terrain requires good upper-body strength and conditioning – something you'll quickly realize the first time you give it a try.

What You'll Need

The core piece of equipment necessary to begin your cycling adventure is of course a bike. As we mentioned earlier regarding footwear, don't skimp on price. The biggest mistake many novice riders make is to go to a department store and buy the cheapest bike they can find. Not only will this cost you more money in the long run, but also it's downright dangerous. Cheap bikes can't stand up to the rigors of mountain terrain. Cheap cycles are also mass-produced and designed to fit the "average" person. Unfortunately not everyone is the average person. A more expensive bike can be tailored to suit your individual bodytype. When you buy a cycle a little bit of tweaking will be required, from adjusting the seat height and distance to the position of the handlebars and size of the frame supports. Be prepared to spend $400 to $500 for your mountain cycle. As time goes on and you find yourself becoming competitive in the sport, you may decide to invest $1000 or more for a professional job.

Two other items are an absolute must – a helmet and a patching kit. You can purchase a good helmet for $60 to $80. A patch kit and pump will set you back about $25. As for footwear, be prepared to spend $100 or more. Many biking experts suggest you hold off on the footwear until you are sure mountain biking is for you. A good sturdy pair of hard-soled shoes will suffice.

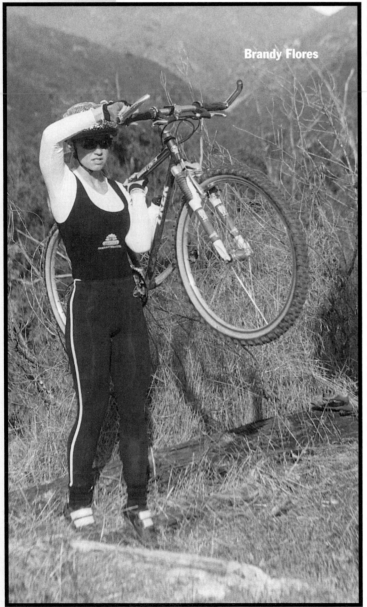

Brandy Flores

Other items you might want to place in a knapsack and take along are: sunglasses, sunscreen, food, first aid kit, notepad, Swiss Army knife, water bottle and windbreaker.

Get Off the Road!

Part of the appeal of mountain biking is that, no matter where you live, you don't have to travel a huge distance to find an old dirt road. Contrary to the name, you don't need to find a mountain either. Any stretch of dirt road or wide trail will do. As time goes on and your riding skills and conditioning increase, you can seek out the more challenging routes. Many ski resorts are open to mountain bikers in the off-season. These trails (downhill slopes) are not for the faint of heart.

Mountain biking is allowed within 47 US state parks. Many states and mountain biking clubs work together to develop and maintain trails. In fact for those new to the sport we suggest making contact with a local biking club. Such clubs are very receptive to new members and will show you the ropes. Like joining a gym for the first time, you learn most of your exercises from an instructor or by watching others. The same holds true for mountain biking. Learn the do's and don'ts from someone who's been there.

Rules of the Road

To make the sport safer for all involved, the International Mountain Biking Association has drawn up a set of "rules of the road." Please follow them to the best of your ability.

1. Ride on open trails only. Respect trail closures, private property, and requirements for permits and authorization. Federal and state wilderness areas are closed to cycling and some park and forest trails are also off limits.
2. Leave no trace behind. Don't ride when ground will be marred, such as in muddy conditions after a rain. Never ride off the trail, skid your tires, or litter. Pack out more than you pack in.
3. Control your cycle. Inattention for even a second can cause disaster. Excessive speed frightens and injures people, gives mountain biking a bad name, and can result in trail closures.
4. Always yield. Make your approach known well in advance. Show your respect when passing others by slowing to a walking speed or even stopping, especially in the presence of horses. Anticipate that other trail users may be around corners or in blind spots.
5. Never spook animals. Give them extra room and time to adjust to you. Running livestock and disturbing wild animals is a serious offence. Leave ranch and farm gates as you find them, or as marked.
6. Plan ahead. Know your equipment, your ability, and the area in which you are riding. Be self-sufficient at all times, keep your bike in good repair, and carry necessary supplies for changes in weather conditions. Keep trails open by setting an example of responsible mountain biking for all to see.

Success at New Heights

In the 1960s Kenyan long-distance runners emerged from relative obscurity to start dominating their sport. Then at the 1968 Olympics in Mexico it was found that those athletes who trained at higher elevations were achieving more success. To this day no one has a precise answer to the phenomenon, but few can dispute the results.

The Adapting Body

When you engage in high-energy aerobic exercise at higher altitudes, your cardiovascular system is taxed to the limit in supplying oxygen to the muscles. The higher the elevation the less oxygen is contained in the air. That's why the average person will pass out at elevations above 10,000 feet. You body, however, is a remarkable machine when it comes to adapting. If there's less oxygen in the air, the body compensates by increasing levels of hemoglobin, the reddish-colored oxygen-carrying pigment found in blood. It also elevates levels of oxidative enzymes (the ones your cells use to produce energy from the oxygen in blood). Over time the body has adapted to the point that it can function at altitude almost as efficiently as at sea level. But what happens if people whose bodies are adapted to use less oxygen at altitude suddenly start exercising at sea level? As expected their ability to use less oxygen gives them an advantage. The increased hemoglobin allows them to carry the additional oxygen to the body cells where the increased levels of oxidative enzymes put the cells in a state of "supercharge." All things being equal, such individuals will perform better in endurance sports.

Now before you break out the climbing gear, a few cautionary points are in order. You can't just climb to any height and start exercising. It isn't easy to train at a higher altitude. With less oxygen in the air your body's ability to exercise is impaired. Both your VO2 max and maximum heart rate can drop due to the reduced oxygen level. This means your workouts will lack the intensity you are used to. The goal is to select an altitude that still allows you to train with intensity but at the same time forces the body to adapt. Over the years researchers have discovered the best altitude to be 1800 to 3000 meters.

A popular training technique is to follow the live-high/train-low philosophy. This theory allows athletes to train with normal intensity at low altitudes but by living higher in elevation, their bodies will automatically make the biological changes that give them a competitive advantage. Studies have shown this setup to result in significant improvements in well-trained endurance athletes.

What About Me?

Most readers are probably not Olympic endurance athletes, and may wonder what all this has to do with you? For the average fitness buff, training at altitude provides a method by which training adaptation is stimulated without necessarily increasing the amount of work you have to do. It's often a way to get away from the hustle and bustle of the daily schedule to concentrate on your workouts.

When training at altitude, always consider your diet and hydration habits. At higher elevations the air is usually drier and leads to dehydration faster. Make it a point to consume extra fluids. Higher elevations also place increased nutrient demands on the body, especially protein and iron (one of the main constituents of hemoglobin). Try not to overdo it the first couple of days. You need up to four days to adapt to the acute demands of altitude exposure. It also takes at least three weeks to maximize the benefits of high-altitude training.

Benefits of high-altitude training:
• increased performance in exercise at low altitudes
• increased red blood cell count
• increased levels of oxidative enzymes
• increased aerobic levels without an increase in training volume
• a way to get away and concentrate on nothing but training

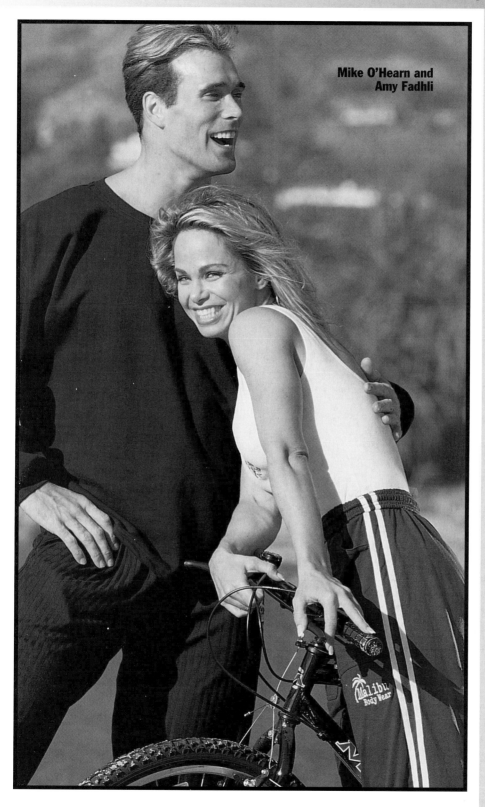

Mike O'Hearn and
Amy Fadhli

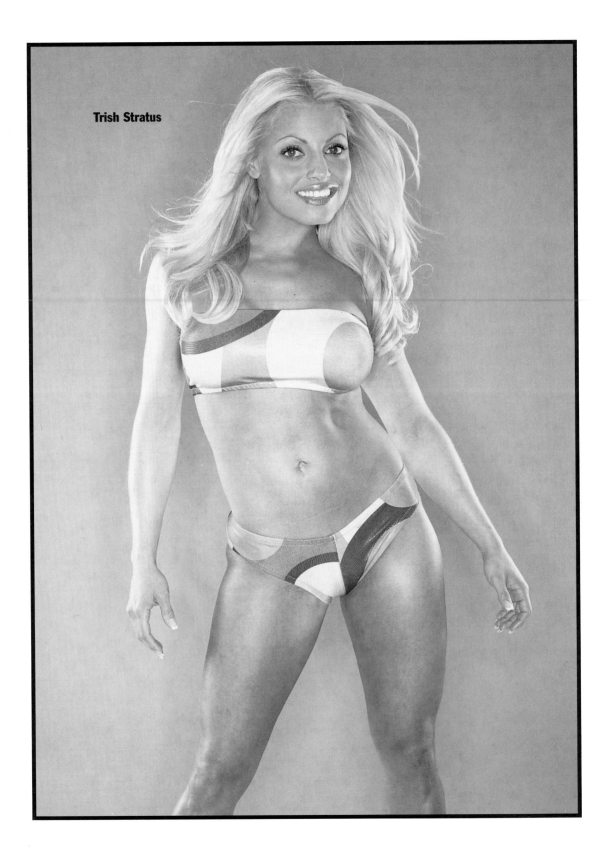

Trish Stratus

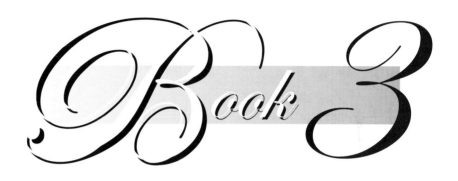

CHAPTER TWENTY-FIVE

Special Considerations

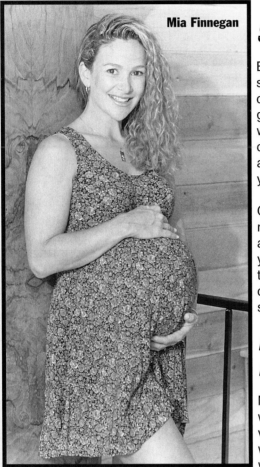

Mia Finnegan

Strength Training for Two!

Before we go any further perhaps the first thing we should say is congratulations on your pregnancy! Although exercise may not be recommended for every pregnant woman, generally it is beneficial to most. Before a pregnant woman decides to start, or in your case continue an exercise program, it is essential that a physician be consulted and clearance received. This is to ensure safety for both you and the baby.

The American College of Obstetricians and Gynecologists (ACOG) recommends women who currently participate in regular exercise can continue their activity during pregnancy. As your pregnancy advances, you will naturally decrease exercise duration and intensity. However, women who have not participated in exercise prior to pregnancy should begin with very low-intensity, low-impact activities such as swimming and walking.

Benefits of Exercise During Pregnancy

Not that long ago the notion of exercising while pregnant was discouraged and downright condemned. The prevailing attitude was "It's bad enough women are lifting weights, but now they want to do it while pregnant!" Well, we're glad such attitudes have changed, and while there are still a few holdouts from the '50s, most physicians now encourage pregnant women to perform moderate exercise. They key word in the previous sentence is *moderate*. Your goal while pregnant is maintenance – not improvement.

Benefits of Strength Training While Pregnant

There are a number of benefits you can realize through prenatal exercise. These include: increased aerobic and muscular fitness, decreased severity of low-back pain associated with pregnancy, better control of weight gain, faster recovery from labor, and an enhanced sense of well-being. Research has shown that women who participate in prenatal exercise return to their prepregnancy weight, strength and flexibility levels faster than those who do not.

Despite the benefits, most pregnant women are hesitant to continue a strength-training program during their pregnancy. But by improving their level of muscular fitness pregnant women can compensate for the typical postural adjustments that occur. This in turn tends to lessen the severity of low-back pain that is sometimes experienced. If pregnant, you should still consult your physician and follow the guidelines set forth by ACOG as they relate to your exercise program.

Postpartum women can also benefit from the proper execution of strength exercises. Women are all eager to return to their prepregnancy shape, and can begin with exercises designed to tighten the abdominal area and improve posture. Certain exercises, namely Kegel and pelvic tilts, are usually prescribed not long after an uncomplicated delivery. Once again, your physician should be consulted before engaging in any rigorous activities.

The growing numbers of women participating in strength training only supports the fact that it is a necessary component for a well-balanced fitness program. Research also suggests that if performed properly strength training has been shown to serve the health and fitness needs of women through the different stages in their life. While strength training is fairly safe, there are a few precautions to be aware of. After the fourth month of pregnancy you must avoid exercise that places you in a supine position (lying on the back). These exercises should be modified to a seated or standing position. Also, emphasize continuous regular breathing throughout each repetition. Exhale on effort, inhale on relaxation, and avoid holding your breath.

Continuing research shows that pregnant women can benefit from safe exercise if they follow certain guidelines. A medical checkup and authorization is required and can help determine what exercise program is right for the mother as well as the baby. Safety is of paramount importance.

The participant should always maintain control of the body. Movements should be made slowly. Throughout your entire pregnancy maintain a neutral spine position. Exercising during pregnancy will be more difficult. The participant should not try to maintain the same workload and performance as before. As the pregnancy advances, it will become increasingly harder to maintain the same strength. Allow the workload to decrease in intensity and duration. The participant should listen to her body and be aware. During pregnancy the center of gravity and body alignment change, balance decreases, and joints loosen and may become unstable. Limit movements to the basic low-impact variety, avoiding sudden changes in direction. Weights and rubber tubing are not recommended for the pregnant trainer.

Your goal while pregnant is maintenance – not improvement.

The safety of doing abdominal work after the first trimester remains controversial, but is not recommended. Train before pregnancy to help with the pushing stage of labor. The elastic memory of strong ab muscles will help speed up your return to prepregnant condition.

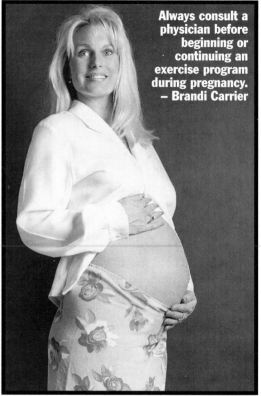

Always consult a physician before beginning or continuing an exercise program during pregnancy. – Brandi Carrier

Upper-back exercises will counter the stooping effect of heavier breasts. Please remember this: During pregnancy is not the time to get into shape. The goal should be to simply stay in shape. Before the pregnancy is when conditioning and strength training should be accomplished. It's like training for an event. You wouldn't wait until race day to start training.

During the first trimester women can usually perform the same abdominal exercises as nonpregnant trainers. A supine position (lying on the back) is considered safe. It's still best to check with your doctor because opinions and understandings change with ongoing research. In all cases, use common sense and listen to your body.

During second and third trimesters you'd be best to limit abdominal work to less than five minutes. In an organized exercise session, women in the later stages should rest sitting up or lying on their left side for a few minutes while other class members complete abdominal work. Again, your doctor should be setting the guidelines during all phases of pregnancy. Overall, the best exercise during pregnancy is walking.

Exercises

Pelvic tilts *(first trimester only):*
• Start on the hands and knees.
• Head in alignment with the spine.
• Keep back straight.
• Contract the abdominals and point the tailbone toward the floor.
• Hold for a count of three and release.
• Relieves low backaches and strengthens the abdominals by maintaining proper alignment of the pelvis.

Crunches *(up to second trimester):*
• Crunches with a pillow support (shoulders elevated above the heart).

Let-backs *(up to second trimester):*
• Sit with knees bent and hands around the knees for support.
• Contract the abdominals and curl the spine while leaning back
as far as your arms will allow.
• Alternate with oblique curls using pillow support.

C-curves *(up to third trimester):*
• Kneel on the floor on all fours or with elbows on a chair seat for support.
• Inhale and contract the abdominals while creating a "C" shape with the spine.
• Exhale and release.

Side C-curves *(up to third trimester):*
• Lie on the left side with the upper hand on the floor for support.
• Contract the abdominals and bring the knees to the chest.
• Exhale and release.

Nutrition

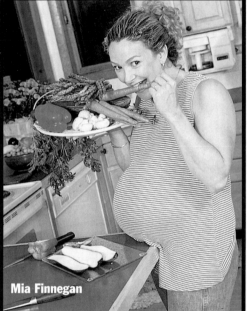

Mia Finnegan

In addition to your doctor's recommendations:
• Eat a small easily digested snack (such as crackers) prior
to exercise.
• Drink plenty of water before, during and after exercise to
prevent dehydration.
• Wear loose comfortable clothes, preferably cotton to help
absorb perspiration.
• Wear a cotton support bra with wide straps.

Exercise Guidelines During Pregnancy

The following exercise guidelines are recommended by the ACOG for activity
during pregnancy:
• Exercise at a low to moderate intensity (55 to 75 percent of max heart rate).
• Exercise to the point of fatigue, not exhaustion.
• Avoid exercising in the supine position (on your back) after fourth month of
pregnancy.
• Drink plenty of water before, during and after exercise.
• Always consult a physician before beginning or continuing an exercise pro-
gram during pregnancy.
• A strength-training workout consisting of a single set of a series of exercises,
collectively involving all of the major muscle groups, should be performed twice
per week.
• Strength training on machines is generally preferred to using free weights
since machines tend to require less skill and can be more easily controlled.
• If a particular strength exercise produces pain or discomfort, it should be dis-
continued and an alternative exercise performed.

And Finally ...

A pregnant woman should immediately consult her physician if any of the following warning signs or complications appear: vaginal bleeding, abdominal pain or cramping, ruptured membranes, elevated blood pressure or heart rate, or lack of fetal movement. Authorities on the subject, however, are quick to point out that strength training is not advisable for all pregnant women. Current research suggests that the previous recommendations are appropriate, but until more data is available, women should immediately consult their physicians if a problem occurs. Finally, as each individual has special needs, training programs for pregnant women should be specialized.

Is There a Risk?

Does moderate strength training during late pregnancy compromise the well-being of either mother or baby? This question was addressed by Dr. Larry Wolfe and his research team at Queen's University, with the results published in the *Canadian Journal of Applied Physiology.* In their study they compared cardio-vascular responses in 12 pregnant women and their unborn offspring, to a typical session of strength/conditioning exercises consisting of hand-grip, single-leg and double-leg extensions.

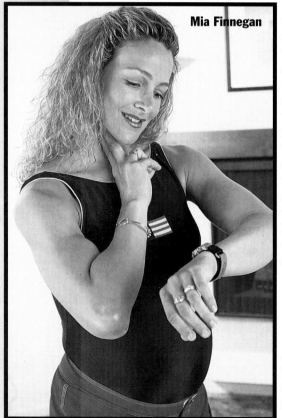

Mia Finnegan

For the mothers, heart rate increases during the exercise were slightly more pronounced, and blood pressure responses were similar, compared to the responses of a group of women who were not pregnant. Decreased fetal heart rate, which may be a sign of decreased oxygen availability to the fetus due to blood redistribution to working muscles, was not generally observed during the exercise. The exception was when exercise was performed in the tilted supine position, as opposed to sitting, and the authors suggest this posture be avoided when performing this type of exercise. On the other hand, the authors found evidence that exercise in this position actually promotes fetal arousal and activity.

Lose Postpregnancy Pounds

As you might expect you don't shed all your pregnancy weight right after delivery – the average weight loss at birth is 12 to 17 pounds. In addition it takes about four to six

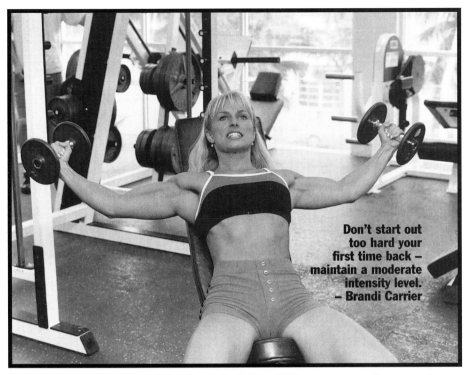

Don't start out too hard your first time back – maintain a moderate intensity level.
– Brandi Carrier

weeks for the uterus to shrink back to its original size, so don't expect to get your old midsection back right away.

Before returning to exercise, make sure you get a doctor's clearance. It usually takes four weeks to be cleared to exercise after a vaginal birth, six to eight weeks after a C-section. This postponement is to enable the pelvic floor to regain some of its strength and for the internal bleeding to decrease.

Don't start out too hard your first time back – maintaining a moderate intensity level is important because you still need ample blood flow going to your core to help the uterus shrink back to prepregnancy size. Plus, your hormones are still causing a good amount of joint looseness, putting you at greater risk for injury.

Aerobic Exercise

Even those who exercised throughout their pregnancy are going to find aerobic recovery challenging to say the least. Your body is tired from childbirth and breastfeeding, and you've lost quite a bit of your cardiovascular capacity. Don't crank up the treadmill to 10 when starting out; work your way up in increments, adding short high-intensity intervals to boost your threshold. Breastfeeding mothers should note that babies sometimes reject postexercise milk because your body's lactic acid can alter the taste.

Warmup duration should be 10 to 15 minutes while maintaining good posture, body alignment, and a neutral spine position. Heart rate checks should start at 5-minute intervals for the beginner and 10-minute intervals for the more experienced trainer. Intensity should be limited to 60 percent of the maximum

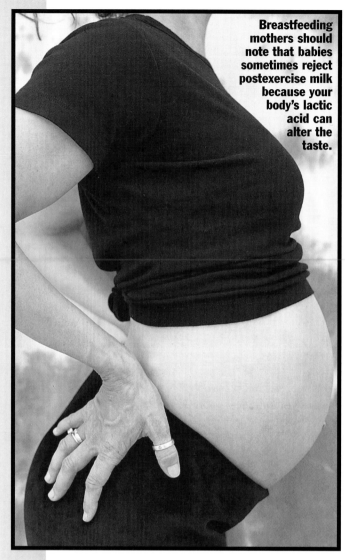

Breastfeeding mothers should note that babies sometimes reject postexercise milk because your body's lactic acid can alter the taste.

heart rate for beginners and 75 percent for the experienced exerciser. Range of motion should be kept to shorter movements rather than full range, followed by static stretches. Pay particular attention to areas such as shoulders, neck, calves and hip flexors. Emphasize relaxation more than extension and flexibility for the lower back.

Overhead arm stretches assist in breathing and allow the entry of more oxygen into the lungs opening up the thoracic cavity. Be careful not to over stretch. Concentrate on slow, sustained stretching. Avoid adductor stretches as these place undue stress on the pelvic bone area.

Target heart rates and ratings of perceived exertion are reached more quickly than in nonpregnant women. This is not the time to challenge the cardiovascular system. Next time challenge the system ahead of time to get into shape for the pregnancy.

Strength Training

If you did some strength training during pregnancy, you can start back pretty much where you left off – at least with regard to the specific exercises. You won't be able to use the same weight as before your pregnancy, but since strength gains are lost more gradually than aerobic ones, a couple of weeks of regular training will bring you close to your prepregnancy condition.

Golden Years Strength Training

Besides helping women look slimmer and more toned, lifting weights – also called strength training – can prevent or slow the progression of osteoporosis in women of all ages, according to health experts. Osteoporosis, or loss of bone density, affects an estimated 20 million older American women and is an underlying cause of more than 90 percent of all hip fractures. Osteoporosis, or porous bone, is a disease characterized by low bone mass and structural deterioration of bone tissue, leading to bone fragility and an increased susceptibility to fractures of the hip, spine and wrist.

Throughout your lifetime, old bone is removed (resorption) and new bone is added to the skeleton (formation). During childhood and teenage years, new bone is added faster than old bone is removed. As a result, bones become larger, heavier and more dense. Bone formation continues at a pace faster than resorption until maximum bone density and strength is reached at around age 30. After 30 bone resorption slowly begins to exceed bone formation. Bone loss is most rapid in the first few years after menopause but persists into the post-menopausal years. Osteoporosis develops when bone resorption occurs too quickly or if replacement occurs too slowly. Osteoporosis is more likely to develop if you did not reach optimal bone mass during your bone-building years.

Now for the good news. Numerous studies have found that post-menopausal women who lifted weights just twice a week preserved their bone strength and improved their muscle mass, muscle strength and balance – reducing their risk of falling and/or suffering an osteoporosis-related fracture.

In terms of recommended training routines, ask ten different experts and you're likely to get ten different answers. There are numerous routines for increasing strength depending on your specific goals. Working out "hard and long" may elicit greater improvement in strength, but it also increases your risk of injury. So why not take a sensible yet effective approach.

Most older individuals are well aware of the need for regular aerobic exercise, such as walking, swimming or running, to strengthen their heart and lungs and tone their bodies, but many dismiss weight training (also called resistance training) as an activity predominantly for the young or the vain. However, it is the only type of exercise that can substantially slow – and even reverse – the declines in muscle mass, bone density and strength that were once considered inevitable consequences of aging. Unlike aerobic (endurance) activities which improve cardiovascular fitness and require moving large muscle groups hundreds of times against gravity, weights provide so much resistance that muscles gain strength from just a few movements.

For those new to strength training, here's what the experts tell us is needed to combat osteoporosis.
• Frequency of training: minimum of twice per week.
• Number of repetitions: 8 to 12 per set.
• Number of sets: minimum of one set per muscle group.
• Number of exercises: 8 to 10 exercises which focus on the major muscle groups.
• Movement speed: slow to moderate.
• Amount of weight: enough to fatigue your muscles by the last few reps (8 to 12 reps for strength training, 15 to 20 reps for endurance training).

Isn't it great! You don't have to spend hours in the gym to significantly improve your strength. You can be in and out in as little as 20 minutes. Now, that's a schedule we can all live with!

Remember, you don't have to be in perfect shape to work with weights. Strength training is now considered an important component of a weight loss program – along with diet, aerobic exercise and behavior modification – and is recommended for people suffering from certain types of arthritis and chronic back pain. Once believed dangerous for the elderly, research has confirmed that a low to moderate resistance strength-training program is safe for the older population and people with high blood pressure or heart disease. Of course, if you happen to be one in less-than-perfect shape, make sure to get your doctor's okay before you start lifting away!

Anorexia Nervosa

Even though most people associate anorexia nervosa with eating, there is a great deal of overlap with exercise. Often sufferers of the condition also exercise to the extreme in an attempt to shed those "extra few inches of fat." Given this important point, we thought it appropriate to discuss the subject of anorexia in a bit more detail.

Anorexia nervosa is an illness that mainly affects adolescent girls, although it can occur in both boys and girls, younger or older than adolescence. The most common signs are loss of weight coupled with a change in behavior (one of the behavior symptoms being excessive exercise). The weight loss is slowly progressive and often starts with a seemingly normal weight-reduction diet. Only after this has continued for several months does it seem cause for worry, usually because by then the weight loss is extreme. As close friends and relatives see the individual on a regular basis, often those who have not seen her in a few months first pick up on the problem. If one word could define the condition it is *determination.* Any attempt to frustrate their efforts is generally met with anger or deceit or a combination of both. Confrontation, rational discussion, bullying or bribery will probably fail to cause more than a very brief change of eating behavior. Continuing weight loss will lead to increasing concern by the family.

The personality changes she may experience will be those of increased seriousness and introversion. She will become less outgoing and less fun. She will usually begin to lose contact with her friends and may appear to lose interest in everything other than food and academic work. She may show increased obsessional behavior, especially in the kitchen where she may become concerned with cleanliness, orderliness and precise timing of meals.

Causes of Anorexia Nervosa

Let us first start by saying no one knows the exact cause of anorexia, but numerous theories have been put forward. From what we do know it seems to be a disorder of many causes that come together to produce the illness. The recognized ingredients include the nature of the personality of the girl herself, aspects of her family members and relationships, and stresses and problems occurring outside home, often at school. There is an increased risk in families in which there are other anorexics and this probably indicates a genetic predis-

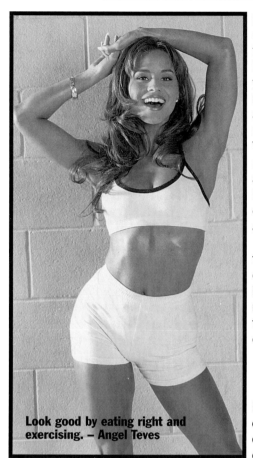

Look good by eating right and exercising. – Angel Teves

position also. Finally the fashion and entertainment industries haven't helped things with their portrayal of what the ideal female should look like. Every year the Emmy and Academy Awards bring forth a selection of 100-pound actresses who unfortunately become role models for millions of teenage girls. When they see such skinniness being rewarded with increased acting roles and strings of "gorgeous hunks of man-hood," is it any wonder many girls stop eating and try to burn off 2000 calories a day?

We could write a whole book on the fashion industry and what it considers the "right look." Suffice to say, a large percentage of the top female models look more like heroin addicts than appropriate role models for girls to emulate.

The Dangers

Even though we touched on this in the chapter on overtraining, the subject deserves repeating here. During the extreme period of weight loss the body tries to conserve energy as best it can. Inessential functions are gradually lost. The menstrual cycle stops as the weight falls, and scalp hair becomes very thin to the point of baldness. The circulation diminishes with coldness of the hands and feet that often become reddened. The heart rate slows and blood pressure falls. Danger from a failing heart becomes a risk at a very low weight if the weight loss is extremely rapid, or if the chemistry is distorted by an extreme of vomiting, purging or diuretic (water tablet) abuse. It is hard to assess a danger-ously low weight but sudden death will more frequently occur once the weight has fallen by 40 percent of normal. Prolonged weight loss during adolescence may eventually lead to permanent failure of normal growth, but this is common only when the illness begins early in adolescence and lasts for several years. A similar severity of anorexic symptoms may lead to the problem of osteoporosis, thinning of the bones, later in life.

Treatment Options

Most girls will be taken first to their general practitioner or school doctor. He or she may well have a good knowledge of the local possibilities for appropriate treatment, but more drastic steps are sometimes needed. It often takes intervention by numerous disciplines (nutrition, psychology and medical) to impart effective treatment.

Success in regaining a normal weight is an essential component in the process of recovery, but it's not the only element. The course of this illness is closely linked with development and maturation. Recovery is often associated with the continuation of maturation after a period of emotional regression therefore involves several stages. Regaining normal bodyweight with a normal eating pattern is the first priority, and may require admission to hospital for its achievement. The return to normal eating unmasks the underlying psychological issues so that they may be explored. These issues will need to be managed according to what problems arise in practice, a task that varies from one patient to another. Finally the individual will need to begin to lead a normal life again, a task that may be slow and tentative as a result of the profound loss of confidence that is so characteristic of the illness.

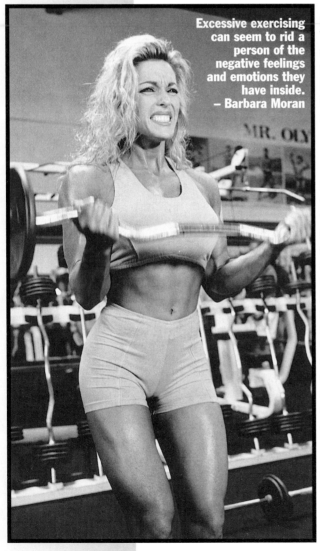

Excessive exercising can seem to rid a person of the negative feelings and emotions they have inside.
– Barbara Moran

Some girls have mild illnesses and may regain a normal weight successfully at home. The underlying issues may be fairly straightforward and easily resolved. Over a period of a few months everything may have returned to normal. But the illness is often more severe than this and several months' hospitalization will be needed to regain the weight.

Compulsive Exercising

Compulsive exercising or "overexercising" is a common characteristic among those who are victims of eating disorders. On the surface the sole purpose of exercise seems to be to burn calories and lose weight, but it is really much more profound than that. People who binge often engage in vigorous exercise in an attempt to burn off calories that may result in weight gain and also to relieve feelings such as guilt, disgust and fear. The person is so fearful of gaining weight, exercising becomes compulsive and obsessive. Many eating disorder victims will exercise in privacy, when they are alone. As the eating disorder progresses, a person could be excessively exercising as much as 3 to 5 hours a day in the quest for weight loss and to eliminate those negative feelings they have inside. Even at some point if they do realize that their exercising has become too much or if someone else confronts them, they often feel their behavior is "okay" and rationalize that their actions are actually healthy for them.

It is important to remember that while an eating disorder victim is using exercise as a way to control weight or lose weight, she is also gaining something inside from it. For example, often sufferers will feel more powerful and in control. They almost always gain a sense of self-respect and self-worth. As mentioned above, excessive exercising can seem to rid a person of the negative feelings and emotions they have inside. You may wonder to yourself how someone who is perhaps sick and underweight can possess the desire and energy to do this, but I can tell you, this behavior can be highly compulsive and is driven by fear. Like fuel that fills a car to keep it moving, fear is what fuels the person to exercise and keeps them going. Individuals will sneak around to exercise and may even have an agenda set up for themselves. Some will go to great lengths to continue. Maybe they sneak away quietly to a private room and have even found excuses to be dismissed from school or their job, or leave a social gathering just so they can find time and/or privacy to engage in training. Even if a sufferer has been hospitalized due to poor health, compulsive exercisers have often attempted to train against medical advice.

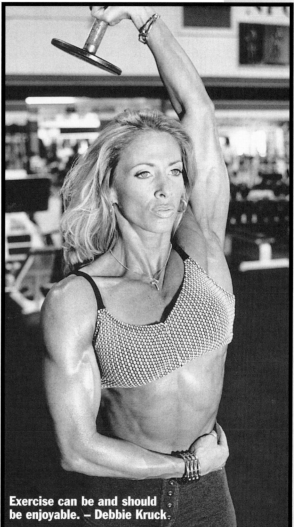

Exercise can be and should be enjoyable. – Debbie Kruck.

While compulsive exercising is not an actual disorder, it can be very dangerous for anyone, even the average person. For those with eating disorders excessive exercising can lead to excessive sweating, resulting in dehydration. Exercise can be and should be enjoyable, but most people who compulsively exercise do not enjoy it and it can be an asset to keeping fit and staying healthy. If you or a loved one is showing symptoms of compulsive or excessive exercising, this can be due to an eating disorder or could possibly lead to one. An athlete may also be more likely to engage in too much exercise that is beyond the limits of safe.

While the total elimination of exercise isn't beneficial for anyone, there are different levels and needs, and appropriate times in which it is safe. Always discuss your concerns about the importance of a healthy balanced diet and safe physical fitness with a professional or your health care provider who will advise you and recommend a safe program that is right for you. Those who have an eating disorder or who are working toward one are usually advised against exercise, and should always seek professional help for additional information.

CHAPTER TWENTY-SIX

Competition – Putting It All on the Line

We assume most readers bought this book to learn how to get in shape. Competing in a fitness contest is probably the furthest thing from your mind. First we offer our sincere thanks for buying our humble literary efforts. Second, give yourself a pat on the back. No doubt you'll get in the best shape of your life. You're all winners in our minds. A few readers, however, may decide to take the next logical step and put their new bodies to the test. What we are talking about here is entering a fitness contest. Although males tend to get the most attention when it comes to competitive sports, we'll be the first to admit that females these days are becoming just as competitive. There's something primordial about stepping onstage and pitting your physique and athletic talents against others. Even though the next few chapters focus on getting ready for a fitness contest, we would like to think there's something here for everyone, regardless of whether or not you decide to compete.

Is Competition for Me?

You may be surprised to learn that competing has many advantages. One of the primary benefits is that you'll get in the best shape of your life. Months if not years of training often leaves individuals stuck in a rut, making little or no progress. But as soon as you shift gears and start preparing for a contest, the change in your physique can be dramatic. Bodyfat percentage will drop into the single digits. Muscle tone and shape will take on a totally new look. Flexibility, an issue you may have overlooked in the past, will improve dramatically when you begin to design and practice your fitness routine.

Besides the changes in your physique in the months leading up to the show, you may see equal improvement during the months after the contest. For those trying to add some quality muscle to their physique, the months following a show are a hard-gainer's paradise. The spartan diet and high-rep training in the months before a show leave the body just begging for nutrients and a change in training

Katie Uter

style. Many bodybuilders and fitness athletes put themselves through the rigors of competition solely to reap the benefits of the postcontest growing period.

Another reason to compete is that the whole process is one giant learning period. Lowering bodyfat percentage to single digits, and holding on to muscle mass while putting together a posing routine, is not done in a weekend. Every day will be spent consulting books, magazines, and other competitors, in an attempt to fine tune your physique and look your best onstage. Nobody can do it alone. That's why all the top fitness stars have coaches and choreographers to help them prepare for the big contests.

One little-known advantage of competing is social. Months if not years of slaving away wondering if you're the only one with such interests will suddenly be erased by attending your first show. You'll discover you're a member of a very large and loyal fraternity. Sometimes the backstage banter with the other contestants and coaches makes the whole thing worthwhile.

Besides contacting the other contestants, you'll also be "selling yourself." If you want to climb the ladder of fitness success, you'll need plenty of magazine coverage. All the movers and shakers in the industry will be there, and as we said earlier all it takes is one of them to think you have the "right look" and away you go.

A final reason to compete is because it's fun! In nearly ten years of following the fitness industry, the authors have yet to talk to one competitor who didn't enjoy the whole experience. There were a few who felt robbed or cheated by the judges – every sport has the same – but no one was disappointed with the actual show itself.

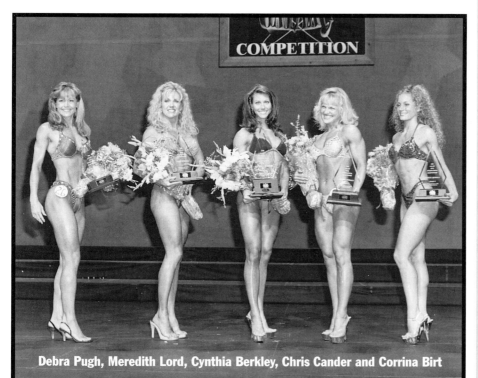

Debra Pugh, Meredith Lord, Cynthia Berkley, Chris Cander and Corrina Birt

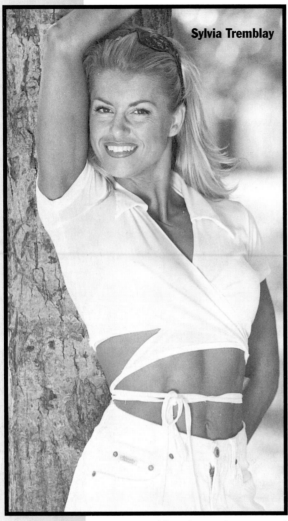

Sylvia Tremblay

Where Do I Start?

Your first show should not be the one you compete in. Stepping up onstage in front of hundreds or thousands of people is not something you do cold turkey. You want to get a feel for the whole shebang by attending a couple as a spectator. Buy tickets to both the prejudging and the evening show. The evening show may be more professional and entertaining, but it's the prejudging where most of the actual decision making takes place.

While you're sitting in the audience pay close attention to the judges, competitors and spectators. The role of the judges and contestants is straightforward, but the fans are something altogether unique. Few sports have such loyal or devoted fans. Within minutes of the beginning of the judging you'll quickly realize that this is definitely not a night at the opera. The audience will be hooting and hollering for their favorites, and *shy and bashful* is certainly not the order of the day.

As a future competitor you'll want to focus on how the contestants present themselves onstage. We are not just talking about the fitness routines either. Little things such as how to stand in a lineup, smiling and turning have made the difference between first and second place. With contests becoming so competitive these days you should spare no attention to detail.

So Many Choices

To list every fitness contest out there would take a whole book. Instead we'll give you general guidelines as to how to select your first show. Competitive fitness evolved from bodybuilding and is organized in a very similar manner. For those new to competition usually the first place to start is the city event. Win (or in many cases place in the top three) and you're eligible to compete in the state or provincial championships. From there you can jump straight to your country's National Championships. Another route is to go from the state or provincial show to an event such as the Atlantic, Western, Southern or Midwest Championships. Competing in these multi-regional shows not only gains you more experience, but it certainly builds your reputation and résumé if you win or place high. Such a title carries a tremendous amount of weight at the national level. It means you are one of the favorites, and unless you are way off in appearance, holds you in higher esteem in the eyes of the judges. This alone will give you an edge over rivals.

If you win the Nationals, you're off to the World Championships to strut your stuff with the best fitness competitors in the world. Win or place high and you earn your pro card, which enables you to compete on the pro circuit and accept cash prizes. We should add that you don't need to win the World Championships to earn your pro card. Most fitness federations allow you to turn pro once you win the Nationals. Keep in mind that, with the explosion of women's fitness over the last decade, it seems there's a new show created every week.

For those select few who have what it takes to go all the way, the top fitness shows include the Fitness International, Fitness Olympia, Galaxy Fitness, Fitness USA, the Jan Tana Pro Fitness, Fitness Universe, and the Fitness World.

In a "Roundabout" Manner

Like their bodybuilding relatives, fitness shows are divided into sections or rounds. Each round is set up to highlight a particular aspect of the contestant's physique and fitness level. The following is a brief description of each round. A few shows such as the Galaxy Fitness also include an obstacle course. You don't necessarily have to win every round to win the contest. In fact, depending on how the other contestants perform, you may not need to win a round, just place high in all.

1. Evening gown round – The judges are looking for beauty, poise and projection. This round is designed to give the judges a general impression of the competitors. Wearing evening gowns, the competitors will introduce themselves and give a brief biography and their philosophy on fitness, within a time limit of 30 seconds at the microphone. The judges' objectives are: a) beauty; b) general impression – overall grooming and cosmetic appearance; c) poise – self-assurance, composure, carriage; and d) projection – speaking clearly, confidently, distinctly, meaning of speech.

Please note competitors are permitted to speak in their native tongue but must submit a handwritten copy to the judges in English. Choice of attire is important and should be both tasteful and elegant. You want to select something that will highlight your physique but at the same time look good on a night on the town.

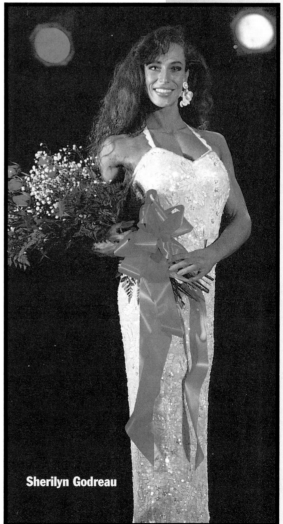
Sherilyn Godreau

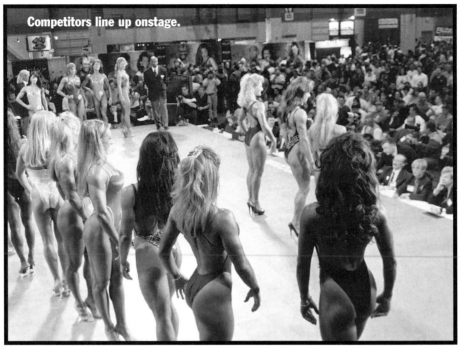
Competitors line up onstage.

2. Swimsuit round – Competitors will present themselves onstage in numeri-cal order, in a straight line or semicircle facing the judges: assuming a semi-relaxed stance with ankles touching. The head judge will instruct the group to execute a series of quarter-turns to the right, allowing the judges to view them from the front, left, back, and right sides before returning to the front position. The judging is based on overall symmetry and muscle definition. Competitors should have good to excellent muscle tone and appear to have a reasonable level of bodyfat. The judges are not looking for muscle mass, "ripped to the bone" extreme striations, or the vascularity of a bodybuilder. No jewelry, gloves, hats, etc. are permitted.

Judging objectives are: a) the competitors should have good to excel-lent muscle tone with reasonable levels of bodyfat; and b) the physique should appear evenly developed with a high degree of attention to symmetry, propor-tion and overall appearance including complexion, poise and overall presenta-tion. The lean muscularity of the upper and lower extremities should flow aes-thetically when viewed from all sides, creating a balanced sculpted appearance. Make frequent eye contact with the judges and audience, and while it's easy for us to say, try to appear calm and relaxed.

3. Fitness routine – Competitors will present a fitness routine for a maximum of 90 seconds (for national and international events maximum two minutes). They will emphasize strength, flexibility and endurance. The routines are meant to give the judges some idea of the competitor's physical condition and abilities. It also gives the competitor the opportunity to express her creativity, personali-ty and interests. Competitors are encouraged to include any talent or interest they may have such as dance, martial arts, jumping rope, baton, gymnastics, aerobics, etc. – and props may be used. Please note, competitors are not expected to be gymnasts. Although routines are to be high-energy movements demonstrating strength, flexibility and endurance, gymnastic tumbling and/or acrobatics is not required, and judges will not penalize competitors who do not display gymnastic ability.

Judging objectives: a) high-level execution of movements, including full extension (execution of movements should appear effortless); b) difficulty and diversity of routine elements; c) clean and fluid transitions; d) adequate use of props – if props are used they should be properly incorporated into the routine; e) projection of audience awareness – this also includes audience participation and stage presence; and f) projection of personality and creativity.

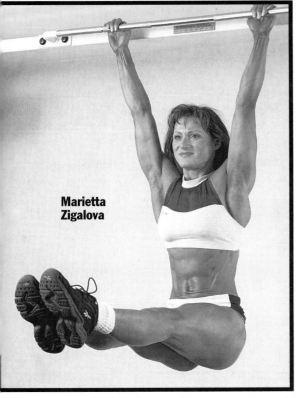

Marietta
Zigalova

Preparation

Preparing for a fitness show can be subdivided into three areas: physical conditioning, diet and stage preparation. As most of this book focuses on physical conditioning, we'll limit our comments here to changes you should make in the months leading up to a contest. Likewise the chapter on diet and nutrition covers your year-round eating habits, so we'll say only a few brief words on precontest dieting. The section on preparing for contest day is very extensive.

Precontest Training

Given the evolution of this sport from female bodybuilding, it's not surprising that fitness competitors follow similar training styles in the months leading up to a contest. During the off-season (from a week or two after a contest up to about three months out from the next show) most competitors focus on balancing out their physique. By this we mean taking a good look to see which bodyparts are lagging behind in terms of proportion and development. Weights are kept medium to heavy, reps usually in the 8 to 12 range.

About three months out from the contest a change in training style is in order – for three primary reasons. For starters the reduced calorie intake and extra cardio will reduce your *energy reserves.* Most people find they can't train as hard or as heavy in the months leading up to a contest. Another reason for modifying your training is *safety.* Again it relates to precontest dieting and conditioning. Most competitors border on, if not actually enter, a state of overtraining during the months before a contest. This is the worst time to try training

"When I get real close to a contest, like the last 10 days or so, the weight I use is so light I can do hundreds of reps. I keep lifting heavy until the last two weeks or so, then I go extremely light. During the last five days I stop lifting weights altogether. Instead I practice my routine and do some cardio to give my muscles a break. It also lets them separate a bit prior to the show."
– top fitness competitor Cynthia Hill, outlining her precontest training strategy.

heavy – the risk of injury is just too great. How many times have you heard of a bodybuilder or fitness star sustaining a major injury just before a contest? Although bad luck sometimes plays a role, the usual cause is trying to push things too hard when the body can't handle it.

The third reason for modifying your training style before a contest is *refinement*. You've pretty much done all you can to balance out your physique for this year. You goal now is to refine it for the show – firm the muscles and add separation between each muscle. The foundation has been built, now it's time to add the finishing touches so to speak.

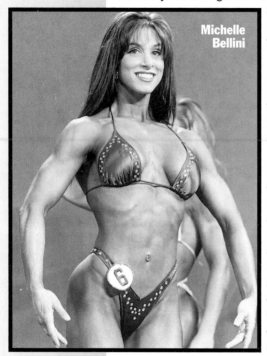

Michelle Bellini

The two big changes you'll make to your training style relate to reps and exercises. Instead of heavier weight for lower reps, you'll decrease your workout poundages and increase the reps. Although it varies, most fitness competitors go from an off-season rep range of 8 to 12 up to 15 to 20 reps per set.

The other change is the types of exercises. During the off-season more emphasis is placed on compound movements that work more than one muscle. Precontest many of the compound exercises are replaced with isolation movements. Doing so helps bring out each muscle's unique detail and shape. Isolation exercises also require you to use less weight, which helps reduce the risk of injury. We should add that most competitors keep at least one compound exercise during the precontest season, but the bulk of their routines consist of isolation exercises. Here are some compound movements and substitute isolation exercises.

	COMPOUND EXERCISE	ISOLATION EXERCISE
Legs	Squats and leg presses	Leg extensions
Chest	Barbell and dumbell presses	Dumbell flyes and cable crossovers
Back	Barbell rows and chinups	Straight-arm pushdowns and dumbell rows
Shoulders	Barbell and dumbell presses	Front and side raises
Traps	Barbell shrugs	Dumbell shrugs and machine shrugs
Biceps	Barbell curls	Cable and dumbell curls
Triceps	Narrow presses, lying extensions	Kickbacks, dumbell extensions

Here's a final change many fitness competitors make to their training. They reduce the rest period between sets. Instead of the usual one to two minutes, most rest only 20 to 30 seconds between sets. The primary aim is to keep the heart rate elevated. That way you get a good cardio workout while weight training. The increased stamina will come in handy when preparing and executing your fitness routine. It also means you'll burn more calories for the same time period – and more calories burned means more fat lost.

Precontest Dieting

Precontest dieting is hard, especially for the drug-free athlete. How many times have you seen a bodybuilder who is huge in the off season, reduced to a mere shadow of himself or herself by contest time? To the novice, the concepts may seem simple: "Just cut back on the calories and lose weight, right?" or, "As long as I keep working out I won't lose muscle." Unfortunately it just doesn't work that way.

Your brain is the problem. No, I'm not referring to your intelligence. Your brain uses only carbohydrates (not fat) as a source of energy, and your body will protect the brain at all costs. During a diet when blood sugar levels can be very low, the body will release the hormone *cortisol.* Cortisol is a catabolic hormone that converts muscle proteins to carbohydrates to feed the brain. This leads to the loss of muscle mass often seen with precontest diets. But don't despair. The answer is a logical, conservative approach to dieting, along with daily collection of precise data.

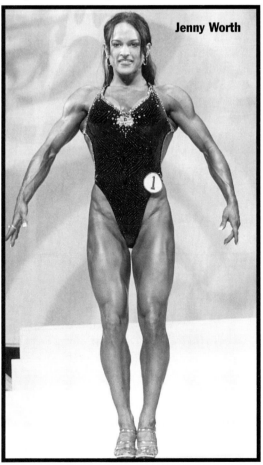

Jenny Worth

You will need an accurate scale, a notebook, a good tape measure, a food scale, a food nutrition content guide, a mirror and a pair of skinfold calipers. The dieting process should begin at least three to four months before the contest. This may seem like a long time, but you must take a more conservative approach.

Assessing Body Composition

First get an honest and accurate assessment of your body composition. Have your bodyfat percentage measured at a health club, a local university (by the exercise physiology department) or local hospital, or do it yourself with skinfold calipers. You will be aiming for 5 to 8 percent bodyfat by contest time, so you must determine how much fat you have to lose.

Calories Needed for Your Weight

Next, determine how many calories you need to maintain your current body-weight. Record everything you eat for at least one week (two is preferable). Use your food scale and nutrition content guide to determine the calorie, fat, carbohydrate and protein content in all the foods you eat that week. Calculate the average number of calories you consume daily (number of calories total divided by number of days).

Now apply some math. Assuming that 3500 calories is one pound of fat, multiply 3500 by the number of pounds of fat you need to lose. Let's say you intend to lose 30 pounds of fat (far too much to have gained during the off-season, but let's use it as an example anyway). That works out to 105,000 calories (3500 times 30 pounds). In simplified terms, you need a caloric deficit of 105,000 calories by contest time in order to lose the 30 pounds of fat. If there are four months before the contest, divide 105,000 by 120 days and you'll discover you need a deficit of 875 calories per day. However, since every calorie you burn is not guaranteed to be a fat calorie, it gets a little more complicated. You must be very careful of what you eat and you must be strict about measuring your body composition.

"Don't keep bad foods around or you might be tempted. Get photos of people you want to look like, and those you'd rather not resemble, and tape them to your fridge. The best preparation for a competition is to 'diet' year round so it isn't a struggle when you decide to enter a contest. You'll look better for any surprise appearances too!"
– top fitness competitor Debbie Kruck, offering advice on precontest and off-season eating habits.

What to Eat

The next step is to determine what to eat. The most important nutrient in our precontest diet is *protein*. Muscle is made primarily of protein and water, and without adequate protein, muscle mass cannot be maintained. Research has shown that the requirement for hard-training athletes is probably somewhere between .5 and 1 gram per pound of body-weight. Let's assume 1 gram to keep it simple.

Going back to our hypothetical example, let's say someone typically eats 3500 calories per day, and she wants a deficit of 875 calories. She now wants 2625 calories per day. Since she weighs 130 pounds, she needs about 130 grams of protein. At 4 calories per gram, this gives her 520 calories. The remaining 2105 calories should come primarily from complex carbohydrate. Fat intake should be kept to a minimum, say 10 to 15 percent.

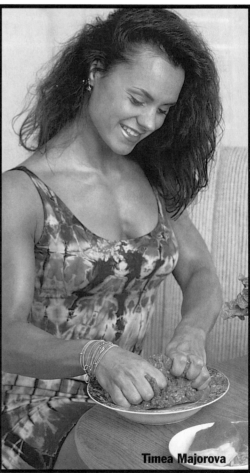

Timea Majorova

Monitoring Your Progress

It is very important to monitor your progress accurately. Track your weight with a scale, your measurements with a tape measure, and your bodyfat percentage with skinfold calipers (all bodybuilders should have a pair of calipers and know how to use them).

Even if you are doing everything right, your body doesn't always behave the way you want it to, so it is crucial that you continually monitor your progress. You may find that the fat is not coming off as quickly as you'd like. If so, add aerobic exercise to your routine (three or four times per week initially). Or perhaps the weight is coming off too fast with an accompanying muscle loss. In this case you would slightly increase your protein and carbohydrate intake. Any changes should be made in small increments and recorded carefully.

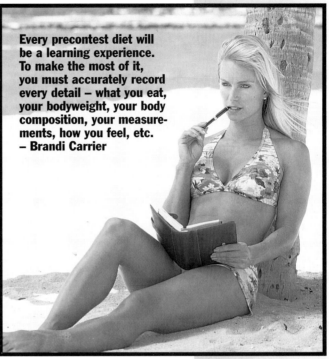

Every precontest diet will be a learning experience. To make the most of it, you must accurately record every detail – what you eat, your bodyweight, your body composition, your measurements, how you feel, etc. – Brandi Carrier

Every precontest diet will be a learning experience. To make the most of it, you must accurately record every detail – what you eat, your bodyweight, your body composition, your measurements, how you feel, etc.

If this process seems simple, that's because it is! Dieting is not supposed to be mystical. If you track your body composition weekly during your diet, you will have a good assessment of your progress and avoid the panic dieting that can strip you of your hard-earned muscle mass.

Stage Preparation: The Fitness Routine

If you've never performed a fitness routine before, we suggest you start getting prepared at least six months before your contest date. You want to be well prepared and ready when the day arrives. First pick up some high-energy fast-paced music that fits your personality. Listen to it constantly and play around with dance and strength moves to see if they will work. One of the best ways to select your music is to have the radio on every chance you get. Visualize yourself performing a routine to the latest upbeat dance song. Another place to preview music is an aerobics class. If you train at a mainstream gym there are probably literally dozens of classes per week. If you've been going to the same instructor's classes, try dropping in on other sessions. Most instructors use their own music and by going to four or five different classes you'll be exposed to a broad spectrum of songs.

The big trend in fitness these days is to splice two or more songs together so you can change the pace of your fitness routine onstage. Use upbeat music from the high-energy tumbling and power movements, and use a slower tempo for the stretching and flexibility movements.

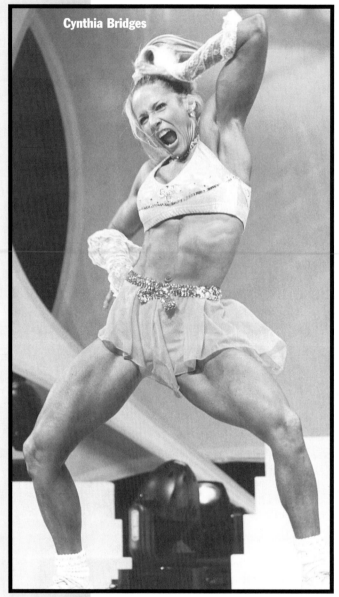

Cynthia Bridges

Once you have a good idea of what music you'll use, your next step is to hire a choreographer. There are very few fitness stars these days who develop their own routines. You need someone who is both knowledgeable and who's not afraid to give you corrective criticism. You may be tempted to rely on close friends, but odds are they'll hold back on their comments in the interest of friendship. A neutral third party will call things as she sees them. It's like learning to drive for the first time. Remember how much fun it was with Mom or Dad sitting in the passenger's seat giving you tips? The same thing holds true when putting together a fitness routine. You want someone who both knows what to look for and, perhaps more important, will give you the feedback you need.

If hiring a choreographer has a down side it's cost. In many respects choreographers are like personal trainers – they usually charge by the hour – and that can be $50 or more. Depending on how much work you need, and the quality of the person you hire, you can expect to invest $500 to $1000 preparing for one contest. On the surface this sounds expensive, but keep in mind what you are up against. Fitness shows these days are highly competitive – and you can be sure that just about every other contestant will have hired a choreographer.

One of the first things you and your choreographer should do is sit down together and watch videos of fitness contests. Pay close attention to both the static poses and perhaps more important how the contestants move from one skill to another. In bodybuilding moving from pose to pose is called transition, and the same philosophy is applied in fitness. You want to combine both grace and power all within two minutes or less.

Just as bodybuilders draw up a list of their best and worst poses, so too must you make an objective analysis of your best and worst skill events. The goal is to present the best package to the judges, so to speak. If your tumbling skills are limited, don't despair. Work in additional flexibility and power movements. Conversely if you have a gymnastics background, go for broke. Nothing looks as impressive onstage as a tumbling run combined with power and flexibility movements. You and your choreographer can make these decisions in the months leading up to the contest.

Now you know why we said start preparing six months in advance. You can't just slap something together and call it a fitness routine. Well, you can, but the judges and audience members will see right through it. Not only will you place near or at the bottom, but also it's somewhat embarrassing to have to follow someone who's done her homework and has an outstanding routine. It's sort of like the regional bodybuilding champ having to go out onstage after Arnold Schwarzenegger in his prime. You get the picture.

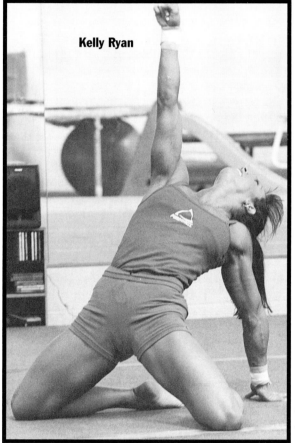

Kelly Ryan

Kelly Ryan Describes the Mandatory Moves

Even though your routine will be designed to show off your individual physique to its advantages, there are six moves that most organizations, including the IFBB and NPC, have made mandatory for all competitors. In fact in addition to your two-minute individual routine, most organizations require you to execute these six mandatory moves in a shortened 45-second routine. This mandatory round has replaced the strength round where contestants had at one time to battle it out on exercise equipment.

The following is a brief description of the six moves, and training tips for executing them, from top fitness competitor *Kelly Ryan.*

Move #1: One-arm pushups – Both a right- and left-arm pushup are required. The key to this exercise is to keep the torso tight. Most competitors lose points by pushing their butts too high in the air or letting their bodies sag down toward the floor. Just as you would in a regular pushup, keep the body parallel with the floor. It doesn't matter how far apart your legs are as long as it's comfortable for you.

Training tips – As expected Kelly recommends lots and lots of pushups to strengthen your core muscles. Another exercise Kelly finds beneficial is to lie on her back and place her hands above her head. She then exhales and raises both her legs and upper body until she's forming a V-shape. Inhale and slowly lower both legs and torso.

Move #2: Straddle presses – Sit on the floor and adopt a splits stance. From there lift the body off the floor by pushing downward with the hands. The judges look for the height of the feet, which must be kept off the floor at all times. Also keep the legs straight and toes pointed outward.

Training tips – Again the abdominals play a big role as you are pulling in and upward with the hips, abs and torso. Even though you are balanced on your hands, the real lifting is surprisingly done with the midsection.

Move #3: Right or left split – You are given a choice with this move – you can have either the right or left leg forward. Judges look for how close you can get to the floor. Try to minimize any space or gaps between your legs and the surface. Upright spinal alignment will give your split a finished look. They key to impressing the judges is to appear to be in control and not as if you are struggling.

Training tips – According to Kelly you have to "sit on your splits on a daily basis." She goes on to say, "There's really no secret. It just takes practice. Directly after cardio sit in your splits for five to ten minutes per side." Kelly finds having a training partner push down on her shoulders helps too. If you can't hold for five minutes, hold for as long as you can comfortably. Add a few extra seconds each session and it won't be long before you can easily hold for five or ten minutes.

Move #4: Straddle split – Adopt a standard splits position with each leg pointing outward at exactly the same angle. Your legs should form a symmetrical 180-degree angle with the floor (as opposed to the right or left split where one leg is slightly forward and the other slightly behind your torso). Kelly adds vari-

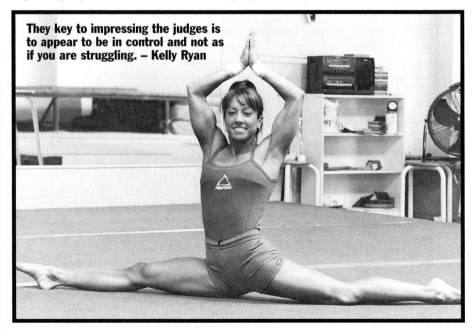

They key to impressing the judges is to appear to be in control and not as if you are struggling. – Kelly Ryan

ety to her splits by leaning forward with both hands on the floor, but sitting up straight is all that is required.

Training tips – No secrets here, just practice, practice, practice. Kelly recommends at least half an hour a day, more if weight training is a regular part of your routine. While great for strengthening and toning the muscles, weight training contracts the muscle and may reduce flexibility in some movements, especially those requiring a wide range of flexibility like splits.

Move #5: L-presses – Sit on the floor with your torso straight, legs together and straight out in front of you. Now press down on the floor with both hands and raise your body off the floor. Once again the judges check the distance between your feet and floor. Once the move is started no part of your body other than the hands should touch down. The ideal position is legs parallel with the floor.

Training tips – Again Kelly recommends V-ups for preparing for this move. The primary movers are the abdominals and other midsection muscles so strengthening this region is an absolute must.

Move #6: Right and left kick – You will need to do two kicks per leg in the mandatory routine. You can do either two kicks with one leg then switch to the other, or alternate back and forth – the choice is yours. The key to getting high points on this move is to keep your torso perfectly straight. Start the kicking leg slightly behind the other and raise it up as high and as straight as possible. Try not to let the torso bend forward at any time.

Training tips – Kelly suggests you alternate holding each leg in position for a few minutes of static stretching, with walking across the floor doing actual kicks.

Hair Today, Gone Tomorrow

You've just spent months if not years developing that great physique of yours. It only makes sense to show as much of it as possible to the judges and audience. Most women don't have the same problem with body hair as men, at least not in terms of amount, but nevertheless getting rid of it will take some creativity.

Besides the actual contest implications, unwanted facial and body hair can ruin your confidence. There are many different methods to remove facial and body hair. Some of the techniques are temporary, like creams and waxing, but there are also more permanent methods such as electrolysis and laser hair removal.

There are pros and cons to every method of hair removal because of skin irritation, risks, expense, time involved, or hair growing back too quickly. Besides the most common method of hair removal, shaving with a safety razor or electric shaver, consider the following brief descriptions of various other methods.

Shaving – Shaving is the most popular method of hair removal for two reasons; it's cheap and it's quick. A pack of razors will set you back only $5 or so, and you can shave your legs in less than 30 minutes.

There are two primary types of razors – straight and electric. As mentioned straight-edge razors are very cheap and easy to obtain. They also give you the closest shave. Most straight edges these days have two or three blades embedded in the plastic head. The heads are designed to both lift the hair out of the skin and snip it off. The end result is the hair is cut off just below the skin surface, giving the appearance of never having been there in the first place. But here's the downside to straight edges: In some respects they are too efficient. Cutting the hair below the skin often irritates the surrounding area and leads to a rash. Likewise dragging a sharp metal object over the skin can also leave a rash. This is why we suggest you do any major shaving at least a week or more before the contest. This gives time for any rash to clear up. You can then do a touch-up a few days before the show.

Electric razors usually eliminate the risk of developing a rash, but it's a trade-off as they don't cut the hair quite as close to the surface. You'll only get a day or two before the hair has grown out enough to give you a "5 o'clock shadow." Still, for quickly removing a large amount of hair a week or so before the contest, nothing beats an electric razor. If you don't have one yourself, check with a boyfriend, your husband, or dare we say it, your brother!

Mechanical epilators – Mechanical epilators pull out the hair and should not be used on sensitive skin areas such as the face, genitals or armpits because the method tends to be painful. In addition, the hair must be about 1/4 inch long to work, and the epilator can still miss some hair. Mechanical epilators cost anywhere from $50 to $100. Results last about a week.

Depilatories – Depilatories have been described as chemical shaving. Chemical warfare is another way of putting it. Depilatory creams and lotions contain chemicals that dissolve the protein structure of hair and cause it to separate from the skin. Some depilatories can increase acne and skin irritation or chemical burns if the formula is too strong or the cream left on too long. Test the cream on a small patch of skin before smearing the whole body. It's better to discover you're allergic to the ingredients on a small area than on an entire leg! Depilatories cost $5 to $10. Results last about a week.

Tweezing – Tweezing pulls hair out from its root, but is a very laborious method since each hair must be removed individually. For a couple of stray hairs tweezing is a viable option, but for most normal hair growth tweezing is a time-consuming process. As expected there is some pain, skin irritation, and inflammation of the hair follicle once it's pulled out. Tweezers cost anywhere from $3 to $30. Results last about three to eight weeks.

Waxing – Waxing pulls sections of hair out from the root. This method can be very painful and pain-reducing gel is often recommended before applying the wax. Some skin irritation can occur from pulling off the wax as well as inflammation of the hair follicle. Wax should not be on skin that is chapped or sunburned, or on the face if you are using a facial product such as Retin-A or Differin as these weaken the skin and tearing of the skin could result when the wax is pulled off. If a professional performs the waxing, treatment cost is $25 to $50 for legs. Do-it-yourself waxing products can be purchased. Hair needs to be at least 1/8 inch long for waxing to be effective. Results from waxing last three to eight weeks.

Electrolysis – Electrolysis is a very laborious method since each hair must be treated individually. With electrolysis a needle is inserted under the skin and an electric current is passed through the hair follicle to damage it. Only qualified professionals should perform needle electrolysis and it can be very expensive since it is time-consuming and multiple treatments are needed. Electrolysis can be painful and there is a risk of scarring and infection. Estimated cost for complete treatment is $1000 to $3000 for legs. Results are long-lasting, but some hair may grow back. As with tweezing, electrolysis is perhaps viable for minor hair growth, but expensive and very time-consuming for larger areas.

Lasers – Laser hair removal is FDA approved. Working with small areas of the skin, the laser beam destroys hair follicles and impairs hair regrowth. There is less pain and it is less time-consuming compared to electrolysis, but there can be redness or pigmentation changes of the skin. Laser treatment works best on people with light skin and dark hair. In addition, laser treatment will not work on deeply embedded hair follicles such as the underarm or the bikini line. Only licensed professionals should perform laser hair removal. It is very expensive and multiple treatments are necessary. The estimated cost for complete treatment is $500 to $1000 for facial hair removal and $2000 to $3000 for legs. Results are long-lasting, but some hair may grow back. If so, it is sparse and finer.

Photo epilation or pulsed laser – Photo epilation is also FDA approved. This treatment uses an intense pulsed light to destroy hair follicles instead of the steady laser beam. Photo epilation will work on underarms, bikini lines, light- and dark-skinned people since the device can be adjusted to skin type, location and depth. The photo epilation beam is broader than the laser, so the treatment can be done in less time. Only licensed professionals should perform this treatment. There are minimal side effects, but a series of treatments are necessary and the estimate for total cost is high – $2000 to $3000 for legs. Results are long-lasting, but some hair may grow back. If hair grows back, it is sparse and finer.

As a final word of warning, there are precautionary guidelines to follow before and after using any hair-removal technique. Follow the directions carefully, or discuss the details with a professional. If you've had skin problems in the past a visit to a dermatologist may be in order.

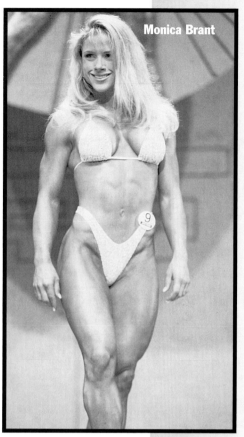

Monica Brant

The Perfect Posing Suit

When it comes to posing suits, female bodybuilders have it much easier than fitness competitors as they only have to buy one outfit, a two-piece posing suit. Fitness contestants, however, need a two-piece posing suit, an evening gown, and an aerobics outfit. Perhaps the best advice we can give you in this regard is to flip through the contest section of a recent copy of *Oxygen* magazine, or watch a video of a recent show. Take a look at what everyone is wearing. Pay close attention to colors, styles and cuts. You may think something as simple as

"My costumes are ready at least two weeks before the show. If you don't know somebody who makes good costumes, go to a place that makes cheerleader outfits. They know how suits need to fit during a routine. I practice my routine – both fitness and physique moves – in the outfits to make sure nothing falls out."
– Fitness Olympia winner Monica Brant, offering advice on where to get a good fitness costume made.

choosing a color is a quick decision, but it's not. African-American competitors should not wear dark colors as they blend in with the skin. Also light colors tend to draw attention to the midsection, making it appear larger than it really is. Light colors also tend to highlight stains more readily. Keep this in mind if you are using copious amounts of artificial tanning dyes.

As to style, you must take your bodytype into account. If you have short legs, then a high-cut design is appropriate as it creates the illusion of length. Those with long legs can wear a lower-cut design, but not too low as long legs are a much-desired physical trait. If you've got 'em, show 'em.

A final word concerns the size of the posing suit. Most fitness federations have rules governing how much of the physique can be "revealed," so to speak. As much as the audience members may love to see you parade onstage in a thong, there are rules to follow. Check with your federation to get a precise set of rules and restrictions as they apply to posing suits.

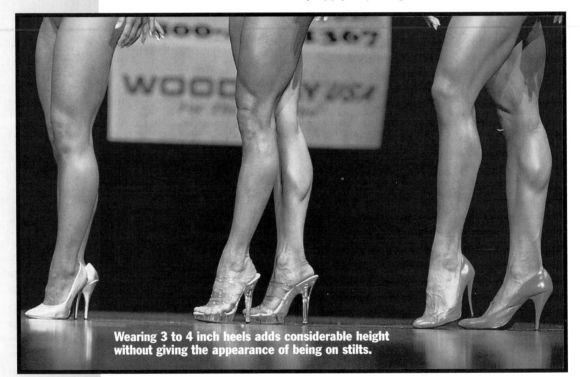

Wearing 3 to 4 inch heels adds considerable height without giving the appearance of being on stilts.

Best Foot Forward

The final piece of "equipment" you'll need to complete your posing suit is footwear. During the comparison round contestants are required to wear high-heel shoes. Once again an issue that seems trivial must be given careful consideration. Many competitors match the color of their shoes with their posing suits. Others opt for black or white as they go with any color. Finally you can take the route used by Mia Finnegan and other fitness stars and wear clear shoes – the so-called Cinderella glass-slipper look.

Besides color there's the heel height to consider. Most women stay in the range of 3 to 4 inches as this adds considerable height without giving the appearance that they are on stilts. For those not used to high heels, one thing you must do is practice walking in them. High heels take a bit of getting used to and the last thing you want to do is walk out onstage and turn an ankle. Not only would it ruin your entrance (to put it mildly) but it twisting an ankle from three or four inches up could leave you with a severe sprain, or worse, a broken bone. Take a few weeks and get a feel for your new footwear.

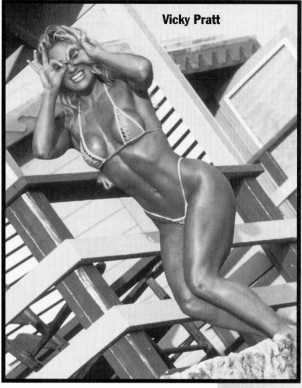

Vicky Pratt

Glasses – To See or Not

Readers with 20/20 vision, please feel free to skip over this topic. For those with corrected vision, a few words are in order. If you wear glasses in your day to day routine, you may want to give them a pass at the contest. True, there is nothing in the rule book that says you can't wear glasses, but you'll never see them worn at a show. Glasses not only distract from a great physique, but they are very cumbersome to wear, especially during your fitness routine. Try doing just one tumble or summersault and you'll see what we mean. Besides the practical limitations, the hot stage lights will make it such that your glasses will be constantly sliding off your face due to sweat.

There are a number of ways to get around the problem. The simplest is to not wear them in the first place. This may seem foolhardy, but with the exception of the free posing round you'll be constantly surrounded by other contestants. Unless you are severely visually impaired you can probably see the contestants on each side of you. As the judges call out the moves for comparison, simply follow the lead of the other competitors.

Perhaps the best solution to the whole problem is to invest in contact lens. For $50 to $100 you can buy soft contact lenses that will give you perfect vision. Put them in when you get up in the morning and remove them before bed at night. For a few dollars more you can buy hard contact lens that you can wear 24 hours a day. Contacts have two primary advantages over glasses. For starters no one can see them unless they're up close and staring into your eyes. And even then it's difficult to spot them. The other benefit is convenience. Unlike large glasses, which just sit on your face, contacts actually rest on the eye. You can jump up and down, tumble, and do practically anything you want and never have to worry about losing them. With the exception of swimming underwater with the eyes open, contacts allow you to engage in just about any athletic endeavor.

If you plan on making fitness a major part of your life, and you have a few dollars to spare, the best alternative is laser eye surgery. With the average price for the procedure dropping into the $1000 range, you can have your eyes restored to near perfection for the investment of a few minutes of your time.

The procedure is usually done on an outpatient basis and generally performed with local anesthetic eye drops. This type of refractive surgery gently reshapes the cornea by removing microscopic amounts of tissue from the outer surface with a cool, computer-controlled ultraviolet beam of light. The beam is so precise it can cut notches in a strand of human hair without breaking it, and each pulse can remove 39 millionths of an inch of tissue in 12 billionths of a second. The procedure itself takes only a few minutes, and patients are typically back to daily routines in one to three days.

Before the procedure begins, the patient's eye is measured to determine the degree of visual problem, and a map of the surface of the eye is constructed. The required corneal change is calculated based on this information, and then entered into the laser computer.

There is little if any discomfort during surgery because the cornea and eye are anesthetized by drops. Some patients experience a "scratchy feeling." After the anesthetic wears off, the amount of discomfort varies with each individual, but any irritation is minor and usually disappears within a few hours. The patient may be sensitive to light for a few days.

Most people can return to work one to three days following surgery, but a rule of thumb is to wait until you feel up to it. Most return to normal activities as soon as the day after surgery.

Laser treatment itself takes only about 15 to 40 seconds, based on the degree of correction necessary. Recovery is minimal, and usually the patient

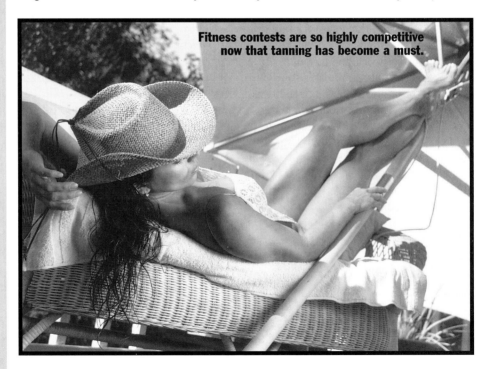

Fitness contests are so highly competitive now that tanning has become a must.

can be driven home after about 30 minutes, and typically will notice improved sight within three to five days of treatment.

According to the results of the US clinical trials and results reported internationally, this treatment appears to be permanent. As people age, however, their eyes change and retreatment may be necessary.

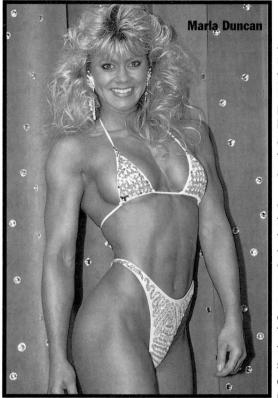

Marla Duncan

Tanning

As with wearing glasses, there's nothing in the rule book that says you must darken the skin, but fitness contests are so highly competitive now that tanning has become a must. Go to any show and you'll see that, with few exceptions, all the top placers have dark and healthy-looking skin.

The primary reason for darkening the skin is to protect you from the intense stage lights. By *protect* we don't mean from skin damage, we mean to prevent the lights from "washing out" your physique. Intense lights have a habit of blurring muscularity and hiding the curves that separate the muscles. The effect is more pronounced if the competitor has light-colored skin. All things being equal, a dark-colored competitor will appear much more muscular and toned than a light-colored competitor. Even though the two may be in identical shape, the darker person appears to be in better physical condition.

Here's a second reason for tanning: The process tightens the skin and makes your muscles and muscularity stand out better. It may also help get rid of a few pounds of water that is trapped just beneath the skin. Once again the end result is sharper muscularity. African-American women may not consider tanning for the darker color aspects, but they should consider it as a way to improve muscularity.

"I'm not a big advocate of tanning beds, but if you do have a medium to dark skin tone, tan a few times before you put your base on. If you are really fair skinned, tanning is not going to do you any good because you are just going to turn red. So you need to experiment with a lot of different tanning products."
– champion fitness competitor and regular Oxygen *magazine contributor Marla Duncan, offering good advice on darkening the skin before a contest.*

Tanning – the Good, the Bad, and the Ugly

Doing it Naturally

By far the easiest and cheapest way to darken the skin is with natural sunlight. There's nothing as relaxing as lying out in the backyard or on a beach to "catch a few rays." Unfortunately *tanning* has become a bad word these days and a few words of caution are in order. Sunlight doesn't contain just tanning rays – it contains the full electromagnetic spectrum. This means while your skin is absorbing rays that will release pigment, it is also being subjected to radiation that causes skin damage.

Humans have not helped matters either with the amount of pollutants pumped into the atmosphere over the last 150 years or so. The atmosphere is in many respects a large filter and helps block out most of the sun's radiation. With the advent of the industrial revolution, humans have been slowly destroying the atmosphere, particularly the ozone layer, and more harmful radiation is getting through. Lying out in the sun for extended periods of time can cause skin cancer and other skin-related problems. So despite its easy access and cost, natural sunlight does have long-term health implications.

"And for women of color, if you think you don't need to tan or use paint, you are so very wrong. Once you get onstage, the lights are going to wash you out and you'll look grey. Even though you have darker skin, you still have to bring out the richness in your skin tone."
– top fitness competitor, suggesting why even African-American women need to darken their skin before a contest.

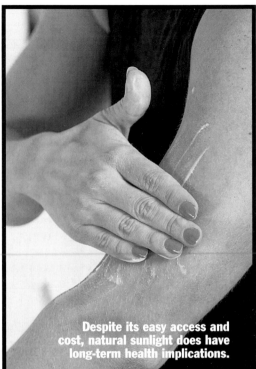
Despite its easy access and cost, natural sunlight does have long-term health implications.

If you decide to go the natural tanning route, make sure to wear a good sunblock. For most people that means nothing less than a *"15"* on the sunblock scale. One application is usually not enough either, especially if you are swimming or playing sports.

Fake Bake

For those who want to keep exposure to sunlight at a minimum, or live in northern climates where lying out in the snow for much of the year doesn't appeal to you, there's the option of artificial tanning beds. These large waffle iron-like contraptions use artificial light sources that will cause the skin to release pigment just as effectively as natural sunlight. Of course any light source that causes a pigment release is also harmful to the skin (pigment is in fact a defense mechanism against harmful radiation). Some of the newer sunbeds are advertised as having the harmful rays removed, but this is just creative advertising. The manufacturers may have tweaked with the light source and cut down on harmful radiation, but no tanning bed is risk free. It's like the food industry saying "calorie-reduced" or "fat-reduced." The question is – by how much? If something is very dangerous to begin with, reducing it can still leave it at a dangerous level.

We hope we have not frightened you too much. Tanning beds are probably safer than natural sunlight for the same period of time, and using one for a few weeks before a contest is probably not going to cause you any harm. Of course if you have a history of skin cancer in your family then you might want to check with your dermatologist before using artificial tanning beds.

There are two primary types of tanning beds. The most popular are the waffle-iron versions mentioned above. You lie down on a glass bed and lower the top half down so you are enclosed in a cylinder of light. The advantage here is comfort. Put on some easy-listening music and relax for 15 to 20 minutes. The disadvantage to such beds is, before long you are lying in a pool of sweat. Granted, it's your sweat, but it's still uncomfortable.

The other type of tanning bed is actually a tanning booth. Instead of lying down you stand up, naked, in a small room decked out in long florescent light tubes. There's no lying in sweat and no need to worry about what the previous user may have had. Also, stand-up booths usually use a more intense light source. Instead of 20 to 30 minutes you're in and out in 10 to 15 minutes. You've probably guessed the downside by now. A more intense light source is harsher on the skin. Still, for a few weeks of usage you probably haven't statistically increased your odds of causing skin cancer.

One of the lesser known advantages of tanning beds is, they enable you to tan the entire body – and we mean *entire* body. Unless you frequent nudist beaches, a scarcity in North America, tanning on a beach means keeping the naughty bits covered. The end result is tan lines that may become visible during your posing and physique rounds. Tanning beds allow you to tan in the nude and get rid of the tan lines. It doesn't sound like that big a deal, but you'd be surprised at the little things competitors sometimes get docked points for.

"I go to a tanning bed maybe six to ten times prior to a competition, to make sure I don't have any strap lines from the beach. Plus, if you can darken your natural tone by a shade or two, it evens you out and gives you a less flawed appearance."
– fitness competitor Mocha Lee, suggesting why tanning beds have their place in pre-contest tanning.

Painted Ladies and a Bottle of Wine

If tanning by light, either natural or artificial, frightens you, then you have one final option – *dyeing.* There are numerous tanning dyes and lotions on the market that will darken your skin without the risk of skin damage (and for those who are allergic to the lotions). They can be divided into two categories – overnight and instant. Overnight dyes work by reacting with enzymes in the skin (much the same as cutting an apple in half and exposing it to air eventually it browns). Smear the lotion on, wait a few hours (overnight is best), and there you have it – instant tan. The downside to such lotions is that they often produce more of a dark yellow color than a natural brown. Depending on your skin type you may end up looking like someone with jaundice! Also keep in mind these lotions will stain everything they come in contact with. If you go the overnight approach, make sure you use an old set of bed clothes.

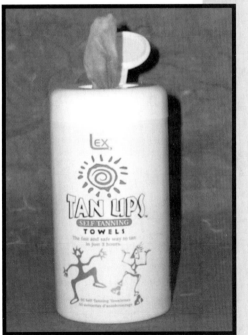

These new self-tanning towelettes will give you a healthy and luxurious golden brown tan without the mess.

The second type of dyes are instant. They are really nothing more than body paint that darkens the skin right on the spot. The quality of such skin dyes has reached the point that the palest of individuals can walk onstage sporting a chocolate brown skin color. As with hair-removal, test the product out on a small

"I'm 100 percent for body paints you can use a few days before an event and then shower the morning of the competition. It prevents color from coming off on your suit, and ensures you won't melt onstage. I always recommend two coats. If I'm competing on a Saturday, I'll paint on Wednesday night, and Thursday too. That way Friday night I don't have to worry; I can just relax."
– top fitness competitor Tanya Carlson-Merryman, commenting on the benefits of instant tanning paints.

area of skin before coating the whole body. Better to have a small localized allergic reaction than over the entire body. Unless you have dark skin to begin with you'll probably need a couple of coats to completely darken the skin. Given the ease with which you can use such products, you might want to conduct a trial run a few weeks before the actual contest just to see how many coats you'll need.

Now in Pill Form!
As expected, modern pharmacology has made available *a pill* that will give you a tan. The tan is produced when such organic pigments as beta carotene (from fruits and vegetables) and canthaxanthin (from marine organisms) accumulate in the skin. The effect can last for weeks and in some cases months. Seems there are no side effects, although, a few cases of anemia have been reported from long-term use. As with the overnight tanning lotions you might want to experiment well ahead of time to see exactly what color you'll end up. Yellows and oranges seem to be more frequent than browns but it depends on the individual. Winning the contest because the judges figure you're dying of some liver disease is not gonna happen in the fitness industry!

Which Will it Be?
As in the proverbial machines versus free weights debate, most people will probably benefit from using a combination of tanning methods. If possible get a good tan foundation from light (natural or a tanning bed) in the weeks before the contest, then do some touching up with one of the tanning dyes in the days before the show. You may even want to give the tanning pill a try, although to be honest it rarely produces that much-desired brown look.

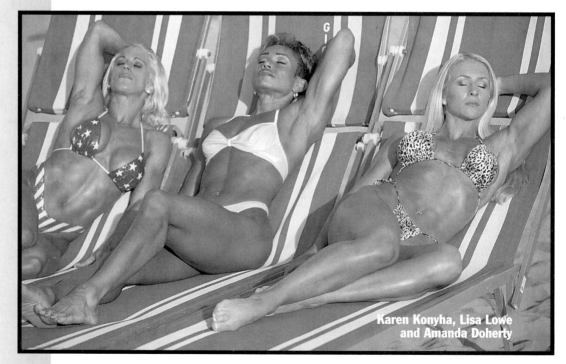

Karen Konyha, Lisa Lowe and Amanda Doherty

Contest Weekend

Well, you're just about there. In a few hours all those months of preparation will start paying off. If you've done your homework you are in the best shape of your life, and perhaps more important, you know how to present yourself. Before we go any further, let us be the first to say *Congratulations!* You are now in better shape than 99.9 percent of the population. Whether the judges place you first or last, you've accomplished far more than most people accomplish in their entire lives. Take pride in knowing you've joined a select group of individuals who've made fitness a part of their life and not just as a means to an end. We tip our hats to your determination and success!

One of the simplest ways to describe the weekend of the contest is *organized confusion.* And no matter how prepared you think you are, there will always be something you missed. Don't panic as all the other competitors are going through the same internal struggles. To make the weekend go a tad smoother, we've put together the following checklist of things to do. It is by no means complete, but it will help you arrive at the show feeling a little bit more prepared.

Schedule of Events

Perhaps the most important tick on your checklist is knowing exactly when and where each part of the contest will take place. You can have the best physique and routine in the world, but it means nothing if you arrive late or miss one of the segments entirely. Most contests have a preliminary weigh-in and registration the night before the show. In most cases this is Friday evening. If you're lucky the weigh-in is at the same location as the contest, but don't assume that. A combination of cost or scheduling conflicts with the venue may mean the promoter had to book another site for the weigh-in.

The prejudging, the first part of the actual contest, usually takes place Saturday morning. The time often depends on the number of contestants. Between 9 a.m. and 10 a.m. is the usual starting time, but once again confirm this in advance with the promoter. Most prejudgings are over by noon, but a big show with a large number of contestants could go until 1 p.m. or 2 p.m. Keep in mind these times are the actual judging times. You want to arrive at the venue at least one hour in advance. It's possible the organizers will tell you to arrive even earlier than that. As we said, it's organized confusion and it's better to be too early rather than not early enough.

Once the prejudging is over the next segment of the contest weekend is usually the seminar put off by the guest poser. Most promoters hire a well-known fitness star (or bodybuilder as most fitness and bodybuilding contests are held together these days) to draw in bigger audience numbers. Besides the posing routine during the contest, the star often conducts a seminar between the prejudging and evening show. If you feel up to it (your energy reserves may be low due to strict dieting and rigors of the prejudging) we encourage you to take in what the guest star has to say. It's one thing to read about someone's training and dieting in a book or magazine, but something else entirely to hear it in person.

"When you head up onstage you shouldn't have any coulda's or woulda's. I have a mantra that I say backstage and also repeat to myself in the weeks prior to a show – kick butt and take names. All of your work is done ahead of time, so have fun. It's time to jam – light it up!"
– top fitness competitor Kelly Ryan, revealing her mental framework before she steps onstage.

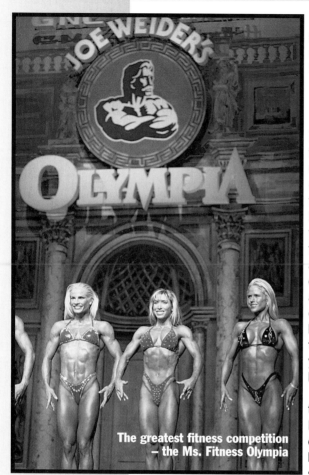

The greatest fitness competition – the Ms. Fitness Olympia

The final part of the contest is the evening show, which in most cases starts between 7 p.m. and 8 p.m. Again confirm the times with the organizers and be there well in advance.

The Out-of-Towners

For those who live in the same area as the contest, the next few paragraphs will seem redundant, but for those from out of town a few pieces of advice are in order. After all your hard work and time it would be a shame to be disqualified simply because you couldn't find the contest venue or you were late. But it has happened and will continue to happen. So much effort goes into the actual preparations for the contest that many competitors forget to *locate* the site of the show in advance – the importance of which becomes even more pronounced in an urban setting. Most big cities come alive on Friday nights. The registration and weigh-in usually starting at 7 p.m., so you'll have to deal with traffic surrounded by get-homers and get-downtowners.

Our advice to competitors from out of town is to scope out the place a day or two in advance. Find the shortest route from the hotel (or wherever you are staying) to the contest venue. Wouldn't hurt to make a dry run on Thursday evening to see how long it will take to drive that distance (if you are relying on a taxi you have other issues to deal with). The traffic on Thursday and Friday evenings will be similar, and your dry run will give you an idea of how much time to budget.

"Well, before I leave for a contest I put all my costumes in plastic baggies and place them in my carry-on luggage. By putting them in baggies you are protecting them from oily things in your luggage like face creams."
– *fitness competitor Debi Lee Stern, offering a tip on how to prevent damage to your fitness costumes.*

The Fitness Contest Travel Kit

Secure in the knowledge that you'll find the venue on time, your next step is to put together your backstage competition kit. The following will serve as a checklist of what you'll definitely need backstage as you prepare for your big debut. Some items will seem redundant but in the excitement of the preparing for the contest you may forget the obvious. Write them down and check them off your list as you pack.

Gym Bag or Travel Bag
To hold all your travel attire you'll need a gym bag of some type. It can be a standard workout gym bag, or an over-the-shoulder piece of luggage that you'd carry with you on a plane. Rather than buy the first thing you see, assemble your travel items first, then select a carry-on bag just large enough to hold

everything. Most contest organizers allow competitors to take bags backstage, but there is a limit. Most won't allow large suitcases or multiple items backstage so your goal is to *minimize.* In no order of importance, here's what to put into your carrying bag.

Competition clothes – As a fitness contestant you'll be required to compete in three different types of uniform. As we went into each in detail earlier in the chapter, suffice to say you'll need to pack your evening gown, bathing suit, and aerobics uniform. If you have the extra money, it wouldn't hurt to have two of each. We know this gets pricey but anything can happen backstage from staining to tearing. It doesn't hurt your chances either if you wear one style and color for the prejudging and another for the evening show. *Overkill?* Maybe that's taking it a bit far, but as we said earlier the state of fitness competition has reached a stage where point scores and placings are often down to single digits. A change of color between the rounds may give you the edge over the other competitors.

Tanning lotion – Even with the perfect tan there will be areas of your body that will fade or streak because of sweating and toweling. Pack a bottle of instant tan to make quick touch-ups between rounds.

Towels – Even at the pro level towels are few and far between. The combination of exercise and hot stage lights will have you sweating up a storm. Go backstage every chance you get and dry yourself off. You are not doing this just for the sake of appearance either. You need good traction onstage to perform your fitness routine. Pools of sweat can be death traps for a fitness competitor in the middle of a tumbling run. Even though most organizers have stage hands to continually mop up, it helps when contestants take the initiative and keep dripping sweat to a minimum.

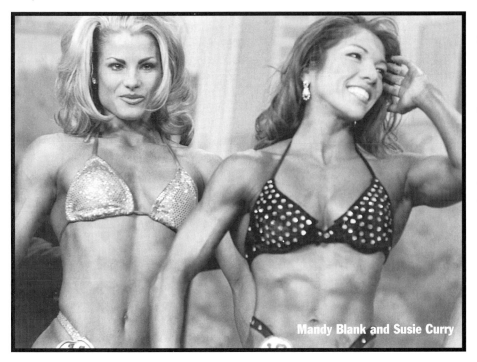

Mandy Blank and Susie Curry

Warmup suit – We could have put this item under "competition clothes" but it's a slightly different topic. Although heat won't be an issue onstage, it may be a concern backstage. Even the biggest and most modern of contest facilities have a reputation for being drafty backstage. Diving straight into a fitness routine without the body properly warmed up is a prescription for disaster. Take a look at sprinters before their race. They're all insulated by one or two layers of clothes. Your fitness routine is just as intense and requires the same degree of preparation. Bring along a track suit or heavy sweatshirt and track pants to keep the body warm before going onstage.

Posing music – Another item you will need is posing music – at least two copies for backup purposes. Posing music should be done on a high-bias recording cassette tape and labeled with your name and competitor number if possible. The label on the tape should also indicate which side to play. Try to make playing your music as easy as possible for the DJ. Music should begin at the beginning of the tape on side A.

Posing oil – Pack at least one bottle of posing oil, preferable two. Things get spilled easily backstage in the confusion and for what a bottle costs, have a backup. If you don't need the second bottle you can give it to someone who has forgotten hers. Little things like that help you win congeniality awards. Laugh if you may but winning such an award will get you extra coverage and attention. And as we keep saying, there's no such thing as too much coverage when it comes to helping your career. A simple act of kindness backstage may win you the whole contest next year (assuming you don't win this year!).

Food – Odds are you are going to be too nervous to eat when you get up in the morning. Chances are, however, by the end of the prejudging you'll be famished. The goal on contest day is to eat just enough to satisfy your appetite without going overboard and bloating yourself (besides the appearance, a large meal may make you lethargic). Save the pigging out for after the show. (You've earned it!) Popular backstage snack foods include bran muffins, granola bars, fruit, rice cakes, etc. Later in the day you can afford to eat something more substantial.

Water – You are over 90 percent water by volume and you are going to lose a lot of it during the next few hours. At the expense of a few dollars, pack a couple of bottles of distilled water. Sip on it throughout the day to replenish lost fluids. You may be tempted at times to gulp it down, but resist the urge to do so. As with food, an excess of water can leave you bloated in the midsection.

Toiletry kit – This item is really a collection of smaller items, which will come in handy throughout the day. You may think of others.

1. toothbrush and toothpaste
2. soap
3. shampoo and conditioner
4. deodorant
5. brush or comb
6. hair spray
7. small mirror
8. small hair dryer
9. tampons or sanitary pads (if need be)

Money

Even though we wouldn't suggest leaving money backstage in a gym bag, it's something you should bring with you. If there's any doubt as to its safety, leave it with your husband, boyfriend, etc.

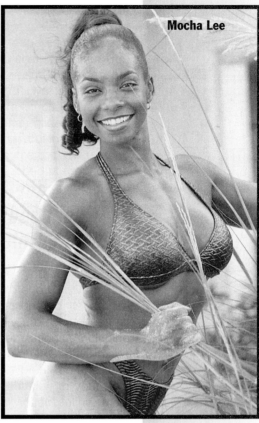

Mocha Lee

These days contests are usually well organized, but occasionally mistakes happen. What if you arrive for the weigh-in and you are told there is no record of your registration? Somehow in the shuffle your paperwork got lost. Whether it's the fault of the promoter or post office, who knows? But there you are at the registration desk and people are telling you you can't compete unless you pay your registration fee. You now have two choices – walk out the door, or take out your wallet.

You probably feel like cursing everyone in heaps, insulting their ancestors, and calling it a day. But what about all that hard work? You'll be wasting months of preparation, not to mention perhaps years of training. And using the vocabulary of a sailor will not win you any friends. The fitness industry is similar to bodybuilding in that usually it's run by the same judges and promoters year after year. The last thing you want to do is develop a reputation as being "a hard case." What supplement manufacturer wants a model or spokeswoman with "an attitude." Our advice is to smile, accept that a mistake has been made and pay the registration fee. Don't be shocked either if the fee is more than what you initially paid. Most contests have late fees and paying on the night of the weigh-in is definitely late (even though it's not your fault).

If you still feel wronged you can always state your case a few days after the show. In all probability the mistake was legitimate (i.e. paperwork), or perhaps your application did not arrive. The odds that the promoter is singling you out are slim. He or she has a reputation to uphold as well. In any case bring along a couple of hundred dollars as an emergency back-up. If you don't need it, so much the better.

The Eye of the Storm

If you liken a fitness contest to a hurricane, then the prejudging is the front and the evening show is the back edge of the storm. Both sides of a hurricane have high winds, but the center or "eye of the storm" is relatively calm. Fitness contests are much the same with the time period between the prejudging and evening show being relatively quiet.

Once the prejudging is over, there are a number of options open to you. You may want to take in the guest poser's seminar we mentioned earlier. You may want to go out somewhere for a quick meal, or maybe go back to where you are staying and crash for a few hours. Odds are you didn't get much sleep the night before. By early afternoon fatigue may be setting in and you still have an evening show to do. Find a place to take a nap for one to two hours to recharge your batteries. Limit yourself to a couple of hours, though, as crashing for three hours or more will make it that much harder to "wake up." The goal is to sleep long enough to recharge your batteries without putting yourself into a deep sleep.

Here's one suggestion to help refocus yourself on the upcoming evening show. Lie back before getting dressed and visualize the night's events. You already have an idea of what's in store having gone through the prejudging. The evening show will be much the same only more formal with a larger audience.

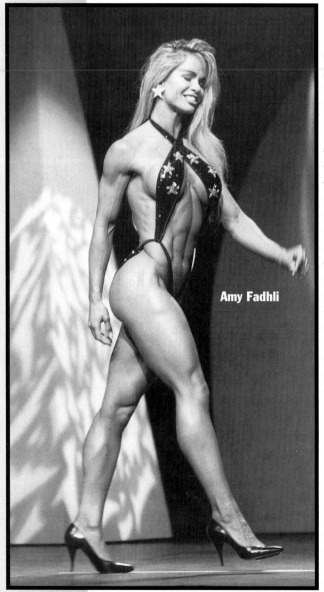

Amy Fadhli

Postcontest Festivities

Once the winners have been announced, our advice is to accept the results as they stand. This won't be a problem if you win the whole show, or place higher than you expected. Problems arise, however, when contestants who thought they had the whole show "in the bag" fail to live up to their expectations. Someone who placed second for a couple of years in a row may figure this is her year. That may be true but then again maybe some other contestant came out of nowhere to win the whole shebang. Or maybe some competitor who regularly failed to make the top ten suddenly got her act together. In any case she won and you didn't.

Fitness contests are like small fraternities, as we said earlier, with the same judges and organizers turning up year after year. Even if you and the majority of the audience feel you were robbed, don't make a scene by throwing trophies and insulting ancestors. Be gracious and accept the judges' decision. Keep in mind that judges are like baseball umpires – while they occasionally miss one, replays show they are usually right. The same holds true for fitness judges as in most cases the winner deserved to win. Your friends may be telling you the show is yours, and you may be blessed with copious amounts of confidence, but let's face it, both of you are a tad biased. The judges call it as they see it.

If you are the victim of a bad call (or worse, politics), simply smile, accept your placement, and wave to the audience as you exit the stage. Trust us, the fans – and more important, the magazines – will let everyone know over the next few months exactly who really should have won the show. Great sportsmanship will always pay bigger dividends down the road.

Win or lose, you have a number of options after the show. If you are fatigued by the day's events, then head back to where you are staying and slip into a coma. If you are like most people, however, you will be too excited to sleep. In this case take advantage of the postcontest party.

The better promoters usually finish off the weekend's proceedings with a big free-for-all bash after the evening show. Some rent clubs, others convert the venue itself into a huge banquet hall and dance floor. No matter where it is held the first order of business is pigging out. Let's face it, you've spent the last couple of months depriving yourself of the really great-tasting foods. No matter how many precontest cookbooks you buy, few contain anything that compares to a large bowl of Häagen Dazs ice cream. We could write a whole chapter on the pleasures of chocolate, but we think you get the point. There's nothing like a good overindulgence in food to wind down a fitness contest. Even if you qualify for a bigger contest within the next week or two, one night of letting loose will not hurt your physique.

Besides worshipping at the food altar, postcontest parties are a great place to meet people. The pressure of the last few days probably meant you didn't get to know the other contestants as well as you would like. Some of the best friendships in the industry got started after a contest. Find out how other contestants prepared for the show. Touch base on training strategies. See what dieting tips you can pick up. Just think of how much knowledge is collectively held by 25 or 30 fitness contestants. Try to tap in. Something you hear at this year's social gathering may win you the whole show next year.

In addition to other contestants, don't be afraid to strike up a conversation with the judges. After all they are human and odds are many of them will be judging you at some future contest. If you didn't place as well as you hoped, be polite and ask for some corrective criticism. Most judges are only too happy to let you know where improvements can be made. Resist the urge to argue with the person, no matter how strong your convictions. This is after all supposed to be a social gathering (besides ruining the atmosphere you run the risk of alienating someone who once again may be evaluating you down the road). If you find that by talking to most of the judges independently they all say much the same thing, odds are you do have room for improvement. The Oliver Stones among you may cry "conspiracy," but realistically the judges are simply telling you your physique or routine still needs a bit of work. Even though your feelings may be hurt, the judges are doing you a favor. They are telling you what you need to work on to place higher next year. To quote Robin Williams in the movie *Dead Poets Society,* "Seize the moment." Make those improvements and you stand a good chance of having those same judges hand you the winner's trophy next year.

CHAPTER TWENTY-SEVEN

Supplements

The current world consumption of natural health products (NHP), supplements, nutraceuticals and functional foods is estimated to be between $70 and $250 billion annually depending upon the product categories that are included in the statistics. In the US, the sale of nutrition products consisting of natural health products (including dietary supplements and herbs), natural and organic foods, functional foods and natural personal-care products generated $44.5 billion in consumer purchases in 1999 *(Nutrition Business Journal, NBJ, 2000).* According to 1999 statistics published by the *NBJ,* 2000, the supplement market generated $15.4 billion in the US.

Why are so many people turning to supplements? Many feel that their health is being badly affected by the modern Western diet. Others have concerns about the loss of nutrients in the processing of foods, the use of genetically modified plants and animals, and the presence of environmental toxins. Despite rapid advances in medicine and food technology, there is a widespread belief that somehow we are being deprived of those substances necessary for life. And that imbalance is leading to illness.

Many people are overweight, and suffer from related conditions such as heart disease and diabetes. Medicine has not come up with a "magic bullet" that can cure those conditions. Much like the old-time snake oil salesman, supplement makers have a tendency to bend the truth in an effort to sell *hope in a bottle.* Some supplements, such as creatine, deliver exactly what they promise. Others remain controversial.

The information we present in this chapter is referenced, but often it is the supplement manufacturer who has sponsored the research. Accept the contents here as informed opinions. Before using a supplement, speak with your doctor and your pharmacist – and use the following guidelines:

1. Always use standardized herbs, preferably approved by the German Federal Agency (Commission E), the body responsible for approving medicinal use of herbals in Germany.
2. Never use more than one herb or supplement with another without approval from your physician or pharmacist.

> **"Believe nobody.
> Trust nobody."**
> – Detective Pembleton,
> to a young offender on
> the TV show Homicide,
> Life on the Streets

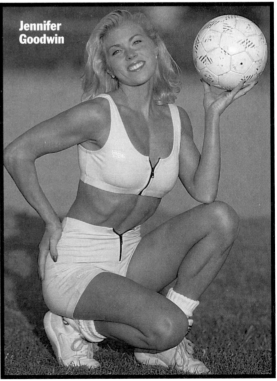

Jennifer Goodwin

3. Be aware that prescription drugs and supplements can have interactions. Speak to your doctor and pharmacist about what you can take, and when you can take it.

4. If you start to feel ill, stop, pick up your supplement, and go seek medical attention.

5. Do not take supplements with prescription or over-the-counter drugs without first checking with your doctor and your pharmacist.

6. Do not give a supplement to a child without first checking with your doctor and your pharmacist.

7. If it sounds too good to be true, then it probably is.[9]

Herbs

"I am a single male, 31, and I have the problem of immature ejaculation. For the past seven years, I am in sexual contact with a woman who is 15 years older than me. I ejaculate one or two seconds before or after intercourse. The problem is getting worse since past two years but before that I used to have sex for more than 10 minutes. Because I am getting married in next month, this must be treated before it and the cure should be permanent for life. Please also suggest any cream or lotion for the penis strength and power. I don't want to use unnatural ways of making longer duration sex like Viagra. I am now looking forward to hearing from you soon." – question sent to "Ask the Herbalist." We think the writer meant "premature ejaculation."

Herbs are distinguished from plant-derived drugs. In contrast to single-molecule plant-derived drugs, herbs are the chemically complex products made from plants or plant parts that are utilized in their dried or extracted forms. The quality of herbal preparations may be affected by the plant's age and growing environment, season of harvest, and postharvest processing.

Herbs have become big business in pharmacies across the United States. Changes in consumer attitudes and preferences push sales of herbs to new heights. Herbs are perceived as safer, gentler, and less expensive than conventional pharmaceutical drugs. The online retailing of dietary supplements and natural foods was expected to hit three billion by year 2002. Consumers are turning to a new wave of herbs for self-treatment and personal well-being. The "active ingredient" many health professionals seek in herbs is usually a relatively low level of a complex mixture of many naturally occurring phytochemicals, often working synergistically.

Under the Dietary Supplement Health and Education Act (DSHEA), the Food and Drug Administration (FDA) chose to classify herbals and vitamins as *dietary supplements* and not as drugs or medicine. Dietary supplements are not required to possess proven medical efficacy prior to marketing. While drug manufacturers must spend millions of research dollars in order to

Lisa Uzzle

market a drug for medical use in USA, the supplement companies are free to focus resources on marketing but none of it on the quality or efficacy of the product.

To ensure consistent purity and potency, a dietary supplement should be standardized to its active ingredients, which is supported by available clinical literature. Great variations in the concentration of active ingredients can exist among different lots of the same plant species because of constituents of a plant and different manufacturing techniques. In the USA the government has not established a standard of quality for herbal products. In contrast, herbal products in Europe must adhere to strict guidelines such as those established by German Federal Agency (Commission E).[1]

Because herbs are not well regulated in the US, there is no oversight of herbal product manufacturing, distribution or labeling. Therefore, unlike in some European countries, the contents and potency of any herbal product in the United States cannot be guaranteed. There have been many cases where herbal products were found upon chemical analysis to differ greatly from what is stated on the label. In some cases these products were found to contain dangerous toxic compounds. Some were even found to contain no herbs at all but were composed of standard prescription drugs such as benzodiazepines (a class of tranquilizers including Valium and Xanax), nonsteroidal anti-inflammatories and corticosteroids. Therefore, the use of an unregulated substance, such as the following herbs, is at your own risk.[37]

Aloe vera – Aloe vera is commonly used topically as a wound-healing agent for sunburns, psoriasis, and skin inflammation.
Side effects – Aloe vera has no side effects reported when applied externally.
Dosages – Aloe vera is applied topically two to four times daily.
Ingredients/dietary sources – Aloe vera contains acemannan (responsible for the emollient effect), sterols, triterpenoids and saponins. Aloe vera has some antibiotic effect with overall skin-moisturizing properties that can prevent excessive drying of the wound and relieve irritation.[2,3]

Bitter melon (Momordica charantia) – The extract of the fruit of Momordica charantia, a member of the Cucurbitaceae family, has been traditionally used to maintain blood glucose levels. Laboratory experiments and clinical trials using an extract of the dried fruit indicate that it promotes healthy blood sugar levels. The precise mechanism of action is unknown.[4]

Black cohosh (Cimicifuga racemosa) – Black cohosh is used for PMS complaints such as vaginal dryness, hot flushes and painful menstruation. Black cohosh is widely used and approved in Germany for treating menstrual complaints. This herb exerts a strong influence on the female reproductive system, normalizing menstruation and relieving menstrual cramps. Black cohosh is a powerful relaxant that is used in the treatment of rheumatic pains, osteoarthritis, muscular and neurological pain.
Side effects – Stomach upset, weight gain and dizziness are rare. But overdose can cause nausea, vomiting, reduced pulse rate, plus headache and visual disturbances.

Dosages – Standardized to 1 mg of 27-deoxyaceteine.

Take 20 mg twice a day of standardized extract.

Ingredients/dietary sources – Black cohosh contains triterpenes, flavonoids, methylcystine, caulosaponin and phytoestrogens.[2]

The active ingredient methylcystine (it closely resembles nicotine) increases intestinal mobility and blood pressure. Caulosaponin constricts blood vessels and causes high blood pressure. Black cohosh may reduce symptoms of PMS by relaxing uterine muscle. Studies have shown black cohosh reduces luteinizing hormone levels, which have been implicated in causing PMS.[5]

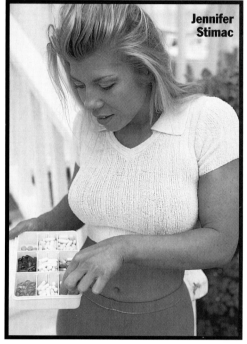

Jennifer Stimac

Black tea – According to the results of a large-scale Dutch population study, consumption of black tea (Camellia sinensis [L.] Kuntze, Theaceae) may decrease the risk of developing atherosclerosis, a hardening and narrowing of the coronary arteries that can contribute to heart attack, stroke, and other serious cardiovascular disease. The study showed that people who drank one to two cups of black tea a day had a 46 percent lower risk of developing severe atherosclerosis, while those who drank four or more cups a day had a risk reduction of 69 percent (Geleijnse et al., 1999). Tea drinking had no statistically significant effect on the development of mild or moderate atherosclerosis, and it appeared to be more protective for women than for men.

Tea drinking among Westerners is associated with an overall healthier lifestyle and diet, and in general, the intake of tea in the Dutch study was higher among participants who were lean, were educated, smoked less, and consumed less alcohol, fat and coffee. However, even after the data were adjusted for these and other possible confounding factors, the inverse association between tea consumption and severe atherosclerosis in this study remained statistically significant.[45]

Blueberry (Vaccinium myrtillus) – Blueberry is used traditionally to treat arthritis, diarrhea and circulatory disorders. Blueberry can also be used to treat eye conditions like night blindness, poor adaptability to bright light, and poor vision due to diabetes.

Side effects – No known side effects are reported.

Dosages – Take 20-60 g of dried fruit daily.[3]

Take 80-240 mg daily or in divided doses.[4]

Ingredients/dietary sources – Blueberry fruits contain anthocyanins, tannins and flavonoid glycosides.[6]

Marijuana (Cannabis sativa) – Many may be unaware that cannabis sativa (L., Cannabaceae) was once a widely accepted medical treatment for the prevention and relief of migraine headache, and listed in the United States Pharmacopeia from 1860 to 1941. In this review article, the author presents an overview of historical use, modern research, and safety data that supports the potential utility of cannabis in migraine, which affects an estimated 23 million Americans [Russo, 1998]. Currently available migraine medications are not always reliable and may cause significant side effects.

Historical information shows that cannabis was held in high regard for the treatment of migraine by American and British physicians for at least eight decades, from the latter half of the 19th Century until the early 1940s. According to Russo, in 1915 " … Sir William Osler, the acknowledged father of modern

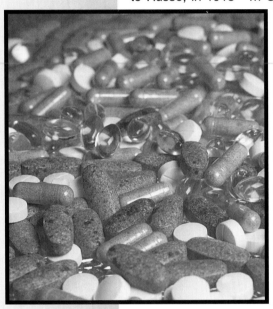

medicine, stated of migraine treatment, 'Cannabis indica is probably the most satisfactory remedy.'" Despite vigorous protest by the American Medical Association, Cannabis was made illegal in the United States in 1937, and the plant was dropped from the United States Pharmacopeia in 1941. Nonetheless, the following year, the editor of the *Journal of the American Medical Association (JAMA)* continued to recommend Cannabis for the treatment of menstrual migraine.

Although no modern clinical studies have specifically investigated the use of Cannabis in migraine, a number of small pain-relief studies have reported positive results in chronic headache pain and improvement of pain tolerance. A study investigating the effects of oral doses of the Cannabis compound delta-9-tetrahydrocannabinol (THC) in patients with cancer demonstrated a trend toward pain relief with escalating doses. The analgesic properties of Cannabis are believed to be unrelated to opioid mechanisms. Recent studies have pointed out some possible mechanisms of action for cannabinoids in migraine, including antinociceptive effects (interference with pain transmission) in an area of the brain that is considered a likely area for migraine generation.

In 1988, after an extensive review of testimony, US Drug Enforcement Agency administrative law judge Francis Young concluded that, "By any measure of rational analysis marijuana can be safely used within a supervised routine of medical care." In a 1995 editorial, the editor of the *British Medical Journal* called for "moderation in the drug war," and a supportive commentary was published by *JAMA* during the same year.[43]

Cascara sagrada (Rhamnus purshiana) – Cascara sagrada is a laxative with a long history of use in the US. Cascara sagrada should not be used regularly for more than one or two weeks without medical supervision.
Side effects – Abdominal cramps, nausea, vomiting and brown discoloration of urine. Long-term abuse can lead to electrolyte imbalances which affect the heart, and a nonfunctioning colon.

Dosages – Cascara sagrada fluid extract is five times more potent than cascara sagrada aromatic fluid extract. Take 5 ml of aromatic fluid extract or one 325 mg tablet at bedtime as needed for constipation.

Ingredients/dietary sources – The active ingredients of cascara sagrada contain anthraglycosides or anthraquinones like cascarosides A, B, C, D, chrysophanol, barbaloin, aloe-emodin-type anthranoids.[7]

Cat's claw bark (*Uncaria tomentosa*) – Traditional uses of cat's claw by the Ashaninka Indians of Peru were for treatments of inflammatory diseases, stomach ulcers, viral infections, menstrual disorders, contraception, arthritis and cancers. Cat's claw has been an important herb in Peruvian Indian folk medicine for many centuries and its properties are now being investigated to better understand its unique nutritional contribution to our current health needs.

People use cat's claw to treat almost anything, and it is recommended by many herbalists as a "cure-all" medicine. A highly effective immune system stimulant that fights viral infection and diminishes chemical sensitivity, it has been used to treat arthritis, intestinal disorders, allergies, and to ease the side effects of chemotherapy.

Side effects – Diarrhea may happen during the first ten days of use. Cat's claw is not recommended for pregnant women or those planning on becoming pregnant. Cat's claw is traditionally used to induce abortion. Cat's claw should not be taken with organ-transplant medications.

Dosages – Traditional Peruvian medicine: use 20-30 g of finely chopped bark, boiled in a liter of water for 20 to 30 minutes. Liquid is cooled at room temp and it is taken three times per day. The Peruvian Indians always use cat's claw by boiling it in water to make an extract.

Ingredients/dietary sources – The bark contains oxindole alkaloids, plant sterols, triterpenes, quinovic acid glycosides, proanthocyanidins and polyphones. Oxindole alkaloids are immunostimulants that may explain the anticancer activity of cat's claw.[8]

Cayenne (*Capsicum spp.*) – Cayenne can be used for painful muscle spasms. Cayenne is also externally useful for the treatments of shingles, headache, arthritis, diabetic neuropathy or numbness in the lower limbs. Cayenne is used internally as a stomach protectant.

Side effects – The active ingredient capsaicin, is highly irritating, especially to mucosal membranes such as eyes, lips and tongue, and may cause inflammation and swelling upon contact. It is one of the active ingredients used in pepper spray. Stomach upset, diarrhea and burning sensations during bowel movements occur on rare occasions.

Dosages – Take 30-120 mg capsule three times a day.[3]

Ingredients/dietary sources – Cayenne fruit contains 0.1-1.5 percent capsaicinoids or capsaicin, carotenoid, fats, vitamins A and C, and protein.[9]

Chamomile (*Chamomilla Recutita, Anthemis Nobilis, Matricaria Recutita, M. Chamomilla*) – In North America chamomile is one of the most highly recognized and popular herbal teas. Chamomile is used for stomach upset, including spasms and inflammation. It can also be used for mouth irritation and minor gum infection. This herb is also used for hiatal hernia, peptic ulcer, Crohn disease and irritable bowel syndrome.

Chamomile is used in creams and lotions to treat bacterial skin infections, in baths for skin irritation or inflammation, and as an inhalant to relieve lung irritation. This herb is an excellent nervine that relaxes and tones the nervous system and is especially useful in treating digestive problems such as gas, colic or ulcers due to anxiety. Chamomile is a sleep aid, a mild anti-microbial, and helpful in removing excess mucous in the sinuses.

Dosages – Approximately 1.5 to 3 g liquid extract or tincture three or four times per day.

Ingredients/dietary sources – The primary biologically active ingredient of chamomile is a light blue essential oil containing tiglic acid esters. This oil can relieve spasm and inflammation in the stomach.[10,48]

Chasteberry (Vitex agnus-castus) – Chasteberry is used in Germany to treat acne, menstrual disorder, and premenstrual breast pain.

Side effects – Allergic reactions such as shortness of breath, rash, itching, wheezing and red eyes may be experienced on the rare occasion. Chasteberry is not recommended for pregnant women or those who want to become pregnant because of the possibility of miscarriage.

Dosages – At a low dose (120 mg per day) of chasteberry, prolactin production is stimulated. At a higher dose (240-480 mg per day) prolactin production is decreased.

Ingredients/dietary sources – Standardized to 5000 ppm agnuside and 6000 aucubin.[11]

Cocoa (Theobroma cacao) – Although cacao is most often used as a food (the raw material for chocolate), it also has therapeutic value as a nervous-system stimulant. In Central America and the Caribbean the seeds are taken as a heart and kidney tonic. The plant may be used to treat angina and as a diuretic. Cocoa butter makes a good lip salve, and is often used as a base for suppositories. Central Americans have used cocoa for centuries to treat fever, coughs and complaints of pregnancy and childbirth. They have also rubbed cocoa butter on burns, chapped lips, balding heads and the sore nipples of nursing mothers. For internal use, they prescribed hot cocoa for asthma and as a nutritive for invalids and persons convalescing from acute illness. In 1994 Argentinean researchers showed that cacao extracts counter the bacteria responsible for boils and septicemia.

Chocolate naturally contains a drug substance, theobromine, which is chemically similar to caffeine and has a similar mild habit-forming, stimulating effect on humans. Its action on muscle, the kidneys and the heart is more pronounced. It is used principally for its diuretic effect due to stimulation of the renal epithelium. It is also employed in high blood pressure, as it dilates the blood-vessels. Many people are "addicted" to this drug and humorously refer to themselves as "chocoholics." Although chocolate is as mildly addicting as is coffee and other caffeine-containing drinks, its effect is relatively innocuous.

There is no evidence that chocolate causes acne, kidney stones or infant colic. However, chocolate does contain chemicals (tyramines) that trigger headaches in some people, particularly those prone to migraines. Many people find a cup of hot chocolate soothes their stomachs after meals. The problem is, cocoa and chocolate may cause heartburn. The herb relaxes the valve between the stomach and the esophagus.[46]

Cranberry (Vaccinium macrocarpon) – Cranberry juice is used to prevent and relieve the symptoms of urinary-tract infection. The juice is used in incontinent people to reduce urine odor. Cranberry juice can prevent the adhesion of bacteria to the human cell surface, which explains its ability to inhibit E. coli colonization in the urinary tract. In addition to cranberry's benefits against infection, cranberry is very nutritious. It contains vitamin A, C, B complex, as well as the minerals phosphorous, manganese, iron and calcium.

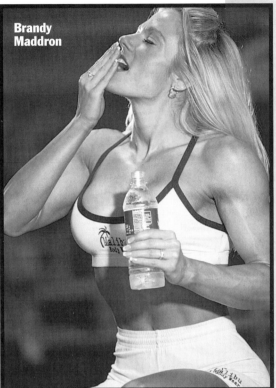
Brandy Maddron

Antibiotics can be used for urinary tract infection but they also destroy body-friendly bacteria and are normally not advised for pregnant women. Cranberry extract appears to be a good alternative because it is both safe and effective.

Side effects – Drinking too much cranberry juice (more than 2 liters per day) may cause diarrhea and stomach upset. No known side effects for people who consume the juice on a regular basis.

Dosages – Drink 360-960 ml cranberry juice daily.[4]

Ingredients/dietary sources – Cranberry contains anthocyanins, triterpenoids, flavonol glycosides, citric, malic and quinic acids.[12]

Dandelion (Taraxacum officinale) – This common garden pest was introduced to North America by the Pilgrims, who enjoyed dandelion wine. Dandelion contains choline, large quantities of minerals such as calcium, sodium, sulfur and, in the fresh leaves, a high content of potassium. The bitter compounds stimulate the appetite and promote digestion. Choline affects the gallbladder and the intestines, often stimulating the mucous membranes of the large intestine resulting in a laxative effect. Choline also has a relationship to the liver's lipid metabolism. Our daily requirement of choline is 2 to 3 grams and a lack of it increases fatty degeneration of the liver. The root has been successfully used to treat liver diseases such as jaundice and cirrhosis, along with dyspepsia and gallbladder problems. Its use as a diuretic is favorable because it replaces the potassium that most diuretics remove. It's the herb of choice for treating rheumatism, gout and heart disease, as well as regulating hormonal imbalances. Fresh latex removes warts if applied several times daily. Recent research shows a wide number of possibilities using dandelion. Its diuretic property can make dandelion useful for relieving the bloated feeling of PMS and help with weight loss. One study shows dandelion inhibits the growth of the fungus responsible for vaginal yeast infections. It also prevents gallstones. There is a German preparation, Chol-Grandelat (a combination of dandelion, milk thistle and rhubarb), prescribed for gallbladder disease. Traditional formulas: dandelion and barberry; dandelion and parsley; dandelion and purslane.[46]

Devil's claw (Harpagophytum procumbens) – Devil's claw has anti-inflammatory properties which may help some cases of arthritis with inflammation and pain. One double-blind, randomized trial concluded that devil's claw root was as effective in relieving pain and safer than diacerhein (known as a symptomatic slow-acting drug for osteoarthritis, or SYSADOA). The study participants (122 people with active osteoarthritis of the hip or knee) were randomly assigned to take either six 435 mg capsules of devil's claw powdered extract plus two placebo capsules, or two 50 mg capsules of diacerhein plus six placebo capsules for four months. Results showed that the two treatments were equally effective in relieving spontaneous pain. However, by the end of the study, significantly fewer people in the devil's claw group needed to take additional analgesics for pain relief. The frequency of side effects was also significantly lower among people in the devil's claw group. The most commonly reported adverse effect was diarrhea, reported by 8.1 percent of the devil's claw group and 26.7 percent of those who took diacerhein. The devil's claw used in the study was a French product marketed under the trade name Harpadol.

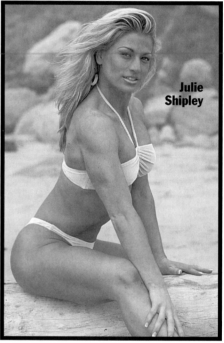

Julie Shipley

Side effects – None reported.

Dosages – For loss of appetite: Take 0.5 g of root three times daily.
For back pain: Take 6 g of dried root (equals 50 mg harpagoside) per day.

Ingredients/dietary sources – The active ingredient is 0.5 to 3 percent harpagoside. Harpagoside is the ingredient accountable for digestive action but not anti-inflammatory effects. However, it relieves pain when combined with other ingredients in devil's claw.[13,41]

Dill (Anethum graveolens) – Dill seed improves digestion and appetite and sweetens the breath. The oil kills bacteria and relieves flatulence. It is frequently used in Ayurvedic and Unani medicines for indigestion, fevers, ulcers, uterine pains, and kidney and eye problems. Ethiopians chew the leaves along with fennel to treat headaches and gonorrhea. In Vietnam it is used to treat intestinal diseases. Contemporary herbalists recommend chewing the seeds for bad breath and drinking dill tea both as a digestive aid and to stimulate milk production in nursing mothers. The herb helps relax the smooth muscles of the digestive tract. One study shows it's also an antifoaming agent, meaning it helps prevent the formation of intestinal gas bubbles.

Historically, injured knights were said to have placed burned dill seeds on their open wounds to speed healing. A mixture of dill, dried honey and butter was once prescribed to treat madness.[46]

Dong quai (Angelica sinensis) – Dong quai is a women's tonic in traditional Chinese medicine. Women use it for menstrual disorders such as painful, absence of, or abnormal menstruation. Dong quai is also used for PMS, and menopause symptoms like hot flashes and vaginal dryness. Dong quai can be used for anemia, dizziness, increased heart rate, abdominal pain or arthritis for both men and women.

Side effects – People may experience diarrhea or become photosensitive. Excessive bleeding and occasional fever are typical allergic reactions. People on blood-thinning therapy should not be on dong quai because it contains coumarins, a blood-thinning substance, unless under medical supervision.

Dosages – Take 4 to 9 g daily. Take 0.5 g of extract tablet twice daily for treatment of painful menstruation.

Ingredients/dietary sources – Dong quai contains ferulic acid, ligustilide, a significant quantity of vitamin E and B12, and phytoestrogens. Dong quai has a high level of the photosensitizing chemical, umbelliferone. Avoid exposure to sunlight, as a bad burn is possible.[14]

Echinacea (Echinacea purpurea, Echinacea angustifolia, Echinacea pallida) – Echinacea is a popular herb in United States and has a long history of medicinal use in America and in Europe. Originally consumed by Native Americans, at least 14 tribes used Echinacea for coughs, colds, sore throats, infections, toothaches, inflammations, tonsillitis and snake bites, among other things. It was used by the Dakotas as a veterinary medicine for their horses. In 1885 the Lloyd brothers of Cincinnati, Ohio introduced Echinacea products primary as an anti-infective, and by 1920 these products were the firm's most popular plant drugs. The development of sulfa drugs in the 1930s caused this plant to fall form conventional medical use, but it has continued to remain an active part of folk medicine. Europeans began growing and using Echinacea, especially the Germans, and to this day have produced the best scientific documentation of its value. The popularity of this extract in the US grew rapidly during the 1980s, and the plant is now again among America's best-selling herb extracts.

The most common anecdotal reports about the use of Echinacea are from people who begin taking the extract at the first sign of a cold. Often to their surprise they find the cold has disappeared, usually within 24 hours, sometimes after taking the extract only once. The most consistently proven effect of Echinacea is in stimulating phagocytosis, or the consumption of invading organisms by white blood cells and lymphocytes. To prove this fact, scientists incubated human white blood cells, yeast cells and Echinacea extract. They examined the blood cells microscopically and counted the number of yeast cells gobbled up by the blood cells. Extracts of Echinacea can increase phagocytosis by 20 to 40 percent. Another test, called the "carbon clearance" test, measures the speed with which injected carbon particles are removed from the bloodstream of a mouse. The quicker the mouse can remove the injected foreign particles, the more its immune system has been stimulated. In this test Echinacea extracts excel, confirming the fact that this remarkable plant increases the activity of immune system cells so they can more quickly eliminate invading organisms and foreign particles.

Echinacea causes an increase in the number of immune cells, further enhancing the overall activity of the immune system. Echinacea also stimulates the production of interferon as well as other important products of the immune system, including "Tumor Necrosis Factor," which is important to the body's response against cancer.

Echinacea also inhibits an enzyme (hyaluronidase), which is secreted by bacteria and helps them gain access to healthy cells. Research in the early 1950s showed that Echinacea could completely counteract the effect of this enzyme, and this could help prevent infection when used to treat wounds. While Echinacea is used internally for the treatment of viruses and bacteria, it is also being used externally for the treatment of wounds. It kills yeast and slows or stops the growth of bacteria, and it helps to stimulate the growth of new tissue. It combats inflammation, too, further supporting its use in the treatment of wounds.

Research in 1957 showed that an extract of Echinacea caused a 22 percent reduction in inflammation among arthritis sufferers. That is only about half as effective as steroids, but steroids have serious side effects. Steroids also strongly suppress the immune system, which makes them a poor choice for treating any condition in which infection is likely. Echinacea, on the other hand, is nontoxic, and adds immune-stimulating properties to its anti-inflammatory effect.

Side effects – Echinacea has an excellent safety record. After hundreds of years of use, no toxicity or side effects have been reported except rare allergic reactions in sensitive individuals. In individual cases, allergic reactions such as rash, itching, fever, swollen tongue and face have been recorded. People allergic to sunflowers, or plants in the daisy family like ragweed, chrysanthemums or asters, should be aware of a possible allergy to Echinacea.

Higher chances of infection because of long-term use of Echinacea may result from a depression of the immune system, possibly through over-stimulation and reduction of the herb's effects. People with chronic infections such as HIV/AIDS or autoimmune disorders such as lupus should not take Echinacea.

Dosages – This is not proven but Echinacea should not be used for more than eight weeks. Take 250 mg up to four times a day during cold or flu season. The dosage form should be standardized to 4 percent echinacosides (angustifolia) or 4 percent sesquiterpene esters (purpurea). People should be on a schedule of three weeks on and one week off for prevention.

Ingredients/dietary sources – Contains 1.2 to 3.1 percent cichoric acid in the flowers, and other caffeic acid derivatives; acid flavonoids, namely rutoside;

alkylamides; alkaloids, including glycine betaine, polysaccharides and glyco-proteins. This herb is thought to boost the immune system by increasing the number and activity of white blood cells.[15,38]

Feverfew (Tanacetum parthenium, Chrysanthemum parthenium, Tanacetum valgare) – Feverfew's name comes from the Latin *febrifugia,* or fever reducer. Feverfew preparations can be used to prevent and control migraine headaches. This herb has been used since the middle ages to treat fever, menstrual disorders, rheumatoid arthritis and headaches. When the wife of a Welsh doctor ended her 50-year history of migraine with a course of fever-few, a detailed scientific investigation of feverfew got under way. In clinical trials in Britain during the 1980s the herb was demonstrated to be an effective remedy for migraine. No fewer than 20 headache patients ate fresh Feverfew leaves daily for three months and stopped using headache-relieving drugs during the last month. After they were given capsules of .37 grains of freeze-dried leaf every day, they experienced less-severe headaches and fewer symptoms (including reduced nausea and vomiting) than observed in a placebo group. As an added benefit, the subjects' blood pressure went down.

Despite extensive research, the exact nature of its action is not yet understood. The constituent parthenolide appears to inhibit the release of the hormone serotonin, which is thought to trigger migraines. The parthenolides in Feverfew do not work by the same method as salicylates. While many herbalists prefer to use the fresh leaves, or an extract made from them, results have been seen with fresh, freeze-dried and air-dried leaves, although boiling Feverfew tea for 10 minutes instead of steeping it did reduce its activity in one study. As a preventative it should be taken in small quantities (three leaves a day) regularly. The herb can relieve arthritic and rheumatic pain, especially in combination with other herbs.

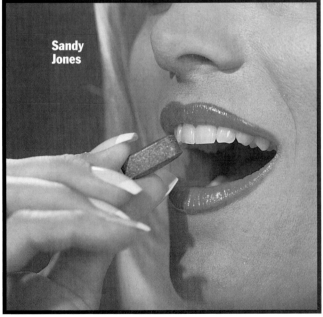

Sandy Jones

This herb has been used since Roman times to induce menstruation. It is given in difficult births to aid expulsion of the placenta. In South America where Feverfew is naturalized, it has been effective for colic, stomachache, morning sickness and kidney pains. In Costa Rica it has also been employed as a digestive aid. Mexicans used it as a sitz bath to regulate menstruation, as well as an antispasmodic and tonic.

Side effects – Eating or chewing fresh or dried Feverfew may cause mouth ulcers, dry or sore tongue, swollen lips or stomach upset. Otherwise it is generally very well tolerated. It has not been shown to cause uterine contractions, but because of its history in promoting menstruation, pregnant women should probably not use it. Individuals taking Feverfew with medical supervision for over six years have reported no adverse effects.

Dosages – Adult dose is 125 mg dried leaves with parthenolide content no less than 0.2 percent once or twice per day. Drug equivalent to 0.2 to 0.6 mg of parthenolide daily.

Ingredients/dietary sources – Chemical ingredient concentration in commercial products varies. The sesquiterpene lactone parthenolide is an active substance responsible for Feverfew's effectiveness.[16,47]

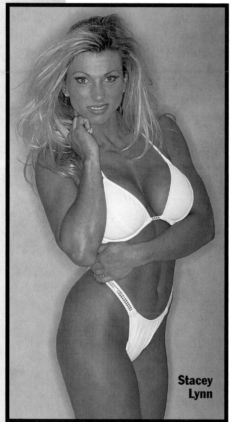

Stacey
Lynn

Garlic (Allium sativum) – Garlic is used to reduce cholesterol and triglycerides, inhibit blood clotting, and lower blood pressure. Compounds derived from garlic also have been shown to have potential immune-enhancement, antibacterial, antiviral and antifungal properties.

The ability of garlic to help promote healthy levels of cholesterol, triglycerides, LDL, HDL, platelet adhesiveness and fibrinolytic activity renders this healthful herb the potential capability to significantly support a heart-healthy lifestyle. A study published in the May issue of *Atherosclerosis* showed that a garlic powder supplement (Allium sativum L., Liliaceae) can help prevent and in some cases even reverse plaque buildup in the arteries (Koscielny et al., 1999). Researchers have long associated arterial plaque with an increased risk of heart attack and stroke. The study was conducted using rigorous controls (randomized, double-blind, placebo-controlled) and took place over a four-year period, making it the longest clinical trial to evaluate the effects of a dietary supplement on reducing heart attack risk.

For the four-year study, 152 men and women were randomly assigned to take either placebo or 900 mg of standardized garlic powder daily (brand name Kwai, Lichtwer Pharma, Berlin). From the beginning, all participants had advanced plaque accumulation, in addition to at least one other established risk factor for heart disease such as high cholesterol or blood pressure, diabetes, or a history of smoking. Researchers used B-mode ultrasound to measure the progression and regression of plaque volume in the common carotid and femoral arteries, at the beginning of the study and at 16, 36 and 48 months.

At the end of the study, those who took garlic had a 2.6 percent reduction in plaque volume, compared to a 15.6 percent increase in the placebo group. When the effects were analyzed by gender, there was a 4.4 percent decrease in plaque volume in men taking garlic, compared to a 5.5 percent increase in the male placebo group. The results for women took researchers by surprise. While women in the garlic group experienced a modest 4.6 percent decrease in plaque volume, those taking the placebo had a massive 53.1 percent increase.

According to the researchers, the striking difference between the two female groups was due to a predominance of younger women in the placebo group, and more older women in the garlic group by the end of the study. Although the age distribution was relatively even at the beginning of the study, it became unbalanced as a greater number of younger women in the garlic group withdrew from the study, mostly due to "annoyance by odor." Unfortunately, this prevented the researchers from drawing meaningful conclusions about garlic based on the age composition of the study groups. Clearly the double-blind design of the study was also defeated by the odor of the garlic pills, which were easily distinguished from the placebo pills. However, the investigators asserted that the 4.6 percent decline in plaque volume observed in women taking garlic remains a "genuine garlic effect."

Based on this study and more than 20 others conducted on standardized powdered garlic, researchers believe that garlic can have not only a preventative but also a curative role in heart disease. Previous studies demonstrate that powdered garlic reduces total and harmful LDL cholesterol levels, serum triglycerides, and blood pressure, and also inhibits cholesterol oxidation and platelet aggregation (the tendency of the blood platelets to clump), among other positive effects. This study adds more support to the scientific case for garlic as a "pleiotropic" substance, meaning the mild effects of garlic on many different measurements of heart health add up to significant overall benefits.

Side effects – Stomach upset may occur if clove is eaten by individuals not accustomed to ingesting garlic. Burning sensation in the mouth, nausea, vomiting and diarrhea. Body odor and bad breath are normal. A potential interaction between garlic and anticoagulant (blood-thinning) drugs such as coumadin (or warfarin) has been documented. Garlic may affect the anticoagulant therapy.

Dosages – The recommended daily dose of alliin is around 4 to 12 mg, which is equivalent to about 4 g of fresh garlic or 1 clove. Average daily dose: fully dried powder, 400 to 1200 mg; fresh air-dried bulb, 2 to 5 g; garlic oil, 2 to 5 mg. Commercial garlic preparations are variable in content. For the best results products standardized for alliin content are preferred.

Ingredients/dietary sources – Raw garlic contains both alliin and allinase (the enzyme). Alliin must be converted into allicin to be effective. Alliin is responsible for both garlic's characteristic odor and its pharmacological activity. Garlic also contains organic sulfur essential oil (disulfides and trisulfides.) Other constituents include vitamins A, B, C and E, adenosine, phytosterols, flavonoids, lipids, proteins and amino acid. Compounds known as ajoenes that occur naturally in garlic have also been reported to have biological activity.[17,42]

Ginger (Zingiber officinale) – Ginger played an important role in early Asian medicine because of its antinausea effect. It is a soothing herb for the stomach, and may help to prevent motion sickness and vomiting while traveling. It is used as a tonic, for lack of appetite, as a postoperative antiemetic for minor day-case surgical procedures, for vomiting associated with pregnancy or morning sickness. Ginger acts as a circulation stimulant and is also helpful in treating cramps or arthritis pain and is used as a remedy for digestive problems, sore throats and as a promoter of perspiration.

Ginger contains zingibain, a special kind of proteolytic enzyme that has the ability to chemically break down protein. Clinical studies have shown that proteolytic enzymes have anti-inflammatory properties. They also play an additional role in controlling autoimmune disease. They help reduce blood levels of compounds known as immune complexes. Ginger is well-known for its anti-inflammatory properties. Indian and Scandinavian studies have consistently shown that ginger is useful for treating most kinds of arthritis. It also contains more than 12 antioxidants. It can be taken as a tea, tincture or capsule.

Ginger gives other herbs a boost by improving the body's ability to assimilate them. Ginger actually protects herbal compounds from being destroyed by the liver and continues circulating in the blood for a longer time. It also improves intestinal absorption of other herbs.

Ginger helps reduce serum cholesterol levels and the creation of blood clots. It aids circulation (including peripheral circulation). Ginger has long been used in eastern Africa for killing intestinal parasites. Researchers discovered that all 42 components in ginger essential oil kill roundworms, among other parasites. Some of these compounds were found to be more effective than the commonly prescribed drug piperatzine citrate.

Side effects – No known side effect or toxicity. Caution is recommended for those on anticoagulants.

Dosages – Take 0.5 to 2 g of the powdered drug daily in single or divided doses. Ginger helps women who suffer excessive vomiting during pregnancy. Pregnant women taking a dose of 250 mg powdered ginger root four times daily experience a significant reduction in the severity of nausea and vomiting. For many people, 940 mg powdered ginger given 30 minutes prior to travel prevents sickness better than Dramamine, a popular over-the-counter motion sickness medication.

Ingredients/dietary sources – Ginger contains essential oil such as sesquiterpene hydrocarbon zingiberene and bisabolene, and pungent principles (shogaols and gingerols). Ginger standardized to 5 percent total pungent compounds shogaol and gineraol.[18,47]

Ginkgo (*Ginkgo biloba*) – The name *Ginkgo* is Chinese for "silver fruit" or "hill apricot," and *biloba* is Latin for "two lobes," denoting the divided shape of its leaves. Ginkgo biloba, also known as the maidenhair tree, is used around the world as a landscape tree because of its remarkable ability to withstand pests, disease, fungi, viruses, bacteria and pollution. In fact it was the only tree to withstand the atomic blast at Hiroshima. That same tree still lives near the epicenter today, a testimony to its incredible ability to survive. A Ginkgo biloba tree may live as long as 1000 years.

For at least 3000 years the Chinese have successfully used Ginkgo to treat a variety of ailments. It is currently the number one prescribed herb in Europe, and has slowly made its way to the United States.

Ginkgo improves circulation and oxygen transport to the brain and limbs, dilates and normalizes blood vessels and blood flow, increases cellular uptake of glucose, inhibits platelet and red blood cell aggregation, scavenges free radicals, and increases brain activity. Ginkgo does not work by stimulating the central nervous system (CNS). Instead it appears to normalize CNS functions. In Germany Ginkgo leaf extract is licensed for the treatment of peripheral vascular disease and for certain hearing losses and headache. Ginkgo leaf extract helps increase peripheral circulation of the blood, thereby enhancing blood flow to the brain. People use Ginkgo for memory deficits, poor concentration and depression.

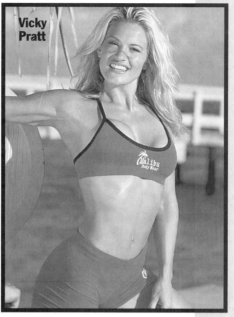

Vicky Pratt

People are now using Ginkgo to overcome the sexual dysfunction sometimes associated with use of antidepressants. Patients taking prescription antidepressants often experience unwanted sexual side effects. In one clinical trial researchers treated 33 women and 30 men experiencing this problem with 80 to 120 mg of Ginkgo extract per day. All patients continued taking their usual antidepressant medication during the trial. (Most were using SSRI-type drugs such as fluoxetine or sertraline.) At the end of the four-week trial, results were assessed through clinical interviews and patient self-reports. Ginkgo was reported to be effective for 91 percent of female patients and 76 percent of males. People suffering impotency also use this herb to lower the needed dose of prescription medicine.

Numerous studies have shown that standardized Ginkgo biloba extract can help improve symptoms of peripheral arterial occlusive disease (PAOD), a circulatory disorder associated with narrowing of the arteries and consequent pain during walking. Based on the positive outcome of an earlier pilot trial, this clinical study was designed to compare the effects of two different dosages of this extract in order to confirm the therapeutic superiority of the higher dose. For the study, 38 people with PAOD took a standard dose of Ginkgo extract (120 mg/day), while 36 were assigned to treatment with a dose twice as high as the standard (240 mg/day). After 24 weeks, both groups had "clinically relevant" improvements in pain-free walking distance, but the increase in pain-free walking distance was statistically significantly higher among those taking the higher dose. Both dosage regimens were reported to be safe and well tolerated. The standardized Ginkgo extract used in the trial was EGb 761 (Rokan), manufactured by W. Schwabe of Karlsruhe, Germany.

Ginkgo biloba has been used to improve cerebral blood circulation and to protect the nerves against damaging free radicals. Both these effects indirectly help in improving mental alertness, awareness and cognition.

Side effects – Side effects include stomach upset, headache, or allergic reactions when taking Ginkgo. Because Ginkgo is a blood thinner, people receiving coumadin, aspirin, Motrin or Aleve should not be taking Ginkgo unless monitored by a physician.

Dosages – 120 to 240 mg native dry extract in two or three doses. People should be advised that it takes about 6-8 weeks to see beneficial effect. Administration for more than three months should be reviewed by your doctor.

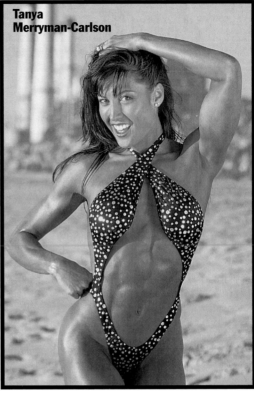

Tanya Merryman-Carlson

Ingredients/dietary sources – The beneficial effects are due to at least two classes of chemical found in Ginkgo:

• 22 to 27 percent of flavonone glyco-sides, determined as quercetin, kaempferol and isorhamnetin. The flavonone glycosides reduce capillary fragility and act as antioxidants, free radical scavengers.

• 5 to 7 percent of Terpene lactones, determined as ginkgolides, bilobalide and ginkgolic acid.

Both substances have an effect on circulation, oxygen uptake and the immune system. It is not really known if the substances found in Ginkgo work separately, or if the combination of these substances produces a powerful synergistic effect.[19,39,40]

Ginseng (Panax [Chinese, Korean or Asian ginseng], Eleutherococcus senticosus [Siberian ginseng]) – Ginseng is widely consumed as a health tonic beverage in Korea and China. Ginseng is used as an adaptogen, which means it helps the body adapt to internal and external stressors and prevent stress-induced damage and illness. Ginseng is a well-recognized root that has been used medicinally for over 2000 years. It helps to increase endurance, stimulate the immune system, fight fatigue and stress, and enhance performance, work capacity and concentration.

Although these effects have not been clearly demonstrated in clinical trials, the use of Ginseng is strongly based on the experiences found in traditional Asian medicine. In animal models, short-term treatment with Ginseng significantly prolonged aerobic endurance.

Ginseng root has a long history of use in enhancing cognitive and physical capacity. The saponins present in Ginseng root, the ginsenosides, are adaptogens which help the body adjust to various types of stress, thereby increasing energy levels and improving physical and mental performance.

Ginseng increases vitality and improves the body's resistance to a wide variety of illness and damaging external influences. Especially helpful to weak and elderly people. Can be used to treat male impotence, and may benefit men and women with stress-induced loss of libido. Suggested dose 100 to 250 mg twice a day, standardized to contain at least 7 percent ginsenosides.

Siberian Ginseng increases resistance to damaging external environmental factors and to illnesses, and increases vitality. People can use it to reduce incidence of flu and acute respiratory disease. It is an excellent general tonic. This herb was taken by Russian and Soviet athletes to improve performance. This herb helps the body deal with stress, facilitates healing, shortens recovery time, increases mitochondria function (energy building blocks of cells), reduces fatigue, and increases endurance and stamina. Siberian ginseng was introduced to the West by the former Soviet Union in the 1970s. Siberian Ginseng became popular because it was a cheaper substitute for Ginseng and due to its official use by cosmonauts and Olympic team members.

Side effects – No known side effects. People with estrogen-dependent cancer should not take Ginseng since estrogenic activity in Ginseng may cause abnormal vaginal bleeding. People with acute illness, high blood pressure, or using large amounts of stimulants such as caffeine-containing beverages, should not take ginseng.

Several studies have shown ginseng products to be mislabeled or mixed with other unwanted ingredients. Ephedrine (a stimulant) and caffeine are sometimes added to Ginseng products to give the patients the energized feeling they want. It is important to purchase extracts from only reputable manufacturers.

Dosages – Chinese or Korean Ginseng: 0.5 to 2 g of root daily or in divided doses.

Siberian Ginseng: 2 to 3 g of root daily or in divided doses.

Ingredients/dietary sources – The active ingredients isolated from Ginseng are saponins, steroid-like compounds. Other isolated compounds are termed ginsenosides.[20,49,50]

Goldenseal (Hydrastis canadensis) – Goldenseal is commonly used in combination with Echinacea to treat cold and flu. Traditionally goldenseal was used for eye irritation and is an eyewash ingredient today. The herb was historically used as an antibacterial, antiviral and antiparasitic medicine for lung, mouth, sinus and stomach infection. People have used goldenseal to try to mask positive results for illicit drugs in urine tests, but the practice does not work. Herbal treatment in some people seems to correct the deficient metabolic process common to liver disorder. Goldenseal is effective in all digestive problems from peptic ulcers to colitis due to its tonic effects on the body's mucous membranes. Goldenseal is a powerful antimicrobial improving all phlegm or mucous conditions, especially those of the sinuses.

Side effects – Goldenseal is well tolerated at recommended doses, but higher doses can cause nausea, vomiting, diarrhea and paralysis. Because goldenseal can stimulate uterine contraction, its use is not recommended during pregnancy.

Dosages – Standardized to 10 percent alkaloids or 2.5 percent berberine and 5 percent hydrastine. Daily dose is 250 mg two to four times a day. At excessive doses, hydrastine may cause central nervous system paralysis by seizure and cause high blood pressure.

Ingredients/dietary sources – Goldenseal's active ingredients have been identified as hydrastine and berberine. Berberine has antibacterial activity and hydrastine exerts astringent properties and reduces inflammation of mucosal membranes. Berberine is able to reduce bacteria such as group A streptococci's adhesive ability to host tissue. This may explain its antibiotic properties.[21]

Gotu kola (Gentella asiatica) – Gotu kola can be used to improve memory, and to overcome stress and fatigue. The herb helps improve circulatory symptoms like numbness and heaviness in lower limbs. Gotu kola extracts are used externally to treat skin inflammation, scar formation after surgery and burns.
Side effects – Rashes and itching occur in allergic individuals. Gotu kola may make the skin photosensitive, and easier to sunburn.
Dosages – Take dry gotu kola leaves 2 to 4 g daily.
Take 60 to 120 mg standardized gotu kola extract daily.
Ingredients/dietary sources – Standardized gotu kola extract contains saponin glycoside such as 40 percent asiaticoside, and 30 percent madecassic acid. Gotu kola also yields 2.2 to 3.4 percent of triterpenes, various concentrations of brahmoside and brahmissoside.[22]

Grape seed (Vitis vinifera, Pinus maritima, Pinus nigra) – The people of France and Italy suffer fewer fatal heart attacks and strokes than people in North America or in the northern regions of Europe. Though they eat a lot of fatty foods, they consume wine on a regular basis. Researchers think a natural substance abundant in grapes, proanthocyanidins, may contribute to the lower fatal heart stroke in Italy and France. It has been demonstrated that proanthocyanidins can protect cholesterol from forming plaque in blood vessels. It is a process thought to be at the origin of many fatal heart attacks. People use grape seed extract to improve venous, cerebral, cardiac circulation, and to reduce tissue injury and inflammation. Grape seed extract is an powerful antioxidant. It is used for diabetic eye disorder and macular degeneration.
Side effects – Very well tolerated. No known toxicity or adverse effects even under high doses.
Dosages – Daily dose is 25 to 100 mg one to three times a day.[4]
Ingredients/dietary sources – The active ingredient in grape seed extract is potent antioxidant bioflavonoids collectively called proanthocyanidins that neutralize free radicals. The extract contains nutritionally useful essential fatty acids, vitamin E and procyanidins. Proanthocyanidins are the most potent free radical scavengers known, and in studies these compounds significantly decrease free-radical generation in the cell. Proanthocyanidins allow migration of red blood cells within tissue and prevent fluid leakage out of the cell body. It also tends to strengthen the blood vessel walls.[23]

Green tea (Camellia sinensis) – People use green tea to prevent cancer and high blood pressure. Green tea is acclaimed for its antioxidant properties, attributed to the presence of polyphenols such as epigallocatechin gallate (EGCG). These compounds promote health by preventing lipid oxidation.
Side effects – None reported. But if too much is consumed, the caffeine content can cause nervousness and restlessness.
Dosages – Green tea can be consumed regularly as a beverage. No maximum dose reported.

Ingredients/dietary sources – Green tea contains polyphenols, flavonols, and methylxanthines such as caffeine and theophylline. Some commercial green tea extracts are standardized to about 60 percent polyphenols. Green tea normally contains 50 mg of caffeine per cup, compared to 75 mg of caffeine per cup of coffee.[24]

Guarana (Paullinia cupanavar) – Guarana is the ground seed kernel of the tropical plant Paullinia cupanavar. For centuries people in the Amazon Basin have used this herb as a stimulant and tonic. These properties are attributed to the presence of tetramethylxanthine (a compound similar to caffeine), high amounts of other alkaloids such as theophylline, and theobromine, tannic acid and saponins. The alkaloids and saponins are believed to contribute to the stimulant effects of guarana.[25]

Hawthorn (Crataegus oxyacantha, Crataegus laevigata) – Hawthorn is used to maintain normal heart function and blood pressure, and possesses antioxidant activity. The herb is a heart tonic in Europe used to reduce the incidence of chest pain, treat increased heart rate or irregular heart beat, and even control hardening of blood vessel. Some people take hawthorn as a sedative.

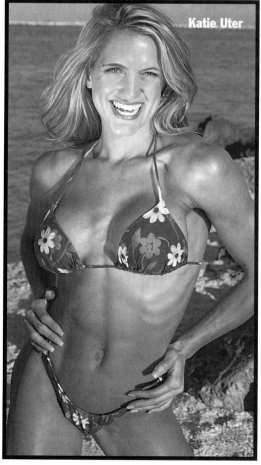
Katie Uter

The leaves and flowers of hawthorn (Crataegus oxyacantha) contain concentrated amounts of antioxidant phytonutrients, especially the oligomeric procyanidins. Hawthorn and its active flavonoid compounds make the heart a more efficient pump, partly by increasing blood supply to the heart muscle and partly by increasing the output of blood from the heart while decreasing the resistance of blood vessels in the body to the normal flow of blood. The result is support of a healthy heart and an efficient flow of blood throughout the body.

Side effects – Although hawthorn is without side effects, it should be used under strict medical surveillance because of its cardiovascular properties.

Dosages – 0.3 to 1.0 g, or by infusion three times daily.[1]

Tincture: 1 to 2 ml three times daily (1:5 in 45 percent alcohol).[1]

Liquid extract: 0.5 to 1.0 ml three times daily (1:1 in 25 percent alcohol).[1]

Ingredients/dietary sources – It contains flavonoids (kaempferol and quercetin) and flavone derivatives, hyperoside, glycosides, procyanidins, proanthocyanidins, cyanogenetic glycosides and saponins.[1]

Proanthocyanidins, one class of flavonoids, block blood vessels constriction in much the same manner as angiotensin-converting enzyme inhibitor or dilate the vessels.

The flowers, leaves, bark and berries of the hawthorn plant contain pharmacologically active pigments called flavonoids. They both inhibit vasoconstriction and dilate blood vessels. The sedative effects of hawthorn are due to a fraction of the flavonoids known as dehydrocatechins. They are central nervous system depressant.[26]

Horse chestnut (Aesculus hippocastanum, horse chestnut seed extract) – Horse chestnut is used to relieve leg swelling due to varicose veins. It doesn't get rid of varicose veins but it seems to help improve symptoms of leg swelling, pain and tension. The extract is thought to work by inhibiting enzymes that weaken the vein and allow fluid to leak out, and improving circulation. It seems to reduce leg swelling about as well as compression stockings. The herb is an astringent anti-inflammatory agent, influencing largely the vessels of the circulatory system. An excellent remedy for fullness associated with hemorrhoids, varicose veins, rectal engorgement, phlebitis and leg ulcers.

Side effects – Consuming the whole horse chestnut can be toxic with symptoms of confusion, nausea, vomiting, dilated pupils and muscle twitching. Horse chestnut seed extract (HCSE) with the toxic ingredient aesculin removed is well tolerated. But people may still experience occasional stomach upset or rash from ingesting this herbal product.

Dosages – People take 300 mg of HCSE or 1 capsule Venastat, which is a brand of HCSE, twice a day. This extract may cause stomach upset and a possible allergic reaction. 300 mg of HCSE is standardized to 16 percent of triterpene glycosides calculated as aescin.

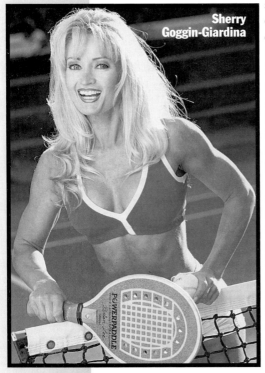

Sherry Goggin-Giardina

Ingredients/dietary sources – The active ingredient in horse chestnut seed extract is a mixture of triterpenoid saponin glycosides called aescin. Aescin reduces edema by reducing the permeability of blood vessels. The whole seeds contain toxic glycoside, aesculin or esculin. The natural horse chestnut seeds are toxic but the extract is purified to remove the toxins.[27]

Kava (Piper methysticum) – Kava root extract is a traditional drink from the South Pacific Islands, where it is prepared and consumed as a religious ceremonial beverage and used socially like alcohol. Recent popularity is based on its potent effect to reduce anxiety and stress, relax muscle, and numb the mouth if you chew the root. Kava is added to Western products as a muscle relaxant and tension reliever, and considered as a herbal alternative to synthetic antianxiety medicines and tranquilizers like the benzodiazepines.

Kava has definite pharmacological activity. Chronic use of kava can decrease anxiety levels while improving cognitive function. Those who use kava for sedation and insomnia may find their muscles relaxed, but their mind clear. According to US statistics, close to 17 percent of the population will experience anxiety disorders in any one year, and the lifetime prevalence is almost 25 percent. Conventional treatment involves benzodiazepine drugs, which can have serious side effects, including dependence, daytime drowsiness, and memory impairment among others. Kava, on the other hand, has demonstrated a remarkable safety profile, with side effects of only 1.5 to 2.3 percent reported in studies of more than 3000 patients.

Kava kava root is a central nervous system depressant and a relaxant of the skeletal muscle, which has no narcotic properties. It also anesthetizes the gastric, bladder mucosa and is useful in treating conditions such as irritable bladder syndrome.

Side effects – Kava is very well tolerated but may cause mild stomach upset for some people. The adverse events reported most often by kava users were gastrointestinal complaints, allergic skin reactions, headache and photosensitivity. Use of kava over several months can cause a scaly, yellowing skin discoloration due to accumulation of plant pigments. This condition resolves once ingestion of kava is stopped.

Dosages – Herb and preparation equivalent to 60 to 120 mg kava pyrones daily.[3]

Standardized extract (70 percent kava-lactones) 100 mg 2 to 3 times daily.[4]

Ingredients/dietary sources – The active ingredients in kava, called kava-lactones, may exert their activities by binding to alpha-aminobutyric acid (GABA) receptors. Small doses are relaxing but large doses are intoxicating. Some of these kava-lactones are not very water soluble, and their content varies from root to root. Maybe that will help explain the variety of effects seen by researchers.[28,44]

Licorice (Glycyrrhiza glabra, Chinese species is Glycyrrhiza uralensis) – Licorice provides soothing benefits for the stomach and digestive tract, has antioxidant properties that help to protect cells from oxidation damage, and can be used as a diuretic, an anti-inflammatory agent, and an expectorant. Licorice is an ingredient in cough drops and syrups, laxatives, and smoking products.

Side effects – People taking too much of licorice can experience high blood pressure, muscle pain, weakness, mental slowness, weight loss and confusion. Potassium loss from licorice will potentiate the side effects of diuretics and cardiac glycoside treatments for heart conditions.

Dosages – Average daily dose is about 5 to 15 g of root that is equal to 200 to 600 mg of glycyrrhizin. Licorice is a potent drug and is effective for a number of medical condition, but it is quite toxic and should only be used in low doses (below 10 g per day) and for less than six weeks.

Ingredients/dietary sources – The root contains glycyrrhizic acid (1 to 24 percent), several flavonoids, isoflavonone derivatives, phytosterols and coumarins. Glycyrrhizic acid activates both glucocorticoid and mineralocorticoid receptors. DGL (deglycerrhizinated licorice) is commercially available licorice with toxic glycyrrhizin removed. But DGL is not as effective as regular licorice.[29]

Ma huang (Ephedra sinica) – Ma huang is used as an appetite suppressant, energy booster, and in the treatment of daytime sleepiness. This herb is also used in alternative medicine for asthma, weight loss, hay fever, allergies, colds and flu, sinus congestion, energy, and sexual enhancement. With respect to weight loss, ephedrine has been shown to be effective in numerous clinical studies. Greater weight reduction has been observed when ephedrine is used in conjunction with caffeine, theophylline or salicylates.

Side effects – The isolated ephedrine in ma huang can increase blood pressure and stimulate thyroid function. People may experience dizziness, confusion, headache or increased heart rate.

Dosages – The maximum dose is 8 mg three times a day.

Ingredients/dietary sources – Ma huang is ephedra. Ephedra preparations can produce the same therapeutic and side effects that are associated with synthetic ephedrine. It can be derived from plants worldwide and has been used medicinally for hundreds of years. Western medicine regards ephedra or ma huang as *ephedrine.* Both ephedrine and pseudoephedrine (Sudafed) have a long history as over-the-counter medications.[30]

Milk thistle (Silybum marianum) – Milk thistle (70 percent silymarin) is used for toxic liver damage, supportive treatment in chronic inflammatory liver disease, cirrhosis and hepatitis. This herb helps maintain healthy liver function through its antioxidant properties. In Germany physicians use it to prevent liver toxicity and cirrhosis from hepatitis, alcohol, and other drugs. The active constituent in milk thistle (Silybum marianum) extract, silymarin, is proven to help in the support of liver health, and also to support detoxification. Silymarin also helps in the maintenance of healthy liver cells and provides protective effects in the liver.

Side effects – Other than a mild laxative effect, milk thistle appears to be safe and relatively nontoxic. Laxative effect or loose stools, may result from increased bile flow or mild allergic reaction.

Dosages – People usually take 200 to 600 mg per day in three divided doses of concentrated silymarin extract, standardized to 70 percent silymarin. Teas are not concentrated enough because silymarin is not very water soluble.

Ingredients/dietary sources – Milk thistle extracts contain silymarin, or silybin, a name collectively given to three compounds: silibinin, silydianin and silychristin. Silymarins are characterized as a new class of substance, flavonolignans. They are mixtures of substances that prevent the uptake of toxins into liver cells, accelerate regeneration of liver tissue, increase glutathione levels, and have antioxidant properties to neutralize free radicals. Silymarin serves as a powerful antioxidant in the liver cells, stomach and intestine, primarily due to its ability to increase the amount of glutathione by more than 30 percent in liver cells.[31]

Nettle (Urtica dioica) – People in Germany use nettle for inflammation of urinary tract and prevention of kidney stones. Nettle has a long history of use for cough, asthma and abdominal cramping.

Side effects – Adverse effects rarely reported but stomach upset or swelling are experienced by some. Skin rash and itching upon contact may last 12 hours or longer. Diabetics should avoid nettle since it may compromise blood glucose levels.

Ingredients/dietary sources – Nettle contains steroids, phenols, flavonoids and vitamins. The active ingredients steroidal and phenolic compounds inhibit prostate enlargement in men.[32]

Rosemary – Rosemary extract is claimed to have antioxidant properties, attributed to the presence of compounds such as carnosic acid, carnosol, rosemarydiphenol and others. These compounds promote health by preventing lipid oxidation by stopping damaging free radicals.[33]

Soya – Soy contains a number of isoflavones; genistein and daidzein have been particularly well studied. Animal tests have provided convincing evidence of improved bone mass following soy consumption. The only completed study investigating effects in humans researched the effects of soy protein on bone mineral density (BMD) in postmenopausal women and revealed significant improvement in lumbar vertebral BMD, but not in femoral or total body BMD.[34]

St. John's wort (Hypericum perforatum) – St. John's wort is a bushy plant with abundant yel-

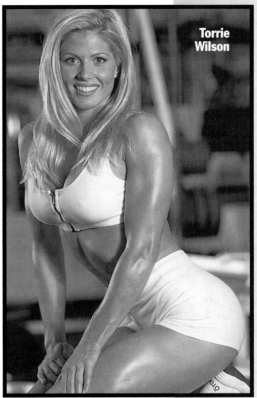

Torrie Wilson

low flowers around June 24, the traditional celebration time of Saint John the Baptist's birthday. St John's wort was thought to possess magical powers in ancient times. Its Latin name refers to the expulsion of evil spirits with one whiff of Saint John's wort.

St. John's wort is used for mild to moderate depression, anxiety, nervousness and healing wounds. It is the most popular prescription drug of any type for treating mild depression in Germany. Standardized extract of St. John's wort has been tested in numerous studies on the relief of mild to moderate depression. The results suggest effectiveness similar to that of prescription antidepressants, but with fewer side effects. It is also used internally for viral infection and anxiety. If used externally, it is good for treating minor wounds, burns and herpes simplex viral infection.

Side effects – People should be warned that St. John's wort can cause photosensitivity, leading to easier sunburn. Given the evidence that St John's wort has at least some monoamine oxidase inhibitor (MAOI) and serotonin-related activity, people should be warned to watch for symptoms: confusion, agitation, fever, sweating, diarrhea, nausea, muscle spasms and tremor. Commonly used doses do not cause an interaction with tyramine-containing foods. It should not be used at the same time with prescription antidepressants unless as directed by your physician, because of potential drug interactions even with a good safety profile.

You should not use St. John's wort as a treatment in preference to a prescription drug at this time. While there are people with good reasons to try

St. John's wort, such as those experiencing sexual dysfunction and other unpleasant side effects from prescription antidepressants the problem of quality and dosage still exists for herbal preparations sold in the US.

Dosages – Extracts of St. John's wort are standardized to 3 percent hypericin with usual recommended dose being 300 mg three times daily.

Ingredients/dietary sources – The herb contains hypericin, flavonoids, phenols, tannins and volatile oils. Hypericin produces a true antidepressant effect, but may not be as strong as other prescription antidepressants. Originally hypericin found in St. John's wort was thought to provide antidepressant activity by acting as a monoamine oxidase inhibitor (MAOI). More recent studies suggest that the antidepressant activity may be due to other ingredients acting by other mechanisms.[35,37]

Tea tree oil (Melaleuca alternifolia) – Tea tree oil can be used for skin bacterial and fungal infection. People have been using tea tree oil for insect bites, burns, canker sores and acne.

Side effects – No known side effects if used externally. May cause allergic reactions. People should test tea tree oil on a small area of skin before full application.

Ingredients/dietary sources – The major ingredients of tea tree oil is terpin-4-ol, accounting for more than 40 percent in concentration. Other ingredients include phenylpropanoids, cineole and eucalyptol.[36]

Valerian (Valeriana officinalis) – Valerian root is commonly used to relieve restlessness, nervousness and disturbed sleep. In Europe valerian has been used as a sedative for centuries.

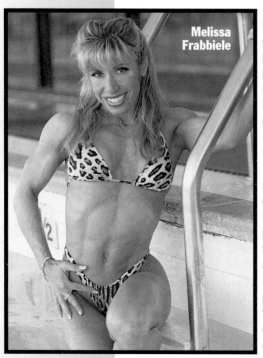

Melissa Frabbiele

One study using valerian assessed tolerability and incidence of side effects; secondary parameters included assessments of sleep quality and well-being. Study participants were 98 healthy volunteers who took either placebo or three tablets of the valerian/lemon balm formula half an hour before going to bed. The test formula was a Swiss product containing 480 mg valerian dry extract (4.5:1) and 240 mg lemon balm dry extract (5:1) (Songha Night) brand name Pharmaton Natural Health Products of Bioggio/Lugano, Switzerland).

Presumably because the primary endpoint was safety, the researchers chose to investigate the effects of the formula in healthy adults who did not suffer from insomnia. Overall tolerability was rated as good by 93 percent of those in the valerian/lemon balm group and 91 percent of the placebo group. The incidence of mild adverse events was similar in the two treatment groups (29 percent in the valerian/lemon balm group and 28 percent in the placebo group). The most frequent of these were sleep disturbances and tiredness; no serious side effects were seen. Interestingly, although none of the study participants reported problems with insomnia, there was a much greater improvement in sleep quality in the group taking the herbal combination. Among those taking valerian/lemon balm, 33 percent reported an improvement in sleep quality, as compared with only 9 percent in the placebo group.

Side effects – None known. People may experience mild stomach upset only. Chronic users can experience headache, excitability and uneasiness. No drug interactions with valerian are known. However, people on valerian should avoid other sedative or hypnotic agents, and central nervous system depressants.

Dosages – Amount equivalent to 2 to 3 g of herb, one to several times per day. Take 150 to 300 mg of valerian extract (0.8 percent valeric acid) 30 to 45 minutes before bedtime. Take 150 mg four times daily for anxiety.

Ingredients/dietary sources – The activity of valerian is attributed to a group of sedatives called monoterpenes, sesquiterpenes, valerenic acid and valepotriates. Valerian has its effects on the inhibitory neurotransmitter GABA, which is the same neurotransmitter affected by the benzodiazepines and barbiturates prescription drugs. Now you know where valerian got its mild sedative or hypnotic properties.[37,43]

Nutraceuticals

Nutraceuticals are naturally occurring dietary substances in pharmaceutical dosage forms. Health Canada defines nutraceuticals as products that have been isolated or purified from foods, generally sold in medicinal forms not usually associated with food, and with demonstrated physiological benefit or protection against chronic disease. Many of the following fall into the grey area of *supplementation* – that is they have characteristics of both food and drugs. In the US, most of the following substances are perfectly legal and sold over the counter. For our Canadian readers some of the following are classified as drugs and are illegal. Without going into the nitty-gritty, suffice to say, as of this writing Canada doesn't have a third category in which to place these so-called grey compounds. The bottom line here is, make sure you are aware of the laws of your country with respect to supplements.[51,96]

Acetyl-L-carnitine – Known as a "smart drug" or "brain booster." Acetyl-L-carnitine (ALC) is a nutrient that helps brain function by triggering the release of neurotransmitters such as acetylcholine. Acetyl-L-carnitine acts on the central nervous system and blocks factors that inhibit the release of acetylcholine. It is therefore helpful in reviving depressed cholinergic systems, thereby promoting memory and cognition.[52]

Alpha-lipoic acid – Alpha-lipoic acid is a potent antioxidant and a coenzyme in metabolism. It is important for the conversion of carbohydrate into glucose, then into energy. This nutraceutical preserves, recycles and protects other antioxidants such as vitamin E, vitamin C and glutathione, aiding in the prevention and treatment of chronic disease.

Alpha-lipoic acid is essential for diabetics. When blood sugar is high, free radicals cause damage that may result in complications such as leg ulcers, cataracts, heart disease, stiffened arteries, diabetic eye disorders and/or nerve damage. This nutraceutical has been used for the treatment of diabetic complications in Germany for over 30 years. In recent years alpha-lipoic acid has been added to creatine products to increase absorption. As with any compound that also affects glucose levels, caution should be taken when using ALA-containing products.[53]

Bioflavonoids – The bioflavonoids are biologically active flavonoids, a special class of plant polyphenolic compounds. They are important nutritional factors, and are found in almost every plant. These nutraceuticals are also important protective and regulatory factors in plant metabolism, and from their widespread distribution are likely to have been an integral part of the human diet throughout our evolution.

This evolutionary relationship is consistent with the many benefits to homeostasis that bioflavonoids offer. Bioflavonoids are found in high concentrations in many fruits. These nutraceuticals are responsible for much of the coloring in such foods as grapes, blueberries and cherries. Bioflavonoids are found in fairly high concentrations in citrus fruits as well. Historically, bioflavonoids were first described as "vitamin P" due to their ability to reduce capillary permeability. Since then their status as a vitamin has been dropped, but the research and use of various bioflavonoids has only increased.

Some important bioflavonoids include quercetin, rutin, hesperidin, and the OPCs found in grapes, bilberries, and pine bark extractions to name a few. Bioflavonoid mixtures are often used in supplements to enhance the effect of vitamins, especially vitamin C.

Bioflavonoids are potent antioxidants, and many also display metal-binding activity, a property which may contribute to their antioxidant effects. Of the over 4000 known bioflavonoids, a number of classes have been distinguished which differ in bioavailability, in antioxidant potency, and in overall safety profile.[54,97]

Choline – Choline is a lipotropic molecule commonly found in lecithin (as phosphatydylcholine), bile, egg yolks, and in a variety of plants. It can also be found in stable salt forms such as choline bitartrate. As a lipotropic agent it is helpful in moving fat out of the liver into the bile. Choline is added as an ingredient in some multivitamin products as well as those specifically designed for the liver or gastrointestinal conditions.

Choline is a precursor for the synthesis of phospholipids, and enhances phospholipid biosynthesis in brain, nerve tissue, and cell membranes. It is important in influencing brain function. Choline is a component of both lecithin and sphingoyelin in the brain and nerve tissue. This nutraceutical is part of the neurotransmitter system that passes messages to and from the brain. The proper functioning of the nervous system depends on choline, which is believed to be involved in producing emotions and behaviors.

As a precursor of acetylcholine, choline accelerates the synthesis and release of this neurotransmitter that is responsible for the transfer of memory messages. Choline is often added to products designed to improve memory or depression. There is evidence that choline phospholipids play a central role in cell-to-cell communication, where hormones and other substances transmit messages from the cell's surface to its interior. This is the mechanism by which a broad spectrum of cell activities such as growth, gene expression, ion transport and energy utilization are regulated.

Supplementing with choline or lecithin might raise blood levels of choline but have no effect on acetylcholine levels or brain function. If choline or lecithin is effective in the treatment of memory loss, they are probably useful only in the beginning stages and then only useful in prolonging the onset of more advanced stages of Alzheimer disease. Both choline and lecithin have been used therapeutically to treat a number of disorders. As precursors to other transmitters, these compounds have proven helpful in treating patients with tardive dyskinesia, a disorder that appears to involve defective nerve transmission.

Side effects – Consuming choline may produce an unpleasant "fishy" odor from the bacterial breakdown of choline in the stomach. In animals choline deficiency has been associated with renal problems, infertility, growth impairment, decreased production of red blood cells, high blood pressure, and memory impairment.

Dosages – Average daily intake is between 400 and 1000 mg of free choline or lecithin. Deficiency symptoms develop when ingestion is less than 500 mg.

Ingredients/dietary sources – The best dietary sources of choline and phosphatidylcholine include beef steak, liver, organ meat, egg yolk, spinach, soybeans, cauliflower, germ, peanuts and brewer's yeast. Small amounts of choline are found in a variety of foods including oranges, apples, potatoes, lettuce and whole-wheat bread.[55,98]

Coenzyme Q10 (Ubiquinone) – Some researchers consider this nutraceutical to be a vitamin because it is a cofactor in several metabolic pathways that help cells produce energy. Coenzyme Q10 (ubiquinone) is a normal component of

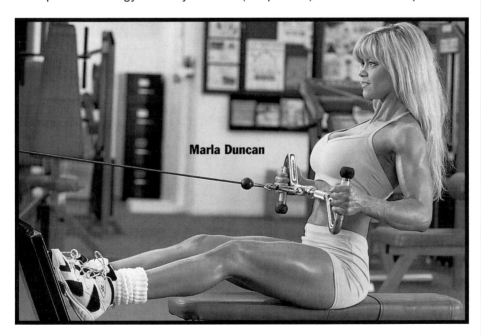

Marla Duncan

the electron transport chain; which allows energy to be converted to ATP during oxidative phosphorylation in the mitochondria. Its ability to transfer electrons has made coenzyme Q10 an effective antioxidant when taken as a supplement. Research has demonstrated the effectiveness of this nutraceutical in the treatment of cardiovascular disease, periodontal disease, breast cancer, hypertension, chronic fatigue, exercise endurance, and AIDS. Some prescription drugs lower the amount of Coenzyme Q10 in the blood. Since this nutraceutical is oil soluble, it is best absorbed when it is emulsified in some form of oil (soft gel).

Side effects – Coenzyme Q10 is usually well tolerated. Some people may experience minor stomach upset or vomiting. This nutraceutical will interact with blood-thinning medication and interfere with blood clotting.

Dosages – Usual doses range from 30 mg (supplemental) to 100 or 200 mg (therapeutic) per day.

Ingredients/dietary sources – Coenzyme Q10 is a natural substance that is made by the body and ingested from foods such as fish, meats and soybean oil.[56,97]

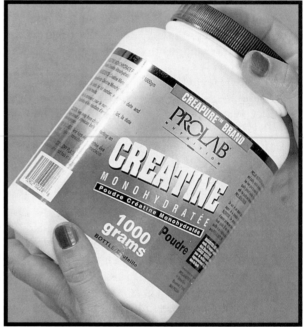

Creatine – Creatine is used in muscle cells to generate energy. Athletes use creatine monohydrate for its performance-enhancing, or ergogenic, properties. It's been shown in numerous studies to be beneficial in activities that are dependent on the anaerobic energy system, including sports such as swimming and field events, which typically involve high-intensity, short-duration movements with short rest breaks during training. The energy comes primarily from stored skeletal muscle ATP and ATP regenerated from phosphocreatine stores. Anaerobic glycolysis is another potential energy source, though its relatively slow rate of ATP production prevents it from contributing to short-duration activities – that is, those of less than 30 seconds.

To date there are no known serious adverse effects associated with creatine supplementation; however, an undetermined percentage of creatine users have reported stomach upset, diarrhea and cramping, which suggests poor intestinal absorption. Increased fluid consumption usually resolves complaints, which are rarely mentioned during the maintenance phase. Anecdotal reports of muscle and tendon injuries appear to be related to inappropriate training and supervision during the initial period of creatine supplementation. Athletes may be susceptible to overtraining, or they may develop or exacerbate an imbalance between muscle groups during periods of accelerated strength and performance improvements.

Creatine monohydrate is typically found in powder form, and manufacturers recommend consuming it in 8 to 16 ounces of water, juice or isotonic sports drink. Begin with a loading phase that consists of four to six 5 gram servings a day for four to six days. A maintenance phase then follows, with the recommended dose of 5 to 20 grams a day. There are some deviations from the recommendations, but there's little evidence to support alternative modes of creatine use.

Side effects – Consuming over 40 grams per day can lead to kidney and liver damage. Be aware that creatine is metabolized to creatinine, meaning people taking creatine may have high serum creatinine even though their renal function is normal.

Dosages – Athletes usually start with a loading dose of 20 g per day for five days, followed by a maintenance dose of 2 to 5 g per day.

Ingredients/dietary sources – People get creatine from their diet, primarily meat and fish. It is also synthesized from amino acids in the liver.[57,94]

Glucosamine – Glucosamine is the monosaccharide glucose with an amino group attached. Glucosamine supplementation has established a very good track record of clinical trials in combating the symptoms associated with osteoarthritis. When compared with ibuprofen, 1500 mg per day of glucosamine was equal in reducing pain after eight weeks. The great benefit to glucosamine supplementation is that it is a precursor to cartilage formation, while ibuprofen and other nonsteroidal anti-inflammatory drugs (NSAIDs) actually prevent the repair of joint tissue while only covering the pain. Glucosamine is both a precursor to chondroitin sulfate (the major glycosaminoglycan in cartilage) as well as a hyaluronic acid (the major glycosaminoglycan in synovial fluid). Glycosaminoglycans are often lost from the body during the progression of aging or injury, leading to weakening of the connective tissues.

Glucosamine can be purchased in salt form, or in acetylated form, N-acetylglucosamine (NAG). The most popular salt forms are the HCl and sulfate versions. Neither form is "better" than the other – they both dissolve and absorb equally and are treated the same by the body. The HCl form contains more glucosamine by weight, since HCl is lighter than H_2SO_4. Both salt forms seem to exceed NAG as a therapeutic agent. Glucosamine is often supplied alone but is commonly mixed with other joint-supporting ingredients such as chondroitin sulfate and bioflavonoids.

Glucosamine sulfate, a sugar molecule, relieves the pain associated with arthritis. This nutraceutical is found within the joints and is responsible for stimulating joint repair.

Side effects – Glucosamine is extremely well tolerated. If stomach upset occurs, you are advised to take glucosamine with food.

Dosages – Take 500 mg three times a day, heavier individuals may require higher dose.[58,99]

Green barley – Barley is a type of green grass that has been used for centuries in maintaining well-being because of its high nutrient content. The part of barley with the highest concentration of nutrients is the juvenile green shoot, before it turns into grain. These young leaves absorb nutrients from the soil at a very high rate and concentration. Young green barley shoots are mainly starch, yet are very rich in vitamins, minerals, high-quality protein, essential fatty acids, enzymes, chlorophyll, several antioxidants, and many unknown substances believed to have powerful properties. Intensively reviewed in the scientific literature, green barley has been shown to lower cholesterol, maintain blood glucose and insulin levels, and may have antioxidant activity.

Ingredients/dietary sources – Barley contains the following vitamins: beta-carotene, vitamins C, E and B, especially thiamin, pyridoxine, riboflavin and pantothenic acid. Barley also contains the minerals phosphorous, potassium, calcium, chromium (an important trace element necessary for insulin to bring sugar from the blood into the cell to be metabolized), and numerous trace elements; protein – 13 percent of barley is protein. There are 18 amino acids present, including eight essential aminos.[59]

Hydroxycitric acid (CitriMax, HCA, Citrin Mg) – CitriMax, also known as hydroxycitric acid (HCA), is a distinctive ingredient derived from Garcinia cambogia, a rare tropical fruit from the jungles of India. Numerous scientific studies show that CitriMax is a safe, natural and effective ingredient for reducing appetite without unwanted side effects such as nervousness, hypertension and insomnia. In addition, CitriMax can be used for extended periods of time with little or no buildup of tolerance. When stopped, there does not appear to be rebound weight gain (the "yo-yo" effect). CitriMax has been found to be as safe as citric acid, which is the principal acid found in oranges, lemons and limes.

The magnesium salt of the product, called Citrin (hydroxycitric acid), helps in weight-loss programs while simultaneously providing magnesium, the mineral element essential for energy metabolism. A number of investigators have reported that serum magnesium levels are reduced in response to endurance exercise, strenuous intense exercise or strength training. The depleted magnesium levels could result in muscle breakdown on account of the sensitive role of magnesium in protein metabolism. Hydroxycitric acid in Citrin Mg helps to increase the metabolic rate through enhanced glycogen synthesis, thereby increasing energy production.[60]

Inositol – Known as one of the B-complex vitamins, inositol is used by the body to complete the synthesis of certain phospholipids, important components of every cell membrane. Inositol is also used to make Inositol Triphosphate (IP3), an important secondary messenger in various cell signaling events. Inositol helps in nerve transmission and regulates enzyme activity. Researchers suggest it plays a critical role in a wide range of physiologic responses in a variety of tissue and systems within the body.

Inositol is also lipotropic, meaning it associates with lipids (fats). Its lipotropic characteristics have been used to help move fatty material from the liver into the intestines, where they can be effectively removed with fiber. Intake of caffeine is known to deplete the body's supply of inositol.

Side effects – Very well tolerated and no toxic effects have been reported.

Dosages – Average daily intake is estimated at 300 to 1000 mg. Some research shows taking 12 g per day of inositol is effective in treatment of depression and panic disorder.

Ingredients/dietary sources – Inositol is found in foods of both animals and plant origin, including cantaloupe, green beans, fish, grapefruit juice, whole-wheat bread, peas, milk and poultry.[61,100]

N-acetylcysteine – N-acetylcysteine (NAC) is the amino (N) terminal, acetylated version of the amino acid cysteine. NAC is a stable form of L-cysteine, an amino acid that participates in several metabolic reactions in the body. The use of this compound in medicine is well researched and documented for a variety of conditions. NAC is a precursor to one of the body's most potent antioxidants, glutathione. Through this action, NAC is used for helping liver support, and has been used to prevent acetaminophen poisoning. Probably its best-known use is as a mucolytic. By breaking (reducing) the disulfide bonds in the mucus of the intestines and especially the lungs, NAC is able to break down the mucus (mucolytic) and make it less viscous. This is especially important during asthma, bronchitis, and bouts of hayfever. As an antioxidant, NAC has a number of scavenging activities that benefit many organ systems and is often used in antioxidant supplements.

Research has revealed the ability of this compound to function as a detoxicant and antioxidant in the body, providing protection against various system dysfunctions by enhancing glutathione production.[62,101]

Pangamic acid – Pangamic acid may act as a stimulant by increasing oxygen uptake in tissues and cells, and may also lower serum lactate concentrations. Pangamic acid, taken before physical exercise, is believed to lower the serum concentration of lactate.[63]

Royal jelly – Royal jelly is a milky white substance secreted by worker honeybees (Apis mellifera L.) to feed all bee larvae for the first three days, but primarily for the queen bee during her entire life. Royal jelly has been extensively studied and its constituents well established. The main "active ingredient" is a substance known as 10-HDA, or royal jelly acid, and can range from 2 to 7 percent depending on how the royal jelly is treated after retrieval. Royal jelly is most often thought of as an anti-aging or energizing ingredient. This comes from the observation that queen bees live longer. Therefore royal jelly must have the same effect in humans. This has never been confirmed by any research. Royal jelly has been traditionally said to prolong youthfulness and improve skin beauty. Modern proponents claim that royal jelly also increases energy, alleviates anxiety, sleeplessness, moodiness and memory loss, and bolsters the immune system. This nutraceutical helps maintain normal blood pressure, lowers cholesterol, and contains natural hormones.

Ingredients/dietary sources – Royal jelly is an extremely nutritious and complex substance. Royal jelly is an excellent source of essential amino acids and fatty acids, as well as acetylcholine. It's also abundant in vitamins including A, C, D, E, and an array of the B-Complex vitamins including B1(thiamin), B2 (riboflavin), B3 (pantothenic acid), B6 (pyridoxine), B12 (cobalamin), biotin, folic acid and inositol – and royal jelly provides important minerals such as potassium, magnesium, calcium, copper, iron and zinc. It is also rich in nucleic acids RNA and DNA. Gelatin, another significant ingredient, is one of the precursors of collagen, which is also a component of royal jelly. Collagen is an anti-aging element that keeps the skin looking smooth and youthful.[64,94,102]

Shark cartilage – Because of the natural, almost disease-free condition of sharks, researchers have studied them looking for clues to their immunity. Substances found in shark cartilage have offered promising clues, and claims have been made that this nutraceutical has significant effects in treating cancerous tumors.

Shark cartilage is tissue that contains no blood vessels because of special proteins that inhibit blood vessel formation. People use it as a cancer therapy by consuming shark cartilage to stop the growth of cancer tumors. In 1983 two researchers at the Massachusetts Institute of Technology published a study showing that shark cartilage contains a substance that significantly inhibits the development of blood vessels that nourish solid tumors, thereby limiting tumor growth. Working independently, medical researchers at Harvard University Medical School found that if one could inhibit angiogenesis – the development of a new blood network – one could prevent the development of tumor-based cancer and metastasis. The substance or substances in cartilage that seem to assist in maintaining good health remain unknown and are currently being studied – however, proteins and carbohydrate mucopolysaccharides are thought to be responsible for the effects.

Ingredients/dietary sources – Shark cartilage is composed of the following: 41 percent ash (mostly calcium and phosphorus used for the calcification of cartilage), 39 percent protein, 12 percent carbohydrates, 7 percent water, less than 1 percent fiber, and less than 0.3 percent fat.[65,95]

Essential fatty acids – Essential fatty acids help in fat transport and metabolism, and in the maintenance of cell membranes, structure and functions. These acids act as components of cholesterol esters and phospholipids in plasma lipoproteins. Essential fatty acids are precursors for eicosanoids, including prostaglandins, leukotrienes, prostacyclins, thromboxanes that regulate the central nervous system, blood clotting, heart rate and blood pressure.

Dosages – Taking 3 to 6 g of linoleic acid daily is adequate to prevent all known symptoms of deficiency.

Ingredients/dietary sources – Four polyunsaturated fatty acids have essential fatty acid activity. They are linoleic acid, arachidonic acid, omega-3 fatty acid and docosahexanoic acid. All other fatty acids can be synthesized in the body from any excess of dietary energy.

Comments: Linolenic acid is found in vegetable oils, flaxseed, soybean and nuts. Research shows combining garlic with fish oil is the best approach for lowering total cholesterol, LDLs and triglyceride levels, which in turn lowers the risk for heart disease.[66]

Evening primrose oil (Oenothera biennis) – Evening primrose oil has always been sought after due to its content of gamma-linolenic acid (GLA). Evening primrose oil (EPO) contains 8 to 10 percent GLA (omega-6), 50 to 70 percent cis-linoleic acid (omega-6), and small amounts of oleic, palmitic and stearic acid. As a source of both GLA and other the omega-6 essential fatty acid, EPO is taken as a daily supplement by many, and used therapeutically for atopic eczema, mastalgia, premenstrual syndrome, and diabetic neuropathy.

Evening primrose oil is an extensively researched dietary supplement and is licensed in England for treatment of skin inflammation, premenstrual syndrome and breast pain. This oil has been shown to dilate coronary arteries and assist in clearing of arterial obstructions. Evening primrose oil can be used to lower serum cholesterol and triglycerides, decrease platelet aggregation, and improve leg sensory function in diabetics.

GLA has been shown to inhibit platelet aggregation and reduce blood pressure. GLA is a precursor to PGE1 prostaglandins, responsible for a number of health benefits. EPO is available in soft-gel capsules containing between 500 and 1300 mg. While the oil is not listed, both flower and root preparations of Oenothera biennis are listed as "approved" for respiratory inflammation by the German Medical establishment. It takes at least three months of consuming evening primrose oil to see improvement. People should be advised of the evening primrose oil long-term treatment.

Side effects – Adverse effects are rare at recommended dose but users occasionally experience mild nausea, softening of stools and headache.

Dosages – These doses are based on a standardized GLA content of 8 percent. For PMS: 3 g daily. For skin inflammation: 4 to 6 g for adults.

Ingredients/dietary sources – The oil is characterized by its high content of essential fatty acids (EFA), particularly cis-linoleic acid (LA) and gamma-linoleic acid (GLA).[1] GLA is obtained from dietary sources or is made by the body from LA which is more common in the diet. Increased GLA consumption helps the other essential fatty acids incorporate into the cell membrane more efficiently and tends to reduce or prevent inflammation.[67,103]

Fish oil (omega-3 fatty acids) – Fish oil lowers triglycerides, improves unhealthy thickening of the blood, helps relieved clogged blood vessels, protects against arterial damage and heart disease, inhibits blood clotting, and may decrease blood vessel inflammation. Docosahexaenoic acid (DHA) is a polyunsaturated fatty acid also known as an omega-3 fatty acid. It has been shown to play a critical role in fetal brain development and vision. The inclusion of DHA in the supplement renders additional support to brain functions.

A recent study suggests that eating 8 ounces of fish a week reduces the risk of a fatal heart attack by almost half. The American Heart Association recommends fish oil supplements only for patients with high triglycerides but they suggest that everyone eat fish two or three times a week. Recent research has linked moodiness among adults – and lack of attention in children – to an imbalance in the ratio of omega-3 fatty acids to omega-6 fatty acids (arachadonic acid).

Any toxin found in the waters they inhabit can accumulate to high levels in a fish's fat tissue. When you consider that fish, particularly fatty fish, act as toxin reservoirs, the potential risks of a high fish diet can outweigh the benefits. For this reason, many nutritionists recommend the use of supplements to boost the body's omega-3 intake.

Side effects – Some people experience diarrhea. Excessive intake of omega-3 fatty acids might result in prolonged bleeding and increased risk of stroke.

Dosages – The British Nutrition Foundation recommends a daily intake of EPA and DHA in amounts corresponding to the intake of 3 to 4 grams of standardized fish oil. Research has found that, at 2000 milligrams per day in the diet, fish oil can help maintain good health. But to achieve this intake level, you need to consume large quantities of fish daily.

Ingredients/dietary sources – Active ingredient for omega-3 fatty acids in fish oil are EPA (eicosapentaenoic acid) and DHA (decosahexaenoic acid). Genetically modified chickens now produce eggs with omega-3 fatty acids.[66,68]

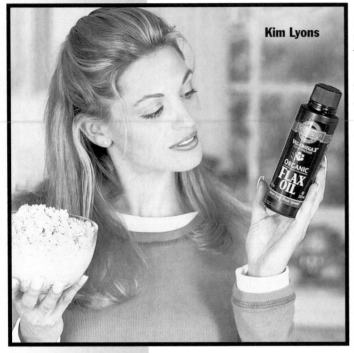

Kim Lyons

Flaxseed – Flaxseed is becoming very popular as a way to get the benefits of omega-3 fatty acids without the fishy side effects. People usually take a tablespoonful a day of ground flaxseed or flaxseed oil. It can act as a bulk-forming laxative similar to psyllium. Flaxseed contains ALA (alpha-linolenic acid).[69]

Phosphatidylcholine – Phosphatidylcholine is a phospholipid that is abundant in nerve-cell membranes and is required for nerve growth and function. In a placebo-controlled study, investigators gave 61 healthy older adults (aged 50 to 80 years) either phosphatidylcholine-rich lecithin or a placebo for five weeks. By the end of the study, memory test scores of the phosphatidylcholine group improved significantly, exceeding those of the placebo group. Memory lapses in the treated group also reduced by 48 percent.[70]

> *"By doing just a little every day, I can gradually let the task completely overwhelm me."*
> – Ashleigh Brilliant

Phosphatidylserine – Phosphatidylserine is a phospholipid that forms one of the large "lipid" molecules that hold together the other large molecules in the membrane system of a cell. The membrane plays a vital role in the entry of nutrients into the cell and phosphatidylserine helps to attenuate these functions. All these effects contribute to the protection of phosphatidylserine on the hippocampus, the seat of memory, and in retarding the loss of connections between the nerves that occurs during aging. Recent clinical studies validate the role of phosphatidylserine in the management of memory loss associated with aging.[71]

Amino Acids

As components of protein, amino acids are important for building and maintaining nails, skin, hormones, enzymes, muscle, neurotransmitters, antibodies, all body tissues and cells. In the absence of adequate carbohydrates or fats, amino acids are used for energy, yielding 4 calories per gram. Amino acids are the second most plentiful substance in the human body after water.

Essential amino acids are those that cannot be manufactured by the body. The eight essential amino acids are isoleucine, leucine, lysine, methionine, phenylalanine, threonine, tryptophan and valine. The 12 nonessential amino acids are alanine, arginine, histidine, aspartic acid, cysteine, glutamic acid, glutamine, glycine, proline, serine, taurine and tyrosine. Amino acids come in three forms: D, L or the combined DL. These letters placed in front of the name, such as D-phenylalanine or L-lysine, describe the direction in which the amino acid is positioned and are called isomers. Some amino acids are only useful to the body in the L or D form, while others can be used in either form or in combinations of D and L.

Side effects – Kwashiordor is the classic protein deficiency condition and is characterized by growth failure, edema, weight loss, impaired immune responses and hair loss. Excessive protein intake can cause kidney stones, especially if insufficient amounts of water are consumed to flush nitrogen byproducts from the kidneys.

Dosages – The daily value is 45 g of protein (source of amino acids). Pregnant or lactating women may need up to 65 g of protein.

Ingredients/dietary sources – The most common dietary sources of protein include poultry, seafood, eggs, milk and extra-lean red meat. A complete protein is a food (such as meat and milk), that supplies all of the essential amino acids in an optimal ratio for growth and repair of tissue.[72]

Arginine – Arginine is synthesized by the human body at adequate levels in adults, but not in children. This amino acid stimulates the production of growth hormone, and is very popular for its musclebuilding and fat-burning effects. Arginine may help in liver detoxification, immune-system maintenance, aid kidney function, slow tumor growth by boosting host defenses, aid in cell regeneration and wound healing.[73]

Aspartic acid – Aspartic acid is a nonessential amino acid that plays a major role in the energy cycles of the body. This amino acid helps to transport potassium and magnesium into the cell. When chemically combined with phenylalanine, it forms aspartame (a synthetic sweetener added to diet drinks under trade name Nutrasweet). Low levels of aspartic acid may contribute to sluggishness or chronic fatigue syndrome.[74]

Carnitine – L-carnitine is found in every cell of your body. It is an amino acid needed for transferring fats into cells where they are burned and turned into energy. For people lacking L-carnitine, supplements may aid in more efficient fat metabolism.[75]

Cysteine – Cysteine is an all-purpose amino acid. It is converted to methionine with the help of vitamin B6. Cysteine helps to protect the liver and brain from free-radical damage caused by alcohol and cigarettes. It works best when taken with selenium or vitamin E together. Along with selenium, cysteine is an important cofactor in the formation of glutathione peroxidase, an antioxidant produced by the liver to neutralize toxins. Cysteine also promotes burning of fat and building of muscle mass.[76]

Glutamine (glutamic acid) – Glutamine can be manufactured from several amino acids, including glutamine. Glutamine is a neurotransmitter. It is also a precursor of glutathione, an antioxidant, and gama-aminobutyric acid (GABA), an inhibitory neurotransmitter. Glutamine has been used to treat personality disorders. Glutamine is a component of monosodium glutamate (MSG) that used in Chinese restaurants as a flavor-enhancer.

L-glutamine is one of the 20 amino acids used to make proteins in the human body. Along with being used to make proteins, it is one of the body's ways of safely carrying excess ammonia out of the body by converting glutamate to glutamine. There are a few clinical applications to high intake of this amino acid. Glutamine (1 gram per day) has been shown in studies to reduce voluntary alcohol consumption in both humans and animals. The mechanism is unknown. Another (better studied) use of glutamine supplementation is in the treatment of ulcers. The mechanism is not completely understood but is thought to stimulate the synthesis of certain mucoproteins which would increase mucin and benefit the ulcer patients. It is considered by some to be an essential component to maintaining a healthy gut wall. L-glutamine is listed in the USP and can be purchased as such.[77]

Glycine – Glycine is a part of many proteins. This amino acid is also an inhibitory neurotransmitter thought to work much like GABA. Glycine is secreted mainly at synapses in the spinal cord. Glycine helps to slow the degeneration of muscle. It is one of the three components needed to synthesize creatine, a chemical crucial to energy flow in skeletal muscle.[78,99]

Histidine – Histidine helps the production of histamine, which is released by the cells as part of the immune response to an allergic reaction. People with histidine deficiency will develop irritability, dry scaly skin, mild skin flushing, and short-term memory lost.[79]

Isoleucine – Isoleucine works closely with other branched-chain amino acids (BCAA), including leucine and valine. Isoleucine is most effective when in balance with leucine or valine. They are important constituents of skeletal muscle. Isoleucine is essential for manufacture of other biochemical factors, including those used for energy production. Research shows isoleucine or other branched-chain amino acids might increase appetite in cancer patients.[80]

Leucine – Leucine is a branched-chain amino acid (BCAA) that helps regulate protein synthesis and degradation in muscle. Leucine is most effective when in balance with isoleucine or valine. They are important constituents of skeletal muscle. All food protein contains leucine. It is important in the optimal growth in infants and nitrogen equilibrium in human adults. Leucine might stimulate the secretion of insulin.[81]

Lysine – Lysine helps in calcium absorption and in the formation of collagen. It is a protein that forms the matrix of bone, cartilage and connective tissue. Vitamin C controls the conversion of lysine to collagen. Recently it has been shown that L-lysine can inhibit the growth of the herpes virus. Herpes virus requires many proteins with the amino acid arginine, and lysine competes directly with arginine in many of these processes. This competition is thought to slow down the growth of the herpes virus. While high doses (500 to 1500 mg per day) are beneficial during the suppression of viral growth, lesser amounts should be taken for long-term use, to prevent an amino acid imbalance problem. Lysine deficiency results in loss of energy, concentration lapse, anemia, irritability and growth retardation.

Dosage – Doses of 1 to 3 g of L-lysine daily are safe when divided among meals.[82,104]

Methionine – Methionine is essential for normal metabolism, growth and maintenance of body tissues. This amino acid functions as a building block for proteins and as a source of polyamines. Methionine is a precursor of SAM (S-adenosylmethionine), which furnishes methyl groups and sulfur to over 100 biochemical reactions. Methionine promotes hair growth and helps protect against skin and nail disorders, prevents fat accumulation in the liver by increasing lecithin production, and is involved in detoxification by chelating heavy metal out of the body.[83]

Ornithine – Along with arginine and carnitine, ornithine triggers the release of growth hormones, producing a musclebuilding effect. Ornithine is produced in the urea cycle by splitting off urea from arginine.[84]

Phenylalanine – Phenylalanine helps in the manufacture of several neurotransmitters such as epinephrine, norepinephrine and dopamine. Many of the observed effects of phenylalanine related to mental functioning. It promotes feelings of alertness and may help in learning and memory. Phenylalanine can be converted in the liver to tyrosine. The artificial sweetener aspartame, or Nutrasweet, is formed by the combination of phenylalanine and aspartic acid. A metabolic condition called phenylketonuria (PKU) results from an inability to process phenylalanine. People with PKU must follow a diet avoiding phenylalanine to prevent mental retardation.[85]

Proline – With the help of vitamin C, proline is essential in the manufacturing of collagen. It enhances skin texture and strengthens joints, tendons and heart muscle. Symptoms of impaired collagen include bleeding gums, bruising, and improper healing of wounds.[86]

Serine – Serine helps in the processing of fatty acids and fat for energy. This amino acid contributes to a stronger immune system by making antibodies and immunoglobulins to fight infection. Serine is utilized in muscle growth and the sheath covering nerve cells.[87]

Taurine – Taurine is an amino acid synthesized in the body from methionine and cysteine. Taurine influences the mineral metabolism in the cells. Most of the supplemental uses of this amino acid are related to cardiovascular or muscle conditions. Taurine is also used to reduce the calcium-triggered response of blood platelets to various activating factors, and to suppress sympathetic nervous system activity while also reducing the responsiveness of vascular smooth muscle cells to vasoconstricting agents. Taurine has also been used as a treatment for epilepsy as is thought to regulate the nervous system. High levels of taurine exist in the retina, bile, white blood cells, skeletal muscles, and the central nervous system. Taurine is important for our healthy vision. In combination with zinc, this amino acid can prevent cataracts. Deficiency of this amino acid is related to seizure, anxiety, hyperactivity and impaired brain functions.[88,105]

Threonine – Threonine is an important building block for collagen, elastin and other proteins. When choline levels are low, threonine acts as a lipotropic agent to help control fat accumulation in the liver. Threonine helps to control seizures and provides a better functioning digestive tract.[89]

Tryptophan – Tryptophan is incorporated into proteins such as hormones and antibodies. It can be converted to energy, niacin or fat when consumed in excess of body needs. Both L and D forms are used by the body. Vitamin B6 is required to produce tryptophan. This essential amino acid is used to make niacin, the neurotransmitter serotonin, and the hormone melatonin.

The mood-elevating effect of tryptophan is well documented. It is the precursor for the neurotransmitter serotonin. This brain chemical helps in the regulation of emotions, sleep, eating, pain and behavior. The amount of serotonin in the brain is dependent on the tryptophan level.

Tryptophan is linked to the metabolism of melatonin, a hormone associated with the regulation of mood, aging and sleep. Tryptophan reduces the time necessary to fall asleep by as much as 50 percent and enhances the quality and length of sleep in some people because of its effects on serotonin production.[90]

Tyrosine – Tyrosine is a nonessential amino acid involved in the production of thyroid hormone, which regulates growth and body metabolism. A low level of tyrosine has been associated with hypothyroidism. Tyrosine is used to produce dopamine and epinephrine. It has been found to promote mood elevation, appetite suppression and reduction of bodyfat.[91]

Valine – Valine is a component of several proteins and functions in concert with other branched-chained amino acids (BCAA). Valine is most effective when in balance with leucine or isoleucine. They are important constituents of skeletal muscle.[92]

REFERENCES

1. www.bayho.com/MM011.ASP?pageno=267
2. www.bayho.com/MM011.ASP?pageno=242
3. www.bayho.com/MM011.ASP?pageno=244
4. www.bayho.com/MM011.ASP?pageno=245
5. www.bayho.com/MM011.ASP?pageno=246
6. www.bayho.com/MM011.ASP?pageno=243
7. www.bayho.com/MM011.ASP?pageno=247
8. www.bayho.com/MM011.ASP?pageno=248
9. www.bayho.com/MM011.ASP?pageno=249
10. www.bayho.com/MM011.ASP?pageno=250
11. www.bayho.com/MM011.ASP?pageno=251
12. www.bayho.com/MM011.ASP?pageno=252
13. www.bayho.com/MM011.ASP?pageno=253
14. www.bayho.com/MM011.ASP?pageno=254
15. www.bayho.com/MM011.ASP?pageno=255
16. www.bayho.com/MM011.ASP?pageno=256
17. www.bayho.com/MM011.ASP?pageno=257
18. www.bayho.com/MM011.ASP?pageno=258
19. www.bayho.com/MM011.ASP?pageno=259
20. www.bayho.com/MM011.ASP?pageno=260
21. www.bayho.com/MM011.ASP?pageno=261
22. www.bayho.com/MM011.ASP?pageno=262
23. www.bayho.com/MM011.ASP?pageno=263
24. www.bayho.com/MM011.ASP?pageno=264
25. www.bayho.com/MM011.ASP?pageno=265
26. www.bayho.com/MM011.ASP?pageno=266
27. www.bayho.com/MM011.ASP?pageno=268
28. www.bayho.com/MM011.ASP?pageno=269
29. www.bayho.com/MM011.ASP?pageno=270
30. www.bayho.com/MM011.ASP?pageno=271
31. www.bayho.com/MM011.ASP?pageno=272
32. www.bayho.com/MM011.ASP?pageno=273
33. www.bayho.com/MM011.ASP?pageno=274
34. www.herbs.org/current/soybone.html
35. www.bayho.com/MM011.ASP?pageno=276
36. www.bayho.com/MM011.ASP?pageno=278
37. www.primenet.com/~camilla/StJohns.FAQ
38. www.ibiblio.org/herbs/immune.html
39. www.herbs.org/current/gnkosexdysf.htm
40. www.herbs.org/current/ginkgohighdose.htm
41. www.herbs.org/current/devilsclawosta.htm
42. www.herbs.org/current/garlicheart.html
43. www.herbs.org/current/valerianmelissa.htm
44. www.herbs.org/current/kavametaanxi.htm
45. www.herbs.org/current/teaheart.html
46. www.herbnet.com/Herb percent20Uses_p2.htm
47. www.herbnet.com/Herb percent20Uses_p6.htm
48. www.herbnet.com/magazine/mag00005_p06–chamomile.htm
49. www.herbnet.com/ask percent20the percent20 herbalist/asktheherbalist_questions percent20on percent20herbs percent20forpercent20athletes.htm
50. www.herbnet.com/ask percent20the percent20 herbalist/asktheherbalist_questions percent20on percent20Sexualpercent20Issues.htm
51. www.bayho.com/MM011.ASP?pageno=313
52. www.bayho.com/MM011.ASP?pageno=302
53. www.bayho.com/MM011.ASP?pageno=303
54. www.bayho.com/MM011.ASP?pageno=304
55. www.bayho.com/MM011.ASP?pageno=305
56. www.bayho.com/MM011.ASP?pageno=306
57. www.bayho.com/MM011.ASP?pageno=307
58. www.bayho.com/MM011.ASP?pageno=308
59. www.bayho.com/MM011.ASP?pageno=309
60. www.bayho.com/MM011.ASP?pageno=310
61. www.bayho.com/MM011.ASP?pageno=311
62. www.bayho.com/MM011.ASP?pageno=312
63. www.bayho.com/MM011.ASP?pageno=314
64. www.bayho.com/MM011.ASP?pageno=315
65. www.bayho.com/MM011.ASP?pageno=316
66. www.bayho.com/MM011.ASP?pageno=236
67. www.bayho.com/MM011.ASP?pageno=237
68. www.bayho.com/MM011.ASP?pageno=238
69. www.bayho.com/MM011.ASP?pageno=239
70. www.bayho.com/MM011.ASP?pageno=240
71. www.bayho.com/MM011.ASP?pageno=241
72. www.bayho.com/MM011.ASP?pageno=192
73. www.bayho.com/MM011.ASP?pageno=193
74. www.bayho.com/MM011.ASP?pageno=194
75. www.bayho.com/MM011.ASP?pageno=195
76. www.bayho.com/MM011.ASP?pageno=196
77. www.bayho.com/MM011.ASP?pageno=197
78. www.bayho.com/MM011.ASP?pageno=198
79. www.bayho.com/MM011.ASP?pageno=199
80. www.bayho.com/MM011.ASP?pageno=200
81. www.bayho.com/MM011.ASP?pageno=201
82. www.bayho.com/MM011.ASP?pageno=202
83. www.bayho.com/MM011.ASP?pageno=203
84. www.bayho.com/MM011.ASP?pageno=204
85. www.bayho.com/MM011.ASP?pageno=205
86. www.bayho.com/MM011.ASP?pageno=206
87. www.bayho.com/MM011.ASP?pageno=207
88. www.bayho.com/MM011.ASP?pageno=208
89. www.bayho.com/MM011.ASP?pageno=209
90. www.bayho.com/MM011.ASP?pageno=210
91. www.bayho.com/MM011.ASP?pageno=211
92. www.bayho.com/MM011.ASP?pageno=212
93. www.ironmanmagazine.com/ironman/nutrition/creatine_monohydrate.htm
94. www.pureroyaljelly.com/info.HTM
95. www.realife.com/whtisshk.html
96. www.nutranet.org/subpages/aboutus.htm
97. www.nutraceuticals.com/glossary.htm#Top
98. www.nutraceuticals.com/glossary.htm#C
99. www.nutraceuticals.com/glossary.htm#G
100. www.nutraceuticals.com/glossary.htm#I
101. www.nutraceuticals.com/glossary.htm#N
102. www.nutraceuticals.com/glossary.htm#R
103. www.nutraceuticals.com/glossary.htm#E
104. www.nutraceuticals.com/glossary.htm#L
105. www.nutraceuticals.com/glossary.htm#T

CHAPTER TWENTY-EIGHT

Thermogenesis

Given that so many people in our society are focused on fat loss, we thought a separate chapter on thermogenics and associated supplements was necessary. The term *"thermogenesis"* refers to an increased production of heat (which is a byproduct of energy metabolism). Thermogenic products increase metabolic rate, which promotes weight loss.

The vast majority of ingredients promoted as thermogenics tend to be stimulatory in nature. Ingredients such as caffeine (guarana and gotu-kola), ephedra (ma huang), and others are included in various levels and combinations as a way to increase energy levels, suppress appetite, induce an "up" feeling, and help consumers burn more calories.

Metabolic rate – Metabolic rate refers to the total of all energy-consuming processes in the body. People with a high metabolic rate burn more calories throughout the day compared to those with a low metabolic rate. This rate is determined by several factors: muscle mass, genetics, sympathetic nervous system activity, spontaneous physical activity, and the body's ability to handle dietary fat.

In general, exercise influences metabolic rate in two ways. The first and most obvious is the direct increase in caloric expenditure that results from actually doing the exercise. For example, running or walking a mile burns about 100 calories. If you complete your five mile run in 40 minutes, then your metabolic rate was elevated during that 40 minutes and the result was an expenditure of 500 calories of energy. A second and equally important elevation in metabolic rate occurs for a period of time after the exercise is over. Depending on the type, intensity and duration of exercise, your metabolic rate might take as long as 12 to 18 hours to come back down to resting level. In general, exercises that use more muscle groups at higher intensity and for longer periods of time are the ones that keep postexercise metabolism elevated.

Nutritional influences on metabolic rate come from the size and frequency of meals, the selection of foods, and the combination of nutrients. Probably the most significant dietary change you can make to increase metabolic rate is to consume smaller meals at more frequent intervals. Compared to eating two or three

Robin Schaefer

large meals each day, spreading those same calories across five or six smaller meals can result in an increased caloric expenditure of 5 to 10 percent. Although it will not specifically have an effect on metabolic rate, it's also a good idea to make sure that each of these smaller meals is a balanced combination of protein, fats and carbohydrates. A balanced intake will tend to suppress feelings of hunger between meals.

To summarize, many factors contribute to your overall metabolic rate. Chief among the factors that you can control are the frequency and intensity of your exercise sessions and the size and frequency of your meals. To boost metabolism your exercise should be intense and often, while your intake pattern should be small, balanced meals consumed frequently (about every three hours).[1]

Powerful Thermogenic Supplements

Caffeine – Caffeine is moderately thermogenic, and raises both core body temperature and resting heart rate. Athletes have been using caffeine as a performance aid for decades – and just about everyone knows that a strong cup of coffee provides a lift when you're fatigued. Caffeine is a central nervous system

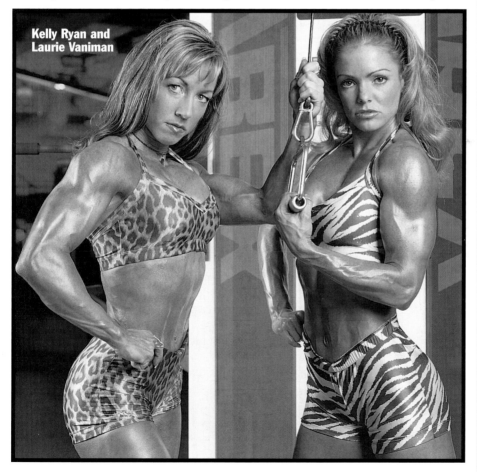

Kelly Ryan and Laurie Vaniman

"Do not allow the body to attain extreme thinness, for that, too, is treacherous, but bring it only to a condition that will naturally continue unchanged, whatever that may be."
– Hippocrates

"I couldn't stop drinking coffee. Finally, I was sent to Maxwell House, and after two weeks, I was completely decaffeinated."
– routine from Saturday Night Live

(CNS) stimulant. This stimulant affects epinephrine and norepinephrine, causing an adrenaline release. Caffeine also mobilizes free fatty acids in the blood, providing a potential fuel source from fat, which allows the body to spare glycogen for later use.

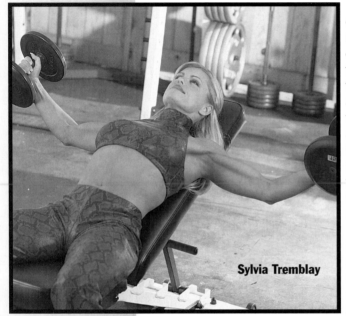

Sylvia Tremblay

Caffeine acts as a diuretic, promoting excretion of water from the body. Diuretics not only dehydrate the body but can also cause bowel movements and gastric distress which would obviously be detrimental to exercise performance. Be sure to take in an equal volume of water for every cup of coffee consumed. Excess caffeine can cause anxiety, irritability, headache and arrythmias. Consult a physician before using caffeine prior to exercise. Even small amounts of caffeine can cause unpleasant side effects. Consuming sugar and other carbohydrates ameliorates these effects.

Caffeine tolerance builds up rapidly. Heavy coffee drinkers can consume a pot of strong coffee and sleep soundly right after. Occasional users may drink one or two cups and be up all night. You can expect your body to reduce all the beneficial effects from caffeine with habitual use. Habitual caffeine users may benefit from caffeine if they abstain from caffeine-containing products for at least three days prior to the event. Even though caffeine does not increase power, it has been shown to reduce the perceived effort at a given workload (so a workout may seem easier for someone using caffeine).

Typical caffeine amounts:
Soft drink: 50 mg caffeine (12-ounce can)
Cup of coffee: 50 to 150 mg caffeine
Cup of tea: 10 to 50 mg caffeine
Guarana: contains 8 to 15 percent caffeine by weight.
Green tea: unless decaffeinated, contains 15 percent caffeine by weight.[2]

Ephedra, ephedrine (ma huang, Mormon tea, Sida Cordifola) – Ephedra is derived from herbs such as ma huang, Mormon tea and Sida Cordifolia (there are about 40 species of plants that contain versions of ephedra). These herbs function as sympathomimetics, meaning that ephedra mimics some of the effects of the body's own sympathetic (stimulant) hormones such as epinephrine (adrenaline) and norepinephrine (either by increasing the levels of these hormones or by reducing their breakdown). Ephedrine is a "non-selective" sympathomimetic, which means that it acts as a general stimulant on many parts of the body simultaneously (lungs, heart, blood vessels, and adrenal glands). It is most often used as a central nervous system stimulant (for alertness or energy), as a decongestant (for asthma/breathing aid) and as an appetite suppressant in a wide variety of weight-loss and "thermogenic" type products.

Research findings on ephedra-containing products are equivocal – some studies show absolutely no beneficial effect, while others show a modest increase in metabolic rate, suppression of appetite and enhanced weight loss. A possible reason for the inconsistent findings is the variable levels of the active alkaloids found in the products. As with many naturally derived compounds, levels of the active chemicals can vary significantly from product to product and from batch to batch.

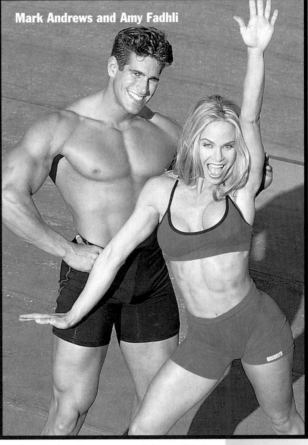

Mark Andrews and Amy Fadhli

Because ephedrine is a stimulant, logic would dictate that either a single dose or chronic repeated use would elevate metabolic rate somewhat (meaning that you would burn more calories at rest and during exercise). One study showed that overweight men and women who were dieting were better able to maintain their resting metabolic rate (which typically falls during a weight loss program) when they consumed 150 mg of ephedrine per day (although no additional weight loss was noted). In the few studies which have been conducted on ephedra-containing products for weight loss, the total amount of ephedrine ingested per day has ranged from 60 to 75 mg (usually in three divided doses of 20 to 25 mg per dose). Keep carbohydrate consumption low while using ephedrine. Insulin counteracts the effects of ephedrine and will ultimately hinder fat loss if carbohydrates remain too high.[3]

Side effects – Women who are pregnant or nursing should avoid using ephedra-containing products. Keep out of reach of children. Avoid using ephedrine-containing products if you have high blood pressure, heart or thyroid disease, diabetes, difficulty in urination due to prostate enlargement, or if taking monoamine oxidase (MAO) inhibitors or any other prescription drug. Reduce or discontinue use if nervousness, tremor, irritability, rapid heartbeat, sleeplessness, loss of appetite, or nausea occur. Serious adverse effects such as seizures, stroke, heart attack, and even death (about 15 to 20 thus far) have been reported but not substantiated.

The FDA has recommended that ephedrine consumption be limited to less than 24 mg per day and that dietary supplements contain no more than 8 mg of ephedrine or related alkaloids per serving. There are a variety of ephedrine-like compounds (alkaloids) present in herbs, including ephedrine, norephedrine, pseudoephedrine, methylephedrine and norpseudoephedrine – and products should be standardized to a total alkaloid content. For example, a product that states 356 mg of a herb per serving is standardized to 6 percent ephedra alkaloids, has 21.36 mg of ephedra alkaloids per serving (356 x 0.06 = 21.36). If the 6 percent strictly refers to ephedra, it is possible that you are risking an overdose of total ephedra alkaloids. Please read your labels carefully, and where possible use German-made herbal extracts or ephedra in pill form.[4]

White willow (Salixalba, aspirin) – White willow tree bark is a source of salicin and other salicylates, compounds which are similar in structure to aspirin (acetylsalicylic acid). Native Americans are thought to have used ground willow bark and bark steeped for tea as a medicinal remedy for everything from pain to fevers. Today white willow bark is often used as a natural alternative to aspirin, and in dietary supplements as an adjunct for weight loss.

By itself white willow bark extract offers no weight-loss benefits. But in combination with other dietary supplements, white willow is thought to extend or increase the activity of several thermogenic ingredients in elevating energy expenditure and promoting fat metabolism.

The primary active compound in white willow bark is salicin. In the body salicin can be converted into salicylic acid, which has powerful effects as an anti-inflammatory and pain reliever. Although synthetic aspirin is clearly a more effective pain reliever and anti-inflammatory agent compared to the weaker natural bark extract, white willow can also serve as a source of tannins, a combination which may provide a synergistic action in elevating energy expenditure through interfering with prostaglandin production and inhibiting norepinephrine breakdown. This effect, when used in combination with other thermogenic supplements, helps promote increased fat oxidation.

Side effects – Stomach ulcers and other gastrointestinal complaints (nausea and diarrhea) are common side effects from prolonged high-dose consumption of either synthetic aspirin of white willow bark extracts. Long-term use of high doses of either salicin source is not recommended, although the natural bark extract is often tolerated much better than the more powerful synthetic aspirin. Individuals with concerns about blood clotting and bleeding time should use aspirin and white willow with caution, as both have a blood-thinning effect.

Dosage – Standardized extracts of white willow bark are available – total salicin intake is typically 60-120 mg per day for relief of acute pain, fever or inflammation. For longer-term consumption as an

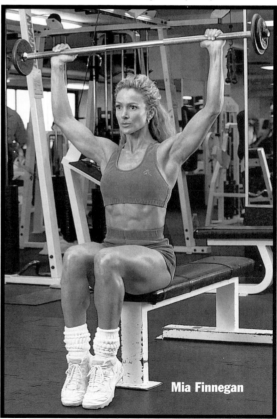

Mia Finnegan

adjunct to weight management and thermogenesis, smaller doses are generally tolerated much better.[5]

The ECA stack – The ECA (ephedrine, caffeine and aspirin) stack is the most popular, and effective, thermogenic combination on the market. This mixture has been shown to be an effective two-phase approach to improving fat loss – as both an appetite suppressant and a stimulator of energy expenditure.

The combination of ephedrine (20 and 40 mg) and caffeine (200 and 400 mg), sometimes combined with theophylline from tea (50 mg) or salicylates from white willow (100 mg), has been found to work better than either agent alone in producing a slight increase in resting metabolism and appears to be about as effective as prescription weight-loss medications such as dexfenfluramine. In another study, ephedrine (30 mg) combined with caffeine (100 mg) and aspirin (300 mg) increased energy expenditure following a meal in obese women.[6]

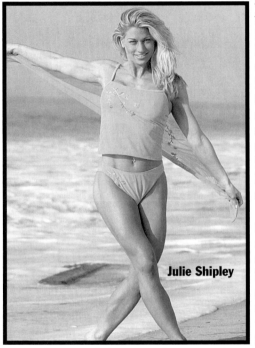

Julie Shipley

In yet another study, the group that received the ephedrine/caffeine combination experienced greater weight loss, as well as a greater ability to maintain their weight loss, compared to a placebo group. Typical combinations include ephedrine at 60 to 150 mg, caffeine at 100 to 600 mg and sometimes even aspirin at 100 to 300 mg. Given in divided premeal doses such preparations have supported weight loss in both lean and obese subjects. In a study of lean and obese monkeys, ephedrine (6 mg) plus caffeine (50 mg) given three times per day resulted in a decrease in bodyweight and bodyfat in both lean and obese animals. Food intake was reduced and energy expenditure was increased by more than 20 percent in both groups. Overall, these results show that the ephedrine/caffeine combination can help promote weight loss by increasing energy expenditure, suppressing appetite, and decreasing food intake.

Researchers in the Department of Human Nutrition, Copenhagen, Denmark investigated the effects of 20 mg ephedrine and 200 mg caffeine mixtures on fat-burning and weight loss. They came to the following conclusion: "We conclude that the ephedrine/caffeine combination is safe and effective in long-term treatment in improving and maintaining weight loss. The side effects are minor and transient, and no clinically relevant withdrawal symptoms have been observed. The combination has shown superior weight-reducing properties when compared with either ephedrine alone (20 mg) or caffeine alone (200 mg) three times a day."

At Harvard Medical School, safety and efficacy of combination of ephedrine (75 to150 mg), caffeine (150 mg) and aspirin (330 mg) was tested for eight weeks. During the study, an average weight loss of 3.2 kg was observed, compared to the 1.3 kg weight-loss average of the placebo group. After five months on ECA, average weight loss was 5.2 kg compared to 0.03 kg gained in the placebo group. The authors concluded:

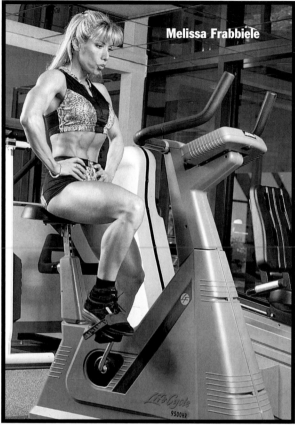

Melissa Frabbiele

"No significant changes in heart rate, blood pressure, blood glucose, insulin and cholesterol levels; and no differences in the frequency of side effects were found. ECA in these doses is thus well tolerated in otherwise healthy obese subjects, and supports modest, sustained weight loss even without prescribed caloric restriction, and may be more effective in conjunction with restriction of energy intake.

"The combination of ephedrine and caffeine significantly improved endurance-prolonging exercise time to exhaustion, compared to placebo. Neither ephedrine nor caffeine treatments alone significantly changed time to exhaustion. The improved performance was attributed to increased central nervous system stimulation."[7]

Overuse of the ECA stack will cause your body to "downregulate" its effects and adapt. Use this stack sparingly. This stack should be taken every other day at most, and for no longer than two to three weeks at a time.

Persons who have any kind of heart disease, high blood pressure, thyroid disease, diabetes, enlarged prostate, or anyone taking MAO-inhibitor drugs for depression or appetite suppression should avoid ephedra and ephedrine containing compounds. Also, children under the age of 18 and the elderly should avoid the use of these products altogether. This stack is extremely powerful, and should be used with caution. Discontinue taking the ECA stack if you experience dizziness, light-headedness, heart palpitations or nausea.[8,9]

Other Weight-Loss Supplements

Chitosan – Chitosan is a dietary fiber derived from chitin. Chitin is an aminopolysaccharide (combination of sugar and protein) that comes from the shells of shellfish. Chitosan is a natural fat magnet that binds to fat 12 times its weight, allowing it to pass through the digestive tract without being absorbed. As a supplement to promote a mild reduction in fat absorption and serum levels of LDL cholesterol, chitosan appears to be effective. As a weight-loss agent, however, chitosan only appears to offer benefits when used in conjunction with a low-fat, calorie-reduced diet. As such, chitosan supplements should not be expected to deliver significant weight-loss effects unless significant dietary alterations are followed.

Unfortunately the fact that chitosan prevents fat absorption also means that it can also cause gas, bloating, and diarrhea (due to fermentation of the fat in the large intestine). Chitosan may interfere with absorption of fat-soluble vitamins (A, D, E and K) and the carotenoids (such as beta-carotene, lutein and zeaxanthin) in a manner similar to the way the "fake-fat" Olestra can reduce absorption of these nutrients. Typical recommendations for chitosan supplements are 2 to 6 grams per day – usually consumed in divided doses of about 1 gram with each meal.[10,11]

Yohimbe (yohimbine) – Although frequently promoted as a "natural" way to increase testosterone levels for musclebuilding, strength enhancement and fat loss, there is no solid scientific proof that yohimbe is either anabolic or thermogenic. Results from a few small trials show that yohimbine can increase blood flow to the genitals (an effect that may occur in both men and women). As such, yohimbe may be effective in alleviating some mild forms of both "psychological" and "physical" sexual dysfunction. In the few studies conducted on the purified form of yohimbine, only about 30 percent of subjects reported beneficial effects in terms of erectile function and sexual performance.

Reported side effects from yohimbe include: headaches, anxiety and tension, and more serious adverse events including high blood pressure, elevated heart rate, heart palpitations and hallucinations. People with high blood pressure and kidney disease should avoid yohimbe. Women who are (or who could become) pregnant should avoid yohimbine due to a risk of miscarriage. It is not recommended to combine yohimbe with other antidepressant supplements or medications.

Yohimbe, in combination with certain foods containing tyramine (red wine, liver and cheese) as well as with nasal decongestants or diet aids with phenylpropanolamine, may cause blood pressure fluctuations.

Typical dosages of yohimbine alkaloids found in commercial supplements (label claims) are in the

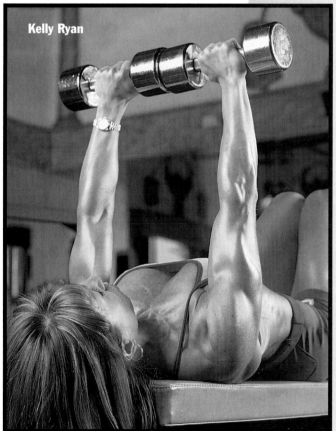

Kelly Ryan

range of 10 to 30 mg. It is reported that more than 40 mg per day of yohimbine can result in adverse side effects such as dizziness, headaches, loss of coordination and hallucinations.[12,13]

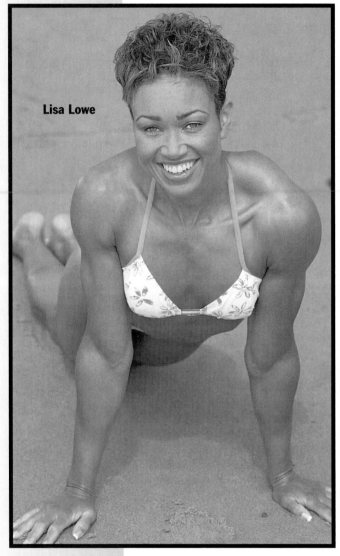

Lisa Lowe

Lesser Thermogenics

Chromium picolinate – Reduces bodyfat, helps build lean, strong body muscle, lowers elevated cholesterol, and reduces elevated blood sugar in diabetics. Chromium picolinate is one of the most popular dietary supplements. Chromium picolinate is used to help reduce bodyfat, increase muscle mass and boost energy levels. Chromium is used in the body for carbohydrate metabolism and insulin function.

Guarana (Paullinia cupana) – South American herb known to assist ephedra in increasing energy, mental alertness and increases metabolic rate. Guarana is a thermogenic herb rich in caffeine and associated alkaloids.

Green tea – Known to help with thermogenesis and aid in metabolism of fat and combats mental fatigue. Studies indicate that green tea may help protect against cancers of the lungs, skin, liver, pancreas and stomach. Green tea benefits the heart by lowering cholesterol levels and reducing the tendency of blood platelets to stick together.

Kola nut – Improves energy aids in reducing mental fatigue, depression and high blood pressure. Kola nut is another thermogenic herb rich in caffeine and associated alkaloids.

Citrus aurantium – Known to help body burn fat more efficiently. Citrus aurantium is derived from citrus rinds harvested while still green. Citrus aurantium provides a rich source of flavonoids and synephrine. Together these two compounds can produce an energizing and stimulating effect in the body.

Bladderwrack – Increases the body's ability to burn fat. Also assists in obesity and normalizing the thyroid gland.

Garcinia Cambogia – Reduces cravings and increases metabolic rate.[14]

The Safest Thermogenic

The most effective thermogenic supplement cannot be found in any dietary concoction – because it's *exercise*. Any physical activity that causes muscles to contract generates substantially more heat and increases in metabolic rate than can be induced by any dietary ingredient or prescription medication. Even moderate levels of exercise can produce increases in metabolic rate and "thermogenesis" to the order of 10 times your average resting metabolic rate – 10 times! No supplement ingredient can claim that.

So the moral of the thermogenesis story is to use regular physical exercise as your primary approach to increasing metabolic rate – and perhaps to judiciously use some of the weight-loss products on the market to help control appetite and maintain energy levels.[15]

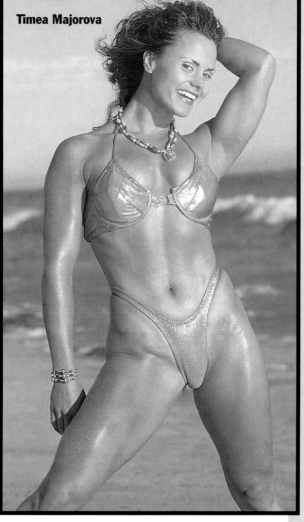

Timea Majorova

REFERENCES

1. www.supplementwatch.com/articles/diet_weightloss/metabolic_rate.html
2. www.supplementwatch.com/articles/sports_nutrition/caffeine&endurance.html
3. www.musclemonthly.com/print/001115-haycock-howz-it-work.htm
4. www.supplementwatch.com/sup-atoz/m/mahuang.html
5. www.supplementwatch.com/sup-atoz/w/white percent20willow.html
6. www.supplementwatch.com/sup-atoz/m/mahuang.html
7. www.dietandbody.com/article1171.html
8. www.athleticnutrition.com/ECA.shtml
9. www.supplementwatch.com/articles/diet_weightloss/thermogenic.html
10. www.supplementwatch.com/sup-atoz/c/chitosan.html
11. www.amazingherbs.com/herforweiglo.html
12. www.supplementwatch.com/sup-atoz/y/yohimbe.html
13. www.dietandbody.com/article1034.html
14. www.doublebarrel2.com/shoppingB/ingredients.asp
15. www.supplementwatch.com/articles/diet_weightloss/thermogenic.html

Hair Care

As we stated throughout the last few chapters, fitness contests are becoming so competitive that you can't leave anything to chance – including your hairstyle. The following chapter will give you tips on how to look your best both onstage and off.

Fashion?

Keeping pace with fashion is not a modern problem. Terms such as formal, business casual, semi-formal, chic and casual "blur" depending on culture, location and age. As long as you wear something that is in good taste, looks good on you, and does not cause other contestants or your coworkers to giggle or shake their heads in disgust – you're fashionable. Hairstyles change on almost a monthly basis, and not always for the better. The 2001 Country Music Awards were marred by female country stars who looked as if they had put their hair through farm machinery. Women who had formerly worn long, thick hair went onstage with bad Beatles-style haircuts. But then that's the fashionable look.

How do bad hairstyles become fashion? Usually one famous person has a bad hair day, and the public imitates it. Here's a classic example. When Raquel Welch was making a film in Paris, one morning she was late and left her hotel without doing her hair. Pictures were taken of Raquel's after-shower tangles, and the French papers published images of the wild-haired

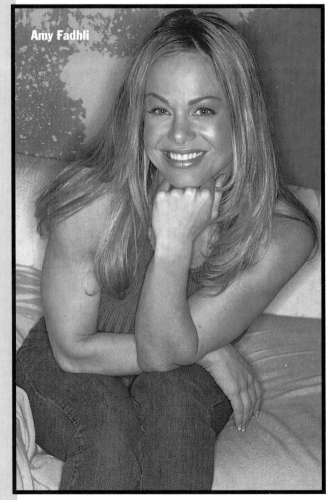

Amy Fadhli

Ms. Welch. Fashionable Parisian women ran for the salons, demanding a similar hairstyle to the sex-symbol "Americaine." The new look was named *L'Animale."* Imagine paying good money to go into a fancy salon and have someone ruin your hair! Is there a lesson to be learned here? Yes! If you find a hairstyle that works for you, stick with it. It might just be back in style next month.

What is it?

Hair is actually dead material when it leaves its root. All that fluff you read about shampoos and conditioners providing badly needed nutrition is not exactly correct. A good shampoo or conditioner acts like an embalming agent. Hair is 88 percent protein. These proteins are of a hard fibrous type known as keratin, which is also responsible for the elasticity of your fingernails.

On a normal scalp there are about 100 to 150 thousand hair fibers. A blonde head of hair has usually much more fibers than red or dark-haired heads. As we said, hair consists mainly of keratin, which is also responsible for the elasticity of fingernails. A single hair has a thickness of 0.02 to 0.04 mm. That means 20 to 50 hair fibers next to each other make one millimeter. Hair is as strong as a wire of iron.

The root of a hair fiber is located in the skin. The fiber grows about 0.35 mm per day, making an average growth rate of 1 cm, half an inch, per month. The growth rate depends on the individual person, her age and her diet. Healthy hair has an average lifetime of 2 to 6 years. After a rest period of three months the single hair falls out, and a new fiber starts to grow out of the skin. The lifetime depends on environment and genetics. The lifetime of hair is responsible for the maximum hair length you can have. Waist length hair takes about six years to grow out from a short hair cut, periodic trims included. If your hair has a life cycle of two years, you had better opt for hair extensions. Hair grows at a faster rate in the spring and summer than in autumn and winter. Not all hair is the same, as the following chart shows:

Growth rate per day:
Scalp hairs – 0.35 mm
Eyebrows – 0.15 mm
Facial hairs – 0.4 mm
Armpit hairs – 0.3 mm
Pubic hairs – 0.2 mm

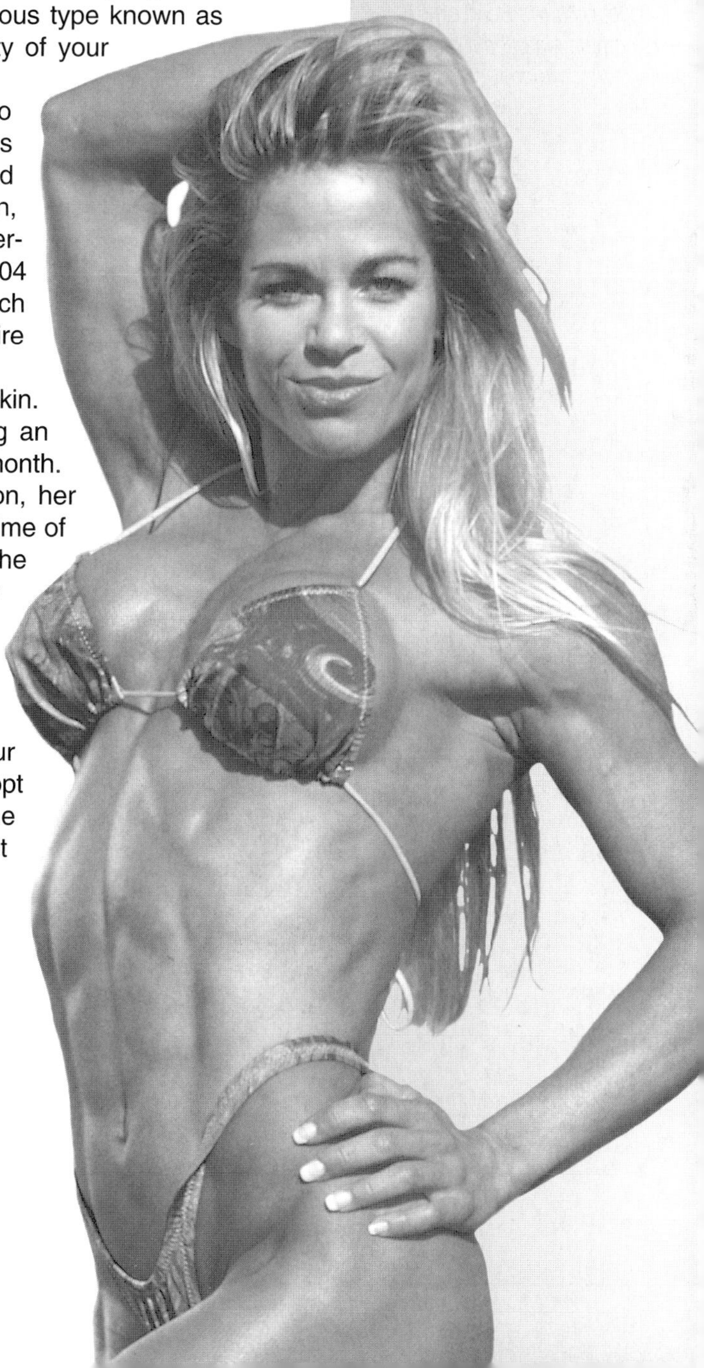

"My second favorite household chore is ironing ... my first being hitting my head on the top bunk bed until I faint."
– *best-selling author Erma Bombeck*

Amy Fadhli

Tools of the Trade

To take proper care of your hair, you need the following:

1. A detangling comb – Designed to be used on damp hair. Start at the ends and work up.

2. A thermal protector – Stops heat damage before it starts.

3. A salon-brand shampoo with a pH of 4.5 to 5.5. … which leads to the proverbial question, "What does pH-balanced mean?" Absolutely nothing. Any company can say its product is *pH-balanced.* The pH of normal hair is between 4.5 and 5.5 (in an aqueous solution). Most companies mean their product fits into this range. However, some companies put "pH-balanced" on the bottle as a marketing ploy. It all depends what they are balancing the pH to: hair, water or sulfuric acid!

4. Acidifying conditioner – Compacts the cuticle, detangles, adds body, and adds natural shine.

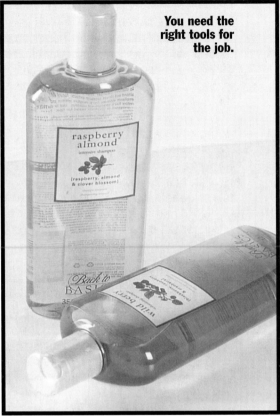

You need the right tools for the job.

5. A conditioner with sunscreen – Sun and tanning beds can adversely affect your hair.

6. A hair dryer with a "cool" setting – Cool air will cause less damage than hot.

7. A good foaming gel or spray gel – Adds body and helps you style your hair.

8. A good "working spray" – Will aid you when blow drying, setting, sculpting or using a curling iron. It is a hair spray that can be applied to damp (if you wish) or dry hair.

9. A good "finishing spray" – Unlike a working spray, a finishing spray will keep the hair or sections of the hair in place all day.

Conditioners

What is a conditioner? Conditioners fall into different groups according to what you want to accomplish. Certain types of hair require specific types of conditioners. Conditioners fall into the following categories.

Acidifiers are acids with a pH of 2.5 to 3.5. This pH compacts the cuticle layer of the hair. This pH range will adjust the molecular bonds in the hair. Acidifiers do not weigh the hair down. Acidifiers create shine and add elasticity. Detanglers are also acidifiers (see above). Most have a pH of 2.5 to 3.5. They close the cuticles of the hair (which cause tangles). Some coat the hair shaft with polymers (polymers are strings of "like" molecules in a chain).

EFAs are oils that are similar to natural sebum, the oil found in hair. If you have dry or chemically treated hair, you must add oil to your hair. EFAs are the closest thing to natural sebum, produced by the scalp. EFAs can take very dry and porous hair and transform it into soft pliable hair.

Glossers make hair glossy. They contain dimethicone or cyclomethicone, which are very light oils derived from silicone. Used in small amounts they reflect light. Glossers also control "the frizzies."

Moisturizers are concentrated with humectants. Humectants are compounds that attract and hold moisture into the hair.

Reconstructors contain protein. Hydrolyzed human hair keratin protein is the best source, because it contains all 19 amino acids found in the hair. Human hair keratin protein has a low molecular weight. This enables the protein to penetrate the hair shaft (cortex). The reconstructor strengthens the hair.

Thermal protectors safeguard the hair against heat. Using a thermal protector is one of the best things you can do if you blow dry, or use a curling iron or hot rollers. Thermal protectors use heat-absorbing polymers that distribute the heat so your hair is not damaged.

How Stress Affects Hair

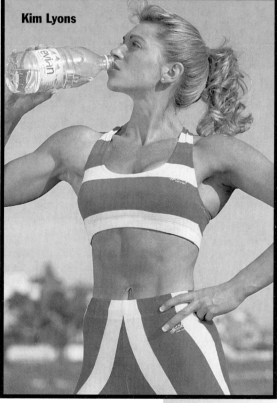

Kim Lyons

"The bride said she wanted three children, while the young husband said two would be enough for him. They discussed this discrepancy for a few minutes until the husband thought he'd put an end to things by saying boldly, "After our second child I'll just have a vasectomy." Without a moment's hesitation the bride retorted, "Well, I hope you'll love the third one just as if it's your own."

It's not uncommon to have a bad hair day (ask Raquel) when you are under stress, because stress causes blood vessels to contract, depriving the hair of nutrients it needs for healthy growth. Stress can also increase sebum production, leading to a greasy scalp and limp hair. Poor diet can also ruin hair. How many strict vegans have you seen with long thick hair? To combat hair stress, you'd be best to do the following:

• Allow hair to air-dry
• Opt for Velcro rollers.
• Drink lots of water.
• Avoid fried foods.
• Don't overdo blow-drying. It can weaken hair, causing it to dry out and break more easily.
• Wait two weeks between coloring and perming treatments. Give your hair enough time to recover.
• Include plenty of fresh fruits and vegetables in your diet.

[Ref. How Stress Affects Hair, pg. 21, 10/12/98]

Perming Techniques

• Body waves add lots of all-over volume and soft waves to fine hair.
• Spiral perms result in all-over corkscrew curls. Hair is wrapped vertically around rod, instead of horizontally.
• Spot perms target specific areas where lift is needed such as at the crown or around the face.
• Stack perms add volume to one-length cuts by adding different-size curls, particularly at the middle and ends of hair for maximum movement.
• Weave perms add waves to selected areas of hair while leaving the rest straight.
• Root perms create volume by adding lift at the roots without curl.
• Curly perms add lots of soft, all-over curls that need little maintenance.

Do's and Don'ts For Permed Hair

1. Don't perm hair that's been colored recently. Wait at least two weeks between processes.
2. Don't shampoo for two days after perming. The solution needs time to settle.
3. Do have split ends trimmed after you perm. Split ends are very noticeable because perming chemicals tend to dry out hair.
4. Blot, rather than rub, hair dry with a towel after shampooing. Rubbing can cause tangles which in turn can lead to breakage.

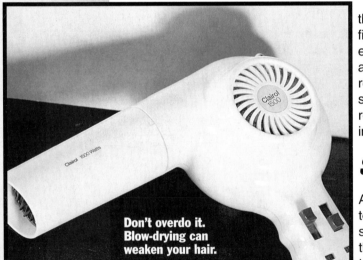

Don't overdo it. Blow-drying can weaken your hair.

If your hair turns out too curly, gently comb through the curls with your fingers to help loosen them. If needed, use your blow-dryer on low speed and direct downward onto curls to relax them. Another option is to wrap small sections of hair around a big round brush, pulling taut while blasting it with heat from your blow-dryer.

Styling Your Hair

A lawyer returns to his parked BMW to find the headlights broken and considerable damage. There's no sign of the offending vehicle but he's relieved to see that there's a note stuck under the windshield wiper. "Sorry I just backed into your Beemer. The witnesses who saw the accident are nodding and smiling at me because they think I'm leaving my name, address and other particulars. But I'm not."

How to Determine and Care For Your Type of Hair

You have fine hair if your hair doesn't style easily, is very limp, straight and often oily. You can increase your hair's volume with a daily protein-enriched shampoo. Thickening shampoos coat the hair's cuticle layer, making it look and feel fuller. To hold the style, apply a lightweight conditioner or a finishing rinse to ends of hair only, where it's needed most.

• For straight hair, brush dry hair back and away from the face. Hold in place with a headband.

• You have medium hair if your hair breaks easily, is straight or wavy, and easy to manage. Use a shampoo formulated with ammonium laureth sulfate, which gently cleans hair without stripping away any essential oils. To maintain your hair's natural balance, apply a conditioner made for normal hair. Leave in for three to five minutes, then rinse well with cool water. If hair still feels dry, use a leave-in conditioner daily for a week.

• For wavy hair, use fingers to brush hair to the side. Use small clips to hold opposite side back.

• You have coarse hair if it's difficult to break, curly, frizzy and rough to the touch. Natural oil buildup is good, lending hair both body and shine. Shampoo every other day with a rich moisturizing shampoo. Coarse hair drinks in moisture, so use a deep conditioner whenever you shampoo. Leave it in for a few minutes and then rinse with cool water to seal in moisture.

• For curly hair, brush dry hair back and away from face. Hold in place with hair combs at crown.

Add Volume

Adding hair volume is a great way to create dynamite hair! And it's not all that hard to do, just try one of the following:

Crimping – Crimp a section of hair from underneath at the nape of your neck and below the crown with a crimping iron. The wrinkled layers are hidden by smoothing hair over from the crown, but add incredible volume.

Switch the part – This trick is typically used at photo shoots. Simply switch the part in your hair to the opposite side for an instant lift.

Flip – Apply mousse to wet roots. Dry hair straight with a round brush, flipping ends up in the back. Rub pomade between fingertips and finger-comb hair behind ears. Flipping works best for shoulder-length hairstyles.

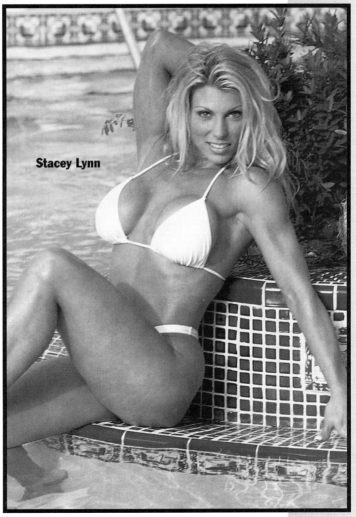

Stacey Lynn

Scrunching – Scrunching adds waves and volume to all hair types. Apply volumizing mousse to wet hair. Blow-dry upside down, scrunching handfuls of hair to create space between strands. This adds bulk.

Hot rollers – As long as you promise not to be seen in public wearing them (we don't want you on the cover of *Trailer Park Monthly)*, hot rollers are the surest way to add volume. Spritz roots with a volumizing spray. Use a blow-dryer, first on warm to activate, then on cool to set. In large sections, wind hair around a hot roller, spritzing each section with hair spray as you roll. Remove rollers as soon as hair cools and style with fingers.

Hair-fattening products – Shampoos enriched with panthenol and wheat protein add volume to hair. Use a mousse that contains a copolymer and alcohol to thicken strands. Chemicals used in hair dyes increase the hair's diameter by penetrating and filling in the follicles, thickening each strand.

Beer: the ultimate hair rinse – Beer not only makes a great hair rinse, it also attracts men. The sugars and protein found in beer thicken the hair. Plus, he'll love the smell!

Let's Get Stylin'!
Enough talk, let's get to work! How can you change your face? Try one of the following Hollywood tricks:

Highlight your cheekbones – Create definition by angling layers around your face. A short crop or bob haircut will make you look more chiseled.

Lengthen your neck – Cut your hair so that it falls just at, or anywhere beyond, your shoulders. Longer hair tricks the eye into seeing a longer neck.

Add softness – A square jaw can be softened by curving layers of hair around the chin.

Cover a high forehead – A style with eyebrow-length bangs or a deep side part can disguise a high forehead, or add visual width to longer, slimmer faces.

Create wide-set eyes – Close-set eyes can be made wider by wearing a style that is swept off the face or worn with a side part.

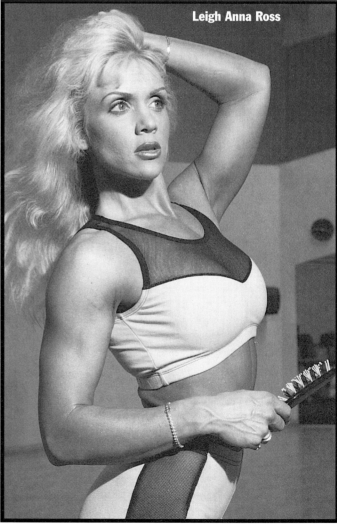

Leigh Anna Ross

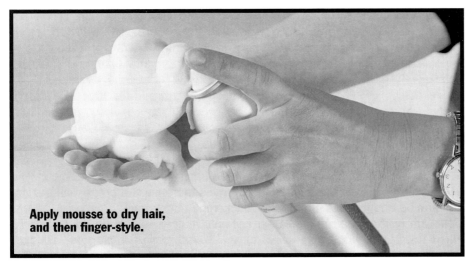

Apply mousse to dry hair, and then finger-style.

Need a Good Bang?

The bangs you choose should depend on the shape of your face.

Round – Use delicately layered bangs. The feathery ends create up-and-down movement on your face, making it look longer and leaner.

Long – Opt for blunt-cut bangs that fall at or below the brow. They make the face look shorter by camouflaging the forehead.

Square – Choose soft, fringy bangs cut just at eyebrow level in the center, but cut a little longer on the sides. These narrow the appearance of the forehead.

Heart-shaped – Temple-length bangs can be easily swept loosely to one side to de-emphasize a pointy chin and help narrow the forehead.

Bang Blowout?

Your stylist picked the wrong week to give up glue-sniffing, and took too much off your bangs. Now what? The answer is to stretch them out! Add a hair straightening product to wet bangs and blow-dry, brushing bangs from left to right and then around a large brush. Pull the hair tightly to stretch out the sections.

Trim Your Own Bangs

Now that your stylist is back in rehab, you've decided to try doing your own bangs. It can be done, but you have to be careful and take your time. But before you do this, try to find another stylist. If you're still determined, use the proper procedure:

1. Make sure your hair is dry. Use two or more clips to hold the rest of your hair back and away from your face. The only loose hair should be your bangs.

2. Tousle bangs with fingers, allowing them to fall naturally. Then, to get that professional wispy look, use a comb as your guide and hold scissors perpendicular to the comb. Snip into the first 1/2 inch of hair that extends beyond the comb.

Hair Curling 101

Curling your hair is a basic method of adding life to your hair. This section covers different techniques and products for creating curly hair.

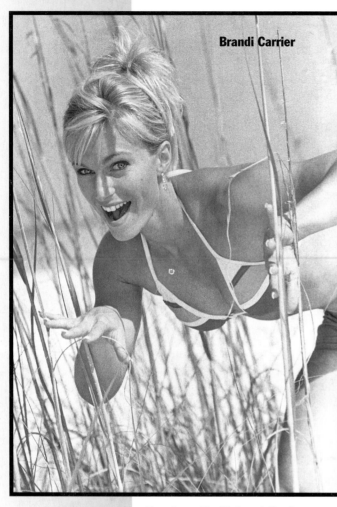

Brandi Carrier

Spare the Rod and Spoil the Curl
Different rods result in different types of curls, consider the following:
Narrow rods – produce tight curls.
Medium rods – produce loose curls.
Concave rods – produce curls that are wavy at the bottom and straight at the roots.
Large rods – result in soft waves through the hair.

Scrunching Made Easy
Using your hands, scrunch hair to form curls while blow-drying with a diffuser attachment. This will result in lots of well-formed curls. For best results, apply a curl-enhancing product to damp hair, then scrunch from ends to roots.

Fight Frizz!
Brushing can cause permed hair to turn into a mass of frizz. To help prevent this from happening, use a wide-tooth comb to distribute a curl-enhancing product through damp hair.

How to Create Soft Curls
Apply mousse to damp hair, then scrunch while diffuse drying. To lock in volume, flip hair over and spray lightly with a finishing product.

Freshen Up Natural Curls
Dampen hair and work in some straightening balm, then blow-dry with a diffuser and gently pull each curl for a natural look.

Make Straight Hair Curly
Spray 2-inch sections of dry hair with a heat-protective holding spray. Wind sections around a medium-barreled curling iron. Finger comb to style.

How to Use Products for Curly Hair
To help make the most of your curls, use one of the following:
Spray gel – Spray on damp hair for added fullness. Works best for fine hair and when making pin curls.
Curl-enhancing gel – When applied to damp hair, it gives curls definition and helps them retain their shape. To use: coat hair, then scrunch while air- or diffuse-drying.
Finishing spray – When applied to dry hair, enhances shine and gives curls staying power.

Frizz-control serum – This silicone-based serum, smoothed over dry hair, repels moisture, controls frizzy ends, and gives hair a glossy finish.

Super-hold gel – Keeps curly, frizzy hair under control. To use: apply to damp hair and style.

Pomade – Makes thick, hard-to-handle hair more manageable. Apply to dry hair and then finger-style.

Mousse – Produces loose, flowing curls with definition and adds body when applied to damp hair.

Specific Styles

How to Create a French Twist
1. Start by gathering dry hair into a long ponytail, giving it a few good tight twists.
2. Slowly lift the ponytail straight up, still twisting your hair to form a tight roll.
3. Fold the ends down and tuck into the length of roll. Secure with hair pins.

Three Ways to Work With a Choppy Crop
Long top layers and shorter underlying layers give this cut lots of versatility.
1. Start by combing mousse through damp hair. Then blow-dry using a vent brush to create volume.
2. Comb dry hair into a side part, secure with a clip. Tease hair at the crown, spritz to hold.
3. Using a flat iron, straighten sections of dry hair. Use your fingers to separate layers.

Two Ways to Work With Long Curls
Long layers help control friz and add lots of bounce.
1. Apply an anti-frizz gel to wet hair. Blow-dry with a diffuser, while scrunching hair with your hands. Leave ends loose for a casual look.
2. Comb a gel through damp hair. Blow-dry in sections using a round brush to smooth.

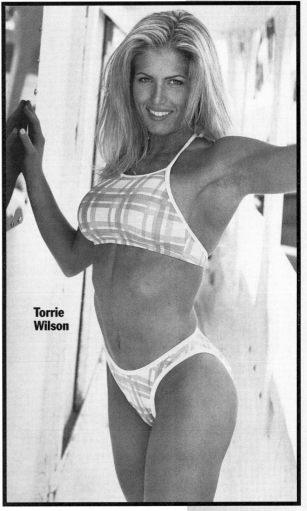

Torrie Wilson

Three Ways to Work With a Basic Bob
This style features long layers cut within the last inch of hair to boost body.
1. Blow-dry hair in sections, using a round brush to smooth. Then comb in an off-center part.
2. With hair dry, comb in a deep side part; brush hair to side. Flip ends with curling iron.
3. Put dry hair into a ponytail and twist until it coils. Secure with pins, leaving ends loose.

Three Ways to Work With a Curly Crop

Long layers at the crown provide versatility for this low-maintenance style.

1. Apply mousse to towel-dried hair, then use fingers to scrunch toward roots. Let it air-dry.
2. Blow-dry, using a round brush to turn bangs under and flip ends. Comb in a side part.
3. Comb some gel through damp hair. Blow-dry in sections, using a paddle brush to smooth.

Three Ways to Work With Soft Waves

Long layers are cut to bring out hair's natural texture.

1. Apply gel to damp hair. Blow-dry with a diffuser, and gently scrunch small sections.
2. Brush dry hair into a high ponytail and secure. Curl ends with a curling iron. Fluff hair with your fingers.
3. Separate hair into two sections and twist each section. Cross the sections over, tuck the ends under, and secure with a pin.

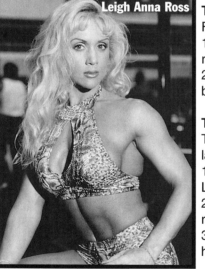

Leigh Anna Ross

Two Ways to Work With Long Layers

Face-framing layers begin below the chin and help out natural waves.

1. Work smoothing lotion into damp hair. Blow-dry, using a large round brush to smooth.
2. Divide dry hair above the ears into two sections. Twist together at back of head and secure.

Three Ways to Work With a Razor-Cut Bob

This cropped bob gets its full, rounded shape from all-over razor-cut layers.

1. Apply gel to damp hair, then direct into place with your fingers. Let it air-dry and tousle with your fingers.
2. Comb some gel through damp hair. Blow-dry in sections, using a round brush to smooth.
3. Work some gel through wet hair. Using fingers to make waves, hold with clips.

How to Create a Braid

1. Gather your hair back into a ponytail, then divide it into three equal sections.
2. Take section at the left and cross it over to the middle (between the other two sections). Then take the piece at the right and cross it over to the middle.
3. Interweave from the left, right, left, right, etc. to form the braid. Secure the end with an elastic band.

Accessorize

A headband can sweep and hold your hair back from your face, which is particularly important if you have oily hair that can rub against the skin and cause pimples. You can play with matching colors and wear everything from a scarf for a day's hike to a tiara for a formal affair.

Hair Color

While there are some jobs that cannot be done badly, a dye-job is not one of them. Before any permanent color can be deposited into the hair shaft, outer layer (the cuticle) must be opened. The insoluble formula then reacts with the cortex, or middle layer, to deposit or remove the color. Hair color is available in a variety of forms – creams, gels and shampoos. These will not permanently change the hair color until they are part of an oxidation chemical reaction. The oxidizing agent is hydrogen peroxide, the catalyst for the chemical reaction which allows the formula to permanently alter the color of the hair.

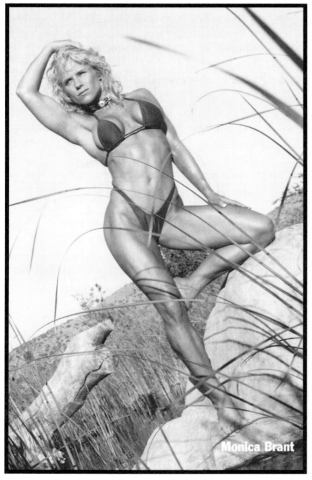

Monica Brant

Black, blonde, red, white, brown and gray. How is natural hair color determined? The answer is the melanophore. The hair roots contain pigment cells called melanin, which creates a black pigment. Melanophore is a chromatophore that sends pigment to new hair. The greater the amount of pigment sent to the hair, the darker the hair becomes. On the contrary, as the amount of pigment sent is reduced, the hair color turns brown and then blonde. As we age, less pigment is sent, and our hair turns gray.

What do you do if you have a bad dye job? Tone down your color with dishwashing liquid – it contains more detergent than shampoo, which softens your hair color. Wash three times with the dishwashing liquid and follow with a leave-in conditioner to restore the softness.

Big Date, Nasty Roots!

Those gray roots coming through and you're just about to head out for a romantic evening? No problem! Grab some mascara and apply it to dry hair. Provided he doesn't run his fingers through your hair (fat chance), the mascara will hold until you hit the shower. But remember to see your stylist soon.

SOURCES

All About Hair. *www.geocities.com/HotSprings/4266/damage.htm.*
First for Women, all volumes, 97-98.

CHAPTER THIRTY

Cosmetics

What is beauty? How do we decide what makes someone attractive? What is the value of being attractive? Physical beauty can best be defined as appearing healthy. Look at pictures of the models in the Victoria's Secret catalogue. Never mind the firm abs and big chests, focus on the faces. They all look well rested. They have faces that you would never see in a doctor's waiting room during flu season. Each model looks as if she's had eight hours of sleep and been blessed with perfect health.

The reality is, she's probably dropping from jet lag and running to the port-o-potty on the beach because of the local food that she ate the night before. She feels like crap and looks like a million bucks! Which makes sense, since that's what she earns every year. But she owes it all to her makeup artist, her personal trainer, and her genetics. This chapter will explain how to use makeup to recreate yourself to be the center of attention, no matter what the occasion.

Back to the subject of beauty. Beauty is best defined by what's not there. No bags under the eyes from fatigue. No blotchy skin, discolorations, pimples, hairs or uneven features. If you look closely at a supermodel's face without makeup, you are often at a loss to identify a single characteristic that makes this face stand out. The individual might appear rather plain. But try looking at the right and left profiles. They're mirror images. That's the secret! Faces are rarely balanced. One eye may be more open than the other, one cheek bone may be slightly higher than the other, there may be a bend in the nose, the eyebrows may be irregular, hairs may appear above the upper lip, and skin tone may vary.

Makeup is used to conceal the things we don't want to show, and balance and emphasize the things we do want people to notice. And with a bit of preparation and a few simple techniques, this chapter will show you how to use makeup to release your inner beauty.

Trish Stratus and Kim Hartt

Keeping It Clean

Keep your skin clean by cleansing twice a day, scrubbing gently only once or twice a week. Make sure to remove all your makeup and wash your face every night before you go to bed. Like you, your skin needs to "breathe." The mind and body are rejuvenated during sleep. Your skin needs to be free of products, which will simply block your pores and inevitably cause breakouts.

Keep your makeup tools clean. Any bacteria, oil or dirt they carry can settle in your pores every time you apply makeup. We recommend washing your brushes and sponges every two weeks in a mild hair shampoo or brush cleaner. Many women experience acne breakouts that are related to their menstrual cycle. It's amazing what a few little hormones can suddenly do to a perfectly clear face!

First suggestion, have weekly facials. The easiest pimples to get rid of are those that never make it to the surface. If you have very oily skin, hydrogen peroxide is amazing at drying up stubborn pimples. You may choose to experiment with the following treatments: benzoyl peroxide, AHAs (like glycolic or lactic acid), BHAs (salicylic acid), or plant botanicals like tea tree oil and lavender.

Benzoyl peroxide is an antibacterial that basically kills the bacteria that causes a pimple. It can be very effective but can also be rather drying to the skin. If you have never used it before, start with a low strength like 2.5 percent and work your way up to 5 percent or 10 percent if you feel your skin can handle it. Benzoyl peroxide products are typically in gel or cream form. They are effective for mild acne, but mediocre at best for more severe types of acne.

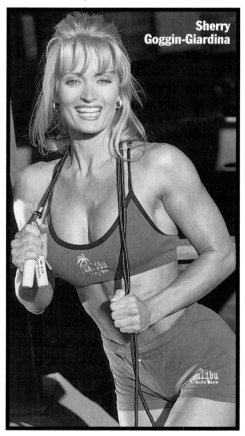

Sherry Goggin-Giardina

AHAs and BHAs work to exfoliate dead skin cells so they don't clog your pores and create a breeding ground for bacteria. Used together with benzoyl peroxide, they can dramatically decrease breakouts quickly. Try using a combination. BHAs penetrate the pores, getting inside to clean out dead cells from within; AHAs exfoliate the top layer of skin, preventing surface buildup.

Botanicals like tea tree oil make a good alternative if you want something nonchemical, but be aware that the antibacterial properties can be a bit strong for sensitive skin. Start slowly to see how your skin reacts.

See your dermatologist, drink plenty of water, get eight hours of sleep a night, have facials regularly, and try one of these treatments. You should be able to reduce or even eliminate your monthly hormonal acne.

"Honey, you could be real pretty if you wore a little makeup."
– cosmetics department salesman to supermodel Cindy Crawford.

"Should we shag now or should we shag later?"
– from the movie Austin Powers: International Man of Mystery.

"Don't torture yourself, Gomez. That's my job."
– Mrs. Addams, from the movie The Addams Family.

If you travel, or if you want something portable for freshening up at the office, in the car or at the gym – or you want to just simplify your cleansing routine at home – the latest generation of cleansing cloths is the answer. You get a complete facial cleanser and makeup remover in a moist cloth that you use once and throw away. They are a bit like baby wipes, but with ingredients like green tea, cucumber and chamomile. The good ones also leave a clean, fresh feel with no oily or soapy residue.

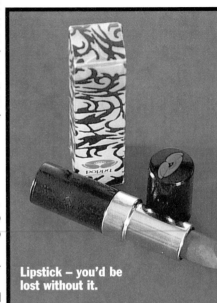

Lipstick – you'd be lost without it.

Organizing Your Tools

To do a job right, you must have the right tools. Stop. Read the first sentence again. Did you do that? Good, because everything else we tell you to do depends on having the following:

• Cotton balls – for applying, blending and removing makeup
• Hydrogen peroxide – for bleaching facial hair and blackheads
• Sponges – for blending in hard to reach places
• Hair pins – to keep your hair off your face while you're working
• Eye shadow brushes – to apply eye shadow (brushes come in small, medium and large)
• Eyelash curler – for curling the eyelashes upward
• Angular brush – used to fill in gaps in the eyebrows
• Eyebrow brush – for controlling the eyebrows
• Blush brush – for applying blush
• Powder brush – for applying powder
• Mascara – for coloring eyelashes
• Fake eyelashes – for special occasions
• Foundation – for laying a base
• Concealer – for concealing blemishes
• Powder puff – for applying powder
• Cotton swabs (Q-tips) – for applying and removing makeup
• Tweezers – for removing hairs
• Pocket mirror – for checking your makeup
• Eyebrow pencil – for touching up your eyebrows
• Lip pencil – used to outline your lips
• Lip brush – for applying lip color
• Lip gloss – to make your lips shiny
• Lipstick – because you'd be lost without it
• Pencil sharpener – those pencils get dull real fast
• Cosmetics case – because if you don't know where it is, you can't use it

So what's the most important piece of equipment? Your cosmetics case. Don't just dump your makeup into your purse with your car keys and loose change. The bristles on your brushes are fragile. Once they're bent and broken, they're pretty much useless.

Would you store your makeup with your dirty underwear? Well, loose change isn't much cleaner, and often worse. There are many compact cosmetic cases on the market that allow you to organize your makeup. Spend the money.

Choosing Your Colors

Here are some basic guidelines to follow when choosing colors:

Foundation – If you apply foundation and it disappears on your skin, then it's the right color.

Concealer – If you apply concealer first, you should cover with foundation that is a lighter shade.

Powder – When applying powder, go with a shade lighter than the foundation.

Blush – Choose a subdued tone. Clown-like cheekbones are all too common a makeup disaster. Pick a color that matches your skin when you blush. If you don't noticeably blush, then pick a tone that is slightly darker than your powder. Try to pick a color that is in the same color family as your lipstick.

Eye shadow – That's a tough one, and is much more a slave to fashion. You can't go wrong with neutral colors. Generally, eye shadow should match your eye color.

Colored contact lenses – Even if you have perfect vision, why not go for a change of color?

Eyeliner pencil – Brown and charcoal are the best colors.

Mascara – Black looks good on everyone. To go for a more dramatic look known as "the sweep," try mascara that matches both your eyes and your eye shadow.

Eyebrow pencil – Choose a shade lighter than your eyebrow hair color.

Lipstick – Choose a color that closely resembles your own natural lip color. For a more natural look, make your lips the opposite of your eyes. If your eye makeup is dark, your lips should be light, and vice versa.

Once you have established these colors, you can choose shades and match them to produce a whole new look. This sort of makeup is an art form, and is responsible for some of the dramatic makeovers seen on TV.

Vivian: "You're late."
Edward: "You're stunning."
Vivian: "You're forgiven."
– an exchange between Julia Roberts and Richard Gere in the movie Pretty Woman.

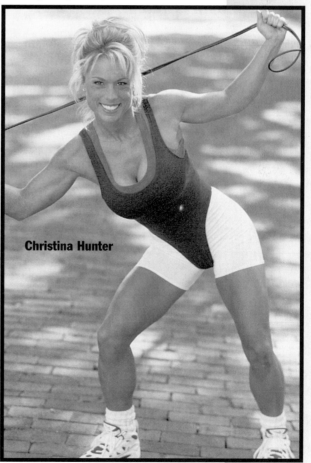

Christina Hunter

Concealer

The name says it all. Concealer is used to cover up flaws that disrupt the symmetry of your face. A common mistake normally made by teenagers is to coat the face with a heavy layer of concealer, and then apply foundation. This results in a plastic, mannequin appearance that is immediately recognizable as artificial. You want to wear makeup so that it accentuates your features. Admittedly, there are cases where a layer of concealer might be called for. If you have a skin disease, an underlying illness, or are undergoing medical treatments that have affected your skin's appearance, then you should consult with a professional beautician about what concealer to use. A common skin problem is acnea rosacea. Use a green tinted concealer to correct the problem. Then cover with foundation.

Acne scarring and injuries can be more of a challenge. The solution is called Covermark. It's a professional-finish foundation especially created to conceal scars, blemishes, injuries, and other flaws. If you visit the Covermark Web site (Covermark.com), you'll find they offer a specially priced foundation set – two tubes of base in your skin tone, which you mix to achieve a precise match for yourself. A similar product is Dermablend, another professionally created crème to cover blemishes. It is sold exclusively at J.C. Penney Department Stores and their subsidiary, Eckerd Drugs. You scoop it from the container with a small spatula, warm it on your hand, and then apply it to conceal. Concealer comes in both water-based and oil-based versions, in the following forms:

Kate: "What do you do, shower once a week?" Doug: "Is that an invitation?"
– exchange from the movie The Cutting Edge.

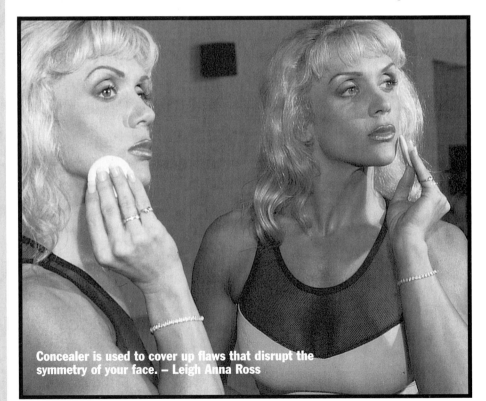

Concealer is used to cover up flaws that disrupt the symmetry of your face. – Leigh Anna Ross

Compact – either powdery or creamy in texture
Pot – creamy in texture
Tube – creamy in texture
Stick – similar to a lipstick
Wand – thinner than a stick, used for difficult to reach spots, or when you want to be very precise in how much concealer you apply.

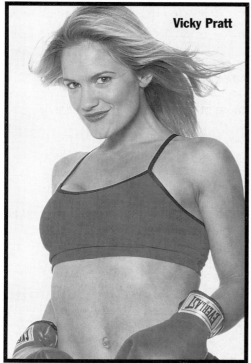

Vicky Pratt

Applying Concealer

1. Wash your face and hands and pat dry. This is the most important step.
2. Using a cotton swab like Q-tips, apply hydrogen peroxide to any blackheads or pimples. Let them air-dry. Other skin conditions do not respond to hydrogen peroxide, so discuss this topic with your dermatologist.
3. Now apply a small amount of concealer to the blackhead or pimple. Use a water-based concealer because it holds on to the skin better.
4. If the pimple still appears raised, you can cover it with a dab of mascara and make like it's a mole!
5. Cover any dark areas with concealer. Common problem areas are around the eyes and the nostrils (during cold and flu season). Use an oil-based concealer for these areas. The larger area requires a concealer with a better consistency than that provided by a water-based concealer. The redness of sore nostrils, and the blueness seen in dark circles around the eyes, can both be neutralized by a yellow-toned concealer.
6. Apply a small amount, make a layer, and then reapply until you have the desired effect. It is always better to start with less. Too much can result in a visibly uneven surface, and is a waste of concealer.
7. Concealer can even be used to help puffy eyes, which are common with allergy sufferers. Apply a yellow-toned concealer around the eyes to neutralize the blue tones. Then apply a second layer of concealer that more closely matches the skin tone. Followed by foundation, the eyes lose their puffiness.

Caffey: "It was oregano, Dave. It was ten dollars worth of oregano."
Dave: "Yeah, well, your client thought it was marijuana."
Caffey: "My client's a moron, that's not against the law."
Dave: "Look, Caffey, I've got people to answer to, just like you do. I'm gonna charge him."
Caffey: "With what, possession of a condiment?"
– from the movie A Few Good Men.

Foundation

Be prepared to spend most of your money (and your time) finding different shades of foundation. Because your skin changes tone, the foundation that worked perfectly this morning looks plain awful on sun-kissed cheeks after a day of skiing on the slopes. Exposure to sun, wind, changes in humidity, your menstrual cycle, certain medications, stress, fatigue, and dehydration can all affect your skin tone.

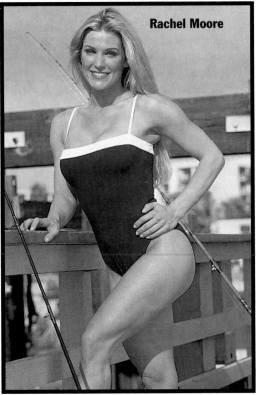

Rachel Moore

So plan ahead. Wear a sun blocker year-round. Protect your eyes with sunglasses, and your face with a large hat. Once you've been in the sun, test your foundation. If it doesn't match, go out and pick up another shade. Foundations are like men, if he hasn't done anything for you lately, chuck him and pick up a new one. Changes in your cycle can cause your skin to break out, so plan accordingly by having both concealer and a matching foundation.

Before spending money, make sure you are drinking enough water. Dehydration is very common. Skin becomes thin and dull-looking. And don't smoke! You can spot a smoker a mile away. The skin lacks vibrancy, a glow that is normally seen in non-smokers. Smoking will increase your wrinkles. That's a fact. Bottom line – smoke, and you grow old faster. That is logical, because smokers die younger.

The shade of foundation you wear may work wonderfully indoors but make you look embalmed in daylight. Be sure to check your foundation under different types of light. Then decide what shade to wear depending on what you have planned.

To select a shade, apply a stripe of foundation on your clean jaw line, not on the back of your hand. The color is *never* the same. Leave it for a few minutes, then check to see if the color has changed, which sometimes will happen if the foundation reacts with your skin's natural oils. Now check the mirror in natural daylight. If the foundation color has disappeared, you have the right shade.

A common skin problem is acnea rosacea. The best color for this particular problem is a yellow-based foundation, as the yellow will cancel out the redness and look much more natural. You can also use a foundation with a pale green tint.

Skin Type and the Right Foundation

Oily/problem skin – Your best bet is a fragrance-free, matte, oil-free foundation. Avoid foundation with oil in it or you'll be looking like a greaseball in no time. Foundations that help absorb excess oil are excellent for oily skins. Two good ones to try are Avon Clear Finish and Clinique Stay True makeup.

Combination skin – Here a light formulation to even out skin tones is a good idea. Opt for sheer coverage and minimal oil for the T-zone. Try the Body Shop Everyday Foundation, Maybelline True Illusion, and L'Oreal Feel Perfecte Foundation.

Dehydrated skin – Any skin type can be dehydrated, even oily skin. For oily to normal, try Avon Calming Effects Foundation, and L'Oreal Visuelle. For drier skin, try Innoxa Skin Perfecting Foundation, and The Body Shop Skin Treat Foundation.

Dry skin – Your skin must need a good drink. Choose a foundation that will nourish and hydrate the skin. Some good ones are Jurlique Moisturizing Foundation, Coral Colors Moisturizing Foundation, and those mentioned above for dry, dehydrated skin.

Foundation comes in four forms:

1. Liquid – Available in both oil- and water-based formulations, this is the most popular, convenient, and easiest form to use.

2. Cream – Great when you're travelling or out for a night on the town. Cream is thicker, and can double as a concealer, saving space in your makeup kit.

3. Tinted moisturizer – If you're into the outdoors then this is the foundation for you. This type of foundation not only moisturizes the skin but often contains a sun-blocker.

4. Dual-finish powder – Also called wet/dry, this is a combination of foundation and powder. It leaves a more professional look when done properly, but it's not something you should do on the run. You want to be sitting down at a makeup table, with plenty of time before you have to go out.

Applying foundation:

1. Pin your hair back so you can easily reach the edges without coating your hair in foundation.

2. Put a small amount of foundation into the palm of one hand. If you have dry skin, or will be outdoors, add a drop of moisturizer.

3. Apply the foundation with your fingertips. If you have long, sharp nails, use a sponge. Gently spread the foundation across your skin.

4. If you are wearing concealer, add layers of foundation until the tone matches the rest of the face.

5. Make sure to blend foundation over the jawbone to eliminate any telltale lines.

6. Apply makeup on one part of your face at a time, blend, then continue.

7. Once you have dotted the area of your face with makeup, use your sponge in downward strokes to blend it in. Your goal is thin, even coverage. Blend all the way down your cheeks and under your jawline and chin, out to your hairline, and around your nose. Use short, light strokes with the sponge taking care not to blend so much that you rub the makeup off.

8. Now that you have an even layer of foundation all over your face, check for any spots that need extra attention. If you must apply more foundation, put a small dot on the area you are adding to and press it lightly into your skin with the sponge until it is blended.

9. Blend a low-watt shimmery nude, bone or ivory eye shadow or a shimmery cream highlighter on the tops of your cheekbones, on the brow bone, and above the bow of the upper lip. This adds fullness and suppleness to the face.

Powder

Powder is the most essential step – it holds your makeup in place. Both concealer and foundation are cream-based products, and that means they can slide. Powder holds the cream-based products in place, and therefore lengthens the lifespan of your makeup application. And no matter how hard you try, different products result in different textures. Powder smoothes out the texture so that the face looks natural. And because both your makeup and your skin can release moisture, powder helps by absorbing extra wetness. If you feel you need oil control, try oil-blotting papers. They look like thin tissues in a matchstick-style envelope. They reduce shine, they don't dry your skin like oil-control lotions, and they don't add extra makeup to your face the way a pressed powder does.

Applying powder:
1. To prevent powder from clumping, blot your face with tissue to remove excess moisture.
2. We can't emphasize this enough, use *very* small amounts. Powder will stay wherever you put it. Put on too much, and you have to wash your face again and start from scratch.
3. Always tap your applicator to shake off extra powder before using.
4. Using a powder puff for large areas (and a sponge for fine-control areas), apply the powder lightly and evenly.
5. Apply powder in a downward and outward motion. An upward motion raises the barely visible hairs on your face, making them stand up, creating a fuzzy texture that is both visible and a tad aging.
6. Use too much translucent powder and it will tend to accumulate in lines and creases, making them more obvious. It should be applied minimally to set your sheer, moisturizing or light-diffusing foundation.

Blush

No one blushes like a teenage girl. Blush represents both innocence and youth. Both are amazingly attractive. The key to using blush is to be subtle. The best test is to have a friend look at you partway through the process. Leave the room, add the blush, and then ask the person to comment. If the answer is "You look better but I don't know what you did," then congratulations, you got it right!

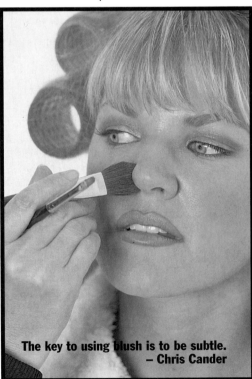

The key to using blush is to be subtle.
– Chris Cander

Albert: *"I want a palimony agreement and I want one now."*
Armand: *"Well, I don't have a palimony agreement on me right now. Is tomorrow all right?"*
Albert: *"Don't use that tone with me."*
Armand: *"What tone?"*
Albert: *"That sarcastic contemptuous tone. That means you know everything because you're a man, and I know nothing because I'm a woman."*
Armand: *"You're not a woman."*
Albert: *"Oh, you bastard!"*
– from the movie The Birdcage.

Blush comes in two forms that we recommend – cream and powder. Gels and liquids are best left to professionals.

Applying blush:
1. Using a blush brush, apply a very small amount of blush to the apples of your cheeks (just smile and you'll see them). With a circular motion, blend upward and outward until the blush is evenly distributed.
2. You can also apply small amounts of blush to other parts of the face to add some color.
3. If you've overdone the color, just add a little powder to cover up your error.

Lips

The lips remain the most alluring part of the face. They are also the most difficult to get right. The wrong color can ruin your whole look. Choosing the right lipstick takes practice, and the shade you choose will depend on the rest of the colors that make up your "look." Here's a guide for most skin tones to help you choose the correct shade of lipstick for you.

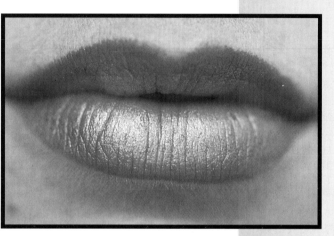

Red Lipstick

Fair skin – Deep plum reds. Soft berry and wine reds with a blue undertone. Avoid reds with an orange undertone. These can make you look washed out and ashy.

Medium skin: Deep reds are most flattering. Blue-reds brighten medium skin with a yellow undertone. Warm brown reds will soften and look warm on medium skin.

Olive/yellow skin – Rich, deep brown reds and deep, dark berry shades are suitable. Stay away from orange/reds and pink/reds.

Black skin – Try reds with a blue undertone, which are deep and rich. Also mahogany, deep plums, and wine reds are worth trying. Avoid orange and pink reds here.

Natural redhead – Soft and/or sheer reds that fall more on a brown shade are flattering, as well as sheer and glossy plum/raisin shades.

Please note reds that are very strong, matte and harsh will make mature skins look older and aging. Berry and plum reds that are soft, sheer and/or creamy are most flattering.

Brown Lipstick

Fair skin – Sheer medium brown with pink undertones or beige lipsticks with a pink undertone will flatter fair skin. Mocha browns and darker brown/pink lipsticks are also flattering for an evening lip look. Extra-pale browns with yellow undertones make fair skin look washed out.

"This woman hates me so much, I'm starting to like her."
– George, in "The Masseuse" episode of the Seinfeld series.

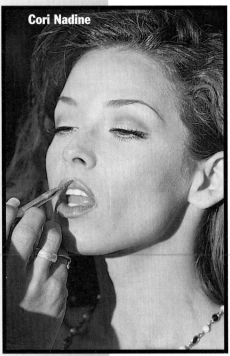

Cori Nadine

Medium skin – Browns that are very pale can make medium skins look ashy and washed out. Stick to rich caramel shades, medium brown with yellow or pink undertones, and creamy coffee-colored browns. Sheer browns in these varying shades can also be very flattering.

Olive/yellow skin – Browns with a red or auburn/mahogany undertone work well with this skin tone. Also, rich browns that resemble coffee, toffee and chocolate colors work well.

Black skin – Almost any shade of brown suits black skin – sheer and shimmery light browns to a rich, dark, coffee brown.

Natural redhead – Browns with a slight red undertone that are sheer, creamy, and/or glossy work well. Browns with a peach undertone are good ones to try as well. The pink browns and light beige shades are not the best choices for redheads who are very fair. These browns may clash with the pink undertones that natural redheads most often have.

Pink Lipstick

Fair skin – Pinks look fantastic on fair skin – sheer, light shiny pink lipsticks with blue undertones work well. Pink with a slight gold shimmer also enhance this skin tone very nicely. Dusty rose with or without shimmer is a good choice. Stay away from hot pink lipstick as it overpowers fair skin.

Medium skin – Rich and deep pinks that lean toward *warm* look best on medium skin. Also pinks with brown undertones enhance and flatter medium skin very well. Sheers, creams and mattes can all be tried and tested with much success using these shades of pink.

Olive/yellow skin – Deep berries, rich rose, and soft to medium plums are very flattering shades to this skin tone, which has very strong yellow undertones. Avoid pinks that are too cool and too light. These pinks can make complexion look drained.

Black skin – Medium and soft sheer pinks are very flattering. A hint of pink in glosses and sheers with a touch of beige can really enhance the skin tone. Berries, deep roses and plums also flatter this skin tone.

Natural redhead – Pinks are not easy for redheads to wear most of the time. With slight red undertones in redheads, good pinks to try would be those with peach and apricot colors in them. Avoid mattes, as these can be too harsh for the delicate complexion. Pink-red sheers and glosses can also enhance lips of natural redheads. The transparency of the glosses and sheers will flatter the natural lip color.

No lip color will look great if your lips are cracked, chapped and dry. The surface must be smooth for any lipstick shade or consistency to look super. Unlike our skin, lips do not produce oil; they have no oil-producing glands. The skin on the lips is actually mucous membrane, so it's a bit of a challenge to keep them smooth and chap free. Here is some good advice on how to treat and keep your lips looking and feeling healthy.

Lips should be moisturized and exfoliated. Exfoliate lips only when minor flaking is visible. Lips that are too cracked and sore will only get worse by exfoliating them. Use a hydrocortisone treatment for severely dry and cracked lips. That's a better option. Exfoliate lips with a gentle facial scrub using a toothbrush or just the tips of your fingers. You can make a paste with baking soda and water to exfoliate lips as well. Work it for a minute and then rinse with lukewarm water. Pat dry and immediately apply lip balm.

Try this as a healing remedy. Apply some pure vitamin E oil and pure aloe vera gel. Lock in moisture with a coating of lip balm like ChapStick or Blistex. In the morning gently rub in vitamin E, aloe vera, and balm with a face cloth. Wash your face as usual, and apply lip balm with an spf 15 or higher to further prepare lips for lipstick, and/or to face the harsh environment outside.

To "build your lips" and make them larger or smaller you need to use a lipstick pencil to draw the outline of your lips. This outline will prevent your lipstick from "bleeding" into the lines around your mouth. Apply lip gloss after your lipstick to make your lips appear moist.

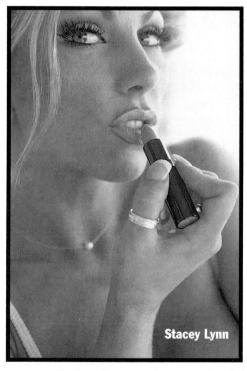

Stacey Lynn

Lipstick comes in five forms:
1. *Cream* – This lipstick provides lips with an opaque texture.
2. *Matte* – This lipstick provides lips with a dull, natural-looking texture.
3. *Sheer* – A shiny lipstick, but more subdued than lip gloss.
4. *Shimmer* – This lipstick sparkles.
5. *Stain* – The toughest and longest-lasting lipstick.

Building Your Lips:
1. Using a lip pencil, draw an outline of your lips. Skip this step if you're looking for a more natural look. If you're going skiing or hiking, and you're not going to be able to carry your makeup with you, color your lips *entirely* with pencil – and forget the lipstick. Your lips will hold the color for hours. Regular lipstick needs to be touched up every hour. Always use a lip liner that matches your lipstick. Darker lip liner with a lighter lipstick will make any woman appear to be older.

2. Apply some powder or apply a coating of lip balm to soften your lips. This step helps to fill in the lines and smooth out the surface.

3. Pout your lips, and apply your lipstick at the center, then work outward.

4. Blot your lips with tissue paper.

5. Stick a finger in your mouth, close your lips around it, and pull the finger out. This will remove any excess lipstick that could find its way onto your teeth.

6. Apply gloss or liquid lip color for a delicious glossed-out finish. Choose a shade that matches the lipstick color for a really intense high-shine look. Opt for

a clear color if you just want the shine without the intensity. Apply most of the gloss to the center of the lips for an enhanced pout, and spread outward.
7. Add powder and you're done.

Eyes

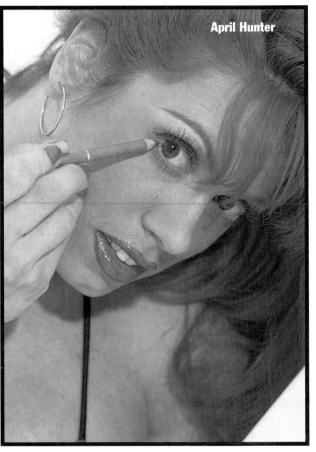

April Hunter

The eyes are the windows to the soul. With a few simple movements your eyes can call a man from across the room or hold him back with an icy stare. Your eyes and lips are the visual anchors on which your face resides. Creating the right look for your eyes is no simple task. It takes time and a lot of experimentation. But the result is worth the effort.

> *"Everything was going so well. She hadn't seen any flaws in me. Now she sees a side."*
> *"What side?"*
> *"A bad side, an ugly side."*
> *"Oh, so what?"*
> *"So what? I wasn't planning on showing that side for another six months. Now you made me throw off the whole learning curve."*
> – Jerry and George, in "The Glasses" episode of the Seinfeld series.

Thanks to colored contact lenses, you can now choose your eye color. You can also choose to have cat's eyes! Yes, contact lenses that give you eyes like a cat. Why would you do something like that? To become the center of attention. For example, you're at a vacation resort and the club is filled with singles. They're all attractive and the competition is fierce. You need an angle, something to make you stand out. Those unusual eyes will draw your object of desire to you like a fly to a flame. Or you may just want a different eye color which will allow you to try a different look. It's still you, but a more exotic and daring you. The experience can be liberating. And there's no rule that says you can't have two differently colored eyes. The possibilities are endless!

Choosing an eye shadow color involves one simple rule, you don't want to "fight" your own eye color or draw attention to your shadow – you want to pull attention to your own shade. Lilac, lavender and hues of brown (such as camel and taupe) will make blue eyes appear bluer than using the same shade as your eyes. For green or hazel eyes follow the principle of complementary colors – pinks, deep mauves, lavenders, rich plums and eggplant shades cause the green or hazel to appear more vibrant. Brown eyes are the easiest to complement – any color lighter or darker than your own brown will attract attention to your eyes, even tints of brown itself. For standout brown eyes, choose shades of blue, steel blue/gray, plum and eggplant.

The safest approach to eye shadow is to choose neutral colors. But why play it safe? If you have brown eyes, try royal blue. What a contrast! If you have blue eyes, try orange, or if that's too daring, try something softer like pale gold or sheer pink-peach. If you have green eyes, try purple or blue. The contrast will make the green in your eyes stand out.

A good base eye shadow brightens the eyes instantly. Try the low-watt shimmers. These add sheen to your eyelids without the frosty look. Your eyes will have a twinkle!

Building Your Eyes

1. Curl your lashes (whether they're natural or artificial) with an eyelash curler. Place the curler over the lashes. Get as close to the base as you can. Squeeze and hold for 20 seconds. Slowly move the curler out, away from the base and repeat.

2. Wipe your eyelash brush with tissue paper to remove excess mascara.

3. Open your eyes wide and apply mascara with your eyelash brush.

4. Create a base of foundation and concealer and apply it to the eyelids.

5. Using an eye shadow brush, begin at the lash line and sweep upward and outward, stopping just after the crease of the eyelid.

6. To widen the eye, use a light shade. To minimize the eye, use a medium color. If you have large eyes, sweep a light beige base color all over the eye area, then apply the darker shade on the lid rather than just in the crease. This works well because the dark shadow on the lid makes the eye appear smaller. If you have small eyes, stick with pale colors on the lid to attract light and make your eyes stand out more.

7. To bring your eyes forward, apply a medium tone to the eyelid crease. Use a darker tone at the corner of the eyes to provide definition. Go too heavy and you'll end up with the New York City street corner "Hi, Sailor. Want a date?" look – and you don't want that.

8. Using an eye pencil, apply a smudged line along the lash lines (never apply makeup to the inside of the eyelid, it smears and can cause infections). Make sure your pencil has a dull point. Touch your pencil against the lash line, do not drag the pencil. To achieve a subtle effect, draw as closely to your lashes as possible to give the illusion of thicker lashes. A sponge is helpful to soften and smudge, as well as correct any mistakes. For extra definition, stipple, or dot, the liner between the lashes

9. Apply powder to set your makeup.

Tweezing

Age, hormonal changes and genetics conspire to place hairs in spots that are just plain annoying. One of the oldest tools for hair removal remains the most effective – tweezers. And always use Anbesol. Rub it into the roots before you start tweezing. No more pain. Okay, some pain, but nothing like before. Then pluck away.

Tweezing the eyebrows takes a bit of planning. Place an eyebrow pencil against the side of your nose. The spot where the pencil touches your eyebrow is where your brow should begin. Mark this with a line. (You can wash your

"So she sees you with hot fudge on your face and she ends it? Do you really think she'd be that superficial?"
"Why not? I would be."
– Jerry and George, in "The Lip Reader" episode of the Seinfeld series.

face later. Tweezing is done before you go to bed, not before you go out!) Place the same pencil diagonally from the nostril to the corner of the eye. This is where your brow should end. Mark this with a line. Repeat for the other brow. You can trace an outline of how you want your eyebrows to arch on both brows. Now you're ready for tweezing.

Tweezing Your Eyebrows

1. Tweeze the hair in the direction in which it grows.
2. Using the lines you drew (as directed in the previous paragraph), tweeze the hairs that don't fit.
3. If you have bald patches in your brows (that's common), use an eyebrow pencil or brow powder to fill in the gaps. To keep your brows from looking fake and overly made up, always use short light strokes of brow color so it looks more like hair than a dark line. Brow powders are preferred over pencils because they are easier to control and look less severe. Although these colors look just like eye shadows, they actually have more pigment, so you need less and the color will last longer. Simply fill in the bare spots of your brows with a small amount of color applied with a stiff angled brush.

Brows should be made up to look polished. The brows are the center of your face and attention to your brows is extremely important in enhancing any look. A *faux pas* many women make is going too dark with the eyebrows. This is very aging. Notice any light-haired woman of any age with very dark eyebrows, and see what the contrast does. Use a light brown or taupe shadow to fill in and subtly extend brows.

In Conclusion

Although there are variations to applying lipstick, eye shadow, and the likes, putting on basic makeup like foundation and concealer is as easy as 1-2-3! Here we go. Always start with a clean moisturized face. Your first step is to apply concealer to areas that need extra attention – like dark circles under the eyes, blemishes, red spots, or broken capillaries. Apply it with your fingers, a clean sponge, or a makeup brush in gentle dabbing strokes, then tap carefully with your fingertip around the edges to blend. You can also apply concealer to your eyelids for a natural look.

Your second step is to apply foundation all over your face or just in the spots you need it. The third step is to apply powder. Even dry skin can benefit from the right powder because it "sets" your makeup for longer wear throughout the day. Apply it lightly with a large powder brush, making sure to dust a little under your eyes to set your concealer (helps prevent creasing). With your basic makeup finished, the rest is really up to your own preference. Here are a few guidelines:

For eye makeup, we recommend you apply your eye shadow first, then liner, then mascara. The mascara will seal in any eye shadow that falls onto your lashes and actually makes them look thicker. Apply your blush after foundation and eye makeup. Then you can adjust the intensity of the color to suit the rest of your face.

Lip liner can come either before or after lipstick, depending on your needs. If you like having an outline to fill in, apply liner first and then lipstick — just make sure to blend the edges with a lip brush or cotton swab so you don't have an obvious line. If you feel confident applying lipstick, we recommend putting your lipstick on first, then liner. The colors last longer this way and the look is more polished.

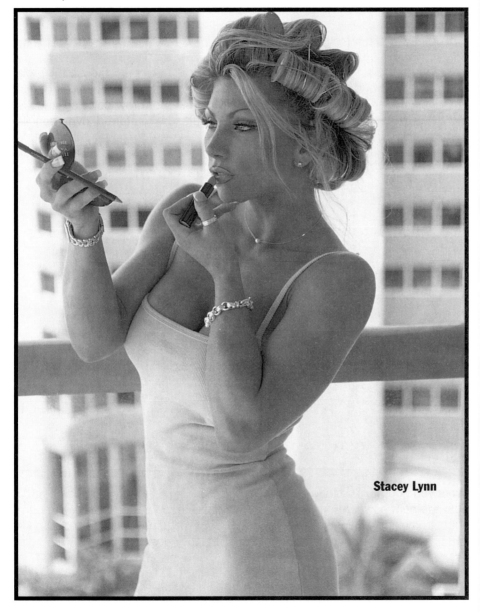

Stacey Lynn

REFERENCES

1. *www.emakemeup.com/tipsheet.html*
2. *www.makeupdiva.com*
3. *www.askariane.com*
4. Crawford, C. *Cindy Crawford's Basic Face,* Broadway Books, NY, 1996

CHAPTER THIRTY-ONE

Fitness Money

For most readers getting in shape and staying there is the primary goal. But a few of you may decide to make fitness a career. The good news is that the explosion in the popularity of health and fitness has created an almost endless list of potential careers. The bad news is that you have to search out the areas where you can make the most impact. Often the greatest challenge is not so much succeeding in an area but actually discovering it in the first place. Let's see if we can wade you through the murky world of fitness money and perhaps help you get started on a new source of income. And if by chance you do make big bucks, the authors will be only too happy to take a small percentage (just kidding of course)!

Prize Money

Even though prize money is perhaps the most well-known source of fitness-related income, it's probably the least lucrative. Attend a show or flip through a copy of a recent fitness magazine and you'll soon discover that, compared to other sports, fitness doesn't pay that well. Think of the hundreds of thousands or millions of dollars available to competitors in other sports – this is just a

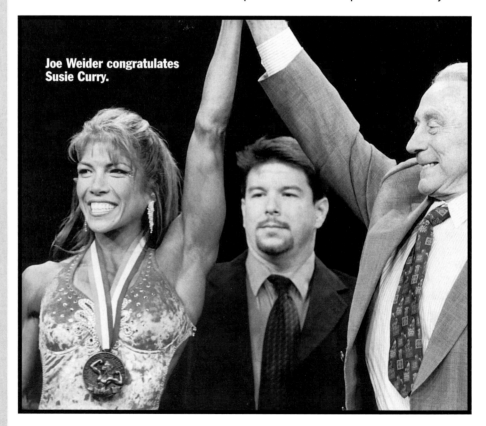

Joe Weider congratulates Susie Curry.

dream for fitness contestants. With the top prize for most contests resembling the registration fee of most other sports, a fitness competitor would have to win just about every show she entered to make what could be called "real money." The other competitors then fight it out for the remaining few thousand which in most cases barely covers their expenses. If placing high in a show does have one advantage, it's that it will get you coverage and publicity, which will in turn draw the attention of the movers and shakers of the sport, the supplement man-ufacturers and magazine publishers. And through these folks you stand the greatest chance of earning the big dollars.

Endorsement Contracts

If prize money is the least lucrative of fitness income, then product endorsement is easily one of the most profitable. A top fitness competitor can earn as much in one year from endorsements as most other contestants earn in their lifetime of competi-tion. With few exceptions the goal of every fitness competitor is to draw the eye of a major sup-plement or clothing manufacturer.

Endorsing is by no means an invention of the fitness industry. Athletes have been endorsing prod-ucts for decades. We need only point you in the direction of Michael Jordan, Wayne Gretzky and Tiger Woods to high-light just how much money an athlete can make by promoting a manufacturer's product.

Fitness competitors can thank the sport of bodybuilding for the phenomenon of supplement endorse-ment. Pick up a 1960s or 1970s edition of Joe Weider's *Muscle Builder/Power* (the forerunner to today's *Muscle & Fitness* magazine) and you'll see Arnold Schwarzenegger hyping the latest Weider protein powder. (There are even pho-tos kicking around of a young Robert Kennedy trying his hand at supplement promotion!) The beautiful young girls surrounding Arnold didn't hurt either, as most of the products were aimed at males in the 15 to 25-year-old bracket.

With the explosion of nutritional supplements in the 1990s manufacturers expanded on the early ads and began courting the top stars to promote their latest supplements. Just as college and universi-ties scout the latest crop of high school talent, so too did supplement man-ufacturers start paying closer attention to the amateur ranks. As soon as the latest pretty face or great body (usually a combination of both) emerged on the scene, out came the checkbooks and business cards. It's reached the point now that if a competitor has the "right look," his or her placing in the competitive ranks is often a secondary consideration. Sure it helps if you can say Ms. or Mr. Such-and-such uses your product, but the look seems to be more important these days than the titles.

Cynthia Ekman

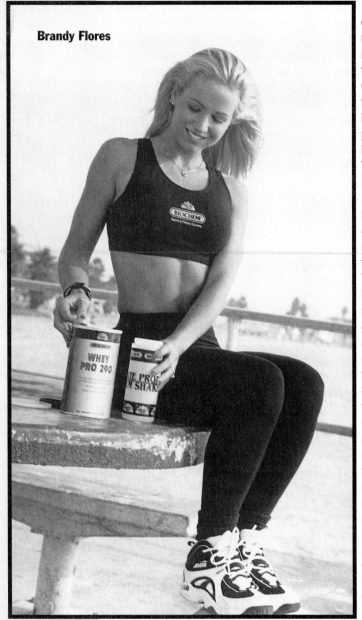

Brandy Flores

The two most popular forms of endorsements these days are for nutritional supplements and clothing. Go to any major contest or trade show (the Arnold Classic and Olympia weekends being two of the biggest) and you'll see display booths of virtually every major supplement manufacturer "manned" by beautiful fitness contestants. The bigger booths, owned by MuscleTech, Twinlab and *MuscleMag International,* are like mini-conventions themselves, with each having three, four, five or more beautiful fitness models there "for your viewing pleasure." The strategy is quite simple. The bulk of supplement consumers are still males in the 15 to 25-year-old category, and there is nothing like a pretty face (particularly if the rest of the anatomy is not displeasing to look at either) to draw them a crowd. The sales people (and to their credit many of these same pretty faces are also highly intelligent women with great business skills) can then start proclaiming the superiority of their products over rivals. It's capitalism at its best (or worst, depending on your point of view).

By now we've either stimulated your interest or prompted you to switch sports. For those in the latter group keep in mind that contest placings are often based on publicity. All things being equal, the contestants more familiar to the judges often place the highest in the shows. And where does this publicity primarily come from? Why, the magazines of course. Frequently magazines push their most important advertisers and their paid athletes. It stands to reason that these athletes are most frequently seen in the various publications.

For those who would love to be "chosen" by a supplement manufacturer, and we're guessing most contestants fall into this category, here are a few tips. The key to being chosen by a supplement manufacturer is *exposure*. In addition to competing in contests you want to make yourself known. Take in as many shows as possible, even if it means just sitting in the audience. Mingle in the lobby and at postcontest banquets with any potential endorsement prospects. The more people who see your face and get to know you, the better your chances of landing that big contract.

Another tip is to have a portfolio put together – a package that contains sample photos, your résumé, and contact numbers (fax, phone, e-mail, mailing address). Besides giving it to potential contractors in person, don't be afraid to mail it to all the supplement and sports clothing manufacturers. All it takes is for it to fall into the right hands and you're in.

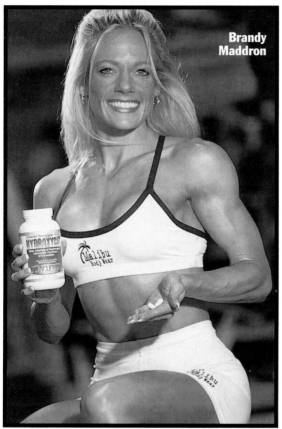

Brandy Maddron

Another suggestion is to not get greedy. Don't turn down a small manufacturer in the hope that EAS, Twinlab or MuscleTech will soon be calling at your door. In a manner of speaking you are like a young actor or actress trying to break into the business. You don't go from high school theatre to the lead in a 100-million-dollar Hollywood production in a single bound. There will be many smaller bit parts in between (Even the old swashbuckling actor Errol Flynn had a one-minute bit part as a corpse in his first movie.) Your primary goal is exposure remember. A small endorsement deal will not only make you a few bucks on the side but will also get your face known throughout the industry. From there it may only be a matter of time before one or more of the bigger companies start knocking on your door.

A final suggestion – and one that can be a double-edged sword – is to get yourself an agent. We say *double-edged* because an agent has the both power to land you that big deal and the ability to prevent you from ever breaking into the industry. Agents are like plastic surgeons and mechanics; many have an outstanding reputation based on quality service, while others leave you wondering how they ever managed to get certified.

The role of an agent is to both get you endorsement contracts and handle most of your business deals. If you have yet to land your first endorsement deal, but your agent keeps playing hardball, odds are you'll never break in. Major supplement manufacturers don't like dealing with small-time agents who think their "stars" are the next Monica Brant or Frank Sepe. Maybe you do have what it takes to emulate these top models, but if your agent starts holding out for more money than you are currently worth, forget landing a deal with the major manufacturers.

Business aside, an agent can also be your best friend. They are popularly called "ten percenters" within the industry as ten percent is the standard fee most agents charge. A good agent will more than earn his or her ten percent. Unless you have a background in business, an agent is almost a necessity when it comes to landing and signing endorsement contracts. Here's one of the ironic aspects of the whole agent/contract thing – most agents won't look at you unless you've landed your first contract, but many supplement companies won't talk to you unless you have an agent! It's the old chicken and egg. The same problem can be found in the literary profession; agents won't represent you unless you have published a book, and publishers only want to talk to writers who have agents.

If you start to get calls from supplement manufacturers, then we strongly urge you to get an agent. You can randomly pick and choose from the yellow pages – or even better, talk to a few fitness competitors who already have one. Like the example we used earlier with the plastic surgeon and the mechanic, you want someone who'll boost your career not hinder it.

Modeling

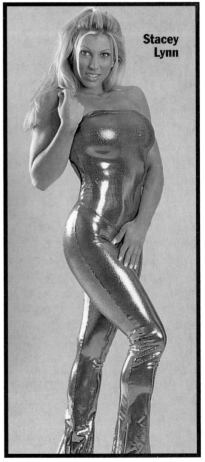

Stacey
Lynn

It only makes sense to follow the topic of endorsements with *modeling* as there is considerable overlap. If there is a major difference, it's that endorsing mainly involves nutritional supplements while modeling usually involves clothes. Most major magazines and supplement companies these days have their own clothing lines – and don't forget the hundreds of smaller companies that focus strictly on clothing. Of course you also have the huge multinational conglomerates that are using fitness models these days to highlight their athletic clothing lines.

Just about everything we said earlier about landing an endorsement contract applies to modeling. You want to get exposure and break into the industry. Your portfolio will be invaluable in this regard. Besides the usual assortment of photos, include images that show you modeling various types of clothing – including swimwear, workout wear, casual and formal attire. The whole nine yards so to speak. The object is to show potential employers how your image and the way you look in clothes will help them sell more products.

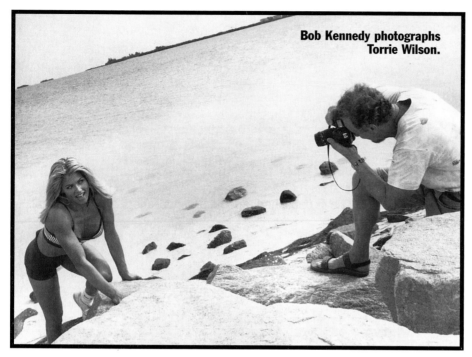

Bob Kennedy photographs
Torrie Wilson.

Photos

Even though we mentioned photos earlier, they serve another purpose besides landing you contracts; they can be a source of extra income. Most of the top fitness stars sell photos of themselves. Many advertise in the pages of *Oxygen, MuscleMag International,* and other fitness and bodybuilding magazines. Go to any large bodybuilding or fitness competition and you'll also see them selling their wares. With the average price of an 8 x 10 glossy going for $5 to $10, it doesn't take many sales to increase your income by a tidy sum.

If you decide to go the photo route, your first major step is to hire a photographer. As with agents, you have the full spectrum of quality choices. Again a referral will go a long way in your attempt to weed out the undesirables. A strong word, perhaps, but the very nature of fitness and bodybuilding – the display of the human body – tends to attract shady characters. Just because some guy (or girl for that matter) comes up to you in the gym and calls himself a photographer, doesn't mean he is one. Anyone can buy a camera and call themselves a lensman (and many do). Even if the individual seems straightforward, request some identification. A business card is a good start, but don't be afraid to ask to see samples of his work, particularly photos of other fitness models. It wouldn't hurt to even check with others in the gym including the employees, to find out if anyone's heard tell of the guy. If everyone draws a blank, avoid him like the plague. If he keeps bothering you, report him to the gym owner.

The previous aside, there are some outstanding photographers to be found. Many advertise their services at local gyms. If your gym has a couple of fitness or bodybuilding competitors, odds are they'll be able to point you in the right direction. If word of mouth doesn't pay off, you always have the yellow pages. Now while the people listed in the phone book might all be accomplished photographers, keep in mind that physique photography is an art form all its own. Shooting a sunset and capturing the human body require different skills. Your best course of action is to shop around. Make an appointment to visit a number of photographers and check out their work.

It's difficult for us to nail down a cost for a series of good quality photos, but like most things in life you get what you pay for. Generally speaking the more established the photographer the higher the cost. Keep in mind that your photos are both an investment and a source of promotion. Putting out a few extra dollars up front for quality work will pay off down the road, in both selling and marketing your physique. All it takes is one photo to fall into the right hands and it could mean hundreds of thousands of dollars in endorsement fees.

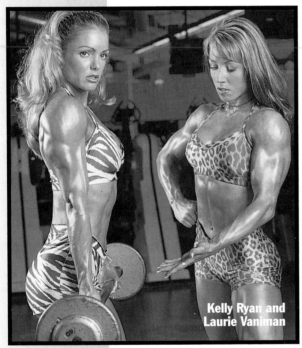

Kelly Ryan and
Laurie Vaniman

Personal Training

Personal training has become one of the biggest fitness-related industries of the last decade. Go into just about any gym and you'll see bodies of all shapes and sizes being led around by enthusiastic trainers armed with clipboards. For the upper eschalon of society having a personal trainer has become a status symbol. Years ago corporate executives hit the golf course for a round and cocktails, now it's off to the gym to "meet my trainer."

As expected of an industry that has evolved so fast, legislation has not kept pace. Anyone can pick up a clipboard and call themselves a personal trainer. As long as no one gets hurt, the trainer may actually build a solid clientele base and make a good income. But as soon as one of their charges gets injured, the first question the prosecutor will ask is, "Can I see your certification?"

Just because someone has built a great physique doesn't necessarily mean he or she knows a lot about fitness and nutrition. Like many aspects of life, genetics is a great equalizer. Granted, all things being equal, the person who spends years working out probably knows more about exercising than the typical coach potato, but there's more to becoming a great trainer than just spending a few years at the gym.

Okay, so you want to be a personal trainer. Your first step is certification. In order to give consumers some level of confidence in their choice of a qualified fitness professional, many certification organizations have been established over the past two decades. Requirements for certification (and prices) vary from organization to organization. Some are self-study courses; others require attendance at a workshop or seminar. Some require candidates to pass an exam; others require a combination of an exam and practical application of skills learned. Content will vary, but generally these programs include:

- Exercise Science (physiology, anatomy, biomechanics, nutrition)
- Health Screening, Exercise Testing and Evaluation
- Principles and Methods of Exercise
- Program Design
- Interpersonal Techniques
- Injury Prevention and First Aid

Most certification programs charge a fee to pay for the examination and optional study materials. The following are some of the most well-known certification organizations in the USA.

ACE – American Council on Exercise
ACSM – American College of Sports Medicine
AFAA – Aerobics and Fitness Association of America
ISSA – International Sports Sciences Association
NSCA – National Strength & Conditioning Association

Besides earning the actual training certification, it makes sense to maintain CPR and first aid status. In fact any certification you can achieve even remotely related to fitness is a feather in your cap. There's probably no such thing as being "overcertified."

No doubt by now you are wondering just how lucrative a career in personal training can be. With the average hourly rate being $50-$100, it doesn't take many clients to earn you a very respectable income. And all of this while being your own boss and setting your own hours of work.

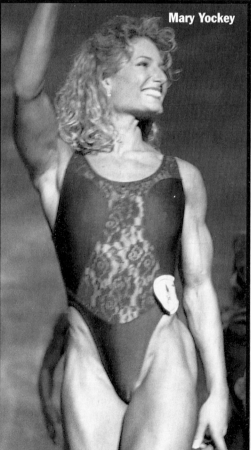
Mary Yockey

Guest Posing

Guest posing probably started with Arnold Schwarzenegger and his good buddy Franco Columbu. In the late '60s and early '70 Arnold and Franco supplemented their income by going to contests and performing short posing exhibitions. For many in the audience, the highlight of the show was watching Arnold display his award-winning muscles. In Franco's case a demonstration of his strength was often included. It wasn't long before many other top bodybuilders jumped on the bandwagon and it's reached the point nowadays that few contests are held without the appearance of a top name guest poser.

When fitness came of age in the early '90s, it was only natural that the top stars would add guest posing to their list of potential sources of income. Many champions of the sport perform dozens of guest spots every year. Although the price varies, the going rate is between $1000 and

$5000 for one or two posing segments, three to five minutes each. Once again do the math and you see how guest posing can be far more lucrative than competing. Of course there is a correlation between winning contests and being in demand for guest posing. With few exceptions the most sought after guest posers are the ones who have won or placed the highest in the top fitness contests. We said "with few exceptions" as a couple of the most popular guest posers had mediocre competitive careers, but made a name for themselves by putting on outstanding posing exhibitions.

You can't just decide to charge $1000 for a guest posing appearance and hang out your sign. Unless you've won one or more of the major fitness contests, you'll have to practically beg for your first exhibition. In many respects you are like an up-and-coming rock band looking for your first gig. In all probability you'll have to do your first couple of spots for free. But remember your goal is to get exposure and develop a good reputation. Provided you make a positive impression, it won't be long before other promoters are calling to ask for your services. If your competitive career improves. Then you can expect your posing requests to also increase in number.

Probably the most important aspect to successful guest posing is performance. It's sad but true – a number of good shows may or may not help your reputation, but one bad one could end it. It's a small world, particularly the fitness and bodybuilding fraternities. Most promoters know each another and often check with one another before employing the services of a guest poser. If you turn up out of shape, you will then have a huge hill to climb to redeem yourself.

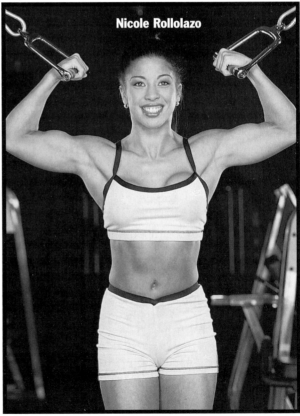

Nicole Rollolazo

The main reason guest posers are hired is to draw additional crowds to the show. Guest posers who have a reputation for consistently pulling off a great exhibition are almost guaranteed to produce a sellout. This in turn means they can charge a higher admission fee. Conversely those who regularly show up out of shape, looking like an advertisement for the Pillsbury Dohboy, quickly lose their marketability.

If you are one of the very lucky few who can maintain near contest condition year-round, then you could easily perform dozens of exhibitions a year. Most, however, can get in top contest shape only once or twice a year. In this case you would have to tailor your guest posing to coincide with these times.

Seminars

Fitness competitors can once again thank bodybuilders for this source of income. After Arnold and Franco popularized guest posing, it wasn't long before those in the audience started asking them questions. It made sense. After all, you have the greatest bodybuilder in the world in front of you, so you might as well ask him how he did it. Arnold wasn't stupid and he quickly expanded his services to include seminars as well as posing. In fact guest posing and seminars often go hand in hand at major competitions, with the top star usually conducting the seminar after the prejudging on Saturday afternoon. The biggest names often appear on Sunday as well. The top stars in bodybuilding and fitness get $5000 or more for a half- or full-day seminar. Again the arithmetic leads to the potential of earning a tidy sum of cash.

As with personal training some of the greatest physiques in the world make lousy public speakers. Conversely some of the most sought after guest speakers have never competed in a contest at any level. Many readers no doubt remember the brilliant university professor who put them to sleep. Then there were others who were so interesting that time flew by. The fitness and bodybuilding industries are filled with characters from both categories.

If you decide to get into the seminar field, our first suggestion is to develop a good base in public speaking. A few readers may have a natural gift for presenting in front of large crowds, but most are it uncomfortable. A few probably find it terrifying. We suggest you take a public speaking course at a local college or university if possible. Some courses merely get you comfortable speaking in front of a large crowd, but others such as the well-known Dale Carnegie course will cover the whole presentation spectrum.

If you are nervous in front of a crowd, then such a course is almost a necessity. Some of the most gifted public presenters were at one time an absolute wreck standing in front of an audience, but with practice and time they mastered the art. Don't let a fear of public speaking stand in the way of an exciting career opportunity. There are millions of people out there just begging for knowledge. To quote Robin Williams in the movie *Dead Poets Society,* "Seize the moment."

Contest Promotion

Note: We have used the terms *bodybuilding* and *fitness* interchangeably because most contests these days feature both disciplines during the same weekend.

In a manner of speaking contest promotion is an example of the old saying "If you can't beat 'em, join 'em." In other words – if you can't win contests, try promoting them! The average person has no idea of what it takes to promote and run a bodybuilding or fitness contest. It has all the complexity of a major conference, and such individuals as Nimrod King and Jan Tana have developed outstanding reputations as contest promoters.

Although not for the faint at heart, if you decide to try your hand at contest promoting, your first step is to become affiliated with a fitness federation –

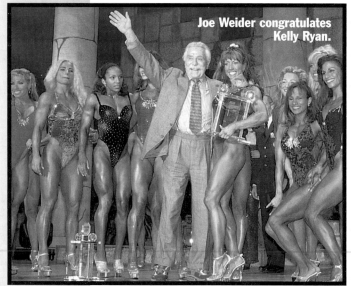

Joe Weider congratulates Kelly Ryan.

and then land the contract. As there will no doubt be other promoters vying for the same honors, the contract usually goes to whoever makes the best impression on the selection committee. If you are a major city vying for the Olympics, you will need years of planning and millions of dollars. Things are not so drastic in acquiring a fitness show, but you still have to do your homework.

Perhaps the best piece of advice we can give is to volunteer your services for a few years to another promoter. He or she can use your help, and in turn you will gain considerable experience behind the scenes. During your apprenticeship learn everything you can about all aspects of running the show, from renting the venue and crowd control, to ticket printing and lining up the judges. For a contest to be successful, everything must run like clockwork.

After a few years of honing your trade, you can make a bid for your first contest. Keep in mind that federations are reluctant to switch promoters if they are doing a good job. If it ain't broke, why fix it? Unless the regular promoter steps down, or hasn't been doing an adequate job over the past couple of years, chances are they'll once again land the contract. But as soon as an opening comes along, be ready to seize the opportunity.

Assuming you land the contract to run the show, your next step is to put your team together. You'll now come to realize how much the previous promoter appreciated your volunteer services. Pick and choose your team wisely, and put the best people in charge of the major areas. Your role is to oversee and make sure each "department head" is getting the job done.

We could write a whole book on what it takes to set up and run a successful contest. Here are a few suggestions we hope will point you in the right direction.

Contest venue – You have to strike a balance between cost, location and size. Generally speaking the bigger the contest the bigger the audience. This in turn means a bigger financial investment. Of course size is not everything and you also want to select a venue that has a touch of class about it. The days of holding contests in high school gyms are over. You want to impress audience and competitors alike. And let's not forget the federation delegate who will be checking up on you to determine whether or not their best interests are being met by having you run one of their contests.

Lighting – Although most venues have their own lighting, you may need to contract out. Lighting a theatrical production and lighting 20 posing bodies are two distinct entities. The next time you're at a contest take a notice of how much light each competitor has on her when standing in a line. Those promoters that take the time to test things out will have all competitors highlighted equally. Conversely if the contestants on the ends are in shadows or flooded out, then you can almost bet the promoter gave lighting a short shift. If possible check your venue's lighting out weeks if not months in advance. In fact lighting will be one of the factors to consider when choosing the venue in the first place. If there's any doubt, hire someone. As with photographers, try the yellow pages, but one or two phone calls to another promoter will point you in the right direction. Try to find someone who has had experience with lighting physique shows.

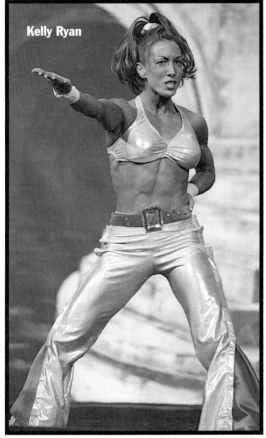

Kelly Ryan

Printing tickets – Setting up the tickets will be one of the least expensive aspects of the show. As a word of caution, print only as many tickets as seats in the venue. The airlines regularly oversell because they know that a certain percentage of passengers won't show up. But fitness and bodybuilding fans are very loyal. You can be sure that 99 percent of those who bought tickets will be there. That last thing you want is a couple of hundred angry (in the case of the bodybuilders, *large* angry) fans at your door. But it happens occasionally especially when people get their wires crossed about the exact number of tickets to be printed.

Most commercial printing shops can run off a couple of thousand tickets for you for a few hundred dollars. Check around to get a good price, then give them at least a few weeks' notice.

Promotion – Probably the most important thing you need to make your contest a success is a large turnout, both audience and competitors alike. And to attract both you need a good marketing scheme. The obvious place to start is the local gyms. The bulk of your potential competitors will train at the various fitness establishments around the city. If it's a state or provincial show, get a list of as many gyms as possible. If you (and your assistants) can visit each in person, so much the better. But if not, put together an advertising package and mail it out. Include a couple of large posters to put on the wall, and a number of contestant entry forms. Keep in mind you are not just targeting competitors by this approach. Most of your potential audience members work out at the same gyms. By the time every relative and friend of the contestants has bought a ticket, your venue will be nearly sold out.

Besides gyms you want to reach the general public as well. If you have a contact in the media, print or TV, so much the better. Let them know about your upcoming contest. If you don't have a media contact, don't despair. Media types are always looking for something different. Suggest to reporters that they cover one of the athletes as they prepare for the show. They do it all the time with athletes from other sports and thanks to Arnold, fitness and bodybuilding shows are taken more seriously these days. Even if they don't want to do a mini-documentary on one of the contestants (or the show in general for that matter), they'll most likely give your show some type of plug.

Helpers – Everyone from the president to Santa Claus has them. They are called helpers, assistants, and they are essential if you want to make your show a success. There is just too much ground for one person to cover. The best corporate executives in the world know how to delegate responsibility – and so must you.

The odds are good to excellent that, as soon as word gets around that you are promoting a contest, people will start coming at you from left, right and center to help out. Many will have had previous experience organizing contests, others will be first timers. No matter what their background – take them all! As you'll quickly discover, you can never have too much help. Payment won't usually be an issue as most volunteers are doing it just to be involved. As a token of gratitude you may want to offer a couple of free tickets for them to give to their friends, but hard cash rarely changes hands. In fact you may get volunteers actually offering you money to let them help out. That's how dedicated and loyal fitness and bodybuilding fans can be.

As we mentioned earlier, set up your volunteers so that each department has a leader and a number of assistants. You can then oversee the whole operation like a general commanding his troops. And just like a general you may want to move your troops around on battle day depending on which area needs reinforcements.

In conclusion, we'll be the first to admit that contest promotion is one of the most difficult ways to earn money from the fitness industry. There are far fewer opportunities than, say, guest posing or conducting seminars. On the other hand making a name for yourself as a promoter is one sure way to make a name for yourself as a "mover and shaker" within the sport.

Writing

Most of the biggest names in fitness and bodybuilding have released their own books, and many have regular columns and articles in the major magazines. Writing is another area where you don't have to dominate competition to be successful. Like guest posing and seminars, it helps to have a proven competitive track record, but some of the best writers never set foot on a competitive stage.

There are different areas where writing can pay off for you. If you do manage to make a name for yourself on the competitive circuit, then writing a series of training courses is a logical step. Once again (we keep saying this but such is the influence of the great one from Austria) you can thank Arnold Schwarzenegger. When Arnold first came to America in the late '60s, Joe Weider had him publish a series of small training booklets which he then advertised through Joe's *Muscle Builder/Power* magazine. Thousands of bodybuilders around the world forked out $5 per booklet to learn how Arnold built his chest, back, arms, etc. To this day Arnold's instructional courses generate him a respectable amount of cash.

Most top fitness and bodybuilding stars these days have their own line of instructional courses. Some are simple booklets of a few pages or less. Others are full-size books of 200 or more pages.

Besides instructional books and courses, you have the whole fitness and bodybuilding magazine publishing world to consider. Every issue of *Oxygen, Shape, Muscle and Fitness,* etc. contains dozens of articles covering topics such as supplementation, training and nutrition. Although many of the articles are the work of staff writers (another career in itself), the magazines also feature freelance work on a regular basis. If you are handy with a pen, write up an article and submit it. Who knows what could happen? Some of the greatest coaches in the world never made it past the amateur level in competitive sports, but because of their knowledge and ability to present it logically, they went on to very successful careers coaching at the professional level. The same holds true in fitness and bodybuilding. Outstanding writers such as Joe Weider, Robert Kennedy and Greg Zulak never made it big on the competitive level, but their names are now synonymous with publishing and writing (in Bob's case over 50 books, thousands of magazine articles, and three monthly magazines).

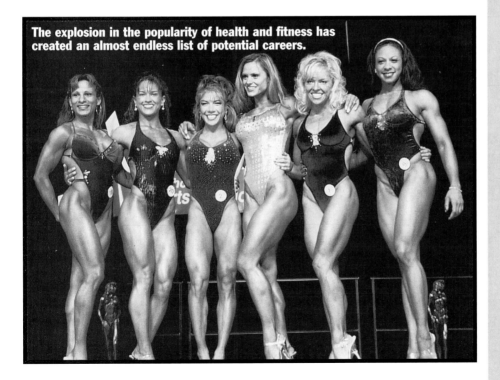

The explosion in the popularity of health and fitness has created an almost endless list of potential careers.

Acting

If the field of contest promotion is difficult to break into, acting is almost impossible – at least if it's landing a leading role you have in mind. We know that sounds blunt, but we have to be honest. As we mentioned in a couple of our previous books, every year thousands of hopefuls arrive at LAX with visions of Hollywood stardom in their eyes. It doesn't take long before reality sets in. A few persevere and do break into the industry, but most end up going back home, or worse get involved in one of the seedier industries that prey on such individuals. There are literally thousands of young hopefuls vying for a part in every Hollywood production. Back home you may have won the state fitness championships, and a pat on the back is well deserved. But Southern California is overflowing with beautiful people. The old cliché of a "small fish in a big pond" is certainly the case in the acting profession – especially for those from a small town and with little or no acting experience. The average person has no idea just how competitive the acting industry is. We know that sounds negative but, as Moms are constantly saying, "It's for your own good."

If you do decide to pursue an acting career, then heed the following advice. For starters, don't take your life savings and head to California. You stand a much bigger chance of landing an acting role back home, or in a city closer to home, than in Hollywood. The reason is simple – less competition. Instead of thousands of other hopefuls it may be only hundreds or even dozens. A great physique combined with a state fitness title will give you an edge over many rivals. Out in California you would be surrounded by rivals with such qualifications.

For those younger readers, we encourage you to start your acting career in high school or junior high. This serves to not only build your résumé, but also to give you an indication if acting is really for you. Watching a profile of Julia Roberts may seem glamorous, but rehearsing the same scene 50 times at 5 o'clock in the morning is not for everyone. If acting does seem to be in your blood then try out for a few local theatre productions. Again you are building your résumé for future directors to review. As with fitness competition, you start at the bottom and work your way up.

With time you may establish a reputation as a quality actress. If you reach this point it's possible you may start attracting offers from directors and producers. Without repeat-

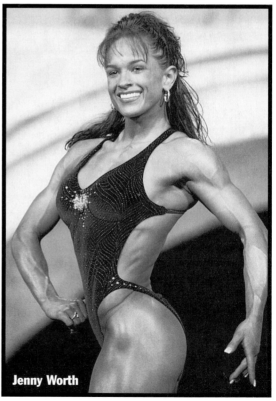

Jenny Worth

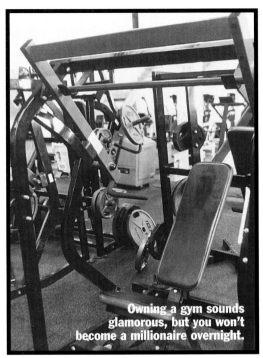

Owning a gym sounds glamorous, but you won't become a millionaire overnight.

ing ourselves, just about everything we said about photographers applies here. Check the individual's credentials before entering into any agreement with him or her. The porn industry is loaded with such predators who prowl gyms looking for new prey.

We should add that, if you have the talent and the look producers are searching for, you won't have to go to them, they'll come after you. *MuscleMag International* and *Oxygen* regulars Vicky Pratt and Trish Stratus started out modeling for Bob Kennedy and eventually wound up costarring in their own TV series. In Vicky's case as Sarge in *Cleopatra 2525*. Trish is now a regular in the WWE (World Wrestling Entertainment). Even though both girls had acting ambitions, it was their regular appearances in *MuscleMag* and *Oxygen* that led to producers knocking on their door.

Only after you've built a decent portfolio and made a few contacts should you think about heading west. At least now you have a fighting chance of being taken seriously as an actress, rather than starting out as just some unknown right off the plane.

Opening a Gym

This is another career option that requires an enormous investment of time and money. Gyms seem to open and close as often as movies these days. We are sure most readers can list off the top of their heads a couple of gyms that have opened and closed in their area over the past few years. In many cases the reason is poor management, but in others it comes down to competition. It's difficult for a small Mom and Pop operation to compete with a huge gym conglomerate that can offer "Lifetime Memberships for $499." Of course many of these huge gym chains go under as well, usually because of their enormous operating costs.

Contrary to popular belief, operating your own gym sounds glamorous, but you won't become a millionaire overnight. For years of sacrifice you may make a comfortable living, but if you hope to retire after five or ten years, forget it. There are far easier ways to make money.

If you do decide to open a gym, the first thing to consider is your potential membership base. If you live in a small town of 500 to 1000, you would need just about every person to buy a membership at your gym just to break even (which for most small gyms just happens to be 500 to 1000). Even if you live in a large area of 5000 to 10,000 you're not on easy street. Only about ten per-cent of the population regularly work out, so once again you'd need to attract a sizeable proportion just to cover your expenses. If your town has another gym operating there, then opening a second makes little sense.

If after carefully sizing up the potential membership base and competi-tion you think you have a good chance of succeeding, then your next decision is what type of gym to open. Unless you live in a large city, your only viable alter-native is the wide-spectrum fitness center. You want to attract as many clients as possible. Hardcore gyms attract only hardcore trainers. Such characters are few in number and tend to keep everyone else away. There's nothing like one 600-pound set of deadlifts to send people to the complaint counter. Likewise upscale health spas mainly attract the high-income bracket. How many of those are found in a small center of population? Not enough to keep a gym going we assure you. No, your best option is to stay middle of the road.

Another decision is where to locate. Do you build from scratch, lease or rent. All three have pros and cons, and this is where your financial advisor comes in. Unless you have a degree in business (or an equivalent background in the area) you will need to seek the advice of someone versed in the art of running a small business. Most towns have financial advisors who specialize in just that – and they are well worth the money they charge.

Let's say you have the gym location finalized, and the financial paper-work complete and out of the way. Your next step is staff. Once again if you have the knowledge you can assume the head position yourself. But if not, you'll need to recruit a gym manager. Try to get someone who has a back-ground in both business and fitness. There are pencil-pushers that make good managers, and fitness buffs that have good business sense, but your best bet is someone who knows a little about both.

With your head honcho in place, you now have to outfit your gym. Again you can buy, rent or lease equipment. It becomes a matter of balancing finances, space and potential clients. In general terms you'll need a combina-tion of cardio and strength training equipment. For cardio you can't go wrong with cycles, treadmills and cross-trainers. For strength training you'll need a line of machines, some barbells and dumbells, and assorted racks and benches.

We could go on outlining the week to week operation of a typical gym but we think you get the picture. Starting and operating a gym takes a lot of planning, organizing and implementing. For the first year or so it will consume just about all your time, and in the end you still may not make a go of it.

Not to leave you on a negative note, we must say there are many advantages to running your own gym. If you've done your homework, and some large chain doesn't steal your members, you can make a comfortable living from the gym business. It probably won't put you on the Fortune 500 list, but there's no reason why you can't slip into the ranks of the middle class!

Another advantage – you are your own boss. No punching a clock for the executive in the penthouse office. No having to worry about job perform-ance reviews. Every minute is your own.

There's still another benefit. You are doing something that in all proba-bility you love. Most people struggle into work on Monday morning, long for hump day on Wednesday, and then can't wait to get out of there on Friday afternoon. Their jobs are nothing more than a rut to follow in order to pay the bills. But making money from something you've done as a hobby for many years is very enjoyable.

Finally, running a gym is very self-rewarding. You are helping hundreds (perhaps thousands) of people improve their lives both physically and mentally. This is a benefit few "normal" jobs can offer. So while owning and operating a gym is a big risk, it does have numerous payoffs. Who knows, maybe you'll be the next Joe Gold!

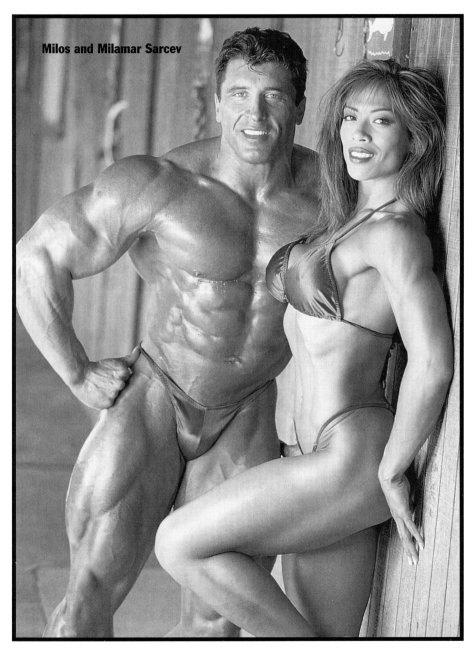

Milos and Milamar Sarcev

CHAPTER THIRTY-TWO

Plastic Surgery

In a culture that equates beauty with success, appearance has become more than just an exercise in vanity. For many it has become as important as a good education and solid references. Long gone are the days when a person could have a career with the same firm for 30 years. The new economy of dot coms (now dot gones), has resulted in a work force that is constantly seeking out new opportunities. Interviews are often a long, drawn out process. The final stage, the face-to-face interview, is the meeting that can make or break a job. And even for those who feel secure in their position, what if you were laid off tomorrow? Does your appearance inspire confidence? Maybe you're a stay-at home mom. If you get divorced tomorrow (just think about how many of your friends that have split up), do you have a look that could sell cars or homes? Your appearance is the spark that first ignites a relationship, whether it's a romantic one or a professional one. Some people are blessed with good looks, but many are not. And some have chosen to reshape their destiny by recreating themselves through surgery.

Many people mistakenly believe that plastic surgery takes its name from the use of silicone and other plastics. The term plastic surgery comes from the Greek word *plastikos,* which means to mold or to give form. Many of the first recorded efforts in surgery were attempts to restore normal form to injured bodyparts. Renaissance Italy was famous for its surgeons who specialized in rebuilding noses lost in sword fighting. Plastic surgery falls into two major subdivisions: reconstructive and cosmetic.

Reconstructive surgery might be defined as a surgical procedure performed on abnormal parts in an attempt to restore a more normal appearance and to improve function. The primary consideration here is the fact that the procedure is carried out on abnormal parts or tissues. The use of tissue expansion and flaps and grafts to repair disfigurement due to burn injury and the transplantation of muscle from the back to a severely injured lower extremity are common examples of reconstructive procedures carried out by plastic surgeons.

Cosmetic procedures are operations done purely to enhance the appearance of bodyparts, which fall within the normal range of appearance and function. Examples would include procedures such as face lifts, nose reshaping done only for

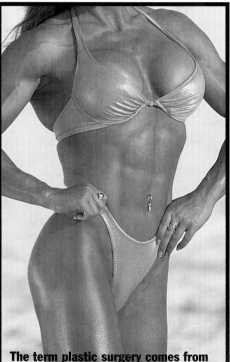

The term plastic surgery comes from the Greek word *plastikos,* which means to mold or to give form.

appearance, and fat suction procedures. The desire of humans to enhance their appearance is not a recent phenomenon. Every culture throughout history has engaged in some form of body modification. The Ancient Britons painted themselves blue and used lime to set their hair. The ancient Egyptians used make-up, and many African tribes use facial and body scarring as a beauty aid. Modern Western society is not all that different. In 1994 alone, Americans spent $16 billion on beauty products. Against that backdrop, cosmetic surgery is a tiny but growing tool in the quest for personal beauty.
[Source: www.surgery.uiowa.edu/surgery/plastic/wips.html]

"A person usually has two reasons for doing something: a good reason and the real reason."
– Thomas Carlyle

Before You Go Under The Knife

With more than a million patients sculpted by board-certified plastic surgeons last year, a 150 percent increase since 1992, cosmetic surgery is no longer solely for celebrities and the super-rich. Many plastic surgeons now offer financing at reasonable rates. California still accounts for the largest slice of the surgical pie with 13 percent of procedures, but Florida is closing the gap with 10 percent. The numbers are conservative because no one keeps track of the estimated 50,000 additional doctors who are allowed to perform the procedures but are not plastic surgeons. That last point should scare the hell out of you. It means the doctor who is about to perform your plastic surgery may in fact not be a plastic surgeon.

A plastic surgeon has gone through rigorous training that is daunting both intellectually and financially, and in the length of time required. In the US a plastic surgeon must have the following:

• At least four years of undergraduate education.
• Four years of medical school.
• Completion of a minimum of three years of clinical training in an accredited general surgery residency. A large percentage of plastic surgeons completed a general surgery residency (duration of five to seven years) and have achieved board certification from the American Board of Surgery (which requires successful completion of the written and oral examinations).
• Completion of an accredited residency program in *orthopedic surgery* (duration of training is five years).
• Completion of an accredited residency program in *otolaryngology* (duration of training is five to six years).
• The resident must then be evaluated by the American Board of Plastic Surgery to

Cosmetic surgery is no longer only for celebrities and the super-rich.

ensure that all prerequisite training was satisfactory prior to beginning plastic surgery training.

• Completion of a residency in plastic surgery (two to three years). After satisfactory completion of a plastic surgery training program approved by the American Board of Plastic Surgery the resident is eligible for board certification. The American Board of Plastic Surgery administers a written examination at the end of the plastic surgery residency, which must be completed satisfactorily.

• An oral exam is then administered two years after completion of the plastic surgery residency, and is based upon the clinical cases collected by the surgeon during the previous two years. If this examination is completed satisfactorily, the surgeon will then be board certified in *plastic and reconstructive surgery*. The entire process of becoming board certified in plastic surgery requires 17 to 20 years of education/training after high school.

Many surgeons will choose to pursue additional subspecialty fellowship training in one of the following areas; hand surgery, craniofacial surgery, burn/critical care, microvascular surgery, or cosmetic surgery. These fellowships are usually one year in length.

Therefore, if your plastic surgeon is 24, there's a good chance he or she is not telling you everything. And you want to know everything about your surgeon before you allow that person to start chopping up your body. With the kind of money plastic surgeons can make, it should be no surprise that less-qualified individuals might try to get a piece of the action. Check out your doctor thoroughly before you go any further. If you don't, you could end up disfigured or dead.

Plastic Surgery After Pregnancy Or Just to Look Better

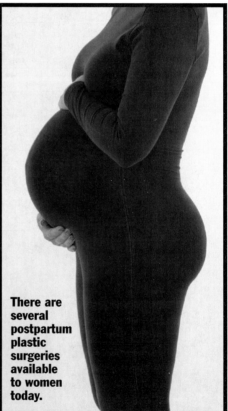

There are several postpartum plastic surgeries available to women today.

Pregnancy causes changes in body shape that are distressing to many women. A protruding abdomen (the "mommy pouch") and sagging bustling can affect a woman's self-esteem. Becoming a mother doesn't mean you can't look as good or better than before pregnancy. Most women enjoy being pregnant and are happy to become a mother. But thanks to modern medicine, today's women have a choice. They can learn to love that postpartum figure, or opt for plastic surgery to help regain (or even improve on) their prepregnancy shape. The following are typical postpartum plastic surgeries.

Breast Enlargement (Augmentation)

Breastfeeding is the healthiest thing you can do for your child. It helps you both to bond with each other, and has been shown to improve sleep patterns in new mothers. Some women have worried that breastfeeding will ruin the shape of their breasts. In fact, changes in the breasts actually occur during pregnancy. As the body prepares to nurture a child, milk glands swell and replace fatty tissue. After childbirth these glands shrink. What's left is a skin "envelope" with little to fill it. This causes the breasts to look less full or sag. Implants can return the breasts to their youthful contour. The small incisions are virtually undetectable, usually made under each breast, around the nipples, or in the armpits. Implants may be inserted just under the gland of the breast or beneath the muscle tissue. Stitches are removed after approximately one week.

The main problems associated with this operation are hardening of the "capsule" around the breast, leakage of the implant, and changes in mammography.

Breast Lift (Mastopexy)

Some women experience extensive swelling in their breasts during pregnancy. In addition to the postpartum loss of fat tissue, swelling can cause the skin to stretch and sag. And no amount of exercise will re-tighten this skin. An outpatient procedure called "mastopexy" can remove excess skin and reduce sagging. Your plastic surgeon can use local or general anesthetic to tighten skin on the lower half of the breasts, which lifts and firms them.

Surgery is determined by the degree of laxity of breast skin. It is common to tighten the skin of the breast by removing the excess. The incision is placed like an upside down T although sometimes it is a Q or L shape. The scars are all on the under surface of the breast and around the nipple. Most of the time this is an outpatient operation and a stay in the hospital is not needed.

The main problem associated with this operation is a long and sometimes heavy scar and loss of nipple sensation. Recovery takes one to two weeks. Most people are back to work within a week or two.

Breast Reduction

Some women have too much breast tissue. The additional mass from pregnancy can be too much. Arthritic necks, bra straps digging into the shoulders, and unwanted attention are all drawbacks that motivate women to seek out this surgery.

There are many ways to perform a breast reduction. A common method of surgery

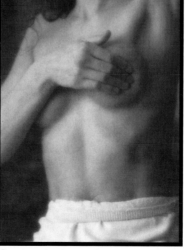

Surgery is determined by the degree of laxity of breast skin.

"Beauty as we feel it is something indescribable; what it is or what it means can never be said."
– George Santayana (1863-1952)

"A narcissist is someone better looking than you are."
– Gore Vidal

is to first mark the new nipple position. Then, with the blood supply of the nipple preserved on a pedicle of tissue, the excess breast is removed. The nipple is moved into its new position and the new breast shape reconstructed. The incision is often around the nipple and on the under surface of the breast, like an upside down T. The operation is done under a general anesthetic. Most of the time this is an outpatient operation and a stay in the hospital is not needed.

If the breasts are not too large and the skin has good elasticity then liposuction may be possible to reduce the size. This is especially useful for women who wish to avoid long scars. It is possible that this technique may preserve feeling and the ability to breastfeed. For many surgeons this method has become the most popular way to perform breast reduction in the patient who is about a DD size. Very large and pendulous breasts still require the more traditional methods, which result in longer scars. The main problem associated with this operation is damage to the blood supply of the nipple and heavy scar. Breastfeeding may not be possible after surgery. Recovery takes one to two weeks. Most people are back to work within a week or two.

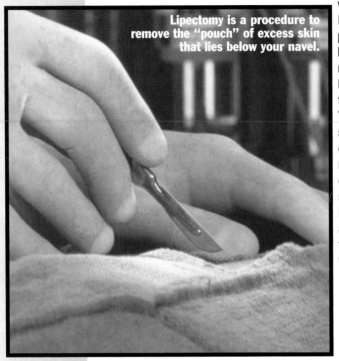

Lipectomy is a procedure to remove the "pouch" of excess skin that lies below your navel.

Stomach Tightening (Abdominoplasty or Lipectomy)

Nowhere else is pregnancy more evident than a woman's abdomen. It was the nine-month home to your infant. It's also the place where stretch marks, C-section scars and loose skin may linger long after childbirth. These "badges of motherhood" can frustrate and depress a woman, even as she rejoices at the life her body helped create. Lipectomy is a procedure to remove the "pouch" of excess skin that lies below your navel. It can get rid of stretch marks and turn a very visible vertical C-section scar into a small bikini line that's easy to conceal. Many women have this operation done at the same time as a tubal ligation or a hysterectomy. Your plastic surgeon may admit patients to the hospital for one or two days. If you have only a small amount of excess skin, you may be a candidate for a mini-lipectomy (a less extensive procedure often done under local anesthetic) that still yields an impressive improvement.

This operation tightens the loose skin of the abdomen and repairs the weak muscles of the abdominal wall (rectus muscle). It is sometimes combined with liposuction to smooth the edges and improve the contour. If the patient is obese, the panniculus of fat is removed at the same time. A mini-abdominoplasty is used when there is localized fullness of the lower abdomen and a less extensive procedure is needed.

Surgery tightens the skin of the abdomen by undermining the skin and stretching it. Excess skin and fat is then removed. The incision is placed across the lower abdomen but sometimes is like an upside down "T." The scars are concealed by clothing. The operation is done under general anesthetic. Often this is an outpatient operation but many patients choose to stay in the hospital overnight.

Patients who are obese or have large amounts of loose skin may need a modification of this operation called a panniculectomy. The main problem (and special concern with this operation) is the long and sometimes heavy scar. The incision is sometimes slow to heal and crusting or scabbing along the scar may occur for several weeks. This is major operation and the risks of major surgery, such as blood clots in the legs, can occur. Recovery takes at least one to two weeks. Most people are back to work within two to four weeks.

Stomach Tightening for Muscle Bulges (Mini-Abdominoplasty)

For many women, excess skin is not the only abdominal change they experience after pregnancy. It's not uncommon for the stomach muscles to separate when holding an expanding uterus. Often those muscles fail to reconnect after childbirth, even with endless situps. This condition can only be repaired with surgery and is sometimes covered by health insurance. Women having difficulty regaining their prepregnancy weight can benefit from the immediate and dramatic improvement a lipectomy can make on their figure. It frequently provides the emotional boost they need to commit to a healthy diet and exercise regimen.

Mini-Abdominoplasty is done to tighten the lower abdominal area and remove the fullness that often develops after pregnancy. It is used when there is localized fullness of the lower abdomen and a less extensive procedure than an abdominoplasty is needed.

Doctors remove an ellipse of skin from the lower abdomen and tighten the muscles beneath that area. Many do liposuction of the abdomen at the same time. The operation is performed under either local or general anesthetic. Most of the time this is an outpatient operation and a stay in the hospital is not needed.

The main problems that are of special concern with this operation are the scar of the lower abdomen and irregularity from the liposuction. Postoperative care: Recovery takes one to two weeks. Most people are back to work within a week or two.

Spot Fat Reduction (Liposuction)

A slower metabolism, less time to exercise (because of the baby), some new mothers complain they just cannot lose fat in certain spots like the thighs, buttocks and upper arms. Your plastic surgeon can resculpt the body, removing fat deposits that contribute to flabby underarms or bulges in the thighs. Liposuction is an outpatient procedure. Small areas can be done under local anesthetic. It

"I base my fashion sense on what doesn't itch."
– Gilda Radner

is not appropriate for large fat deposits or for women who are generally over-weight. However, this procedure can be the impetus to encourage a healthy weight loss.

Labioplasty

During a normal vaginal delivery, many women tear or otherwise damage the labia (the opening to the vagina). Labioplasty can repair this damage and help a woman heal faster from such injuries. Your plastic surgeon may perform this outpatient procedure under local or general anesthetic. Recovery takes only a few days.

Changes in Skin Pigmentation

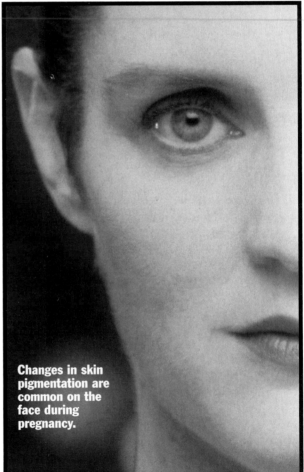

Changes in skin pigmentation, called chloasma, are common on the face during pregnancy. Some studies suggest that up to three out of four women may develop these changes which are characterized by a blotchy brown increase in pig-ment. If the pigment is in the epidermis it is often helped by bleaching agents such as hydroquinone. Maybe now that the biological clock has finished ticking, you have the opportunity to turn back time and regain your youthful fea-tures. The choice is yours.

Changes in skin pigmentation are common on the face during pregnancy.

Cosmetic Surgery

There are numerous tech-niques that can enhance your features. The rest of this chap-ter discusses the various oper-ations available and what they involve. Please remember that all operations have risk. The risks of plastic surgery are divided into two groups. The first group includes those risks that are present in all operations: swelling, bruising, bleeding, infection, a scar and numbness or change in feeling. The second group of risks are unique to the particular operation.

"Like a prune, you are not getting any better looking, but you are getting sweeter"
– N. D. Stice

"The greatest discovery of my generation is that human beings can alter their lives by altering their attitudes of mind."
– William James (1842-1910)

"The nice thing about egotists is that they don't talk about other people."
– Lucille S. Harper

Face Lift

This operation is done to tighten the loose skin of the face and neck. One of the most difficult areas to treat is the nasolabial fold, the crease between the nose and the corner of the mouth. The surgery tightens the skin and the underlying muscles of the face and neck. The incision is placed in the natural creases in front of the ear and inside the ear. It extends above the ear into the scalp and behind the ear on the hairline. The operation is done under either local or general anesthetic. Most of the time this is an outpatient operation and a stay in the hospital is not needed. It is common to perform neck liposuction at the same time as a face lift.

All operations have some risk. The main problem which is special for this operation is damage to the facial or VII nerve. This nerve controls movement of the face. Recovery usually takes one to two weeks. Most people are happy with the result and back to work within a week or two. Others are less than pleased.

"My eyes are not as I would like. They are not raised up at the corners as they were supposed to be. My left eye has a little ridge which seems to give me a hollowed out look under my eye. My neck is very lumpy and feels tight – even after three months. I also have a deeper laugh line on the right side than I do the left. The left side is about what you should have, but the right is more saggy looking." – a 56-year-old woman's comments on her face lift. [Reference: www.talksurgery.com/consumer/stories/story00000012.html]

"Beauty without grace is the hook without the bait."
– Ralph Waldo Emerson (1803-1882)

Blepharoplasty

This operation is done to remove bagginess and tighten lose skin on the eyelids. Surgery removes the excess skin. At the same time it is often necessary to remove the fat pads which have come close to the surface. The incisions are placed in the natural crease lines of the upper and lower eyelids. Some patients are candidates for transconjunctival blepharoplasty. In this operation for lower lid bagginess, the incision is placed on the inside surface (the conjunctiva) of the lower lid. This avoids a visible scar. The operation is done under either local or general anesthetic.

The main problem associated with this operation is ectropion or pulling down of the lower lid. Asymmetry of incision, dryness of the eyes, and inability to completely close the eyelids have also been described.

"Doctors are the same as lawyers; the only difference is that lawyers merely rob you, whereas doctors rob you and kill you too."
– Anton Chekhov

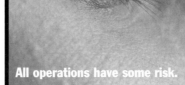
All operations have some risk.

Recovery takes one to two weeks. Most people are back to work within a week or two. And the results are noticeable.

"Didn't look like a lizard any more. People noticed a change but thought it was my hair or something else. Eyeliner and mascara no longer smudge onto my upper eyelids." – a 45-year-old woman comments on her operation. [Source: www.talksurgery.com/consumer/stories/story00000023.html]

Forehead Lift

This operation is done to tighten the skin of the forehead. This reduces lines and raises the brows. The incision is usually placed in the hairline or an inch (2.5 cm) or so back in the scalp. It extends from one side to the other. The operation is done under either local or general anesthetic. In younger patients, the operation may be done using the endoscopic or keyhole approach so that there is less scarring.

The main problem associated with this operation is damage to the nerves of the scalp, which causes numbness behind the incision. This risk is reduced but not eliminated with endoscopic forehead lifting. Also, the scar can stretch and because scar does not grow hair this may be noticeable in those with thin hair.

Recovery takes one to two weeks. Most people are back to work within a week or two.

Skin Resurfacing

This operation is done to remove the fine lines of the face and after scar revision to smooth or sand scars and make them appear more even. When used on scars the most common technique is dermabrasion. The principle of resurfacing the skin is straightforward. Dermabrasion, chemical peeling and laser resurfacing work in similar ways. The top layer of the skin is removed and as the new skin grows there are changes in the remaining skin. Which of these procedures is best for you depends on several factors and your doctor can discuss them with you. There is no incision. The operation is done under either local or general anesthetic, depending on the amount of skin to be resurfaced. Topical anesthetics, including ice and EMLA cream, are occasionally used. Most of the time this is an outpatient operation and a stay in the hospital is not necessary.

The surgeon performs a controlled burn to achieve the beneficial effects. Complications can occur using the laser, as with all resurfacing procedures. In addition, herpes infections after surgery are especially dangerous and require vigorous treatment. The main problems associated with this operation include: prolonged redness, unevenness of the resurfacing, lines of demarcation between the treated and untreated areas, and changes in the pigment (color) of the skin. The initial recovery takes one to two weeks. Most people are back to work within a week or two. The redness may last several weeks or even months. An effective procedure, it is also a painful one, as the following account demonstrates.

"The laser surgery felt like being shot in the face at close range with a pellet gun and burned terribly. After surgery I looked like someone had brutally beaten me in the face with their fists. Ice and petroleum jelly are the only post-op treatments. I was very fortunate that I did not blister and peel. Swelling and bruising subsided slowly [each person is different], as did the pain. Some vessels are still apparent after one treatment and will need one or two more treatments for nearly complete removal." – 30-year-old woman who had dermabrasion for broken blood vessels after a car accident.
[Source: www.talksurgery.com/consumer/stories/story00000046.html]

Rhinoplasty

Commonly known "nose job," the purpose of this operation is to reshape the nose. The procedure can refine the appearance and reduce the size. In some patients who have difficulty breathing, this operation may help them breath more normally. The operation can be performed on all age groups, including teens and the elderly.

The surgeon separates the skin of the nose from the underlying bone and cartilage. The bone and cartilage are then reshaped and the skin redraped over the surface. Patients who have a deviated septum may benefit by correcting this problem at the time of surgery. The incisions are placed inside the nose, unless the surgeon uses an open approach in which case the scars lie across the columella (the tissue between the nostrils). If the nostrils flare sometimes the surgeon may make an incision at the junction between the nose and the skin of the upper lip to narrow the flared appearance. It is not unusual to combine rhinoplasty with chin augmentation to improve the profile. This operation is done under either local or general anesthetic. Most of the time this is an outpatient operation and a stay in the hospital is not needed.

The main problem associated with a nose job is the need for secondary surgery, usually minor, in about 5 to 10 percent of patients. A rare complication is the development of a small cyst (called a mucous cyst). Recovery takes one to two weeks. Most people are back to work within a week or two.

Otoplasty or Ear Pinback

The purpose of this operation is to correct protruding ears. Otoplasty is one of the few cosmetic surgeries performed on children. Although the operation is done on both men and women, it has great appeal for men because many of them wear their hair short and cannot conceal their ears.

Surgery weakens the cartilage of the ear so that it bends into its new shape. At the same time stitches are placed in the cartilage to hold the ear in position until the new shape has formed. The incision is placed in the natural creases behind the ear. The operation is performed under either local or general anesthetic. Most of the time this is an outpatient procedure and a stay in the hospital is not needed.

The main problems associated with this surgery are an abnormal reaction to the stitches and recurrence of the problem. The recovery takes one to

"You'd be surprised how much it costs to look this cheap."
– Dolly Parton

"Happiness is good health and a bad memory."
– Ingrid Bergman (1917-1982)

two weeks. Most people are back to work within a week or two. It takes many months before the final result is seen.

Cheek and Chin Implants

This operation will enhance the shape and appearance of the cheekbones and chin. There are many ways to perform cheek and chin implantation. The method must be tailored to the needs of the individual. The surgeon creates a pocket over the cheek tissue or at the chin, and places an implant into the pocket. There are two types of implant, solid and porous. The incision may be placed in the crease lines outside the eye, under the chin, in the mouth, or on the inner surface of the eyelid (the conjunctiva). The operation is done under either local or general anesthetic. Most of the time this is an outpatient operation and a stay in the hospital is not needed.

The main problems associated with this operation are patient dissatisfaction and movement of the implant. Recovery takes one to two weeks. Most people are back to work within a week or two.

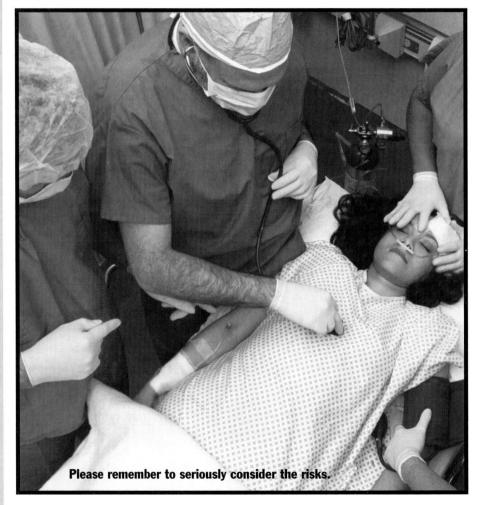

Please remember to seriously consider the risks.

Hair Transplantation

Many women experience hair loss. Transplantation can recreate your hair pattern, but the new hair pattern will not be exactly the same as your hair was before it became thin.

There are several methods of transplant surgery. One is to replace individual hairs or groups of hair. This procedure is called grafting. The surgeon uses small plugs of hair called mini- or micro-grafts. At any one time 250 to 750 miniature plugs are inserted. Another method is to excise the bald area and replace it with flaps of hair-bearing skin – scalp skin with normal hair that is moved into a new position. These procedures are done under either local or general anesthetic. Most of the time these are outpatient operations and a stay in the hospital is not needed.

The main problems specifically associated with hair transplants are the need for multiple operations, scarring, a poor result and numbness. Recovery takes one to two weeks. Most people are back at work within a day or two after hair grafts and a week or two after a flap. The recovery period is much longer following tissue expansion.

Scar Revision

This operation improves the appearance of scars. There are many ways to perform scar revision surgery. The method must be tailored to the patient's individual needs. The operation is done under either local or general anesthetic. Most of the time this is an outpatient operation and a stay in the hospital is not needed.

The scar will not disappear after surgery. All scars are permanent. The aim is to make your scar less noticeable. In most cases there is about a 90 percent chance of improvement. Sometimes the scar looks about the same after surgery and there is minimal improvement. In rare cases the scar can be worse (less than 1 percent). True keloid scars are rarely improved with surgery alone and so it is important to distinguish between hypertrophic scars and keloids. Some surgeons feel that silicone or oil gel sheets applied to the scar after it has healed may improve the appearance. Sometimes steroid injections are used to reduce the amount of collagen in the wound. Recovery after surgery takes one to two weeks. Most people are back to work within a week or two.

Liposuction

This operation has become extremely popular in recent years. It is the permanent removal of bodyfat from localized areas of the body. It does not tighten skin although sometimes the underlying tissue seems pulled tighter by a thin layer of scar tissue (adhesions). Liposuction sculpts areas and is not designed to remove large amounts of fat or to treat obesity. A relatively new technique called ultrasonic liposuction may be able to remove larger amounts of fat. Cellulite is not usually improved by traditional liposuction and in some cases may be made worse.

"If you can't learn to do it well, learn to enjoy doing it badly."
– Ashleigh Brilliant

"The concept is interesting and well formed, but in order to earn better than a 'C', the idea must be feasible."
– university management professor in response to student Fred Smith's paper proposing reliable overnight delivery service. (Smith went on to found Federal Express Corp.)

Surgery involves small incisions through which the fat is removed in individual tubes. Different sized tubes are used to remove the fat and the pattern crisscrosses to reduce the risks of irregularity. The operation is done under either local or general – you can choose – but most patients are more comfortable asleep. Most of the time this is an outpatient operation and a stay in the hospital is not necessary.

The main problems associated with liposuction are surface irregularity and the need for secondary surgery. Ultrasonic liposuction also has complications such as nerve damage, but probably results in less bleeding and surface irregularity. Recovery takes one to two weeks. Most people are back to work within a week.

Ultrasonic Liposuction

Ultrasonic liposuction is a method of removing fat from the subcutaneous space. The fat is first broken up by ultrasound, then removed by suction. At the same time the skin may be tightened. During ultrasonic liposuction, ultrasonic sounds waves are produced by a generator. These waves are transmitted to the tip of a suction cannula (tube) or wand. When this tip contacts the fat cells, the cells are broken up and the fat emulsified. This liquefied fat can then be removed by low-pressure suction, which is less traumatic than traditional liposuction. In certain situations the procedure has advantages over traditional liposuction.

In the original European method of ultrasonic liposuction the fat was emulsified with an ultrasonic wand. Then in a second step it was removed with suction. This two-stage procedure is time-consuming. The method being developed for use in the United States uses a suction cannula which is also a wand. In this way emulsification and suction proceed at the same time.

Complications with ultrasound-assisted lipoplasty can occur but major problems are uncommon. They seem to be more common when large volumes are removed and when the tissue closest to the skin is aggressively suctioned. Many of the risks are the same as for traditional liposuction. These include bruising, swelling, bleeding, infection, and change in nerve function. In addition, surface irregularity can occur in up to 3 percent of patients but only a third of those cases need additional surgery. Brown discoloration of skin may occur in up to 4 percent of patients. The brown pigment is due to hemosiderin (an iron containing material produced when red blood cells break down) and increased pigment due to inflammation. It may be long lasting and seems to be more common when the inner thigh is suctioned.

Another danger is nerve damage, which may occur in up to 6 percent of patients. "Pins and needles" and aching pain are the most common problems. Damage to the nerve that supplies the lower face muscles (VII nerve) has been seen after suctioning along the jaw. It appears to recover on its own and no treatment is needed. The outer sheath of many nerve cells is a fatty layer called myelin and the nerve damage may be due to stripping of this layer.

As if that weren't bad enough, up to 4 percent of patients may experience small lumps and texture change in the skin. Small pieces of fat may break off during suctioning. These may be felt as small sausage-shaped areas deep in the skin, just above the muscle. They may act as trigger points for pain and discomfort.

The patient may have considerable drainage. Drains are sometimes used after surgery but in some patients the drainage may be persistent. It consists of a mixture of the wetting solution, small particles of fat and residual oils. Collection of fluid or serum (seromas) is the most common complication of ultrasonic liposuction.

After surgery the skin may not contract and in situations where large amounts of fat have been removed this may require additional surgery. An advantage of ultrasonic liposuction is that it appears to tighten the skin more than traditional liposuction.

A serious danger is skin necrosis. The ultrasonic probe can damage the blood supply to the skin or cause burns directly. This may lead to the death of a small area of skin. The superwet method is used to reduce the risk of burns in the cavity being suctioned. Also, ultrasonic liposuction should not be used on patients who have pacemakers.

One final caution, a dietary change is recommended following liposuction, because free radicals may be created by the surgery. Some doctors recommend antioxidant medications before and after surgery.

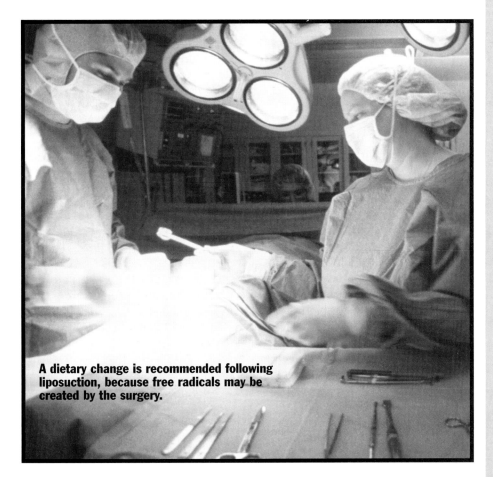

A dietary change is recommended following liposuction, because free radicals may be created by the surgery.

CHAPTER THIRTY-THREE

Questions and Answers

As is becoming the custom, we like to finish off our books with a question and answer section drawn from *MuscleMag International* and *Oxygen* magazines. Every month fitness experts such as Mia Finnegan, Vicky Pratt, Marla Duncan, Amy Fadhli, Monica Brant and Dr. Christine Lydon address the various concerns and issues submitted by readers.

Besides giving you extra information, this section highlights the broad scope of topics both magazines cover on a monthly basis. Some of the questions are geared toward fitness competition, others apply to everyone. Chances are the answer to the very question you had in mind can be found within this chapter.

Q I have noticed in many magazines that women who compete have no hair on their bodies. What is the reason for this? How do they achieve this look?

A There are three main reasons women rid their bodies of hair for a competition or photo shoot. The first is that the tanning products will get stuck in the hair and give the appearance of an unnatural or unbalanced skin tone. Second, during competition you want to look your best – with no flaws. Hairless skin gives you a leaner, tighter look than if your skin has hair on it. Third, if your arms, legs, and other bodyparts have a lot of hair, you will not be able to see the cuts in your muscles. Hair covers them and doesn't allow stage lighting to cast shadows, which is the way your definition is revealed.

How do they achieve this look? There are three easy methods. The first

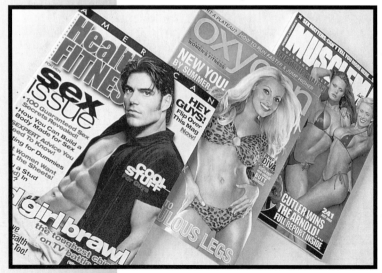

is shaving, but only with a sharp double-edge razor and moisturizing shaving cream. You will need to test this out to see how your body responds. Be prepared to use at least six to eight razors per show to prevent razor burn and nicks. The second method is to apply a topical solution for hair removal. Again, experiment months or weeks before the show. Some products may make you break out or could even cause a rash. The third and most painful way is waxing. Once again, get the facts and experiment in advance.

Q How do you feel about nonfat diets?

A Nonfat diets will make you fat in the long run. Over the years we have grown to think of fat as our enemy, when it is in fact our friend. Fat does more than provide calories for your body.

• Fat protects your internal organs by forming a natural protective layer.

• Fat serves to insulate your body and protect it against heat loss when external temperatures drop.

• Fat is a stored energy source. It is a primary source of energy at rest and provides 50 percent of our energy while exercising moderately. During intense exercise 80 percent of your fuel supply comes from fat.

• Fat-soluble vitamins such as A, D, E and K are not absorbed without it.

• Fats and oils also assist in maintaining a stable blood sugar level.

Q My trainer says I have to drink one gallon of distilled water every day. Is this true – and why?

A While preparing for competition you definitely need to drink more water than normal, up to a gallon a day in most cases. Distilled water, which contains no minerals at all, is actually dead water. I don't recommend it until the last four days before a competition. Then it will limit sodium levels and encourage your body to excrete lots of fluid as you go into your competition.

Some people retain more water in their bodies, but in most cases, cutting sodium the last few days before a competition does the trick. But there is no need to deprive your body of what it needs until it is absolutely necessary for competition. Sodium is important as it helps regulate blood pressure and water balance in the body. Keep in mind, an electrolyte imbalance can be fatal. Be sure you are getting the proper amounts of sodium, potassium, magnesium and zinc, as well as replacing the fluids you sweat out during your training.

Q I have entered in three fitness competitions and each time right before I have to go onstage, I have experienced sweaty palms, a rapid heartbeat, an upset stomach and – believe it or not – an attack of perpetual yawning! Why is this happening to me?

A I'm not surprised at the yawning. The initial symptoms indicate anxiety. Your nervous system is causing these common physiological reactions. The yawning is actually an

Marla Duncan

involuntary way for your body to bring in more oxygen, nothing to be concerned about. Eventually these annoying problems will disappear as you become more experienced and confident about being onstage. You may also want to try some breathing and visualization techniques to relax yourself.

Q I travel quite a bit for my job. The time away from my gym is really affecting me mentally as well as physically. My per diem won't really cover one-day gym visits, which can get expensive. What should I do?

A Most hotels have some sort of exercise facility (no matter how rinky-dink). Even a few sets of exercises with free weights and some lunges can make a difference both physically and mentally. Do an intense arm and shoulder workout if the facility has only a few dumbells. Spend 15 minutes doing some ab exercises. No equipment needed here! If your company puts you up in the cheaper hotels that don't offer the equipment you need, invest in one of those sturdy exercise bands out on the market. They travel quite easily and can be used for a total-body workout.

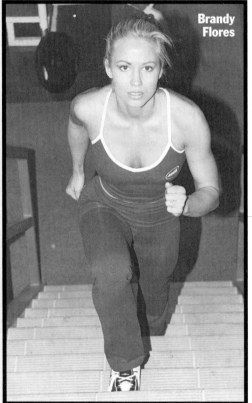

Brandy Flores

Q I'm a 48-year-old mother of three. I was quite athletic prior to the birth of my children, but now my exercise regimen is next to nil. I'm aware of muscle memory and would like to start a weight-training program again. What else would you recommend to help me regain the muscle tone and fullness I once had?

A I would add some *creatine* to your diet. Once thought to benefit only bodybuilders and athletes, studies have proven that daily does of creatine combined with some basic exercise, can drastically increase the rate at which the average woman or man (at any age) puts on muscle. With regular use of creatine you can potentially regain or retain the muscle mass typically lost as our bodies grow older – and you can even add more muscle.

Q I really enjoy the benefits of stair-climbing. I find it really works my lower body as well as improving my overall cardiovascular condition. With the warm weather approaching, I would like to incorporate jogging stadium stairs into my program. Is this a good alternative?

A As you might already know, I'm a huge advocate of changing one's workout, even taking it outdoors, but I do have to warn you about this exercise. Mechanical stepping is preferable over real stair-climbing because descending the stairs can place considerable force on the knees, tendons and joints. I would have to recommend it only once a week or every ten days. If possible wrap your knees for added support.

Q I've just started training with weights. How long does it take to look toned?

A That actually depends on your starting condition. The right diet and exercise program coupled with lots of discipline can show positive changes in as little as two or three weeks. When preparing for a fitness show I know I require about nine weeks of strict dieting and increased aerobic work to get the look I want. This is based on my present condition, which is kept about seven pounds from contest shape at all times.

Everybody is different. You might need more or less time, depending on your present condition and genetic makeup. Hard work and discipline play a major role in the success of any diet and exercise program. Be realistic and patient. Set small goals. When you obtain them you will get the extra motivation you need to continue toward your ultimate goal.

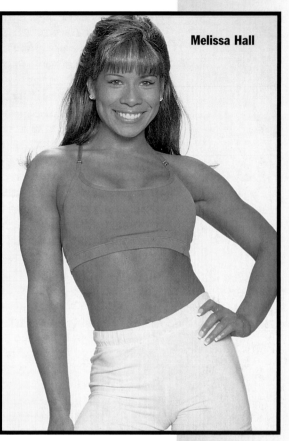

Melissa Hall

Q I have been training for a few years now and have dropped a fair amount of weight. I'm just a little anxious about gaining it back. How do I keep the weight off?

A I'm assuming you used a combination of proper diet and exercise to lose the weight. Congratulations on your success! To keep the weight off the answer is to follow a maintenance diet. You can use the diet that helped you lose the weight, but make a few changes. Two or three times a week don't be afraid to splurge with your favorite lunch or dessert. Don't get carried away and have both! I have found that consistency helps me maintain my weight year round.

Q I have heard so much about circuit training but I don't totally understand it. Could you explain the concept for me? As well, do you ever use it?

A Circuit training is designed to increase muscle endurance, yet is equally good at helping you lose fat and tone your muscles. You can train your whole body or just select muscle groups. A total circuit routine is composed of one exercise per bodypart. The exercises are performed back-to-back, with no rest between movements.

I use circuit training sporadically in my regimen. For example, when I was home for a week during the Christmas holidays, I wanted to spend as much time as possible with my family as well as visit friends and finish my shopping. Therefore knowing I had to exercise I chose a whole-body circuit-training routine. I performed five circuits with only a three-minute rest period between each.

I worked out every other day, giving myself an hour and 15 minutes to complete my routine. Circuit training is a great way to add variety to your workouts. It can be used when time is limited or as a way of getting back into weight training after a brief layoff.

Q I think I am typical in that my hips and thighs are an inch wider than I want them to be. I would really like to minimize the fat stores in these areas, but I'm not willing to incur the costs associated with eating too little. Can it be done?

A Welcome to the club. Probably every second letter I receive addresses this concern. Unfortunately I have both good news and bad news for you.
The bad news – that's life! I know that sounds harsh, but the reason I get so many letters about the hip, buttock and thigh area is because 95 percent of the female population has the same grievance. The reason? That's just where women store bodyfat. Our hormones and genetics are responsible. Until menopause, our fat has the greatest tendency to head south. Men conversely store excess fat in the stomach and chest regions. Now this might be better for thong bikini bottoms but no so good for the heart.

The good news – the picture isn't totally bleak! You *can* change the shape of your body, but it takes hard work. I wish I could give you a simple answer but sculpting the body you want is like creating a piece of art – it takes patience and skill. Here's how you do it:

1. Try lots of cardio and a low-fat diet. These two things go hand in hand as the most important factors for fat loss. Bring your cardio up to five times a week and cut the obvious fats from your diet.

2. Use heavier weights for your upper body. The biggest complaint I hear from women who are successful at losing weight is that it disappears everywhere, not just from their lower half – leaving them looking stringy on top. You can offset this imbalance by building your lats and shoulders.

3. Use higher reps during your lower-body exercises. Skip heavy weights for your bottom half. Try sets of 20 to 50 reps using light weights. This will keep good muscle tone in the area without adding to muscle size.

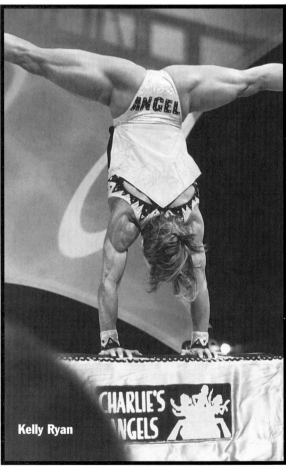

Kelly Ryan

Q I am 22 years old and I have been seriously working out for two years. I want to take my training goals in a new direction and focus on competing in a regional fitness show. My biggest fear isn't training or diet, it's *stage fright.* How am I going to perform a dance routine in front of hundreds of strangers? Do you have advice as to how newcomers can overcome this phobia?

A Every time I compete I feel nervous energy right before I walk onstage. This is a common reaction among competitors, especially when competing for the first time. Practice is your only saving grace when it comes to stage fright. Try to arrange a small group of family and friends to attend one of your practice sessions. This is an easy way to get used to having an audience since they are familiar faces who are there to support you. You could also try going through your routine in front of several gym members. Any practice technique you can come up with will help you feel more at ease onstage.

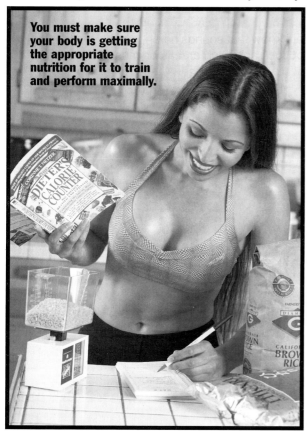

You must make sure your body is getting the appropriate nutrition for it to train and perform maximally.

Q How does a fitness competitor organize her dietary intake when preparing for a competition without sacrificing energy and strength? Should I keep a constant calorie intake from 12 weeks out, or is it better to slowly cut my calories? Should my proportions of carbs, proteins and fat stay the same as I diet down?

A You must make sure your body is getting the appropriate nutrition for it to train and perform maximally. I decided to hire a nutritionist – Cathy Sassin of Intrafit – to help manipulate my competition diet. Not only did Cathy help me get in the leanest shape I've ever been in, but I did it without sacrificing any lean muscle tissue and my energy level was great throughout the entire 12 weeks. It is important to get professional nutritional counseling because every body is different.

As I get closer to the competition date, I slowly increase my calories and my proportions change slightly. The *slow* change allows my body to adjust to the modification so I never shock my body's nutritional needs.

Q I have read that the best method for fat-burning is lower-intensity aerobics for a longer duration. My goal is to lose weight, but I don't always have the time to train for long periods. Do you have any suggestions for those of us on the run?

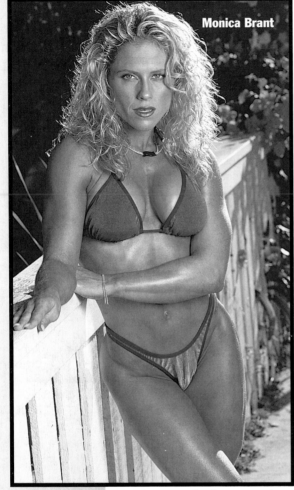

Monica Brant

A If you only have a limited time to train, step up the intensity of your workouts. Turn your jog into a run, walk on an incline, or interval train. By increasing the intensity of your training, you'll burn more calories (therefore more fat) in less time. Lifting weights will also help because it will speed up your metabolism.

Q Do you have any suggestions for preventing weight gain in someone with Graves disease? I recently had my thyroid radiated and now take regular does of Synthroid. Unfortunately the weight just keeps coming on. I eat healthy and exercise, but I am getting very discouraged. Please help.

A Beyond eating a healthful balanced diet and exercising regularly, there is little advice I have to give. Bare in mind that prior to your diagnosis it was probably very difficult for you to maintain your weight. The eating and exercising habits you developed during that period may no longer be appropriate. If you continue to gain weight, consult your endocrinologist to be certain the medication you are taking is sufficient in bringing your thyroid hormone levels to a normal range. It's not unusual for postirradiated thyroid function to continue to decline over the coming years; you may need to increase your Synthroid dose over time.

Q I am planning to start competing in fitness next year. My ultimate goal is to win the Fitness Olympia. What was it like to have your name announced as the winner? What is the best piece of advice for rookies like me?

A It is hard to put into words all the feelings and emotions I went through when my name was called as Ms. Fitness Olympia. I can say that it was the most rewarding experience I've ever had. Success is so much sweeter when you put your whole heart and soul into it.

The best advice I can give to anyone just starting out is to compile a written list of your goals and then design a plan on how to obtain them. Winning the Ms. Olympia does not happen overnight. It is best to establish smaller goals and treat them as stepping stones to your final goal. Remember to reward your-self for each step you've accomplished. Before you know it you'll be on your way to becoming the next Fitness Olympia champion.

Q I'm finding fitness competition very expensive by the time I pay a chore-ographer, have my costumes made, and travel to the events. I sure could use a good sponsor! I know you had a contract with Weider, and are now with GNC. How did you get these sponsors? What do you have to do for them? Do they pay well?

A It is always nice to have a sponsor when training for fitness competitions; however, sponsorships do not grow on trees. If you're just starting to compete, my best advice is to *get noticed.* Go to as many events as you can. Talk to people. You never know, one of these connections could lead to a possible contract. More than likely your first type of sponsorship may be with a supplement company that will provide you with free supplements.

   My best form of advertisement was taking part in the fitness competi-tions. This is where I was noticed. It takes time and persistence to get a large contract like Weider or GNC. I also have an agent who handles negotiations. Remember, your contacts are the key. The more people with whom you asso-ciate in the business the better your chances of being noticed.

   Once you are under contract make sure you are worth your weight in *gold.* Usually you'll be asked to do guest appear-ances, advertisements and photo shoots. All contracts are structured differently so your job description may vary from time to time. Payment and job requirements are all a mat-ter of negotiation.

Q I really admire you as an athlete and fitness competitor. You are a terrific role model for fitness wannabes like me. I was just wondering who your role mod-els were when you were starting out. Did one woman stand out?

A Thank you for your kind words. It has been a goal of mine to be a role model for women and men like yourself. When I first started training for fitness com-petitions my role model was *Mia Finnegan.* I admired her for her strength and athleticism. It is nice to have role models for encourage-ment in your training efforts. Sometimes that picture on the refrigerator or in the workout room can give us the little boost we all need once in a while.

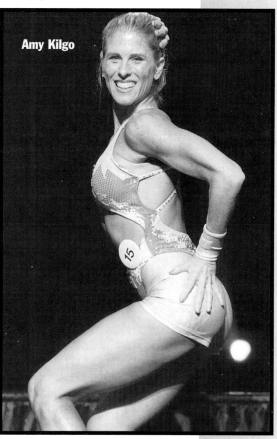

Amy Kilgo

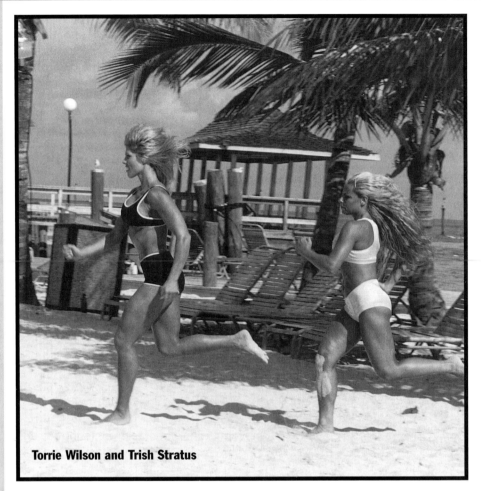

Torrie Wilson and Trish Stratus

Q As part of my cardio I enjoy jogging on the beach. But recently I experienced one of the most dreaded and painful sporting injuries possible – I strained my Achilles tendon. Has anything like that ever happened to you? What do you suggest for recovery? Do you have any advice to help prevent this from ever happening again?

A Fortunately I've never had an Achilles tendon injury. I know this type of setback is considered one of the worst due to the longevity of rehabilitation. The most important advice I have for you is to take it really slow and listen to your body. I would not recommend jogging until you're completely healed. I'm also a big fan of beach jogging; however, as with any high-impact sport, there's a lot of pressure applied to the Achilles tendon.

If you're really enthusiastic about training and will not consider rest as an option, try aqua therapy. Whether you swim for your aerobic training or water-jog laps in a pool due to buoyancy of your body in water, you will experience only 10 percent of your bodyweight on impact, in comparison to 100 percent on land. As far as preventing injuries like yours from occurring, my best advice is to make sure to thoroughly warm up.

Q What type of cardiovascular activity is best for burning fat while preparing for a fitness competition?

A Ask yourself what you like to do for aerobic activity. If you don't enjoy something, you're probably not going to do it. Almost every type of cardiovascular activity will burn fat, as long as it's done with consistency, proper training methods, and paired with a clean diet. The only two activities that will not help burn fat as efficiently are swimming and walking. Yes both burn calories but your body adapts to swimming by holding on to excess fat to help keep the body warm and buoyant. Leisure walking is also great for someone who wants a basic fitness program, but for competition training you need to train the heart muscle by maintaining a training heart rate for fat-burning.

Q I steam all my vegetables but I was told this takes away all the vitamins. Is this true? And if so, should I microwave them instead to preserve the nutrients?

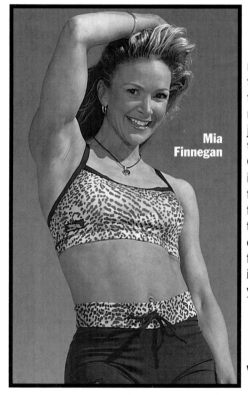

Mia Finnegan

A Whether you steam or microwave your vegetables you're going to lose some of the water-soluble vitamins such as B and C. Microwaving protects the vitamins a bit more, being that they cook more quickly, and with little or no water. Steaming vegetables in a basket just above water level with the lid on is the next best bet, but just until tender. Overcooking vegetables until they're soft is the main culprit in vitamin loss. My favorite preparation method is juicing fresh vegetables or eating them raw, so there is no chance of losing any of the essential vitamins. Be sure to use your fresh vegetables within four days of buying them to ensure no loss of vitamins in your refrigerator.

Q You have awesome abs! Even after having a baby you've got a flat tummy and still carry a six-pack. What's your secret?

A It takes three things to have great abs: regular crunch workouts, low bodyfat and regular cardiovascular training. Train hard, eat well and hop on the eliptical rider and you too can have a six-pack! Abdominal muscles can't show through until your bodyfat is low enough – for women this usually happens at about 16 percent. Think of it as making the perfect protein drink, just the right mixture of all ingredients, perfectly blended – and, *voila!*

Q I am interested in fitness modeling and am wondering how I go about this. I love fitness training and I follow a very strict low-fat, low-sugar diet. I believe you started your career with a Robert Kennedy swimsuit photo shoot. How do I go about getting in on something like this? I desperately want to succeed.

A Actually Bob (Kennedy) took a few test shots with a plain backdrop before he invited me to his swimsuit photo shoot in Nassau. I do know that he gets at least a hundred letters a week from fitness models and fitness model hopefuls. There is no reason why you shouldn't send him a few photographs. They don't have to be professional photos but they should give a clear indication of your body shape and facial appearance. Write Robert Kennedy, c/o of MuscleMag International, 5775 McLaughlin Rd., Mississauga, ON, Canada L5R 3P7.

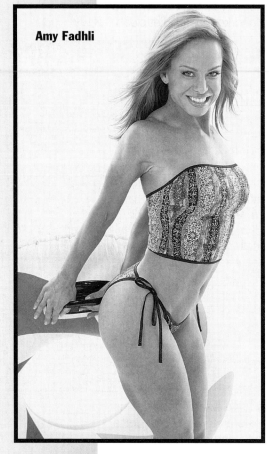

Amy Fadhli

Q I have "high calves." They are balled up just under my knee and I think they look downright ugly. I really want to have diamond-shaped calves. How do I go about it? I already perform loads of standing and seated calf raises but nothing seems to work. Help!

A There is nothing you can do short of implants or oil injections (neither is recommended) that will make much of a difference. Your natural lower leg shape is genetically predetermined. Regular calf raises (with weights) will help build the calf to a larger size, but you will not significantly alter the high calf shape that you have inherited.

Q I recently heard of a study that concluded that deep knee bends (squats) overstretch the tendons. Other people tell me squats will damage my knees and hip area. I have seen pictures of you squatting, so I know you believe in squats. Can you tell me your opinion on whether or not squats are a bad idea?

A Squats are necessary for those women who really need added size in their upper legs. Squats also contribute to building the glutes. Personally I do very few squats these days because my legs grow easily and I feel they are big enough. There are a few rules in squatting. Keep your back flat, head up, and squat down to just above parallel, controlling the weight as you lower. Never squat right down or bounce at the bottom of the exercise. This could definitely cause joint problems. Use common sense and good form and you should not suffer any ill effects.

Q I'm 18, having been athletic all my life thanks to eight years of gymnastics training. Now that I'm no longer competing, just training for fitness, my legs are toning down but still staying hard by using medium weight and high reps. My arms are the problem. They are nicely shaped but I want them to be more defined. My diet is good except for a cheat every once in a while. I would like to be Ms. Fitness America someday and a spokesmodel. I know I can do it if I persevere. I'm wondering if you have any advice to give me on how to do what you do. I think you are absolutely awesome!

A You're so young – and that's great. You have so much time. The fact that you have a gymnastics background will certainly help boost your competition career. The definition you are looking for in your arms will come with time and muscle maturity. Just continue training and keep your diet clean.

Q On a recent visit to my physician I learned that I need more fiber in my diet. What are the best food sources? Should I start to take fiber supplements? Do you have any suggestions?

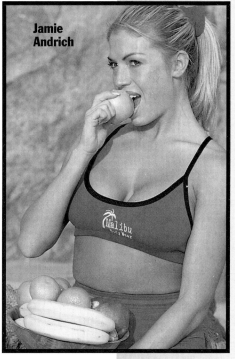

Jamie Andrich

A First of all consult your doctor. The physician who recommended you increase your fiber intake will likely have some dietary suggestions. According to the RDA your daily fiber intake should be 20 to 30 grams. This is not easy. Try to fill this requirement with whole natural foods. Fibrous fruits include: berries, grapefruit, oranges and dried fruit. Vegetables – such as green leafy lettuce, carrots, broccoli, cauliflower and potato skins – are also great choices. As for starchy carbs, go for 100 percent whole-wheat and whole-wheat grain breads and crackers, wheat germ, bran, oat bran, brown rice and beans.

Q I have given birth twice. As a result I have terrible stretch marks across my abdomen. I would like to compete in fitness but the swimsuits are so low cut. Do you have any suggestions for camouflaging them?

A Believe it or not, many top fitness competitors have stretch marks. And it's so easy to remedy. Go to any large department store and ask for a product called *Dermablend*. It is the best for covering scars, burns and stretch marks. There are a variety of shades to match your skin color. It's even waterproof. You can even use it at the pool or beach. Just be sure to match the Dermablend shade to your competition skin color.

Q I first saw you in a *MuscleMag International* swimsuit issue over two years ago. You always look so vibrant. Do you run outside as part of your training, or do you prefer a treadmill? Who among the fitness stars of today actually runs for conditioning (as opposed to using cardio equipment like treadmills or step machines)?

A Most fitness women seem to prefer the machines. They are often kinder to the knees. Actually I was a competitive runner and hurdler for years before I got into a traditional fitness program. Now I prefer to use treadmills and step machines, especially in bad weather, but I have no qualms about street running or beach running. Running in the gym is motivating since so many others are doing it too – but training outdoors in the fresh air is more exhilarating.

Q I need bowling-ball glutes. Right now my backside is too soft and flat. I notice most of the fitness women I see in magazines have nice, rounded firm glutes. Please help me!

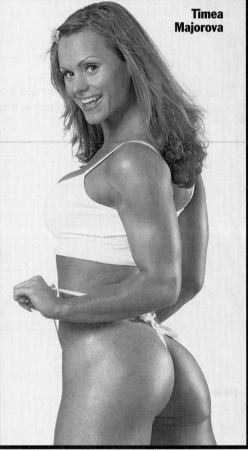

Timea
Majorova

A The best exercise for the glutes is the full squat, but beware of overdoing it. Full squats can build other areas of the hips, which may detract from your appearance (especially if you are inclined to be wide in the hip region). My personal favorite is the walking lunge. Hold a five-pound dumbell in each hand and step into a lunge with your right leg so that your left knee is almost touching the floor. Then immediately step forward with your left leg so that your right knee is only a few inches from the floor. Try 20 reps (10 paces per leg).

Q I am preparing for my first fitness competition. Many of my training mates have stopped eating dairy products for fear of looking smooth. My goal is to get leaner, and I don't want to be at a disadvantage. However I am afraid of becoming deficient in calcium. Other than supplements, do you have any suggestions for supplementing my diet?

A Did you know that calcium is the fifth most plentiful substance in the body? It is crucial for the development of strong bones, prevention of osteoporosis, energy production, and maintenance of a healthy immune system. I'm glad to see you are concerned with getting your daily recommended dosage (FDA recommends 1000 mg per day for men and women between 19 and 50 years of age). My diet doesn't include a lot of dairy so I make sure to eat additional foods that also contain high amounts of calcium, such as tofu, grains, some juices, almonds and green leafy vegetables. However, you should always take a good daily multivitamin.

Q Eight months ago I lost 40 pounds through changed eating habits and exercise. I walk an hour every day, weight train three days a week, and take Tae-Bo classes. My upper body is toned and my calves are hard, but I need to focus on my thighs and glutes. I work out at home, so my equipment is limited. What are your suggestions?

A Congratulations on your amazing turnaround. Losing weight is the hardest part, so you definitely have the motivation to continue the healthy lifestyle you have started. I suggest adding lower-body circuits to your workout. Many movements require minimal equipment – squats, lunges, step-ups, butt-blasters and plies. Keep your reps high (15 to 20), your rest periods short, and make sure you are focused and in control at all times. As you become stronger, increase the reps and the speed of the movements. Not only will circuit training help to define the muscles in your thighs and glutes, but it will improve your aerobic capacity and burn calories.

Q Step classes are one of my favorite forms of exercise. I am usually exhausted when I finish, but I've always wanted to know if "step" is an effective fat-burning workout.

A Group exercise is an awesome way to burn fat. Dancing to great music and feeding off the energy of an instructor and other members can really make your workout time fly by. In preparing for contests I have taken many aerobics classes. Making yourself aware of your heart rate during exercise is the best way to determine how effectively you are burning fat. You should be training at a minimum of 65 percent of your maximum heart rate. My heart rate is usually extremely high in fitness classes, so reaching this minimum is rarely a problem. Avoid overexerting yourself at the beginning of the class so that you can keep your intensity strong throughout.

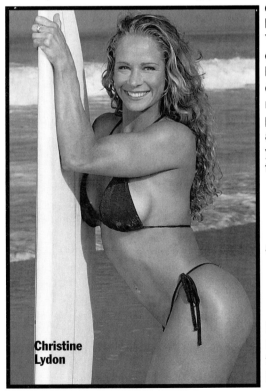

Christine Lydon

Q I have a problem with ingrown hairs due to bikini waxing. How can I solve this eyesore, along with the irritation it causes?

A Understanding why ingrown hairs occur will help prevent them. When waxing the hair is pulled from the root. A new hair must develop, which is weaker at the tip than the cut hair. When the skin is dry, and/or you have dead skin buildup, the hair is not strong enough to come through. This causes it to curl back into the skin, leading to irritation and possible infection. The end result is a red bump that looks like a pimple. To prevent ingrown hairs, regularly use a loofah and/or a fine scrub to exfoliate while in the shower.

Q I've been sticking to a pretty clean diet and training consistently but I think I have hit a plateau with my weight/fat loss. Should I change my diet, my workouts, or both? What do you suggest?

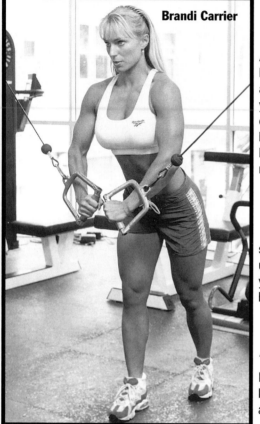

Brandi Carrier

A When you hit a plateau use the process of elimination. Change one factor at a time; that way you'll know which one was causing the problem. Ask yourself the following questions. When and how hard do you train with weights? When and how intense are your cardiovascular workouts? Do you eat before you work out? Are you eating afterward? What are you eating and when? All these factors must be addressed before you can determine why you've hit a plateau and how to move past it. Most of the time nutrition plays the most significant role.

Q Do you believe in the Zone diet and eating the 40-30-30 way? Ever since I started eating this way my bodyfat has risen about 5 percent. I'm now struggling to get my fat percentage down to where it used to be. I do cardio and weights six days a week. Can you please give me some advice on how to lower my bodyfat and lose excess fat in my lower abs and hips?

A No, I don't believe in the Zone diet; and it sounds as if you wish you hadn't either. I shudder to think what would happen to my body if I tried that diet. In order to maintain my shape, I try to adhere to the following: 45 percent carbohydrates, 40 percent protein, and 15 percent fat.

Sounds like you have the training and dedication part down. I'm sorry the Zone diet failed you. I think you know what it will take to get those unfortunate pounds off – continued consistent cardio, and a fat- and calorie-restricted diet for a while.

You want some ideas for toning the hips and lower abs? Try kickboxing. I don't think you'll find another form of exercise that works the entire body so effectively. Most classes end with ab and leg work too.

Q For the past few years I've worked out regularly and tried to keep my diet healthy. Lately I have become interested in competing in fitness. I feel I've been blessed with good genetics to help me build a solid physique. What level of commitment must one make in order to prepare for a fitness show – novice or pro?

A Many people don't realize the time and dedication that goes into preparing for any level of fitness competition until they actually compete. Most think that a competitor must spend hours in the gym. In actuality a large proportion of her time is spent grocery shopping, preparing meals, tanning, manicures, pedicures, selecting a competition suit to best exemplify her physique, working on stage presence, choreography and gymnastic practice. As you can see, if you choose to compete, it is not just a part-time hobby.

Q I am an aspiring fitness competitor and have been challenged by random sports injuries ranging from a sprained ankle to a strained shoulder. How do you deal with these types of setbacks, and have you ever experienced any sports-related injuries?

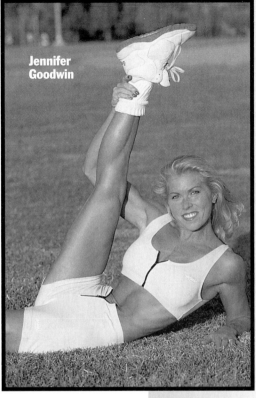

Jennifer Goodwin

A I have been blessed – no major injuries in my lifetime. However, due to all my gymnastics practice sessions, I have developed terrible pains in my wrists. There have been several times when I have had to cancel a private lesson because of pain. It is definitely an overuse problem. Fortunately when I allow myself enough rest, the pain subsides.

One great preventative measure is to allow enough time for stretching. You are less likely to pull or strain flexible muscles than tight ones. During weight-bearing activities, I make sure I lift only the amount of weight I know my body can handle. A gradual increase in weight resistance is a far more effective way of increasing muscular strength. It's also imperative to allow yourself adequate time for a proper warmup and cooldown.

Q I have noticed that several people in the gym are talking about the so-called fat-burner supplements. What is your opinion on these fat-loss aids? And if you recommend them, when and how do you add them to your diet and exercise program?

A Because I'm not a medical professional, I would recommend you consult your physician before sampling any supplements. As far as the general population is concerned, not everybody gets the same benefits from using these stimulants. There is such a large variety, including ephedra, aspirin, guarana root, caffeine and many others. You must be cautious and choose one that's healthy for you. I've found that these fat-loss aids help out when my natural fat loss plateaus. Keep in mind that most of these fat-loss aids are nothing more than appetite suppressants. They keep you from cheating, and may also provide you with extra energy. I have had the most success taking them 30 minutes prior to doing cardio. Make sure you don't take them too late in the afternoon since they might prevent you from falling asleep.

Q I'm getting married this winter and am working hard to get and stay in the best shape of my life. I'm currently weight training three or four days a week. If you could give three helpful guidelines for starting a fat-loss program, what would they be?

A My first piece of advice would be to clean up your diet. Start eating smaller, healthier, more frequent meals. Next, try to include some form of sustained moderate aerobic activity for a minimum of 25 minutes. Slowly increase your aerobic training time by five minutes every third session, but don't exceed 60 minutes. For motivation, go through fitness magazines and choose a mentor who best exemplifies your desired fitness look. Post the photo on your mirror at home. This will remind you of your goals and keep you focused on achieving success.

Q I have been weight training and exercising for over ten years and I always hear women in the gym saying they want to lose just five more pounds. What is your advice for getting rid of the final five?

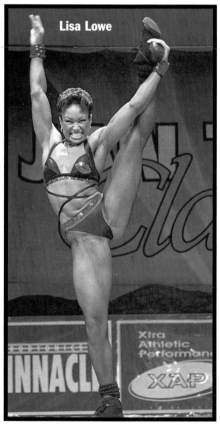

Lisa Lowe

A Losing weight boils down to one simple equation: calories consumed minus calories burned equals *you!* Naturally if you eat more than you burn, then you'll forever be gaining weight. Obviously exercise is the first step to increasing the amount of calories expended. Most people are horrified when they hear the word *diet.* But there are simple methods of reducing your caloric intake without drastically changing the way you eat. For example, serve yourself sauces or dressings on the side, so that you're inclined to use less. Try to reduce the amount of simple carbs you eat, especially in the evening. Instead of eating sugar or flour you might find more success with complex carbs like rice, potatoes, oats or yams. It might take a while before you see changes, but if you make eating healthy a lifestyle, you will find it easier to stay at a consistent weight.

Q I've competed in five competitions within the past year and placed in the top five each time – but I've never won. How do I stay motivated and not let it get me down?

A We are only disappointed when our expectations aren't met. Women who compete must have a realistic understanding of their personal potential. You must go into a competition simply determined to do your best. Remember, you're not competing against anyone but yourself. If your best doesn't place you high, or as high as you wish, you must examine your performance to determine how to make it better. I don't recommend anyone take part in a competition to win. Do it to learn about yourself, nutrition, motivation and goal-setting. Winning is simply icing on the cake.

Q My body lacks shape and definition. I appear big and chunky. When people meet me for the first time they refer to me as "big and strong," but they never say I have a great body. How can I give "eye appeal" to my bod?

A Eye appeal comes from a variety of aspects, not the least of which is your overall deportment. Stand and sit straight at all times. An eye-catching body also comes from shape training. Work your weak points hard. Women who have a low bodyfat percentage also tend to stand out. Diet and exercise your fat away to release the charismatic beauty of your physique. Fat hides curves and it's a women's natural curves that are truly stunning.

Q Is it possible to catch pink eye by touching germy gym equipment?

A Yep, it sure is. Pink eye or conjunctivitis, is characterized by redness, swelling and a mucous or mucopurulent discharge from one or both eyes. The bacteria most commonly responsible for pink eye, haemophilus aegytius, is highly transmittable. Follow a few very simple rules of thumb and you will avoid exposing yourself to contagious gym entities.
1. Never touch your eyes, nose or mouth in the gym.
2. Wash your hands with an antibacterial soap after your workout.
3. Wear flip-flops in the locker room, shower and sauna to "sidestep" fungal infection.

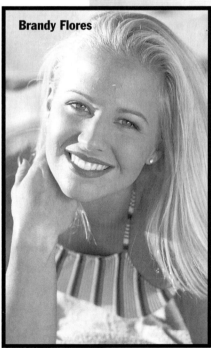
Brandy Flores

Q I'm in the best shape of my life. I realize it's too hard for me to remain this lean (only 10 percent bodyfat) year round. I would like to have professional photos taken so I can remember my lean days. Do you have any suggestions for me in preparation for the photo shoot?

A Doesn't it feel great to be in your best shape ever? Congratulations on some serious hard work. I definitely recommend having your pictures done so you'll always have proof of your dedication to fitness.

Your body will look even better if you have the right tan. If you can't get out in the sun try a tanning salon. Although tanning beds are bad for your skin, using them a few times to get a base is a good idea. The night before a photo shoot I apply a coat of Jan Tana Self Tanner evenly on my body. If I am still not dark enough I use Jan Tana Bronzer. And then at the photo shoot, I'll use Neutrogena Dry Body Oil to give my skin a radiant glow. A good makeup job is also very important for photo success. Make sure your face makeup matches your body color. Depending on the nature of the shoot, I usually go for a fresh, natural look.

Q I am thinking about having collagen injections for my lips. Have you ever had this done? What do you think about it?

A No, I'm proud to say I was blessed with my mom's genes for plump lips. What do I think about it? I've seen a few great results but more bad ones! It seems either the surgeon, the patient, or both have a warped sense of what looks natural. Too much collagen is injected, causing a lumpy, fish-lipped appearance. I'm not opposed to this procedure, I'm opposed to the abuse of it. Research your options. Talk to a woman who's had it done and choose a plastic surgeon whose work you approve of.

Q I need your advice. I know you have a lot of guys always hounding you. I'm sure you know how to deal with the pesky ones. There is a mentally challenged teenager at my gym who constantly bothers me. He'll come over to say hello and then just stand there. It makes me feel awkward since I don't know what to say. What should I do?

A Please have some compassion. The guy probably just has a crush on you. As long as he's not a threat, what is creating a little light conversation going to cost you? Ask him what bodypart he's training, how his day is going, that kind of thing. When you're ready to move on, let him know it was nice seeing him again, but you need to start another set and you're running late. Trust me, it will be good for your soul.

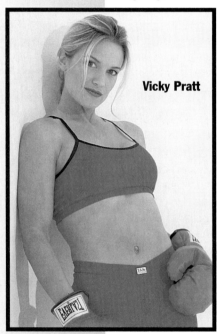

Vicky Pratt

Q I have an artificial leg and have been working out for two years. I am in good shape but since I cannot run on the treadmill, I'm unable to get that slim look. What other types of cardio do you recommend for me?

A There are so many other ways you can tighten your body. Your gym or rehab facility may have an upper-body ergometer. It's like a stationary cycle for the upper body. The pedals are at arms' length and around chest height. Boxing is another awesome cardiovascular workout and it also has toning effects on your arms, chest, back and waist.

Q I have been training for two months now and there's some improvement, but my calves are still too small. How do I increase the size of my calf muscles? Besides calf raises what other exercises can I do? These don't work at all on my stubborn calves?

A Even my best bodyparts didn't respond to training for four to six months. If your calves are your weakest bodypart, two months is not near enough time. To be honest with you, everyone responds differently. I would add some donkey calf raises to your standing and seated raises. Train your calves twice a week for six months and see if they respond. If not, train them every other day for the next six months.

Q I have recently taken up spinning. I really love the workout I get – it's so intense. But I find that my toes go numb halfway through the class. How important are those special cyclist shoes with the clips?

A I love the intense workout of spinning as well. In regard to shoes, they are imperative if you want the full benefits a spinning session can offer. Unlike the cages that are used for a tennis shoe on the pedals, a shoe with a clip helps distribute your weight centrally as opposed to your toe region. Continuous pressure on your toes is what makes them numb. The special shoes also help place more resistance on the outer sweep of the quads as well as the hams and glutes. I suggest you invest in the shoes and spin away.

Q I notice that many of the back programs include chinups and most triceps routines include dips. I see guys are able to do these exercises without difficulty, yet when I try them I can't even do one rep. Do you have any suggestions to help me develop the strength to perform these exercises?

A Women are generally weaker in the upper body than men. But with a friendly hand you'll soon be doing these exercises on your own too. I recommend having your training partner or a person with some spare time spot you by cradling your ankles in his or her hands. This way you can use your legs to help you lift your body doing chins and dips. After a few weeks you'll have built your strength enough to attempt the lifts on your own. You'll be surprised at how fast this technique works.

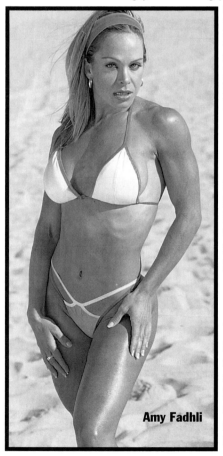

Amy Fadhli

Q This is very much an embarrassing question but because of your well-published history in this area, I figured you would be the perfect person to ask advice from. About a year ago I had my breasts augmented. The incisions were made around the nipples. They became slightly keloid. Is there anything that can be done?

A You can ask your plastic surgeon or dermatologist about laser scar removal. It works quite well but can be expensive. A more conservative approach is the new soft gel-filled silicone cushions that provide topical therapy for the healing of scars. I have seen The Clinical by Life Medical Sciences Inc. widely advertised. You can ask your plastic surgeon to recommend a brand.

Q I have a sweet tooth. What can I do to curb my cravings?

A Believe me I know how you feel! I have sweet cravings too. I sometimes try to satisfy them during one of my meals. For example if rice is part of my meal, I sprinkle Equal sweetener on it. This works great on oatmeal and Cream of Wheat too. If that does not do the trick, I reach for sugar-free Popsicles and eat one for dessert. Another great idea is sugar-free, fat-free instant pudding made with skim milk. If you like yogurt, try the low-sugar, non-fat version that comes in a variety of great flavors. When dining out, if you must have dessert, only eat half. This takes discipline – especially if there's nobody around to eat the other half! If this is the case have the server take away half before you start in on your dessert.

As you can see, you can give in to your sweet cravings, but you still have to show some willpower. If you make the right choices they will pay off in the way you look and feel.

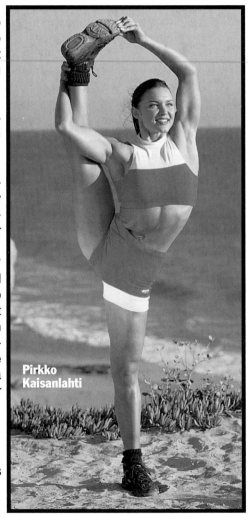

Pirkko
Kaisanlahti

Q I know flexibility is an important element in fitness routines. How can I improve?

A As well as being an important element in fitness routines, flexibility and stretching are vital for your overall wellness. The only way to improve your flexibility is to stretch on a regular basis.

Why is stretching so important? Stretching increases flexibility, which will reduce injuries during training and can also lead to improved athletic performance. It allows for a greater range of motion within the joints, and more flexible joints can withstand greater stress and impact. To improve flexibility, stretch at least three times a week. Here are some points to remember while stretching.
• Never stretch a cold muscle.
• Don't bounce.
• Avoid holding your breath.
• Avoid stretching a muscle beyond its normal range of motion.
• Avoid severe/painful stretching.

Q I am seriously interested in becoming a personal trainer. Please give me some information on where to get the training material and how I go about getting certified.

A There are quite a few personal training certification programs available today. My advice would be to try the yellow pages, ads in health and fitness magazines, and ask other trainers about the organization that certified them and what they thought of the program. Many of the courses consist of at-home study and then an exam is held several times a year in major cities around the country. Keep in mind you need your own transportation to and from the exam and maybe even accommodations.

Q Do I really need vitamin and mineral supplements when preparing for competition? If so, which ones are best for me?

A I am a big advocate of getting most of your vitamins and minerals from whole food sources, but in this day and age there is lots of research indicating that our food supplies are being grown in mineral-depleted soil. Keeping that in mind, food is still my number one choice. But if you're on a restrictive diet, such as the kind followed by bodybuilders and fitness competitors, you'll definitely need to supplement due to the potential lack of nutrients you are ingesting. Vegetarians and those who don't eat meat or dairy foods may also need extra calcium, iron, zinc and vitamin B12.

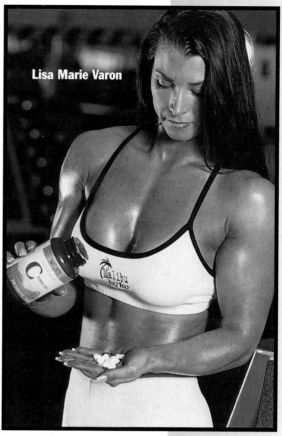

Lisa Marie Varon

Q I have excessive facial hair. What can I do to get rid of it for good?

A You should understand that many women have this problem. According to the AMA, facial hair can be caused by excessive androgen hormone production, which is naturally produced by our bodies. Even with normal levels of androgen some women tend to get stimulated hair growth due to their hair follicles being more sensitive to the hormone.

There are both cosmetic and medical solutions to the problem. Check with your physician for the latest medical treatments. Be sure to ask about any adverse side effects from a medication, and tell your doctor about any allergies you may have just in case.

There are a number of useful cosmetic treatments: bleaching, plucking, waxing, electrolysis and sugaring. These methods will probably handle the problem without any side effects.

Q I really love lifting weights. However, lately my shoulder has been acting up. This is really putting limitations on my workouts. Do you know anything about shoulder therapy?

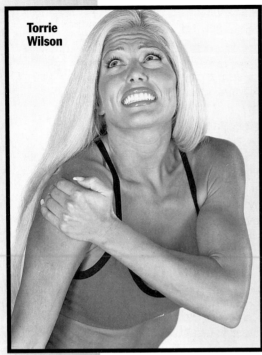

Torrie Wilson

A Shoulder discomfort is quite common when I'm training. Because I am weight training and taking gymnastics lessons, my rotator cuff gets inflamed, causing pain and discomfort in my shoulder. This pain is a signal that lets me know something is wrong and it's time to take action. Usually it starts when you are pushing more weight than your rotator cuff can handle. I treat my shoulder with rest and ice before any severe injury occurs. I also perform specific rotator cuff and scapular strengthening exercises. A good physiotherapist can show you the right moves. The key is to address the problem early before it gets serious and causes further injuries to the shoulder.

Q I have always been so impressed with your smile. How do you keep your teeth so white?

A Years ago when I was a dental hygienist, new home bleaching systems had just been introduced to the general public. I experimented with them and got the results you see today. I suggest you visit your dentist. He or she should be able to get you started on a home bleaching treatment. I do not suggest you purchase an over-the-counter system. They are not prescription strength. If you have any veneers, crowns or bonding on your front teeth, the bleaching will not be effective. There are ways around this, but you will have to discuss them with your dentist.

Q I've been spinning four or five times a week, and while I'm noticing my legs and rear have become firmer, my quads have become very thick. What can I do to maintain the firmness but reduce the thickness of my thighs?

A I cannot stress enough the importance of cross-training. I suggest two days per week to maintain your leg and glute firmness. Try jogging three days a week as well. My legs looked their best when I followed this regimen. They were hard, lean and compact.

Q My boyfriend recently broke up with me and I have been really depressed. I have lost a lot of weight and can't seem to get motivated to go to the gym. I admire your dedication. How do you keep so motivated even when times are hard?

A The best therapy for depression is to focus on yourself. Set a realistic goal to better your body. This requires dedication and forces you to think about what you need to do rather than what you used to do with him. Pursue your goal. This will surely take your mind off your troubles, not to mention your ex will probably be kicking himself when he sees your brand new body and your new aura of confidence.

Q I am planning for my first fitness competition. I eat a fairly clean diet, and my bodyfat fluctuates between 14 and 16 percent. How far out from an event do you start to seriously diet down?

A How far out you start your diet depends on how lean and fit your body is to start with. For me 12 weeks out works best. Crash diets are hard on the body. Three months is long enough to allow my body to healthfully adjust to a decreased caloric intake. As the contest time draws closer, I manipulate my food proportions – protein, carbs, fat – and the amount of calories in order to achieve my desired results.

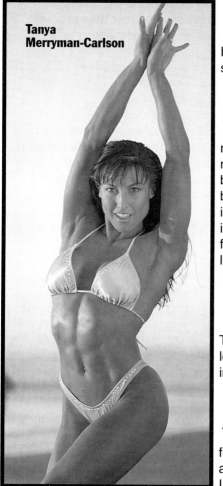

Tanya Merryman-Carlson

Q I started weight training three years ago. I try to vary my workouts, and in doing so have achieved some great results. How much rest do you suggest I take between sets and different exercises?

A Determining your rest time depends on your training goals. Since my focus is to maintain muscle while getting leaner, many of my workouts are supersets with minimal rest between movements. Giving your body less rest forces you to increase the aerobic component of your workout. But if your goal is to increase muscle mass, I recommend taking a longer rest so your muscles have time to fully recover, thereby increasing your ability to lift maximum weight.

Q I'm preparing for my first fitness competition. I have organized everything from my training schedule to outfit design. The only thing undecided is how to style my long hair. Do the judges prefer hair that's flowing or pulled back into an up-do?

A How you wear your hair is definitely a personal preference. Choose whichever style makes you feel beautiful and confident. When I compete I like to wear my hair in a variety of ways. In the 1998 Fitness Olympia I wore my hair in pig tails during the routine round. The most important thing is not to let your hair cover up your beautiful body, especially during the physique round. If you wear your hair down, when the judges ask you for your half- and quarter-turns, remember to pull it away from your back and shoulders so they can get a full view of your musculature. Also, try to keep your hair out of your face during your performance. The crowd likes to see your smile, don't cover it up.

Q Why does creatine supplementation require a loading phase? Wouldn't five grams postworkout be effective without the five to seven days of loading?

A Creatine requires a loading phase in order to rapidly raise intracellular levels to a threshold amount, which has scientifically been proven to have a significant impact on muscle metabolism. Even without the loading phase you would eventually enjoy the same results; but it would take a couple of months, rather than a week, to complete the intracellular saturation process and start building muscle.

Q I've had stretch marks on my inner and outer thighs since I was 12 years old. I've never been overweight; in fact I was too thin growing up. The stretch marks have faded with age, but they are still noticeable. Is there any way to get rid of them? I want to wear shorts without worrying about what people think.

A We are our own worst enemies when it comes to body perception. I strongly suspect the faded stretch marks aren't noticeable to anyone but you. That being said, there are few treatment options for stretch marks. Creams, lotions and even laser treatments are largely ineffective for long-standing stretch marks. Microdermabrasion is a relatively painless and affordable procedure which may yield more satisfactory results. It's a relatively new technique that utilizes tiny silica particles to exfoliate the first few layers of the dermis. For more information consult your dermatologist.

Q Four months ago I began a more intense workout program and changed my diet. Ever since then my menstrual cycle has varied from eight days early to three weeks late. Could my change in training be the cause?

A Irregular cycles may be a nuisance but they don't necessarily indicate a medical problem. Environmental factors such as stress (physical or mental) are a common cause of elongated cycles and occasional missed periods, so is menopause in middle-aged women. Unless your menses are more than three months apart, you aren't at risk of uterine hyperplasia (an abnormal thickening of the uterine lining) and its associated health risk. If you are troubled by the irregularity, the birth control pill will regulate your cycles.

Q My photos have been sent to all of the major fitness and bodybuilding magazines, but I'm still not getting any calls for photo shoots or guest appearances. I think I have the right look for fitness modeling. Would it help to get an agent or manager? Do you have a manager?

A Persistence is my best advice for fitness modeling. Go to as many competitions and meet as many people as possible. Remember to have your pictures available at all times. The more contacts you make in the fitness industry the better your chances of making the right connection.

Whether or not to hire a manager is your decision. Make sure you interview several candidates to see which one will work the hardest for you. Get references and check them out. Hire a manager with good credentials — somebody who has your best interests at heart. A good manager works for you, not the other way around.

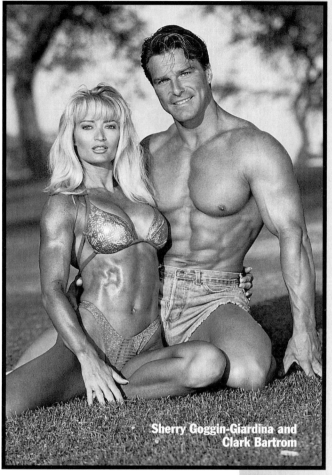

Sherry Goggin-Giardina and Clark Bartrom

Q I recently started going to a gym. I love weight training but I do not want to develop a V-shape back like some of the fitness women I see in *Oxygen.* I think it looks too masculine, and I already have a boyish figure with narrow hips. How do I keep my back from getting that V-shaped tapered appearance without giving up my workouts?

A Exercises that build the latissimus dorsi (lats) which contribute to a V-shape are chinups, pulldowns, seated rows, and barbell and dumbell rows. That said, please reconsider why you are against the tapered appearance. Most fitness women aim to increase their V-taper. I feel that a tapered back, running down to a small waist and tight hips, is extremely attractive. Virtually every man I know thinks the same.

Q I have been trying to lose bodyfat by dieting and doing aerobics. My schedule is crazy so I can't exercise at the same time every day. Will this affect my results?

A I usually do my aerobics first thing in the morning before breakfast. This is a great time for cardio because the body is slightly depleted from not eating anything during the last eight hours. You will burn more fat and get the blood moving for the rest of the day.

Q I can't seem to lose that last five pounds. Do you have any suggestions?

A I am assuming you are on a precontest diet and have been training for some time. Maybe your diet isn't working as well as it was in the beginning. When I diet for competition, my metabolism sometimes hits a plateau. To kick it back into high gear, I shock it by eating anything I want for a day. I know that seems unreasonable, but if you've been dieting strictly for too long, your body adapts to what you're feeding it and stops responding. It merely utilizes the amount of food it is accustomed to and maintains its current state of metabolism. You need your metabolism to fire up and start burning your body's fat stores for fuel instead of the food you are feeding it. It's almost like you are tricking your body. After that day of off-diet nutrition, get right back on your precontest program and your metabolism should start flying again.

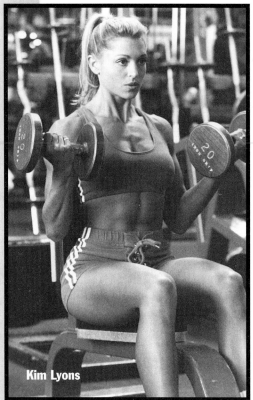

Kim Lyons

Q Due to my crazy work and family schedules, I am only able to go to the gym three times per week. What is the best combination of weight training and cardio to maximize my limited workout time?

A I would suggest dividing your resistance training into three sections – for example lower body one day, chest and arms the next, and on the last day back and shoulders. Perform at least three different exercises for each bodypart, so that you can train each muscle with a variety of grips, angles and movements. Weight training should take you 30 to 40 minutes per day. This allows sufficient time for stretching, cardio and abdominal-training. Continue this pattern for at least six weeks. At this time add variety to your regular routine to prevent your body from reaching a plateau.

You can get results by working out three times a week. Just make sure you maximize your time in the gym, and make every workout as efficient as possible.

Q I'm a workout fanatic! I love to participate in all kinds of sports, but recently I've noticed that my back's been hurting me. What can I do to alleviate the pain?

A Athleticism is great for your body, but you must properly warm up and stretch before any activity. Many people neglect the importance of flexibility. Before I weight train or do gymnastics I make sure my muscles are fully warmed up. I walk or ride the bike for a few minutes and then spend about five to 10 minutes stretching my major muscles. After doing any sport, it's extremely important to "cool down" and stretch all your muscles again. Stretching classes like martial arts and yoga can teach you the different stretches and how to do them properly. I also think it's important to get a sports massage regularly. This type of therapy helps relax tight muscles, and break up any knots you might have developed. Also make sure you take a day off from exercising every week so your muscles can repair.

Q I'm 27 years old and I just started weight training. The changes I'm noticing are exciting but I'm losing a lot of my flexibility. What do you suggest?

A Flexibility is an important element in any fitness program. It should be part of the focus in all of your workouts. Take a few minutes to stretch when you're finished training (when your muscles and joints are warm). If you have a training partner, you can perform deep stretching movements a few times a week. If you don't have someone, taking a yoga or Pilates class on a regular basic will help you stay limber.

Q I heard that rubbing Preparation H onto my thighs and wrapping them in cellophane overnight will make them smaller. Is this true?

A If that were true, sales for cellophane would be booming. Preparation H is a vasoconstrictor used to decrease the swelling of hemorrhoids. If you rubbed it on your legs and covered them with plastic, the vasoconstrictor may pull water from the epidermis, which would make the skin on the legs appear tighter. However, this effect is only temporary. The only way to truly have shapelier legs is to train consistently and eat healthy.

Q I want to compete in a fitness show but the only thing holding me back is having to do a fitness routine. I'm very athletic but I'm not a dancer. I certainly don't want to look stupid. What can I do?

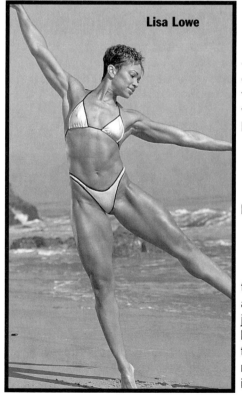

Lisa Lowe

A The best thing you can do is hire a choreographer. Once upon a time I felt the same way you do, then I discovered that working with someone makes a big difference. A choreographer can help you put together a routine featuring your strengths, which will not only make you look your best, but also help release some of that anxiety.

Q I am looking for a new way to fill my daily protein requirements. Are beef jerky and turkey jerky good sources of protein? Are they good for you?

A Jerky can be a good source of protein provided it is used with other whole food sources. But there are so many types on the market — some are good, some aren't. When it comes to choosing the best jerky, read the labels. Whether it's turkey or beef jerky, the first ingredient should be either turkey breast or beef, not some mixture of meat parts. The best place to purchase jerky is from a whole foods or nature store. Jerky is dehydrated meat (just as raisins are dehydrated grapes), so don't eat too much in one serving. The nutrition section on the label will give you the serving size – usually one ounce. This may not seem like enough because all the water has been taken out, but remember, the protein still remains.

Q It's hard to believe you're pregnant with a big belly by now. Do you think you will ever compete again? If so, do you think it will be easy to get back into shape?

A It is hard to say whether or not I will compete again. Until I can adjust to my new role as a mother, I don't feel comfortable making that decision. I will, however, get in shape again for my own benefit. I've always led an active life, and I know I will continue to do so after the baby is born. Because I've been so active during my pregnancy I believe my body will bounce back fairly easily. I plan on taking it one day at a time and giving my body time to readjust. Who knows, maybe I'll bounce back quicker than I expect and be ready to compete by next year!

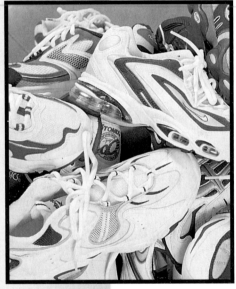

Q What type of shoes are the best to wear during your fitness routine? Do you recommend wearing socks?

A After trying several brands of athletic shoes, I have found that the old-fashioned Reeboks work the best for me. They have all the support and traction I need to execute my gymnastics stunts, as well as the comfort necessary for dancing. Reeboks also allow my foot to extend, making kicks and splits look longer and more exquisite. I always prefer wearing small socks. Not only do they feel better than bare feet, but I like the look. These are, however, just my preferences. Different competitors have their own unique styles. Some wear jazz shoes and others prefer ballet slippers. The best choice is what you feel comfortable in.

Q I hear fitness and bodybuilding experts telling us to consume high levels of protein – levels that far exceed the RDA. Why is that? Is it safe?

A The RDA values were set to give an average American a nutritional guideline. For people who get their exercise reaching for the remote control those seemingly low protein values are fine. If you are an athlete, your body has different needs. Protein is the building block of muscle. Every time we train we break down muscle protein. It only stands to reason that active people need more protein in their diets. How much more? I try to eat 1 gram of protein for every pound of my bodyweight. Some athletes eat more. Some less. The best way to figure it out is to experiment. The byproduct of protein breakdown is uric acid and must be flushed from the body. When consuming high levels of protein, you must drink lots of water. If your urine is light to clear you're okay. If it is bright yellow and pungent, drink more.

Q Should I do my cardio before or after my weight workout? I never know what order to follow.

A There is no right or wrong answer here, but I would recommend doing your weights first. By weight training when you are fresh, you'll be able to lift heavier and longer since your body still has lots of glycogen stored in your muscles. If you perform cardio first, you may not have the energy you need to get a great weight workout. When you do your cardio last, you give your muscles a good cooldown, which helps prevent injury. My only exception to this rule is leg day. By doing cardio first I really warm up my legs. If I wait until afterward, I am too tired. Besides, I don't want to lift heavier to build size on my legs.

Q I like to wear makeup when I exercise. I feel unattractive without it. However, I've been told that it's not good for my skin. What do you recommend?

A Exercising without makeup is definitely the way to go. Sweat and dirt mixed with foundation, powder, and blush is a nasty combination. Talk about clogging your pores! Luckily there are some great tinted moisturizers and light foundations on the market. They contain sunscreen, which is a must for outdoor exercise as well as clubs and gyms. Did you know that fluorescent lights are also damaging to the skin? These new protective concealing moisturizers can be found at better department stores. No matter what you wear, always cleanse your face after a workout!

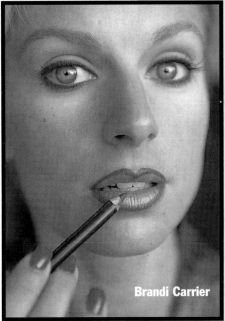

Brandi Carrier

Q How often should I train my abs? Some trainers say twice a week. Others suggest working them more often. You have great abs. What do you do?

A In my early training days, when I was trying to build a strong base, I used weights for all my abdominal exercises. I worked them every other day. After a few years of this I felt I had the thickness I needed so I lost the weights and now train abs daily with lots of reps and various types of crunches. I don't believe you can overtrain your abs. Who doesn't want a tighter, leaner, smaller waistline?

Q My trainer recommends I train through a cold or the flu. He suggests I can sweat the virus out of my system. Is this true?

A Your trainer is wrong. People develop colds or the flu because their resistance levels are low. Using extra energy to work out will reduce your ability to fight the bacteria or virus, exacerbating the illness. Also, colds and the flu can cause muscle weakness, which increases the risks of injury while weight training. The best advice a trainer can give a client with an illness is to rest and allow the condition to subdue before continuing an exercise program.

Q I would like to take up swimming as part of my workout program. My only concern is how the chlorine will damage my hair. I've been told it can be pretty harsh. Any help you can offer would be appreciated.

A I had to swim laps as part of my preparation for the Maui Super Fitness show. We were required to freestyle 100 meters for time. The best advice I have about hair care came from some of the girls on the swim team. Most facilities require you to rinse off before entering the pool. Wet your hair completely. Then comb through a large amount of cheap conditioner and put on a swim cap. The conditioner will not only help you put your cap on, it will temporarily coat your hair, preventing chlorine from doing as much damage.

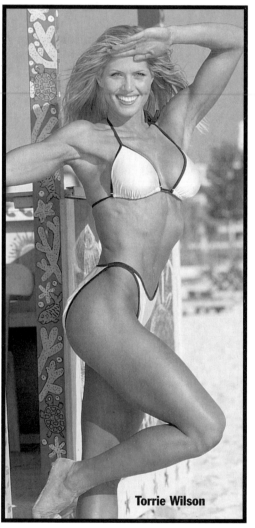

Torrie Wilson

Q I recently began an exercise program to lose ten pounds. I do 45 minutes of aerobics every day. I've lost the excess weight but my body feels soft. I lack the curves I thought would "come out" after the fat was gone. What can I do?

A You're probably suffering from what I refer to as "skinny-fat syndrome." You might be the right size now, but unless you start a regimen of resistance training, your physique will maintain its soft, shapeless form. Not only will weight training the individual muscle groups add shape and fullness in the right areas, but you will also notice a taught, firm feel to your body. Never underestimate the benefits of weight training.

Q I notice so many people at the gym using wrist straps. Are they really necessary?

A Straps are a great invention. I use them all the time for my back workouts, although they are probably most widely used by those who are trying to lift very heavy weights. If you are like most people, the limiting factor in your back workout is your grip strength (or lack thereof). Your poor hands and forearms get maxed out long before your back has reached its max. That's where straps come in. They improve your grip strength, letting you hold onto, and ultimately lift heavier weights. My advice? Buy some and get an experienced trainer to help you use them properly. They can be a little tricky at first.

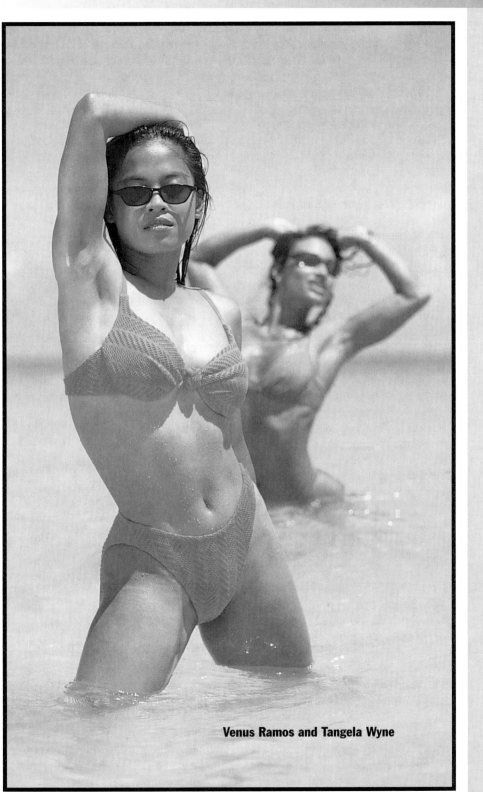

Venus Ramos and Tangela Wyne

Glossary

This glossary provides definitions and sometimes discussions of words and terms found in this book as they relate specifically to women's health and fitness, and in reference to exercise and training in general.

L. [Latin]; G. [Greek]

A

Abs, abdominals – the muscles in the front of the stomach that give the "six-pak" look in people with sufficiently low bodyfat. Their function is to draw the base of the rib cage and the hips toward each other, as occurs when performing crunches. Note that conventional situps are performed largely by the iliopsoas muscles of the hips.

Abdominoplasty – surgery of the abdomen for cosmetic purposes.

Abduction, abductor – abduction is movement away from the central axis of the body, an abductor is a muscle whose contraction results in this movement.

Accessorius [L. *accessorius,* to move toward] accessory or supernumerary. Also denoting specific muscles.

Acetaminophen – a common over-the-counter analgesic (pain reliever) that is not a nonsteroidal anti-inflammatory drug, sold under the brand name Tylenol and many others. It may be used when a pain killer is desired which will not inhibit clotting or produce gastric upset, though it will not provide any anti-inflammatory effects, nor may it be substituted for aspirin in the ECA stack.

Acetone – strong solvent used in nail polish remover. Appropriate only for natural nails. Contained in some astringents/toners/fresheners.

Acetylcholine – an ester of choline found in many tissue, synapses and neuromuscular junctions where it is a neural transmitter.

Acetylcholinesterase – an enzyme at the motor end plate responsible for rapid destruction of acetylcholine, a neurotransmitter.

Achilles tendon – the tendon connecting the lower end of the calf muscle to the back of the heel.

Acid perm – a permanent wave with a pH from 6.5 to 8.0. A milder perm than an alkaline perm, it produces softer curls.

Acne – skin disorder caused by blocked follicles, leading to inflammation of the sebaceous glands.

Acrylic – sculptured nail material. Combination of a liquid and powder that is mixed to form the artificial nail.

Actin – a contractile protein of muscle.

Actin filaments – composed of the contractile proteins called actin, plus some regulatory proteins which play a role in allowing (or preventing) myosin head binding to actin.

Actinic – pertaining to changes caused by the ultraviolet rays in sunlight.

Acupuncture – in acupuncture, fine needles are inserted at specific points in the body to stimulate, disperse and regulate the flow of Chi, vital energy, through the body and to restore a healthy energy balance. Often used in the US for pain relief, acupuncture is also used to improve well-being and to treat acute, chronic and degenerative conditions.

Acute vs. chronic – *acute:* occurring over a short period of time, or lasting a short time; *chronic:* persisting over a long period of time, or recurring. Allopathic medicine is good at treating acute illness, but abysmal at treating chronic illness.

Adduction, adductor – *adduction:* movement toward or beyond the midline of the body in the frontal plane; *adductor:* a muscle whose contraction results in this movement.

Adductors, thigh – several muscles located in the upper part of the inner thigh whose function is to pull the legs toward the midline.

Adhesion – a fibrous band which abnormally connects structures within the body cavities. Adhesions are usually the result of inflammation of at least one of the structures involved.

Adipose – the tissue in your body that stores fat cells.

Adrenoceptor – a receptor that responds to hormones (such as epinephrine [adrenaline]) produced by the adrenal gland.

Aerobic – requiring oxygen when describing exercise, refers to extended sustained levels of exertion during which metabolic processes that provide energy are dominated by the complete oxidation of nutrients.

Aerobic exercise – any extended physical activity that makes you breathe hard while using the large muscle groups at a regular, even pace. Aerobic activities help make your heart stronger and more efficient. They also use more calories than other activities. Some examples of aerobic activities include: brisk walking, jogging, bicycling, swimming, aerobic dancing, racquet sports, rowing, ice or roller skating, cross-country and downhill skiing, and using aerobic equipment (treadmill, stationary bike, etc.).

Aesthetician – professional who works to clean and perfect skin.

Agonist – a chemical agent that stimulates, activates, accelerates or enhances a process in the body (compare antagonist).

Alae [L. *ala,* wing] – relating to a muscle of the nose, and others.

Alanine – an amino acid. BCAAs are used as a source of energy for muscle cells. During prolonged exercise, BCAAs are released from skeletal muscles and their carbon backbones are used as fuel, while their nitrogen portion is used to form another amino acid, alanine. Alanine is then converted to glucose by the liver. This form of energy production is called the alanine-glucose cycle, and it plays a major role in maintaining the body's blood sugar balance.

Algisium complex – natural marine-derived complex which functions as an anti-inflammatory agent.

Alkaline perm – a permanent wave with a pH from 7.5 to 9.5. Produces a tight curl.

Allantoin – known for its gentleness. A very healing, soothing and anti-irritating ingredient. Often used in antiacne products, after sun products, and clarifying lotions.

Allograft – an organ transplanted from one human body to another.

Almond, sweet oil – emollient used in lotions and creams. Known for its mildness.

Aloe vera – plant from which aloe gel is extracted. Known for its gentle soothing properties. Especially good for burns and moisturizing the skin. Promotes healing and cellular renewal.

Alpha-hydroxy acid – any one of several natural acids (glycolic, lactic, citric, malic) obtained from fruit which assist in shedding dead skin cells. They provide the benefit of chemical exfoliation of the skin, making skin appear clearer. Solutions vary from 2 percent to 15 percent (you need a prescription for anything higher). The 8 percent formulas are generally recognized as being quite effective with minimal irritation. Glycolic acid is thought to be the most effective exfoliant of all the alphahydroxy acids. (See special information section for how to make a homemade AHA solution.)

Alpha-lipoic acid (ALA) – a sulfur-bearing phytonutrient with antioxidant properties; amplifies effects of other antioxidants. It is an insulin potentiator that may be, in some respects, the very best insulin mimicker. Here's an analogy of what ALA does. If ALA were a person, he would be the one who yells at the muscle cells to pick up the key, open the door, and help bring in the creatine. ALA plays a role in energy metabolism. ALA amplifies the ability of other antioxidants to combat free radicals and enhance recovery. Also may enhance insulin sensitivity, improving the body's ability to add lean mass and reduce fat.

Amino acids – nitrogen-bearing organic acids that are the building blocks of protein. The branched-chain amino acids are leucine, valine and isoleucine.

Aminophenols – phenol derivatives used in combination with other chemicals in permanent (two-step) hair dyes.

Ammonia – alkaline ingredient used in some permanent hair color. It works with the developer, sending a chemical action which decolorizes the hair.

Ammonium hydroxide – used to stabilize and adjust the acids in skin peels and hair waving and straightening.

Anabolic – the genesis or construction of lean muscle tissue. Certain supplements said to be anabolic contribute to a metabolic environment that is conducive to muscle growth and repair. Steroids are the most commonly known anabolic supplement. Of course they are illegal, but prohormones that have flooded the market in the past few years work in a similar fashion by influencing hormone levels (and hence the term "prohormone"). The prohormones androstene and DHEA fall into this category.

Analgesic – tending to reduce or eliminate pain.

Androgenic – producing or accentuating male sexual characteristics (body hair, deepened voice, male pattern baldness). One of the characteristics of steroids, whether synthesized in the lab or naturally in the body is their anabolic-androgenic ratio. If a certain amount of "steroid x" produces the same anabolic effects as a given amount of testosterone, how do the androgenic effects compare to those produced by that quantity of testosterone?

Androstenedione – androstenedione is a hormone and a precursor to testosterone, one step removed. It can be converted to a select number of other hormones including estrogen, but its effect on free testosterone levels (as opposed to serum levels) is well documented and occurs during a specific time interval following ingestion.

Antagonist – a muscle that relaxes or stretches during the performance of a movement.

Anterior – before or in front of.

Anterior tilt – forward tilt of the pelvic girdle.

Antibiotic – a drug that fights infection from bacteria (immunosuppressant drugs make transplant patients more likely to get infections).

Antibodies – proteins made by the body's immune system that help the white blood cells fight off foreign "invaders" like bacteria, viruses or transplanted organs.

Anticatabolic – preventing or lessening catabolism.

Anticoagulant – delaying or preventing the process of the clumping together of blood cells to form a clot.

Anticus [L. *anticus,* anterior] – designating a muscle as placed anteriorly, e.g. serratus anterior.

Antifungal – a drug that fights infections from fungus (immunosuppressant drugs make transplant patients more likely to get infections).

Anti-inflammatory – substances that can soothe irritation of the skin. Also can be the property of a substance that prevents irritation causing swelling and ill effects of toxic cosmetic ingredients.

Anti-irritant – substances that soothe the localized/superficial inflammation of the skin that is due directly to one or more external substances.

Antioxidants – vitamins or substances which impede oxidation or spoilage promoted by oxygen or peroxide.

Antiperspirant – a product, usually containing aluminum salt, used to prevent perspiration and the odor it causes. May contain an additional deodorant, but not necessarily.

Antiviral – a drug used to fight infections from viruses (immunosuppressant drugs make transplant patients more likely to get infections).

Apple juice and pectin – clarifying agent, emulsifier, and thickener in shampoo.

Applied kinesiology – a diagnostic system using muscle testing to augment normal examination procedures.

Apricot kernel oil – similar to almond oil, used as an emollient in lotions, creams, etc. Ground seeds are often used in facial scrubs and masks.

Arch [L. *arcus,* a bow] – any structure resembling a bent bow or an arch.

Areola – the circular area of different (usually darker) pigmentation around the nipple of the breast.

Arginine – a conditionally essential amino acid with anabolic and immune system supportive effects. It is required for growth, immune function, wound healing and many aspects of protein metabolism. Arginine is necessary for the production of growth hormone. It is also a precursor for nitric oxide, a critical substance that helps regulate the function of cardiovascular, nervous and immune systems and which is essential for muscle growth.

Aromatase – an enzyme responsible for (among other important duties) converting testosterone into estrogens.

Aromatherapy – use of essential oils fragrance for therapeutic benefits.

Articulationis [L. *articulationes,* the forming of new joints of a vine] – pertaining to muscles that insert into a joint capsule.

Arytenoid [G. *arytenoideus,* ladel-shaped] – pertaining to muscles attached to the laryngeal cartilage.

Ascorbic acid – also known as vitamin C. A water-soluble vitamin, and an antioxidant. Your body cannot store vitamin C, so you must supplement regularly. It is not resistant to heat, so cooking will destroy it. Vitamin C functions primarily in the formation of collagen, the chief protein substance of your body's framework. It also helps in the production of vital body chemicals. Vitamin C also is a detoxifier (helps cleanse your body of toxins).

Ash – a cool or green-based shade when referring to makeup or hair color.

Aspirin – originally a brand name, *aspirin* is a generic term for acetylsalicylic acid (C 9 H 8 O 4), a common over-the-counter non-steroidal anti-inflammatory. Side effects include inhibition of blood clotting (may increase internal bleeding and/or the extent of bruising if used when injury is fresh).

Assistant mover – a muscle that aids the prime mover to effect joint movement.

Astringent – a solution which removes oil from the skin; usually used after washing the face to remove any remaining traces of cleanser. Designed to dry and shrink superficial tissues by reducing water content and sometimes promotes healing of inflamed skin.

Atlanto- [G. *Atlas,* in Greek mythology a Titan who supported the world on his shoulders] – relating to muscles attached to the second cervicle vertebra, the atlas.

ATP – adenosine triphosphate, the compound that is the primary source for intracellular energy.

Autonomic nervous system – a part of the nervous system that we cannot control voluntarily (the brain cannot control the way it works). Divided into the sympathetic and parasympathetic nervous system, it is what is commonly called our "fight or flight" response to stress. For example, some of us may feel uncomfortable speaking before a large audience. We cannot control our sweaty hands, flushed cheeks and perspiration.

Avocado – oil from seed and pulp used in creams, lotions and hair preparations. Found to significantly increase the water-soluble collagen content in the dermis.

Avulse, avulsion – tearing away a bodypart or structure such as tearing a tendon or ligament away from a bone.

Axillary [L. *axilla,* armpit] – pertaining to muscles that are found in the region of the armpit, e.g. axillary arch muscle.

B

B-complex vitamins – a group of 11 known vitamins that work together in your body. All play vital roles in the conversion of food into energy. Essential for the normal functioning of the nervous system and the maintenance of good digestion. Helps promote healthy skin, hair and eyes. These are water-soluble vitamins, which means they cannot be stored by your body and must be replaced every day.

B1 (thiamin) – a vitamin which maintains energy levels, supports brain function (memory). Aids in digestion. Necessary for metabolism of sugar and starch to provide energy. Maintains a healthy nervous system. Alcohol can cause deficiencies of this vitamin and all B-complex vitamins.

B2 (riboflavin) – a vitamin which helps with energy production and amino acid production. Helps body obtain energy from protein, carbohydrates and fats. Helps maintain good vision and healthy skin.

B3 (niacin) – a vitamin Important in carbohydrate metabolism, formation of testosterone and other hormones, formation of red blood cells, and maintaining the integrity of all cells. Helps body utilize protein, fats and carbohydrates. Necessary for a healthy nervous system and digestive system. It also lowers elevated blood cholesterol levels when taken in large amounts of more than 1000 milligrams a day.

B5 (pantothenic acid) – a vitamin which supports carbohydrate, protein and fat metabolism; hemoglobin synthesis. Helps release energy from protein, carbohydrates and fat. Needed to support a variety of body functions, including the maintenance of a healthy digestive system.

B6 (pyridoxine) – a vitamin which supports glycogen and nitrogen metabolism, production and transport of amino acids, and production and maintenance of red blood cells (hemoglobin). Essential for the body's utilization of protein. Needed for the production of red blood cells, nerve tissues and antibodies. Women taking oral contraceptives have lower levels of B6.

B12 (cobalamin) – necessary for carbohydrate, protein and fat metabolism. Important to amino acid and fatty acid synthesis; essential for hemoglobin and nerve cell growth and maintenance. The antistress vitamin, sometimes prescribed for stress reduction.

Ballistic – a movement due to momentum rather than muscular control. Ballistic stretching involves "throwing" a bodypart in order to stretch a joint beyond the range of motion attainable through controlled muscular contraction such as when "bouncing" at the bottom of toe-touches.

Barbell – a straight or curved bar typically five to seven feet in length, designed to hold weights loaded onto the ends.

Barbicide – brand name of sanitizer used to disinfect salon implements.

Basal metabolic rate – the rate at which the body burns calories while awake and at rest. Usually measured in calories per day.

Base – also known as foundation, a skin-colored makeup used to smooth the surface of the skin and even its coloration. Prepares the face for other makeup. Comes in liquid, cream, powder, cake and stick form.

Basecoat – clear, thick polish applied before nail color to create a smooth and adhesive surface for nail color. Used to prevent staining of fingernails, and to prolong life of nail color.

BCAA (branched-chain amino acid) – leucine, valine and isoleucine are called "branched-chain" aminos due to their molecular structure, and are important essential amino acids well known for their anticatabolic (muscle-saving) benefits. They are called BCAAs because they structurally branch off another chain of atoms instead of forming a line. Studies have shown that BCAAs positively affect skeletal muscle growth, enhance fat loss, help to stimulate protein synthesis and inhibit its breakdown – so BCAAs have powerful anabolic and anticatabolic effects on the body. They may also potentiate the release of some anabolic hormones, such as growth hormone. Regular ingestion of BCAAs helps to keep the body in a state of positive nitrogen balance. In this state your body much more readily builds muscle and burns fat. Studies have shown that athletes taking extra BCAAs have shown a loss of more bodyfat than those not taking BCAAs.

BCAAs are used as a source of energy for muscle cells. During prolonged exercise, BCAAs are released from skeletal muscles and their carbon backbones are used as fuel, while their nitrogen portion is used to form another amino acid, alanine. Alanine is then converted to glucose by the liver. This form of energy production is called the alanine-glucose cycle, and it plays a major role in maintaining the body's blood sugar balance.

Beeswax – wax obtained from honeycombs or resin from bark. Thickener, emulsifier and stiffening agent in ointments, cold creams, lotions, lipsticks, etc. Sometimes used for hair removal.

Benign tumor – slow-growing, nonmalignant tumor that does not spread to other parts of the body.

Bentonite or kaolin – clays found in powders and foundations that may clog pores. These clays are used in facial masks to absorb excess oil. Also known as "China clay." Can promote dryness of the skin if used too frequently.

Benzoyl peroxide – an antiacne medication that kills acnegenic bacteria and inhibits production of oil by the sebaceous glands. Usually available in 2.5 percent, 5 percent and 10 percent formulas.

Beta-agonist – a beta-agonist or beta-adrenoceptor agonist is a drug or chemical that partially mimics the effects of epinephrine, primarily targeting the beta-adrenoceptors which accelerate heart rate and increase blood pressure (beta-1), dilate bronchial passages (beta-2), and release fatty acids from fat cells into the bloodstream (all beta receptors). The most commonly encountered beta-agonists are asthma drugs such as ephedrine and albuterol which target the beta-2 receptor.

Beta-carotene – a phytonutrient carotenoid with antioxidant and provitamin A activity. In addition to providing the body with a safe source of vitamin A, beta-carotene works with other natural protectors to defend your cells from harmful free radical damage. This is an important micronutrient in helping the body with metabolic functions, such as recovery from exercise.

Beta-hydroxy acid – used to exfoliate epidermis of skin and prevent clogged pores. Salicylic acid is a BHA (found in many OTC acne medications and Clinique Turnaround Cream/Lotion).

Beta-hydroxy Beta-methylbutyrate (HMB) – a compound made in the body and a metabolite of the essential amino acid leucine. Studies have found that HMB has a decrease in stress-induced muscle protein breakdown. Studies also found that HMB may enhance increases in both muscle size and strength when combined with resistance training.

Beta-sitosterol – a sterol (plant hormone) derived from crude germ oils. Increases growth hormone and natural testosterone levels in the body.

Biceps [L. *bi*, two + *caput*, head] – two heads. Pertaining to muscles with two heads, e.g., the biceps brachii.

Biceps brachii – the familiar "make a muscle" muscle that flexes the elbow joint. Additionally, the biceps supinates the forearm and helps raise the upper arm at the shoulder.

Biceps femoris – the large, two-headed muscle on the back of the thigh. Contracting this muscle flexes the knee and also extends the hip (only one head of the muscle originates above the hip joint and contributes to this movement).

Bioimpedance – the resistance of a path through the body (typically measured between the feet and/or hands), most often used to estimate bodyfat percentages because fat conducts electricity more poorly than muscle.

Biological value (BV) – the measure of protein quality, assessed by how well a given food mixture supports nitrogen retention in humans. Biological value is derived from providing a measure intake of protein, then noting the nitrogen uptake versus nitrogen excretion. The actually process is much more complicated, though. In theory a BV value of 100 is maximal. Some protein products claim they have a higher BV than 100, but they refer to a chemical score, not the biological value of whey.

Biomechanics – a branch of study that applies the laws of mechanics to living organisms and tissues.

Biopsy – examination of a small amount of tissue by a pathologist who can provide a diagnosis of tumor type.

Biotin – this vitamin is used for fat, protein and carbohydrate metabolism, cell growth, and fatty acid production.

Biventer [L. *bi,* two + *venter,* belly] – muscle having two bellies.

Blackheads – a mixture of dead skin cells, oil, and bacteria exposed to oxygen.

Blepharoplasty – any operation for the correction of a defect in the eyelid; surgery on the eyelid.

Blood-brain barrier – a protective barrier formed by the blood vessels and glia of the brain. It prevents some substances in the blood from entering brain tissue.

Blotting – to remove excess oil or moisture from lipstick or any other creamy makeup to "set" it for longer wear.

Boar bristle – commonly used in natural bristle brushes. Allows for better distribution of natural scalp oils through the hair.

Body (hair) – the volume or springiness of hair.

Body composition – quantification of the various components of the body including water mass, fat mass, bone mass, and bone-free lean body mass.

Body dysmorphic disorder – a psychiatric disorder characterized by preoccupation with some imagined defect in physical appearance when none is actually present.

Boron – a trace mineral. Studies show that boron helps the body retain minerals such as calcium and magnesium. Taking large amounts of boron, over 10 milligrams a day, can be toxic, particularly to the organs that manufacture testosterone. You can find traces of boron in all the food groups, even in wine, with the greatest concentration in prunes, raisins, parsley flakes and almonds. A 1987 study showed that boron could dramatically increase testosterone levels – by the way, this study was for postmenopausal women who had testosterone deficiencies. Once their boron-rich diets brought their testosterone levels back up to normal, those levels stabilized. A lack of boron in your diet may have a negative impact on energy utilization.

Botanical – refers to a product containing plants or ingredients made from plants.

Bovine cartilage – a source of mucopolysaccharides which have anti-inflammatory and joint protective properties.

Bovine colostrum – usually from cows, a dairy product that has similar properties to human colostrum. Adults cannot usually absorb colostrum antibodies and growth factors the way a newborn can. But it still has superior nutritional values that may make it a useful supplement.

Brassy – refers to unflattering warm tones in hair color created by chemicals or damage.

Brevis [L. *brevis,* short, brief] – a short muscle or head, e.g., short head of biceps brachii.

Bromelain – a naturally extracted digestive enzyme that may help accelerate tissue repair.

Bronzer – a makeup which makes the skin appear more tanned. Can be found in powder or cream form, not to be confused with "self-tanners," which are not water soluble.

Brown fat – a type of fat cell with a greatly increased density of mitochondria and a much greater blood supply than ordinary "white" fat. Besides being able to store fat, brown fat cells can convert calories directly into heat through a process known as non-shivering thermogenesis. Brown fat is used by mammals to maintain body temperature and to expend excess calories that are consumed but not stored as fat.

Buccinator [L. *buccinator,* trumpeter] – a muscle of the cheek.

Buckwheat – a plant native to Asia that has fragrant white flowers and small triangular seeds. The edible seeds are often ground into flour. According to animal studies, buckwheat is better than casein (a milk protein) for promoting muscle growth and body growth and decreasing blood lipids. For persons allergic to wheat gluten, it provides a gluten-free food with uses similar to grains. Roasted buckwheat is known as kasha. Buckwheat is usually available as flour.

Buffer – an extremely fine-grit manicure tool used to shine the surface of the nail.

Bulbo- [L. *bulbus,* a bulbus root] – any globular or fusiform structure. A muscle covering a bulbar structure.

Bulking, bulking up – to gain size and mass, preferably (but not always) mostly or entirely muscle and other lean tissue.

Bumper plate – a weight plate (almost always Olympic) with a rubber outer rim to reduce damage to the floor (and the plate) in case it is dropped. These are most commonly used in Olympic lifting where very heavy weights are pressed overhead.

Burn – the sensation in a muscle that comes from the lactic acid and pH buildup resulting from exercising the muscle to failure.

Bursa – a sac or sac-like bodily cavity, especially one containing viscous lubricating fluid. Located between a tendon and a bone or at points of friction between moving structures.

Bursitis – inflammation of a bursa.

Butyl, propyl, ethyl and methyl parabens – synthetic preservatives used in non-protein-based products.

Butylene glycol and propylene glycol – solvents used to dilute.

C

C12-15 alcohols benzoate – emollient and provides a silky feel to dry skin.

Cable machine – an exercise machine in which the lifter pulls on a handle attached to a cable. The main difference between an exercise in which the resistance is transmitted through a cable rather than being done with free weights is that the force is in the direction of the cable rather than always pointing downward. For example, when using a cable machine to perform curls, the cable may continue to provide resistance at the top of the movement – while the resistance the biceps must work against when lifting free weights is minimal when the forearm is at or near vertical.

Caffeine – alkaloid that stimulates and enhances alertness and boosts energy. A herbal compound that fights fatigue. Caffeine increases endurance during prolonged submaximal activity by increasing blood epinephrine (adrenaline) levels, thereby allowing fat cells to break down more readily during aerobic activity. Caffeine also makes a muscle contraction more forceful.

Calcium – most abundant mineral in the body; essential for the formation and repair of bone and teeth, but also essential to nerve transmission, muscle contraction, blood clotting and other metabolic activities as well. Long-term calcium deficiency is linked to degenerative bone diseases.

Calendula (a.k.a. marigold) – used in fresheners, soothing creams and products for sensitive skin. Sometimes used in deodorants. Some adverse skin reactions have been reported in medical literature.

Calf Muscle – the muscle on the back of the lower leg responsible for extending the ankle. The calf muscle has two heads, which connect at the bottom and attach to the heel: the gastrocnemius, the top of which attaches above the knee joint, and the soleus which attaches below.

Calisthenics – exercise performed without weights, or outside resistance designed to develop muscular tone and promote physical well-being.

Callus – patch of dry, dead, hard skin. Particularly found on feet which endure lots of friction.

Calorie – a unit of energy equal to the amount of energy needed to heat one gram of water one degree celsius. In common usage, the "calories" most often refer to kilocalories (also known as Kcal or "food calories"), which are really 1000 calories.

Cambered bar – a barbell with most of the middle portion offset. Used to increase the range of motion in bench pressing. Also very effective for avoiding scraped knees while deadlifting, and for letting the arms hang straight down during shrugs.

Camphor – used as an antiseptic, stimulant and anti-inflammatory ingredient in toner, aftershave, lip balm and after-sun preparations.

Candelilla, carnauba and microcrystalline – waxes used in stick cosmetics such as lipstick and blush.

Canthaxanthin – a carotenoid related to beta-carotene used as a red food coloring. When taken in (relatively) large quantities, it imparts a reddish-orange tone to the skin. Used as a tanning aid. It is nontoxic and has some antioxidant activity, but prolonged use at high doses has been known to cause crystals to form inside the eye.

Cap – the deltoid muscle of the shoulder, which can be divided into front, middle and rear heads for training.

Capitis [L. *caput,* head] – pertaining to the head.

Capsularis [L. *capsa,* a chest or box] – a muscle joined to a capsule as, for example, a joint. Any structure so designated as a capsule.

Carbohydrate – there are two basic forms of carbohydrates: simple and complex. Simple carbs are usually devoid of fiber and include such foods as refined sugars, fruit juices and apple sauce. The problem with simple carbs is that they promote a large insulin surge, which can lead to hypoglycemia. Complex carbs are absorbed more slowly, so they don't cause as great an insulin surge as the simple type. Primary macronutrient source of energy in the body; burned as glucose and stored in muscle as glycogen (excess stored as fat), and includes all sugars (1 gram yields 4 calories).

Carb up – after any period of carbohydrate depletion, particularly as part of a cyclic ketogenic diet, the consumption of large quantities of carbohydrates with the intent of saturating muscle glycogen stores.

Carnitine (L-carnitine) – nonstructural amino acid that transports fatty acids into muscle cells for use as energy fuel. Carnitine is water-soluble and can be made in the body from the amino acids lysine and methionine with the assistance of vitamins C, B6 and niacin, which act as coenzymes in the process.

Carnitine was discovered in meat in 1905, and was once called vitamin T. They thought it was a vitamin at first. About 98 percent of the body's carnitine exists in the heart and skeletal muscles. Carnitine is synthesized in the liver from lysine and methionine, but half of the body's daily requirement for carnitine comes from foods sources including meat, poultry, fish and some diary products. Without supplemental carnitine, some people cannot use fat as energy.

Carnosus [L. *carnis,* flesh or muscle] – pertaining to muscular tissue or dermal muscles.

Carpi [G. *karpos,* wrist] – muscles relating to the eight carpal bones of the wrist.

Carrot oil – primarily used as a fragrance and coloring agent in cosmetics. Thought to be good for both dry and oily skin.

Casein – primary protein found in milk, along with whey protein. Casein is the insoluble protein fraction of milk. It is absorbed more slowly and provides the body with amino acids over an extended period in comparison to whey protein, the soluble protein fraction in milk.

Castor oil – used in lipsticks, concealers, hair pomade, ointments, creams and lotions.

Catabolic – metabolic condition in which muscle is broken down and energy is released.

Catabolism – protein breakdown in muscles.

Cat's claw – herb used in South American folk medicine for its anti-inflammatory and immune system protective properties.

Cavernosus [L. *caverna,* a grotto or hollow] – pertaining to the cavernous tissue of the reproductive system.

Central nervous system (CNS) – the part of the nervous system which in vertebrates consists of the brain and the spinal cord, to which sensory impulses are transmitted and from which motor impulses pass out, and which supervises and coordinates the activity of the entire nervous system.

Cetyl alcohol (fatty alcohol) – a gentle humectant, lather booster and emulsifier. In hair products it is used to smooth and soften the hair cuticle.

Chamomile – used in many products for blonde hair to enhance color. Also used in a variety of cosmetics as an emollient. Anti-inflammatory, soothing agent for tender skin; also provides antioxidation.

Cheat reps – performed by deviating from strict form (leaning, adding extra momentum at the bottom of the movement with whole-body motion) after a lifter has reached the point of failure with a given weight.

Chelating – a deep cleansing process which strips the hair lightly before a chemical service. Also known as clarifying.

Chemotherapy – the use of certain medicines to destroy tumor cells. Chemotherapeutic drugs may be given by mouth or injected through an intravenous line. Sometimes chemotherapy is given directly into the nervous system.

Chick embryo extract – this type of extract contains short amino acid chains called oligopeptides, plus additional essential amino acids and trace elements (iron, copper, cobalt, selenium and zinc). Peptides in the extract possess both cell stimulating and protective properties. The peptides indicated that they were activating growth factor receptors in them. The extract works as a general tonic and stimulates the adrenal gland, normalizing its function. It also acts as a mild stimulant and an antidepressant; and it improves libido, erectile function, spermatogenesis and other aspects of sexual function in men and women. It also improves sleep and promotes weight loss.

Chiropractor – one who practices chiropractic, a method for restoring normal condition by adjusting the segments of the spine.

Chitosan – chitosan is a natural product extracted from chitin (byproducts of crustacean shell extracts). It's a waste product of the crab and shrimp industry. It can be used to inhibit fat digestion and as a drug delivery/transport agent. It has also been used as a cholesterol lowering substance. Chitosan is marketed as a "fat-blocker,"and seems to impede fat absorption by "gelling" with fat in the small intestine. Side effect of chitosan is that, since it is made from seafood, some people have an allergic response to it. Also, you need a high concentration of chitosan for it to gel with fat.

Cholesterol – this is a type of lipid which, although most widely known as a "bad fat" implicated in promoting heart disease and stroke, is a vital component in the production of many steroid hormones in the body. It also plays a vital role in proper cell-membrane structure and functioning. It's a substrate for bile-acid synthesis, as well as sex-hormone and vitamin D synthesis. There are different types of cholesterol – namely, HDL and LDL (HDL being the good form and LDL being the bad form).

Choline – a B-fatty acid involved in the production of neurotransmitters in the brain that regulate mood, appetite, behavior, memory, etc. Most effective in phosphatidyl choline form, it is believed to help concentration and alertness. Studies indicate that choline improves cognitive performance. Blood levels of choline decrease during prolonged exercise.

Chondro- [G. *chondros,* cartilage] – pertaining to muscles that arise from costal cartilage.

Chondroitin – chondroitin is extracted from bovine tracheas or shark cartilage. It is a major component of connective tissue, especially cartilage. Chondroitin can stimulate repair of cartilage cells and also block enzymes that damage joints.

Chromium, chromium picolinate – chromium increases the efficiency of the hormone insulin, which the pancreas releases after you eat carbohydrates or protein. Chromium acts to make the receptors of muscle cells more sensitive to insulin (which allows you to store more carbohydrates in the muscle cells as glycogen rather than in fat cells as lipids). Insulin also helps muscles use amino acids for building protein rather than breaking them down. Exercise increases the excretion rate of chromium.

Chrysin – an antiaromatase, which means it stops a lot of excess testosterone from converting to estrogen. Also, a compound with significant antiviral activity – especially in relation to the HIV. It has an effect on the benzodiazepine receptors (which have a calming, antistress effect). Chrysin taken in the correct dosage could possibly reduce cortisol secretion due to the body sensing less stress. Chrysin may act as an antiestrogen by inhibiting aromatase activity, limiting the conversion of testosterone to estrogen.

Circuit training – a sequence of exercises performed one after the other with little rest between exercises. Somewhere between traditional aerobics and traditional weight training.

Circumduct – the act of moving a limb in a circular manner.

Citric acid – derived from citrus fruit, it maintains pH balance, preserves and stabilizes foam when used in cosmetics. Used in many post-perm ingredients to neutralize odor.

Citrus aurantium – herb containing synephrine.

Clarifying shampoo – slightly more alkaline (higher pH) than ordinary shampoo, used to remove excess buildup of products or water chemicals from hair.

Clavicularis [L. *clavicula,* small key] – pertaining to muscles associated with the clavicle.

Cleansing creams – contain little or no soap or detergent, usually with an oily base. Meant to be applied, then removed with wiping rather than rinsing.

Cleido- [G. *kleis,* clavicle] – related with the clavicle.

Clenbuterol – this drug is classified as a beta-2 agonist, and is used for treating asthma. It is not an anabolic steroid or a growth hormone. Currently it is not approved for sale in the United States, but is sold in Europe under various names such as Spiropent, Monores and Ventipulmin. Researchers in 1987 noted an unusual effect in animals when given this drug. Their muscles grew – while they lost bodyfat! The main side effects associated with this drug include tremors, heart rhythm disturbances, headaches, nervousness, excessive sweating and insomnia. Bodybuilders use it because it mimics the actions of epinephrine. It simulates a process called thermogenesis, which turns fat calories into heat and results in a loss of bodyfat. The side effects start when you use more than 80 micrograms or more. The dosage used to treat asthma is around 20 to 40 micrograms twice a day.

Clove oil – used in creams and lotions as an anti-irritant.

Coal tar colors – most synthetic colors all called such because the first synthetic colors were made from coal tar products. A misnomer because most today are derived from petrochemicals.

Cocamide DEA – either made synthetically or derived from the kernel of the coconut, it gives lather and cleans skin and hair.

Cocoa butter – mainly used as a thickening agent in cosmetics. Well absorbed by the skin and imparts a sheen. Used in many lipsticks, soaps and emollient creams. An acnegenic substance to some.

Coconut oil – used as an emollient in soaps and as a shine enhancer in some hair products.

Coenzyme Q10 – this antioxidant is shown to have heart protective and energy productive properties. CoQ10 is involved in cellular energy production. Several studies have reported improved endurance after taking CoQ10. It is considered one of the best antioxidants.

Collagen and elastin – these are animal byproducts used in many products. As human skin ages, our own soluble collagen becomes inflexible and the skin's connective tissue less moisturized naturally. The use of animal collagen and elastin to replace our own is not possible, although these ingredients have moisturizing properties. Effective in smoothing the hair cuticle.

Collars – any kind of sleeve which may be slipped over the end of a weight bar after the plates have been put on and tightened to hold the plates securely in place. This prevents plates from slipping off the end of the bar, shifting position, or rattling during the exercise. Olympic spin-lock collars typically weigh either 5 or 5.5 pounds each.

Colli [L. *collum,* neck] – pertaining to the neck or the neck of a structure, e.g., longus colli muscle.

Cologne – a toilet water containing alcohol and fragrant oils. Not as concentrated as perfume.

Comedogenic – a cosmetic preparation known to promote acne. Pore-clogging.

Comfrey – root from which allantoin is extracted. Anti-inflammatory, astringent and emollient. Contains mucopolysaccharides.

Communis [L. *communis,* in common] – relating to more than one structure working as one unit, e.g., extensor digitorum communis.

Compound movement – an exercise that targets more than one muscle or muscle group simultaneously; usually the movement involves flexing or extending at least two joints. Lat pulldowns, squats, and bench presses are compound movements – curls, leg extensions and flyes are not.

Compressor [L. *compressus,* to press together] – a muscle that, when contracted, produces pressure on another structure.

Concealer – an opaque makeup used to cover darkness under eyes, redness of the skin, or any irregularity in the skin color or texture. Comes in a waxy stick, cream, or opaque liquid form.

Concentric – done as the muscle contracts. "Concentric strength" is the weight that can be lifted working against gravity (that's what you usually think of as weightlifting).

Concentric contraction – when a muscle overcomes resistance causing the muscle to shorten and the joint angle to be reduced.

Conditioner – creamy hair product meant to be used after shampoo. Moisturizes and detangles hair.

Conjugated linoleic acid (CLA) – occurs naturally in whole milk and red meat. A collective term used to designate a mixture of positional and geometric isomers of the essential fat linoleic acid. It is actually a fat derived from linoleic acid (an essential fatty acid). Studies have shown that CLA can increase lean body mass and decrease fat, inhibit the growth of tumors and enhance immune function. CLA is found naturally in beef, cheese and whole milk.

Contralateral – situated on the opposite side.

Cool – refers to blue or violet-based undertones in hair, skin or makeup.

Copper – active in the storage and release of iron to form hemoglobin for red blood cells.

Cornflower – used in toners, astringents and healing creams. Can cause photosensitivity in some people.

Cortex – middle layer of an individual hair shaft in which the pigment of the hair is contained.

Corticosteroids – catabolic steroids used to reduce inflammation by signalling tissues to break down. While this certainly does have medical uses, corticosteroids will not aid in building muscle.

Cortisol – a catabolic hormone that is released and increases in response to stress when the body is subjected to trauma such as intense exercise, including weight training. Excess cortisol is known to increase catabolism (protein breakdown in muscles). Cortisol leads to muscle breakdown through promoting a release of muscle amino acids for transport to the liver, where the amino acids are converted into glucose.

Cosmeceutical – while the Food, Drug and Cosmetics Act does not recognize the term "cosmeceutical," the cosmetics industry has begun to use this word in reference to cosmetic products that have drug-like benefits. The Food, Drug and Cosmetics Act defines *drugs* as those products that cure, treat, mitigate or prevent disease or that affect the structure or function of the human body. While drugs are subject to an intensive review and approval process by FDA, cosmetics are not approved by FDA prior to sale. If a product has drug properties, it must be approved as a drug.

Cosmetics – "articles intended to be applied to the human body for cleansing, beautifying, promoting attractiveness or alternating the appearance without affecting the body structure or function." Many cosmetics alter their advertising to meet these guidelines, such as antiwrinkle creams, since they would otherwise be considered a drug. For example, "to reduce the appearance of fine lines," whereas a drug such as Retin-A actually does reduce fine lines, and thus is actually affecting the structure of the skin – not just changing its appearance.

Costalis [L. *costa,* rib] – pertaining to muscles attached to ribs.

Cramp – painful, involuntary muscular contraction.

Cranial – refers to the head or skull.

Cream – a preparation for the skin used to impart moisture. Usually thicker and more emollient than a lotion.

Cream rinse – a mixture of wax, thickeners, and a group of chemicals used to coat the hair shaft and detangle after shampooing.

Creatine (monohydrate) – a muscle fuel that is extracted naturally from meat and fish, or synthesized in the lab. Once it is in the muscles, creatine combines with phosphorous to make creatine phosphate (CP), a high-powered chemical that rebuilds the muscles' ultimate energy source, adenosine triphosphate (ATP). CP powers your muscles for high intensity exercise for short periods only. Consequently, athletes who compete in power and sprint events will have an advantage if they take supplemental creatine. More CP in the muscle cell translates into a greater resistance to fatigue. Also, CP helps with the transfer of energy into the muscle cells, thus speeding up the action, which may enhance performances that are aerobically taxing. Reports says people who take creatine supplements may recover from intense activity faster and experience less postexercise muscle soreness.
    Creatine is a naturally occurring compound in the muscle tissue and when converted in the muscle tissue to phosphocreatine during exercise can provide sudden bursts of energy. Insufficient amounts of phosphocreatine could result in a fatigued feeling in the muscle. The creatine monohydrate powder provides enough energy to delay the onset of fatigue. Creatine monohydrate is a synthesized metabolite that is the powerful energizer providing instant energy and strength with better endurance and helps to maintain optimal levels of ATP production during intense exercise.

Cucumber – used in facial creams, lotions and cleansers. Known for its astringent and soothing properties. Also an anti-inflammatory agent (slices placed over puffy eyes can reduce swelling).

Cuticle – outermost layer of skin (a.k.a. epidermis) or the fold of skin at the base of the fingernail. Hair cuticles are the outermost layers of the hair shaft which overlap like shingles. When healthy and lying flat, these cuticles impart sheen to the hair.

Cyclic adenosine monophosphate – important in the regulation of metabolic and neurologic processes and activity, cAMP is generated in response to the activation of cellular receptors and, in turn, the presence of cAMP within the cell activates the process in question. cAMP is broken down by cAMP-phosphodiesterase.

The activity and duration of the process is governed by the rate at which cAMP is produced in response to receptor activation and the rate at which it is broken down. This is why the combination of ephedrine and caffeine produces a greater metabolic response than the sum of their effects when taken individually: ephedrine increases receptor activation, caffeine inhibits cAMP breakdown.

Cyclomethicone (volatile silicone) – solvent used to dilute.

Cytochrome C – a chemical compound composed of amino acids and iron which acts as a carrier of oxygen to the mitochondria. Allows for more oxygen uptake by the cells, thus prolonging endurance.

Cytoplasm – the fluid portion of a cell outside the nucleus.

D

D&C – a prefix designating that the certifiable color in question has been approved for use in drugs and cosmetics.

Dandruff – a condition of shedding dead cells from the scalp. Usually caused by sebhorric dermatitis.

Deep penetrating treatment – a conditioner for hair meant for occasional use. Of greater intensity than ordinary conditioners. Formulations usually contain protein, vitamins and moisture to help dry, damaged hair.

Definition – extremely low bodyfat coupled with superior muscle separation and vascularity; the physical manifestation of "dialing it in." Adjectives that describe this desired state include *ripped, shredded, sliced, cut, striated.*

Deltoideus [G. *deltoeides,* shaped like the letter delta] – the musculus deltoideus, shaped like an inverted delta.

Dentate [L. *dentatus,* toothed] – notched muscles, e.g., the serrati.

Deodorant – a product used to counteract odors caused by the decomposition of sweat on the body. Contains antiseptic substances to kill bacteria and sometimes strong fragrance to mask offensive smell. (Not to be confused with antiperspirants which actually inhibit production of sweat.)

Depilatory – product used to remove hair from the follicle.

Dermabrasion – a surgical procedure for removal of acne scars, nevi (skin blemishes), tattoos or fine wrinkles by using special abrasive tools on the epidermis (outer layer of the skin).

DHEA (dehydroepiandrosterone) – a hormone made by the adrenal glands used by the body to make male (androgen) and female (estrogen) hormones; possible positive effects on mood and energy in older individuals (40+) whose production of DHEA has declined. Has been referred to as the "fountain of youth" hormone because it declines rapidly as we age, and supplementation with this hormone reverses many of the ravages associated with aging. Studies show that men with the highest DHEA levels have better cardiovascular health.

Diabetes – a disease in which the body does not make or properly use insulin, making it difficult to break down sugar.

Dibencozide – the biologically active coenzyme of vitamin B12, necessary in the metabolism of fat, proteins and carbohydrates.

Dimethicone – moisturizing silicone skin and hair conditioner and antifoam ingredient.

Dimethicone Copolyol – complex of natural silica, acts as a spreading agent for easy application of product; also functions as a moisturizer.

Dimethylglycine (DMG) – a substance originally isolated from apricot kernels. Said to increase oxygen uptake and decrease recovery time between workouts.

Diuretic – any agent or compound that increases the flow of urine from the body. Diuretics can range from herbal teas to powerful drugs that flush out electrolytes and water. They are classed based on the location and mechanism of action in the kidneys. Athletes use diuretics to eliminate water weight to further emphasize their muscular definition. Most bodybuilding and fitness federations have banned the use of diuretics and test for their presence.

DMAE (dimethylaminoethanol) – supplement reported to minimize buildup of lipofuscin (age spots) in the brain. Plays a participatory role in acetylcholine synthesis. DMAE has been shown to stimulate vivid, lucid dreams, suggesting possible sleep-pattern enhancement.

DMDM (hydantoin) – preservative, antimicrobial to fight bacteria.

DNP (2,4 dinitrophenol) – the first weight-loss drug ever offered to the public, around 1933. DNP is a yellow crystalline that's slightly soluble in water. After being injected, it increases the metabolism an average of 30 percent over baseline in less than a minute, returning back to normal anywhere from six to 48 hours. However, DNP has way too many side effects, including blindness, and if you take too much it can cook you to death from the inside out. You can lose weight with it, but it is highly dangerous. Street names for DNP include Hexalon.

DOMS (delayed-onset muscle soreness) – the pain and soreness you feel a few days after a heavy workout.

Dorso- [L. *dorsum,* back] – muscles related to the dorsal surface of the body, e.g., latissimus dorsi muscle. Also any structure related specifically to the thorax.

Double process – a hair color treatment which requires two steps to complete. First the hair is lightened and second the new color is added.

Downward rotation – movement of the scapula as the arms are lowered, and the superior border of the scapula moves away from the midline (spine).

Dumbell – a short bar with fixed or changeable weights mounted on each end with enough space in between to grip with one hand. The word *dumbell* comes from the practice of demonstrating strength by lifting heavy cast metal bells (like the Liberty Bell only smaller and not cracked). A "dumb bell" was a bell made without a clapper so that it would not ring through one's show of physical prowess. Eventually any weight meant to be held with one hand was referred to as a *dumbell* and later what we now know as the dumbell shape became standard.

Dysmorphophobia – body dysmorphic disorder, irrational fear that one is deformed or is being deformed.

E

ECA stack – a thermogenic supplement blend of ephedra, caffeine and aspirin that is popular in the fitness and bodybuilding cultures. It is said that these three ingredients give a synergistic effect together which gives better results than any one on its own.

Echinacea – herb with immune protective properties, shown to have some benefit protecting against colds and flu. It can be used as a preventive measure to protect the body against the natural stress the immune system suffers in heavy training.

Ectomorph – thin and linear body type.

Egg protein – source of protein with high protein efficiency ratio (PER), usually in egg white form (albumin) when used in protein powder to avoid cholesterol in egg yolk. Egg protein is the standard by which all other proteins are measured because of its very high ratio of indispensable amino acids (also called essential amino acids because they must be supplied to the body from food or supplements) to dispensable amino acids.

Elasticity – the ability of the hair to stretch without breaking and then return to its original shape. Determines how well it will hold a curl.

Elder flower – used in eye and skin creams for its astringent properties.

Electrolysis – destroys the hair roots with an electric current. This is a permanent means of ridding yourself of unwanted hair.

Electrolytes – minerals such as sodium, potassium, magnesium and calcium used by cells in the creation and elimination of membrane potentials used to propagate nerve impulses and muscular contraction.

Embolism – obstruction (blockage) of a blood vessel by a foreign substance. The foreign substance could be fat, an air bubble, or any of a number of substances. Blood clots are the most common type of embolus.

Emollients – ingredients that soften or smooth.

Emulsifier – an agent used to make an emulsion, which is a mixture of liquids, minute globules of one being suspended in a second that doesn't dissolve the first.

Endocrine – glands that produce chemicals released into the bloodstream. The pituitary and adrenal glands are endocrine glands; salivary glands and sweat glands are not.

Endomorph – rounded body type with small shoulders.

Enzyme – a protein catalyst; enzymes are involved in digestion and both the synthesis and breakdown of proteins, hormones, and other substances in the body.

Ephedra/ephedrine – the active ingredient in the Oriental herb ma huang (Ephedra sinensis); this chemical has been proven to be both a powerful energizer and weight loss aid. Ephedrine is a powerful thermogenic agent: It releases norepinephrine, a brain neurotransmitter that exerts a stimulating effect. This same neurotransmitter signals the sympathetic nervous system, which is called into play during "fight or flight" response. Body temperature rises and promotes the breakdown of fat cells for fuel.

Ergogenic – tending to increase muscular power, endurance or size.

Essential amino acids – amino acids which cannot be synthesized by the body from other amino acids and, thus, must be present in the diet: leucine, isoleucine, lysine, methionine, phenylalanine, tryptophan and valine.

Essential fatty acids – unsaturated fatty acids which cannot be synthesized by the body and are used as the starting point for the biosynthesis of necessary metabolic and hormonal chemicals.

Estrogens – there is no one hormone named "estrogen"; estrogens are hormones that induce or accentuate female sexual characteristics (as well as performing other functions, depending on the specific hormone). Estrogens include estrone, progesterone and estradiol.

Exfoliating – a process of removing the top dead skin layers to reveal healthier, newer skin underneath. This can be done chemically with such acids as AHAs or BHAs, or physically with scrubbing grains such as apricot kernels or baking soda.

Extension – hair extensions are pieces of real or synthetic hair that are woven in close to the scalp to achieve greater length and/or fullness. Nail extensions are synthetic additions which add length to the natural nail, such as nail tips, wraps, gels and sculptured acrylic nails.

Extensor [L. *ex-tendre,* to stretch out] – a muscle that, upon contraction, tends to straighten a limb. The antagonist of a flexor muscle.

EZ-curl bar – a short barbell with a shaft bent like a stretched-out letter W. Typically used for performing curls with the hands turned inward more than they would be using a straight bar, putting less strain on the wrists. A typical Olympic EZ-curl bar weighs around 20 pounds, though there's no "official" standard weight. Standard (takes plates with 1-inch holes) versions would be lighter, typically 10 to 15 pounds.

F

Fat – macronutrient that is a source for long-term energy and energy storage (as adipose tissue); necessary for absorption and transport of fat-soluble vitamins and constituent of hormones and cell membranes. One gram of fat equals nine calories.

Femoris [L. *femur,* thigh] – pertaining to the femur or thigh.

Fiber – the more insoluble the fiber is (fiber that does not dissolve in water), the better it is for you. Insoluble fiber reduces the risk of colon cancer and high blood pressure. Fruit fiber seems to be more beneficial than vegetable or cereal fibers, probably because fruits are loaded with pectin, an insoluble fiber. As a rule, the higher the insolubility the fewer the calories. Corn bran is the best, followed by wheat bran, then oat bran. It is best to eat fiber after you work out to avoid intestinal discomfort.

Finishing spray – a hairspray with medium hold used on a finished style to maintain its style and shape.

Flat – describes muscles that have lost their fullness. Flatness is commonly caused by overtraining, undertraining, or a lack of nutrients and water.

Flavonoids – a group of compounds widely distributed in plants which have a characteristic molecular structure. They have been found to have many beneficial activities, such as anti-inflammatory and anticarcinogenic properties.

Flaxseed oil – flaxseed is an excellent source of the omega-3 fatty acid alpha-linolenic acid (an EFA). Supplementing with flaxseed oil has been shown to lower cholesterol, decrease heart disease, increase satiety and improve cell integrity.

Flexion – movement resulting in the reduction of a joint angle.

Flexor [L. *flectere,* to bend] – a muscle that upon contraction tends to bend a joint; the antagonist of an extensor.

Folic acid – this vitamin is used for red blood cell formation, protein metabolism, appetite, body growth, and reproduction.

Follicle – a pore in the skin from which a hair grows.

Forced reps – additional repetitions of an exercise performed with the help of a partner when you're unable to do any more reps on your own.

Fragrance – any natural or synthetic substance or substances used solely to impart an odor to a cosmetic product.

Fragrance-free – products so labeled may still contain small amounts of fragrances to mask the fatty odor of soap or other unpleasant odors. (There is no official governmental definition for this term.)

Free-form amino acids – separate and isolated amino acids not bound or linked to any other amino acids.

Free-hand movement – any exercise that can be performed without exercise equipment, using only your bodyweight, such as a pushup or squat without weight.

Free radicals – free radicals are highly reactive molecules in the body which can destroy tissues by oxidizing cell membrane lipids and damaging DNA, the body's genetic material. Free radicals are produced through the body's normal process of metabolizing the air we breathe and the food we eat, as well as exposure to tobacco smoke, excess sunlight and environmental pollutants. Antioxidants work in the body by neutralizing free radicals before they can do significant harm.

Free weight – equipment moved in the performance of an exercise which is simply raised and lowered as a complete unit. So called because the weight is free to move in any direction and in any manner the lifter can manage. Free weights include barbells and dumbells.

Freezing spray – a hairspray with the firmest hold. Used to maintain style in hard-to-hold hair.

Fructose – also known as "fruit sugar," even though it is found in many foods besides fruit and it is not the majority of the sugar content in most fruits. Fructose also forms half of the sucrose (ordinary table sugar) molecule. Approximately 50 grams of fructose per day can be metabolized by the liver into glucose; amounts consumed beyond that will be converted into triglycerides using an alternate pathway.

G

Gamma butyrolactone (GBL) – a related product to GHB (gamma hydroxybutyrate).

Gamma hydroxybutyrate (GHB) – GHB is a simple carbohydrate found naturally in every cell of the human body. GHB is both a metabolite of and a precursor to an amino acid called GABA (gamma aminobutyric acid). The FDA has labeled GHB as a "date-rape" drug, and wants to ban it from the market. GHB itself does not cause a person to remain conscious, engage in sex and then forget what they did. These problems occur when you take GHB with high levels of alcohol, since both alcohol and GHB are metabolized by the same enzyme in the body.

Gamma oryzanol – a byproduct of rice bran, which helps increase lean body mass while decreasing fatty tissue. Also shown to help increase testosterone production.

Garcinia Cambogia – fruit from India that contains hydroxycitric acid (HCA), an organic acid influencing carbohydrate and fat metabolism.

Garlic – has properties of being a stimulant, antispasmodic and antibiotic. Also helps lower your total cholesterol level. Expect to spend Friday night alone if you are a heavy user.

Gastritis – irritation of the stomach.

Genistein – a compound thought to protect you against cancer. It is found in soy based food products. It suppresses the production of stress proteins in cells, proteins that otherwise help cancer cells survive destruction by the immune system.

German volume training (GVT) – a training technique in which 10 sets of 10 reps are performed for each exercise. The same weight is used for each set and rest periods between sets are kept to a minimum.

Ginkgo biloba – herb shown to enhance mental acuity. Some research has shown that Ginkgo biloba increases cerebral blood flow to the brain, and to boost brain levels of adenosine triphosphate and scavenge free radicals. Combined with ginger, ginkgo has also been shown to reduce stress-induced anxiety.

Ginseng – a family of herbs with adaptogenic properties affecting energy. There are different ginsengs (Asian, American, Siberian). Some ginsengs have shown to have memory-enhancing effects. Studies show that an individual ginseng component called ginsenoside Rb acts favorably in reversing memory deficits by increasing the secretion of acetylcholine. Studies also suggest that ginseng extract improved learning and retention processes.

Glandulars – supplements derived from animal glands and claimed to boost human gland function. Not true, but a nutritious source of protein and minerals.

Glial cells – cells of the central nervous system that nourish and support the nerve cells and the blood vessels that supply the nervous system. There are several types of glial tissue: astrocytes, ependymal cells and oligendrocytes.

Glucagon – a protein hormone (produced mainly by the islets of Langerhans) that promotes an increase in the sugar content of the blood by increasing the rate of glycogen breakdown in the liver.

Glucomannan – a fiber derived from the Amorphophallus Konjac root, a perennial plant of the Araceae family. The root is low in protein, lipids (fats), calories and vitamins, but, because of its glucomannan content, it can provide many tangible musclebuilding and health advantages. Glucomannan can help mitigate insulin response to high-glycemic carbohydrates, which might allow bodybuilders to add variety to low-carb diets and still accrue the benefits of a strict regimen. Glucomannan may also help remove fat from the body.

Glucosamine – organic compound found in cartilage and joint fluid; relieves joint pain and may help in healing some joint injuries. Glucosamine is a provider of the building blocks of joints.

Glucose (monosaccharide) – type of sugar that circulates in the bloodstream, thus the term *blood glucose levels* or *blood sugar*. All carbohydrates, whether simple or complex, are eventually converted to glucose in the body. Glycogen is many units of glucose together.

Glucose tolerance factor (GTF) – GTF is thought to be a complex of chromium, nicotinic acid, and the amino acids glycine, cysteine and glutamic acid (these aminos are components of glutathione). GTF is thought to be synthesized by the liver. In many people chromium is likely the deficient substrate for GTF formation. GTF is found in foods such as organ meats, whole gains, cheese, mushrooms and brewer's yeast.

Glutamine – an amino acid. Glutamine is the most abundant amino acid in muscle tissue. Studies are beginning to show that having extra glutamine in your body may be important to maximize muscle growth by increasing growth hormone levels. Glutamine is also important to maintain proper health, and is shown to have anabolic and anticatabolic properties. During intense training, the signal for muscle breakdown (which is a bad thing) may be the release of skeletal muscle glutamine. That means each time you train, your muscles release glutamine which in part triggers a catabolic state (a catabolic state is synonymous with muscle breakdown). Documented clinical studies have shown that glutamine will have a significant impact on maintaining a positive nitrogen balance which is essential to muscular development and recovery.

Glutathione – a tripeptide of glutamic acid, cysteine and glycine; fundamentally important in cellular respiration.

Glutes – a shortened version of *gluteas maximus,* the largest of the muscles forming each of the human buttocks.

Gluteus [G. *gloutos,* buttock] – pertaining to the muscles of the buttocks.

Glycemic index – the glycemic Index (GI) measures only the rise in blood sugar elicited by various foods and drinks. It is not like an index of factors like nutrient density or vitamin or fiber content. The GI can help you if you want to avoid a spike in blood sugar, and insulin.

Glyceryl monostearate – emulsifier; also pearlescent agent.

Glycogen – it is a term for many units of glucose strung together. The body stores glycogen in two areas, the liver and the muscles. Only about 5 grams (20 calories) worth of glucose flows in the blood. Liver stores about 75 to 100 grams, or 300 to 400 calories; an hour of aerobics can burn up half the liver glycogen content. The muscles store about 360 grams, 1440 calories. Carbohydrate loading is one technique used to increase muscle glycogen content. By not consuming enough carbohydrates, you deplete both liver and muscle glycogen reserves. While complex carbs are considered to be more desirable than simple carbs, simple carbs are more efficient after a workout for replacing muscle glycogen. Simple carbs are absorbed faster, and promote a greater insulin output. A carbohydrate drink with at least 50 grams of carbs will do the trick.

Glycogen (liver) – liver glycogen is a fuel reserve that helps maintain blood glucose levels. Most importantly, the brain relies on a constant supply of glucose to function properly.

Glycogen (muscle) – muscle glycogen is extremely important, since it's the primary fuel that powers anaerobic training, such as lifting weights. Glycogen that's stored in a muscle is available only to that muscle because muscles lack a certain enzyme (glucose-6-phosphatase) needed to release glucose into the blood. Muscles can absorb glucose without insulin, which is why exercise helps prevent diabetes.

Glycogenesis – the formation and storage of glycogen.

Glycogenolysis – the breakdown of glycogen to glucose in the animal body.

Goldenseal root – a stimulant that increases your body's tonic properties. Stimulates secretion of bile. A key component of the emulsion of your body's fat.

Gracilis [L. *gracilis,* slender or delicate] – musculus gracilis of the thigh.

Green tea – perhaps most notable, recent research has shown that green tea reduces the risk of developing stomach cancer by 50 percent and esophageal cancer by 60 percent. No one knows for sure, but scientists think that polyphenols in green tea protect health by combating free radicals. The main constituents of green tea are polyphenols, caffeine, vitamins, minerals, amino acids and other nitrogenous compounds. It also contains small amounts of carbohydrates and lipids. Also, green tea contains polyphenols, theanine and catechins. The greater the theanine content in green tea, the higher the price.

Grit – the texture of a nail file ranging from coarse to medium and fine.

Growth hormone – known in the medical community as somatotrophin. It is a powerful anabolic hormone that affects all systems of the body and plays an important role in muscle growth. It is a peptide hormone composed of many amino acids (191 of them) linked together. It is rapidly metabolized by the liver and has a half-life in the blood of approximately 17 to 45 minutes. Because of this, detecting GH in a drug screen is very difficult.

Guarana – source of caffeine. Comes from the seed of a herb found in the Amazon, long popular among Brazilians for its stimulatory effects.

Guggul lipids (guggulbolics, guggulsterones) – the thyroid gland is the major regulator of metabolic rate. When the body senses a reduction in calories (when dieting), there is a reduction in the conversion of the thyroid hormone T4 to T3, thus slowing down the metabolism and reducing the effectiveness of the diet. Guggul lipids in turn increase the conversion of T4 to T3, and therefore restore the metabolic rate so weight loss continues.

Guggulsterone – guggulsterone is a ketosteroid specifically called Z-guggulsterone. It increases the metabolic rate via stimulation of the thyroid gland. Studies indicate that guggulsterone can result in higher levels of T4 (thyroxine), one of the two main thyroid hormones.

H

HDL (high-density lipoprotein cholesterol) – protects against cardiovascular disease. HDLs help to shuttle cholesterol out of the blood and back to the liver, where it's degraded into bile that can then be excreted from the body.

Hemangiomas – a reddish-purple birthmark. Flat types are also known as port wine stains.

Henna – derived from the henna plant, a vegetable dye made from its leaves and stems into a powder. Traditionally it imparts a reddish cast to the hair by coating it. Clear henna enhances shine. Henna cannot be dyed over since it coats the outer hair shaft, affecting the penetration of the chemical colorant.

High-intensity training – a form of training made famous by Dr. Arthur Jones and Mike Mentzer. The theory is based not on doing more or less exercise but rather an appropriate amount of exercise to stimulate optimum muscle growth.

Highlights – the subtle lifting of color in specific sections of hair.

Homeopathic – traditionally a philosophy of therapy in which medical conditions are treated by preparing a solution of a substance which produces symptoms similar to those produced by the condition, diluting it until no molecules of the active ingredient remain in the solution, and then drinking it. The term is often applied to any solution so prepared, and irrespective of whether the homeopathic solution is intended to cure or cause a particular reaction, it is an expensive technique for consuming small quantities of water. While it is not obvious why one would wish to go this route, it does have the advantage of relatively few side effects.

Humectant – an ingredient in skin and hair products that draws moisture from the air to moisturize.

Hydrolyzed keratin – protein for the hair derived from nonanimal sources.

Hydroxycitric acid (HCA) – also known as Citrimax. Acid found in the fruit Garcinia Cambogia that affects fat and carbohydrate metabolism. This compound is a citrate lyase inhibitor. Citrate lyase is an enzyme responsible for facilitating the conversion of carbohydrates into fat. Effectiveness of HCA is fairly well documented. Said to promote additional glycogen formation and result in enhanced aerobic performance, it is further hypothesized that chromium and carnitine potentiate the effects of hydroxycitric acid. Used both as a weight reduction supplement and energy purveyor, though it seems more effective in the latter, especially when used in conjunction with long bouts of strenuous exercise.

Hydroxymethylbutyrate (HMB) – a metabolite of the branched-chain amino acid leucine, HMB is also available in supplement form. Some studies have shown increased growth in cattle given HMB, but evidence of any value for increasing human muscle growth and athletic performance is limited.

Hypertrophy – muscle growth.

Hypoallergenic – cosmetics that are less likely to cause allergic reactions. (There is no official legal definition for this term.)

Hypoglycemia – a term meaning low blood sugar. A set of symptoms that point to irregularities in the way the body handles glucose, the sugar that circulates in the blood. Symptoms of hypoglycemia include sweating, trembling, anxiety, fast heartbeat, headache, hunger, weakness, mental confusion, and on occasion seizures and coma. However, this state occurs rarely because the body has a lot of backup systems to prevent that from happening.

I

Idiopathic – cause of injury unknown.

IGF-1 – stands for insulin-like growth factor. An important hormone for muscle growth. Naturally produced by the body in response to exercise and necessary for normal physiological functioning. Excess of IGF-1 may be associated with an increased risk of breast cancer, and prostate cancer.

Iliac – refers to the area of the hip bones on either side of the body.

Immune system – the body's natural defense mechanism.

Immunosuppressant – a drug that lowers the body's natural defenses, like those responsible for rejecting a transplanted organ.

Inflammation – the way the body reacts to injury or "invasion," like an infection. Signs of inflammation are redness, swelling and high temperature.

Innervation – nerve stimulation of a muscle.

Inosine – a purine nucleotide that promotes oxygen transport and the release of oxygen molecules into the red blood cells. Also promotes production of adenosine triphosphate (ATP) which is essential for muscle function.

Inositol – this vitamin is used for cholesterol and fat metabolism, cholesterol reduction, lecithin formation, hair growth, and retardation of artery hardening.

Insulin – an anabolic hormone that's supposed to take the sugar and transport it into the muscle. Insulin also promotes increased amino acid entry into muscle and increases muscle protein synthesis. Too much insulin can cause sugar to bypass muscle, and be stored as bodyfat.

Insulin resistance – a reduced sensitivity to insulin, meaning that more insulin must be released to cause a given amount of nutrients uptake into the body's cells. Note that the downregulation of insulin sensitivity is likely to be more extreme in lean tissue than adipose tissue, so persons who have developed a high degree of insulin resistance are likely to preferentially store nutrients as fat rather than use them for tissue growth and repair. Type-II (adult-onset) diabetes is an extreme form of insulin resistance.

Intensity – in high-intensity workouts either the pace you keep while you train is higher than normal, as in moving quickly and taking a shorter rest between sets, or the weight you use during those sessions is relatively heavy for you. High intensity can certainly result when the workload within a given time period is increased as well as the extra weight and faster pace.

Inversion – the movement of the foot toward the midline of the body at the ankle joint. Also see supination.

Ion exchange – a technique of separating materials by reversible interchange between ions of like charge.

Ipriflavone – a synthesized compound used to stimulate bone formation. While clinically used as an antiosteoporotic agent, bodybuilders have used it in order to promote gains in lean body mass. Despite numerous studies with humans, no reports of weight gain have been made from scientific sources.

Ipsilateral – situated on the same side.

Iron – mineral essential to oxygen transport in blood (via hemoglobin and myoglobin), enzyme production and immune support. A deficiency can cause the most common form of anemia. Teenagers need additional iron during their years of maximum growth; women need extra iron during the years they are menstruating and during pregnancy.

Iron oxides – inorganic pigments approved for cosmetic use, including the eye area.

Ischemia – localized anemia or lack of oxygen.

Isoflavones – phytonutrient antioxidants, including genisteine and diadzein, that act as estrogen receptor protectors (minimize PMS, menopause side effects) and lower cholesterol levels.

Isokinetic contraction – accommodating or variable resistance. Movement of a bodypart through a range of motion at a constant speed.

Isolation exercises – defined as exercises which involve only one muscle and one joint. These are different from the many exercises which are multi-joint in nature and typically involve several different muscles and are referred to as structural exercises.

Isoleucine – an essential branched-chain amino acid found abundantly in most foods. Especially high amounts found in meats, fish, cheese, most seeds and nuts, eggs, chickens and lentils. In the human body isoleucine is concentrated in the muscle tissues. This and other BCAAs are popular with bodybuilders looking to restore muscle mass traumatized from excessive overtraining. While research is inconclusive, most users of products containing these BCAAs attest to its worth.

Isomer – a molecule with the same chemical composition as another (same number of atoms of each type), but with a different chemical structure (arrangement or configuration of those atoms). Two chemicals which are isomers of each other may produce effects on the body that are similar or completely different.

Isometric contraction – muscular contraction that does not result in a change in the length of the muscle.

Isopropyl Lanolate, Myristate, Palmitate – synthetic moisturizers.

Isotonic contraction – muscular contraction that overcomes resistance, resulting in a change in the length of the muscle.

J

Joint – the articulation of two or more bones.

Joint cavity – the space between bones that is encapsulated by a synovial membrane and articular cartilage.

Jojoba oil – contains superior properties to keep skin soft. It is beneficial to acne-prone skin and dry hair.

Juice – meaning anabolic steroids. Other slang words for steroids include *gear, sauce* and *roids*.

K

Kaolin – a white clay used for absorbing impurities from the skin.

Ketogenic – producing or causing the body to produce ketones.

Ketogenic diet – a diet involving the restriction of carbohydrates to the point of inducing ketosis (buildup of significant levels of ketones in the bloodstream). Usually this requires keeping carbohydrate consumption below 20 grams per day. Ketosis reduces appetite and some studies (but not all) have shown ketogenic dieters to lose relatively more fat and less lean body mass than nonketogenic dieters. Note, however, that ketogenic diets are not usually well suited for actually gaining muscle.

Ketosis – a condition brought about by the restriction of carbohydrate intake, resulting in excessive acetones or other ketone bodies being secreted by the body; stored fat becomes more available for energy.

Kombucha – a tea made from a fungus/yeast fermentation with high nutrient level. Used by people for immune protection, increased energy, and other positive effects. Sometimes called a Kombucha mushroom. It is two life forms, a yeast culture and bacteria living in symbiosis, from Manchuria. *Very dangerous* because local bacteria and molds can move in and produce a variety of toxins. Stay away from this one.

Krebs cycle – a sequence of chemical reactions occurring within the mitochondria of living cells in which acetic acid (produced from foods) is oxidized to produce high-energy phosphate bonds (converting ADP to ATP) to be used to power the body's other metabolic processes. Also known as the citric acid cycle.

L

Lactate threshold – the point during a graded exercise test at which the blood lactate concentration suddenly increases; a good indicator of the highest sustainable workload the individual can perform.

Lake colors – dyes that don't dissolve in water. These water-insoluble forms of certifiable colors are more stable than straight dyes and ideal for products in which leaching of the color is undesirable (coated tablets and hard candies, for example).

L-alanine – used as body fuel by tissues of the brain, nervous system and muscles. Important in converting energy to stored energy in the body's Krebs energy cycle. Important nitrogen quality for postinjury states. Builds up the immune system, producing immunoglobulins and antibodies. Metabolizes sugars and organic acids.

Lanolin – a natural extract of sheep wool used as a moisturizer which is a common cause of allergic reactions, but is rarely used in pure form.

Lateral flexion – flexing the trunk or neck to either side in the frontal plane.

Laterals (side raises) – your target zone is the *side delts*. Stand with two dumbells at your sides, palms facing in toward your thighs. With your elbows slightly bent, slowly raise the dumbells away from your sides. As the dumbells reach shoulder height, make sure your little fingers are level with or higher than your thumbs. Lift the dumbells up to about shoulder height, but no higher than that. Pause at the top for a contraction and then return to the starting position.

Lats – a term which is abbreviated jargon for the latissimus dorsi. This Latin term translates roughly into "lateral muscles of the back." When viewed from the rear, and relaxed, the lats form the shape of large inverted cones.

Lavender extract – soothing anti-inflammatory agent.

Lean body mass – fat-free body tissue, comprising mostly muscle. Lean mass is the primary determinant of the body's basal metabolism (calories you burn at rest). In healthy women bodyfat (bodyweight minus lean body mass) ranges from 18 to 22 percent; in men 8 to 12 percent.

Lecithin – a phospholipid containing glycerol, fatty acids, phosphoric acid and choline. Serves as a structural material to every cell in the body. Important to the brain and nerves.

Leptin – this protein was been portrayed as the way to a cure for obesity. Leptin was first described as an apiodocyte-derived signaling factor, which, after interaction with its receptors, induced a complex response, including control of bodyweight and energy expenditure. It could be quite a fat-burner. Research shows that people who used high doses of leptin for six months lost weight, most of it bodyfat.

Leucine – an essential amino acid which cannot be synthesized by the body but must always be acquired from dietary sources. Leucine, and the other branched-chain amino acids (BCAAs), isoleucine and valine, are frequently deficient in the elderly, and increased body requirements can occur after trauma or surgery. These branched-chain amino acids may prevent muscle-wasting in these conditions, but no studies have been done to determine if extra intake will help in muscle-building in healthy individuals. While research is inconclusive, most users of products containing these BCAAs attest to its worth. Because leucine cannot be made by the body from other sources, it's important to maintain adequate amounts in the diet.

Lever – a rigid bar (like a bone) pivoted on a fixed point. Used to transmit force, as in raising a weight at one end by pushing down on the other.

Ligament – the connective tissue that joins bone to bone.

Limiting factor – a characteristic that determines the upper limit of performance on a particular task, exercise, etc. (muscle fiber type, cardiac output, and oxygen uptake).

Liposomes – microscopic sacs manufactured from natural or synthetic fatty substances which include phospholipids (components of cell membranes). When properly mixed with water, phospholipids can "trap" any substance that will dissolve in water or oil. Manufacturers say that liposomes act like a delivery system, depositing product ingredients into the skin. When the liposomes "melt," ingredients such as moisturizers are released.

Lipotropic – applies to substances essential for fat metabolism, promoting the physiologic utilization of fat.

M

Macronutrient – a nutrient (such as protein, carbohydrate or fat) used in large quantities to provide energy for life and/or raw materials for synthesis or tissue repair.

Ma huang – herb that yields the stimulant ephedra.

Magnesium – mineral necessary for energy metabolism, protein and fat synthesis, neuromuscular transmission, ammonia scavenging and binding of calcium to teeth, etc. This mineral aids in bone growth, and is necessary for proper functioning of nerves and muscles.

Maltitol – this is a sugar alcohol that is used as a sweetener. It has half the caloric value of sucrose because it is not completely absorbed by the body.

Maltodextrin – a long chain of glucose molecules (carbohydrates) that provides sustained energy without sharply increasing insulin levels. Essentially a chain of molecules of the simple sugar glucose linked together. An average of seven glucose molecules link together to form a maltodextrin molecule.

Mammogram – X-ray of the breast.

Mammoplasty – cosmetic plastic surgery of the breast.

Manganese – needed for normal tendon and bone structure.

Mastopexy – correction of a pendulous breast by surgery. A pendulous breast appears droopy and positioned lower than normal.

Maximal aerobic power – the most oxygen that can be taken up and used by the body during maximal work. Relates directly to the rate at which the heart can supply the muscles with oxygenated blood.

Maximal heart rate – the highest heart rate attainable. Estimated by subtracting an individual's age from 220.

Medium-chain triglycerides (MCT) – MCTs are technically fats, but they have very unique properties. The difference between them and other fats lies in their molecular structure. MCTs are shorter than other fats, which allows them to be burned rather quickly by the body for energy. MCTs enter the mitochondria – the powerhouse of a cell – without assistance, and do not require the usual transport mechanism. MCTs are an attractive supplement because of their calorie density. They have 9 calories per gram, like fats, but lack the disposition to be stored as fat. All fats are not created equal. Research shows that animals maintain a lower bodyfat when they use MCTs in place of traditional fats.

Melanin – the pigment which naturally colors the hair and skin.

Melatonin – hormone produced by the pineal gland that regulates circadian rhythms; helps induce sleep and acts as an antioxidant.

Mentoplasty – surgery of the chin, whereby its shape and/or size is changed.

Mesomorph – body type with thick muscles and heavy bone structure.

Metabolite – a chemical produced by the body from some other chemical such as a component of food, a supplement, or a drug.

Methionine – a sulfur-bearing essential amino acid important in hair, nail and muscle production, liver maintenance (lipotropic effects), and production of creatine and other aminos.

Methoxyflavone – also called 5-methyl-7-methoxyisoflavone. A synthetic isoflavone that is highly anabolic, yet free of any androgenic effects. It halts the muscle-wasting and increases lean tissue growth. It increases calcium phosphorous, potassium and nitrogen retention to a significant degree.

Micronutrient – a nutrient (such as a vitamin or mineral) needed in small quantities for the normal functioning of the body.

Military press – pressing either a barbell or dumbells straight overheard from shoulder height to full arm extension with an erect torso. Performing this exercise while seated puts less strain on the lower back than if it is done standing.

Mineral – inorganic substances necessary for good health as an ingredient or a catalyst.

Mineral (chelated) – a chelated mineral is generally attached to a protein transporter molecule with the intent of improved transport across the gut to the bloodstream. Although some of the minerals are well absorbed in this manner, this is not necessarily always indicative of the best form for absorption.

Mitochondria – cellular organelles found outside the nucleus that provide energy for the rest of the cell by oxidizing nutrients to produce ATP.

Monounsaturated fats – an essential fatty acid (EFA) that seems to reduce the risk of cardiovascular disease. This is considered a type of "good fat." Olive oil and canola oil contain EFAs. You need approximately 2 percent of your daily calories as EFAs.

Motor unit – the functional unit of muscular contraction consisting of a motor nerve and the muscle fibers it innervates.

Muscle confusion – a technique to counteract the cessation of growth that occurs when muscles adapt to the training demands placed upon them. To keep the body growing and getting stronger, a trainer needs to vary the number of sets and reps, the poundages, rest, and exercise angles during each workout.

Muscle group – a group of specific muscles responsible for a particular movement or action at the same joint.

Myofibrils – contractile organelles found in the cytoplasm of muscle cells.

Myosin – one of the principal contractile proteins found in a muscle.

Myosin filaments – made mostly of bundled molecules of the protein myosin, but they also contain ATP and enzymes which split ATP to generate the power for muscle contraction.

Myositis – inflammation of a muscle.

N

N-acetylcysteine – a stable form of the essential amino acid L-cysteine. Cysteine is a precursor for glutathione, an important antioxidant in the body. Cysteine also serves as a major sulfur source for many body components.

NADH (nicotinamide adenine dinucleotide) – also known as coenzyme 1. It is the coenzymatic form of vitamin B3. NADH is involved in the production of energy in every cell. It supports healthy neurotransmitter functions.

Natural – ingredients extracted directly from plants, earth minerals or animal products as opposed to being produced synthetically. In the context of cosmetics there is no regulation for the use of this word.

Negatives – training technique that results in the lengthening of the working muscles. Emphasizing the negative portion of the movement, the lowering of the weight. Specifically, resisting gravity by lowering the weight slowly and under control.

This is an advanced training strategy whereby the lifter allows the working muscles to lengthen under control. Associated with muscle damage and delayed-onset muscle soreness and should therefore not be performed very often.

Nettle – a botanical additive used in hair and skin products, particularly eye creams and treatments for the scalp.

Niacin (vitamin B3) – a vitamin important in carbohydrate metabolism, formation of testosterone and other hormones, formation of red blood cells, and maintaining the integrity of all cells. Helps body utilize protein, fats and carbohydrates. Necessary for a healthy nervous system and digestive system. It also lowers elevated blood cholesterol levels when taken in large amounts of more than 1000 milligrams a day.

Noncomedogenic – substances that are less likely to clog pores or promote acne. (There is no official legal definition for this term.)

Norandrostenedione – naturally occurring prohormone that works in a manner similar to androstenedione, however, results can be much better, and side effects less.

Norepinephrine – a hormone produced by your adrenal glands. Important for many bodily activities including brain function.

O

Oat-derived polysaccharide – natural complex derived from oats that functions to assist the body's immune system to maintain healthy skin.

Oat oil – powerful antioxidant and emollient. Provides deep antioxidant activity.

Octasanol – a naturally derived wheat germ oil concentrate that has been clinically proven to increase oxygen utilization when exercising.

OKG – a natural chemically bonded compound that combines the amino acid ornithine along with alpha-ketoglutarate, a Krebs cycle intermediate. It is used as an anticatabolic agent and fat-loss promoter. Not a whole lot of research available.

Olestra – a fake fat substitute that will save you calories, but may also deplete your body of nutrients. If you use this product, or products containing this substance, make sure you get your full 2 percent dose of essential fatty acids (EFA).

Omega-3 fatty acid – essential fatty acid (EFA) that seems to reduce the risk of cardiovascular disease. This is considered a type of "good fat." Sources include fish, salmon, mackerel and sardines. You need approximately 2 percent of your daily calories as EFAs.

One-rep max (1 RM) – your absolute strength in a given movement. Powerlifting competitions are a test of 1RM strength. For many trainers, especially beginners, attempting a 1RM is harmful because of the higher risk of injury. A weight with which you can just complete 10 reps is a good approximation for most people of 75 percent of their 1RM.

Organelle – any identifiable specialized part of a cell that is, to an individual cell, much like the heart or liver is to the body. Examples of organelles include mitochondria and the nucleus.

Origin – the point of attachment of a muscle closest to the body's midline or center.

Ornithine – made from the amino acid arginine and in turn is a precursor to form glutamic acid, citruline and proline. When combined with arginine it helps release a growth hormone that metabolizes excess bodyfat.

OTC (over-the-counter) drugs – products that intend to treat or prevent disease, or otherwise affect the structure or functions of the human body, are considered drugs. Over-the-counter drugs are those that can be purchased without a doctor's prescription. Examples of over-the-counter products are fluoride toothpastes, hormone creams, sunscreen preparations, antiperspirants and antidandruff shampoos.

Otoplasty – surgery of the ear.

Overtraining – training beyond the body's ability to repair itself. This state can be caused by training the same bodyparts so frequently so that the body does not have time to recover before the next workout; when workouts are consistently harder than the body is able to recover from fully; or impairment of the body's normal recovery ability due to nutritional deficiencies, illness or stress. Besides impairing athletic performance, overtraining can increase the risk of injury and disease. Symptoms of overtraining include fatigue, reduced performance, and increased resting heart rate.

P

Paba (para aminobenzoic acid) – important for the formation of red blood cells. Aids in the conversion of protein into energy. Necessary for healthy skin, and hair pigmentation.

Pantothenic acid (vitamin B5) – a vitamin which supports carbohydrate, protein and fat metabolism; hemoglobin synthesis. Helps release energy from protein, carbohydrates and fat. Needed to support a variety of body functions, including the maintenance of a healthy digestive system.

Pectin – a soluble fiber found in the skin of fruits (apples and peaches) and vegetables. One study found that eating pectin will make you feel full longer. Researchers speculate that pectin may slow digestion and keep food in your stomach longer.

Phaseolus vulgaris – an ingredient found in white kidney beans which has been shown to effectively prevent the body from absorbing up to 35 grams of unwanted starch per meal.

Phenylalanine – an amino acid, one of the main ingredients to enhance brain function. It has also been used to relieve stress.

Phosphatidylserine (PS) – a phospholid. An ingredient which may block cortisol (a hormone that breaks down muscle cells into fuel). Also reported to increase levels of glucose, the energy source of the brain.

Phosphorus – mineral that is structural component of all cells (including muscle). Necessary for energy metabolism, protein synthesis, and growth/maintenance of all tissues.

Pituitary gland – an endocrine gland situated at the base of the brain. Supplies hormones that control many vital processes.

Polyphenols – polyphenols are potent and wide ranging in their physiological properties. They are antioxidants, cancer preventatives, dental cavity and gingivitis preventatives, prebiotics and even internal deodorizers.

Potassium – mineral that helps maintain cellular integrity and water balance, nerve transmission and energy metabolism. Necessary for muscle contraction. Potassium helps to lower blood pressure, lower risk of stroke, maintain muscle balance and prevent muscle cramping. Potassium helps to reduce the amount of sodium in the body.

Pregnenolone – steroid hormone from which most other steroid (sex) hormones are made, including DHEA. Has beneficial neurotransmitter effects.

Proanthocyanadins – potent antioxidant phytonutrient found in some pine needles (pycnogenol) and grape seeds and skin (grape seed extract). Especially synergistic with vitamin C, making them more powerful antioxidants together than by themselves.

Prohormone – chemicals produced by the body (or close "chemical cousins" of such chemicals, as is the case with the nor- varieties). The "pro-" part is used because rather than themselves being the hormone one is actually interested in supplementing, they are instead used by the biochemical pathways of the body to produce the hormone of interest.

Protein – primary macronutrient for growth and maintenance of the structural parts of our body (including muscle). Cannot be stored – must be replenished through diet (1 gram equals 4 calories).

Protein (soy) – soy protein does not offer much benefit in promoting growth. Soy protein does not form a good curd in the stomach, thus making it a fast protein. The amino acid pattern in soy is inferior to that of milk proteins, and not as favorable.

Protein (whey) – dairy source of protein (other than casein) known for high levels of BCAAs and high nitrogen retention. Made from milk curd, whey protein is the Rolls Royce of proteins because it has a superior amino acid composition (including high levels of leucine, arguably the most important branched-chain amino acid), superior biological value (meaning that more of what you eat gets digested and into your system) and is very low in lactose (a milk sugar that most adults have difficulty digesting).

Protein (whey hydrolyzed) – when you hydrolyze whey protein, you permanently modify the native protein structure – the protein has been denatured. A denatured whey protein has little or no biological activity. The hydrolysis process breaks apart peptide bonds, which destroys the protein structure and the vital whey protein biological activity. However, you still get the amino acids of whey proteins from the hydrolyzed whey protein.

Protein (whey ion-exchange) – this special process revolved around the positive and negative charges or ion properties of whey protein. It features the use of a resin to isolate the protein material from the whey, followed by ultrafiltration methods to further concentrate the protein. This contains 90 percent protein, and less than 1 percent lactose. True ion-exchange whey protein is clear in a solution.

Protein (whey microfiltration) – microfiltration whey protein features filtering membranes with microscopic holes. Sometimes called cross-flow filtration, or nanofiltration, depending on the size of the holes of the filtering membranes.

Pseudoephedrine – an isomer of ephedrine that is a far weaker stimulant and bronchodilator and is used primarily as a decongestant. It is not a suitable substitute for ephedrine in the ECA stack.

Pulmonary – concerning or involving the lungs.

Purslane – an edible weed that is sometimes put on salads, mostly in Europe. Loaded with linolenic acid, and omega-3 fatty acid that may help reduce the risk of heart attack, as well as improve the health of cell membranes in the eyes and brain. It is also an excellent source of vitamin E, providing six times as much as spinach.

Pycnogenol – source of proanthocyanadins.

Pyridoxine (vitamin B6) – a vitamin which supports glycogen and nitrogen metabolism, production and transport of amino acids, production and maintenance of red blood cells (hemoglobin). Essential for the utilization of protein. Needed for the production of red blood cells, nerve tissues and antibodies. Women taking oral contraceptives have lower levels of B6.

Pyruvate – a key energy metabolite for the breakdown of fuel (glucose, fatty acids, amino acids, etc.) to energy in the body, pyruvate can give increased energy, assist in burning fat as fuel, and have anticatabolic effects (such as producing alanine). Pyruvate acid is alpha-ketopropionic acid. Studies have shown that pyruvate can help decrease fatigue, and increase vigor with only six grams per day. The human body breaks down carbohydrates for energy though a process called glycolysis. As these sugars and starches are metabolized, pyruvate (pyruvic acid) is produced, which readily enters the mitochondria of cells to create vital energy fueling the muscles and other parts of the body.

Q

Quadratus [L. *quadratus,* square] – more or less square-shaped muscles.

Quadriceps, quads [L. *quadi-,* four + *caput,* head] – the large muscle of the front of the thigh, composed of four heads: the vastus lateralis, vastus intermedius, vastus medialis, and rectus femoris. All of these join at a common tendon attached to the kneecap, and all are involved in extending the knee joint. The rectus femoris attaches to the pelvic girdle (above the hip joint) rather than to the femur. In addition to extending the knee, it also flexes the hip. Exercises targeting this muscle include leg extensions, squats (any kind), deadlifts and lunges.

Quercetin – a bioflavonoid that occurs in many plant foods. Quercetin has a synergistic effect with ephedrine and caffeine, increasing and prolonging their properties.

R

Radio- [L. *radius,* ray] – pertaining to muscles associated with the radius of the forearm.

Renal – having to do with the kidney.

Repetition, rep – movement through one full range of motion of an exercise.

Rest-pause system – a method of training that employs near maximal repetitions (1RMs) for multiple repetitions. This is accomplished by resting 10 to 15 seconds between repetitions.

Retin-A – vitamin A derivative that acts as a topical antiacne treatment. Additionally found to be beneficial in removing fine lines from facial skin. Creates photosensitivity. Available by prescription only.

Retinol (vitamin A) – a vitamin with antioxidant properties, important for eye protection and bone growth, protein and hormone synthesis (including GH and testosterone), and supports tissue maintenance. Helps reduce susceptibility to infection. Essential for healthy skin, good blood, strong bones and teeth, kidneys, bladder, lungs and membranes.

Retraction – backward movement of a part.

Rhinoplasty – surgery of the nose to improve appearance and/or function.

Rhombo- [G. *rhombos,* a rhomb] – resembling a rhomb, an oblique parallelogram of unequal sides. Relating to two superficial muscles of the back.

Rhytidectomy – a procedure to reduce wrinkles and sagging skin on the face and neck. Commonly referred to as a face lift.

Riboflavin (vitamin B2) – a vitamin which helps with energy production and amino acid production. Helps the body to obtain energy from protein, carbohydrates and fats, and to maintain good vision and healthy skin.

Ribose – ribose is a simple sugar that is extremely important in many processes in the body. Ribose is found in all living cells. It is the backbone of genetic material, and the starting point for production of ATP. Ribose effectively increases ATP and TAN (total adenine nucleotide) recovery, while improving performance in heart and muscle cells. Ribose also fortifies muscle ATP but through a different pathway than creatine. Ribose also bolsters muscle recovery after you train. Ribose promotes a more efficient salvage pathway, thus allowing better ATP recycling and consequent increased muscular recovery after training. If the body does not use the salvage pathway, when ribose is insufficient, it must make ATP from scratch.

Rosemary extract – natural antioxidant.

Rotation – movement of a bone around its long (longitudinal) axis.

S

Saccharin – an artificial sweetener. Nearly 700 times sweeter than sugar, yet leaves an aftertaste. It is not metabolized by the human body. It is useful in diabetic diets in which the patient must lower sugar intake. The FDA has listed saccharin as an "anticipated" human carcinogen, meaning, in certain individuals the sweetener may increase the risk of cancer.

Salatrim – this is a calorie-reduced fat that has only five calories per gram, as opposed to the usual nine.

SAM-e (S-adenosyl-L-methionine) – a naturally occurring molecule in virtually all body tissues and fluids. Fundamentally important in a number of biochemical reactions involving enzymatic transmethylation, contributing to the synthesis, activation and metabolism of such compounds as hormones, neurotransmitters, nucleic acids, proteins, phospholipids and certain drugs.

Sarcomeres – chains of tiny contractile units which are aligned end to end along the length of the myofibrils.

Saturated fats – fats comprised of fatty acids in which all possible bond positions along the carbon backbone are filled with hydrogens. Saturated fats are solid at room temperature, stable at high temperatures, and have a long shelf life. Overconsumption contributes to heart disease.

Saw palmetto – herb shown to have protective properties for the liver. It is also shown that saw palmetto reduces the size of epithelial tissue in the prostate, especially in the transitional zone.

Sclerotherapy – a way of treating varicose veins by injecting a solution into the vein.

Sebum – natural oils in the skin and scalp that lubricate and protect.

Selenium – trace mineral with potent antioxidant effects. Component in sulfur-bearing amino acid production and fetal development during pregnancy. Recent clinical evidence of cancer preventive properties.

Set – a group of a desired number of repetitions of an exercise or movement.

Silica (silicon dioxide) – absorbent, anticaking, abrasive.

Silicone – a compound of silicon used in shine-enhancing hair products to seal the cuticle of hair and in many oil-free cosmetics.

Smilax – a chemical substance derived from the sarsaparilla plant said to boost natural testosterone levels in the body.

Sodium – also known as *salt*. Regulates body fluid volume, transports amino acids to cells, and plays a role in muscle contraction and nerve transmission. Sodium is an important mineral found in our bones, in the fluids surrounding our cells, and in the cardiovascular system. Sodium, with potassium, assists nerve stimulation and regulates water balance. It is also involved in carbohydrate absorption.
    The average person requires a minimum of one tenth of a teaspoon of salt a day. Any athlete who sweats needs more. A teaspoon a day of salt does not cause problems, nor does eating fresh foods high in natural salt such as fish, carrots, beets and poultry. Eating processed and junk foods can lead to high potentially dangerous levels of sodium intake.

Sodium lauryl sulfate – a white powder used as a detergent, emulsifier and surfectant in cosmetics. A very strong degreaser. Also used as a water "softener."

Somatotrophin – known in the medical community as GH or growth hormone. A powerful anabolic hormone that affects all systems of the body and plays an important role in muscle growth. A peptide hormone which is composed of many amino acids (191 of them) linked together. It is rapidly metabolized by the liver and has a half-life in the blood of approximately 17 to 45 minutes. No wonder detecting GH in a drug screen is very difficult.

Spot – to "stand guard" while someone performs a set with heavy weights. The spotter's main duty is to prevent injury in case that someone cannot finish safely.

Squalene – shark-liver oil.

St. John's wort (hypericum performatum) – a plant herb used to relieve mild depressive symptoms, sleep disorder and anxiety, although probably not effective against serious depression. In large doses it may be unsafe as it can make the skin and eyes extra sensitive to light.

Stearic acid, stearyl alcohol – used for its emollient properties and as a moisturizing ingredient.

Steroids – steroids are synthetic derivatives of the hormone testosterone that allow the user to gain muscle mass and strength rapidly. In addition to their musclebuilding effects, anabolic steroids increase the oxidation rate of fat, thus giving the user a more ripped appearance.

Sterols – plant hormones usually isolated from crude germ oils, which aid the body in hormone production in fat metabolism.

Stevia – herb from Brazil and Paraguay that is a good substitute for sugar and artificial sweeteners. You can also bake with it.

Stevioside – an artificial sweetener. Extracted from the herb Stevia. It is 300 times sweeter than sugar, but has a strong aftertaste.

Succinates – vital nutrients and important metabolic activators, especially in the production of ATP.

Sucralose – an artificial sweetener. Approved by the FDA in 1998. It is 600 times sweeter than table sugar, it is made from a process that begins with regular sugar. You can bake with it. Sucralose was discovered in 1976. Derived from sugar through a patented multistep process that selectively substitutes three choline atoms for three hydrogen oxygen groups on the sugar molecule. The tightly bound chlorine atoms create a molecular structure that is exceptionally stable and is about 600 times sweeter than sugar. The body does not recognize it as sugar or another carbohydrate. The sucralose molecule passes through the body unchanged – it is not metabolized and is eliminated after consumption. Sucralose has no calories. The acceptable daily intake for sucralose is 5 mg per kg of bodyweight.

Sugar alcohols – this group of sweeteners includes mannitol, sorbitol and xylitol. Although found in fruit, they are commercially synthesized and not extracted from natural sources. Sugar alchohols provide a reduced glycemic response (no steep hikes in blood sugar). Sugar alcohols are absorbed slowly, but incompletely, which can cause diarrhea in some people.

Sulfur – this mineral is used for body tissue formation and collagen synthesis.

Superficial – external, located close to or on the body surface.

Superior – refers to the head or upper; higher.

Superset – one set of an exercise immediately followed by a set of a different exercise, *with no rest between sets*. Traditionally this method of training has been used for resistance exercises. You can superset antagonistic movements (such as the bench press and the barbell row). Another application would be to superset two exercises for the same muscle group (maybe bench press and cable crossovers). Some newer techniques even incorporate resistance exercises with non-resistance exercises.

Supination – *foot:* inversion combined with adduction of the forefoot; *forearm:* rotation of the wrist and hand laterally.

Supine – refers to the body lying face up, as opposed to prone.

Synephrine – a nervous system stimulant with properties very similar to ephedrine. Has equivalent thermogenesis properties but doesn't give the "buzz" effect of ephedrine. Becoming more popular as an ingredient for fat-burner products.

Synergist – a muscle cooperating with another to produce movement that could not be performed by either muscle individually.

T

Talc – a soft mineral, magnesium silicate, used as a powder to absorb excess moisture. Scrutinized as a possible carcinogen because of its close relation to asbestos.

Taurine – an essential amino acid. Plays a role in cell-membrane stabilization, calcium balance, growth modulation and the regulation of osmotic pressure in the body (water transfer). It is also a key component of bile, which is necessary for fat digestion, absorption of fat-soluble vitamins, and control of cholesterol levels. A link has been shown between deficiency in this amino and retinal dysfunction (serious eye problems).

Telangiectasia – an increase in the number and size of blood vessels in an area of the skin. It is often caused by overexposure to sunlight.

Tendon – a tough cord or band of dense white fibrous connective tissue that connects a muscle with another bodypart (such as a bone) and transmits the force produced by the contraction of the muscle to produce movement in the bodypart in question or to use that part as an "anchor" from which to induce movement in another part of the body.

Tensor [L. *tendere,* to stretch] – pertaining to a muscle whose function is to make a structure to which it is attached firm and tense.

Teres [L. *tero,* round or smooth] – denoting certain muscles that are round and long.

Testosterone – the primary natural androgenic and anabolic steroid hormone found in the body.

Theanine – a unique amino acid found in green teas. The greater the theanine content in green tea, the higher the price. Theanine increases GABA levels in the brain and counteracts high and even toxic doses of stimulants, such as caffeine. Sleep time is improved, spontaneous physical hyperactivity is decreased and toxicity reactions are markedly reduced. Theanine can help offset the length and intensity of the stimulatory effects of alpha and beta-agonists and caffeine. It goes beyond helping you relax and sleep well for one night. By reversing the excitatory state quickly and safely and promoting relaxation and restoration of your brain chemistry, you are in effect priming your body for stimulation once again the following day. That should allow you not only to grow, but also to get even better results from your supplements.

Thermogenesis – the generation of heat, usually through biological processes. Thermogenic drugs such as ephedrine and caffeine increase the rate at which the body produces heat internally, generally through the mechanisms used to maintain body temperature.

Thiamin (vitamin B1) – this vitamin maintains energy levels and supports brain function (memory). Aids in digestion. Necessary for metabolism of sugar and starch to provide energy. Maintains a healthy nervous system. Alcohol can cause deficiencies of this vitamin and all B-complex vitamins.

Tibialis [L. *tibia,* a pipe or flute] – pertaining to muscles attached to the tibia.

Tissue – a group of similar cells and fibers that form a distinct structure.

Tocopherol (vitamin E) – antioxidant vitamin, emollient and moisturizer.

Tonic – the state of being in a consistent state of muscular or neural activity (tone).

Torque – the effect of producing a force through rotation. The product of force times length of the force arm.

Toxic shock syndrome (TSS) – a rare but potentially serious disease that has been associated with tampon use. TSS is believed to be caused by toxin-producing strains of the staphylococcus aureus bacterium. The warning signs of TSS are: a sudden fever of 102° F (38.9° C) or more, vomiting, diarrhea, muscle aches, a rash that looks like sunburn, dizziness and fainting, or near fainting, when standing up.

Trans-fatty acids – unsaturated fatty acids that have a "z" shape caused by unsaturated bonds being on alternate sides of the molecule. Naturally formed unsaturated fatty acids are usually in the "cis" configuration, with the unsaturated bonds on the same side of the carbon chain. The transconfiguration is typically produced by the partial hydrogenation of polyunsaturated fatty acids, which is done to increase shelf life, heat stability and thickness.

Transparent soap – superfatted soap with a high glycerin content. Usually used for sensitive and normal-to-oily skin (e.g. Neutrogena, Pears).

Transversus [L. *trans,* across + *vertare,* to turn] – denoting muscles that lie across the long axis of an organ or a part.

Trapezius – a kite-shaped muscle of the back with the points of the kite at the base of the skull, the shoulders, and the center of the lower back. The trapezius is primarily visible as the pair of bulges on either side of the neck.

Tribulus terrestris – herb for sexual deficiency or as a mild aphrodisiac. It may increase libido and serum testosterone.

Triceps [L. *tri,* three + *caput,* head] – denoting a muscle with three heads, e.g., musculus triceps.

Triglyceride – chemical name for *fat,* usually used when referring to fats in the bloodstream rather than in food. The name comes from the three fatty acid chains that together with the glycerol "backbone" make up the molecule.

Tryptophan – an essential amino acid known for its calming and mood-enhancing effects. A naturally occurring ingredient in turkey that mellows you out and makes you want to take a nap after the Thanksgiving feast. Tryptophan can also be called 5-HTP (5-hydrotryptophan), which is made with a slightly different compound than regular tryptophan.

Tyrosine – A nonessential amino acid that is synthesized in the body from phenylalanine. Like phenylalanine, tyrosine is involved with the important brain neurotransmitters epinephrine, norepinephrine and dopamine. Its primary use in supplementation is mood related. Not likely to produce any effect on physical strength or appearance.

U

Ulcer – an open sore, lesion of the skin, or mucous membrane accompanied by sloughing off inflamed dead skin. Canker sores are an example of an ulcer commonly found in the mouth.

Ulcerations – to form an ulcer (ulcer: see above).

Ulnaris [L. *ulna,* elbow forearm] – pertaining to the larger and more medial of the two bones of the forearm.

Umbilicus – the navel, the site where the umbilical cord was once attached.

Unsaturated fats – fats containing fatty acids with some carbon-carbon double bonds. Saturated fats, however, have all possible positions that could be occupied by a hydrogen atom filled, leaving no double bonds in the carbon chain.

V

Valine – one of the amino acids the body cannot for manufacture itself but must acquire from food sources. Valine is found in abundant quantities in most foods. Valine has a stimulant effect. Healthy growth depends on it. A deficiency results in a negative hydrogen balance in the body. Used by bodybuilders in conjunction with leucine and isoleucine for muscle growth, tissue repair, and as an energizer. To date there is little scientific evidence to support this use, though studies have shown that these three substances might be able to help restore muscle mass in people with liver disease, injuries, or who have undergone surgery. Studies on healthy people have shown them to be ineffective. While research is inconclusive, most users of products containing these BCAAs attest to its worth suggesting that more research is needed. Because valine cannot be produced by the body, healthy people should ensure that they are obtaining at least the recommended amount in their diet.

Vanadyl sulfate – source of trace mineral vanadium. Helps optimize glycogen storage to yield more energy. Vanadyl is supposed to help you attain a little more muscle and inhibit fat storage by controlling insulin release. In theory vanadyl works inside the muscle cells by bringing carbohydrates into the muscle without the assistance of insulin. If there is less insulin, there is less chance of carbohydrates being converted to stored bodyfat.

Varicosities – the condition of being varicose (varicose: distended, swollen, visible veins).

Vascular – pertaining to or composed of blood vessels (blood vessels: commonly refers to arteries, veins and capillaries).

Vasoconstriction – the narrowing of blood vessels.

Vasodilation – the widening of blood vessels.

Vastus [L. *vastus,* huge] – a large muscle of the thigh, musculus quadriceps with three vasti and a rectus.

Vein – a vessel that carries blood away from tissues and toward the heart.

Velocity – the rate of motion of a body traveling in a particular direction.

Venous – pertaining to the veins or blood passing through them.

Ventilation – the process of oxygenating the blood through the lungs.

Ventricle – a small cavity or pouch. Chambers of the heart that push blood out to the tissues.

Vertigo – a feeling of dizziness, as though the environment were revolving.

Viagra – brand name of sildenafil, a selective type 5 cGMP phosphodiesterase inhibitor, which enhances nitric-oxide-dependent vasodilation in the corpus cavernosum, thus increasing erectile response in males suffering from impotence. Note that Viagra does not initiate or increase sexual drive or desire, or affect testosterone levels.

Viscosity – the state of being sticky or thick.

Vital capacity – the total volume of air that can be exhaled following a maximal inhalation.

Vital signs – signs of important body functions like pulse, blood pressure, temperature, etc.

Vitamin – a micronutrient that is a complex organic molecule essential for the biochemical transformations necessary for proper metabolism and disease prevention.

Volume, training volume – number of repetitions done in a training routine; training is high volume if many repetitions are done, whether in many individual sets, circuit training, or just spending all day pumping away at the weights.

Voluntary muscle – skeletal muscle; muscle under one's control.

W

Warm – refers to yellow, red or orange-based undertones in hair, skin or makeup.

Warmup – a light to moderate physical activity performed prior to exercise.

White blood cells – cells produced by the body that help fight infection.

Willow bark – white willow bark is a source of salicin, a chemical relative of aspirin. The effects of willow bark are mild pain inhibition, with increased blood flow to the skin, and greater heat loss.

Work – the movement of force through a distance.

Work rate – power or work generated per unit of time.

X

Xyphoid process – the smallest and lowest division of the human sternum that is cartilaginous early in life but becomes more or less ossified during adulthood.

Y

Yohimbe bark – a chemical substance derived from the yohimbe, said to boost natural testosterone levels in the body.

Z

Zinc (Zn) – mineral important as a cofactor in energy metabolism, amino acid and protein synthesis; antioxidant effects to protect the immune system. Essential for growth, tissue repair, and sexual development. Plays an important role in healing. Since animal proteins are the best sources, vegetarians are often deficient in zinc.

Zinc oxide – an oxide of zinc, an astringent.

Zinc stearate – used in powder to improve texture and to lubricate.

ZMA (zinc magnesium aspartate) – This compound has been found to increase muscle strength.

Contributing Photographers

Jim Amentler, Alex Ardenti, Garry Bartlett,
Reg Bradford, John A. Butler, Paula Crane,
Ralph DeHaan, Bob Delmonteque,
Francis Faulkner, Skip Faulkner,
Rich Finnegan, Irvin Gelb, Eric Jacobson,
Robert Kennedy, J.M. Manion,
Ricky Marconi, Jason Mathas, John Mulazzi,
Mitsuru Okabe, David Paul, Dan Peterson,
Rick Schaff, Rob Sims, Zach Taylor,
Rafael Tongol, D.J. Wallis,
Dennis Warren, and the late Art Zeller.

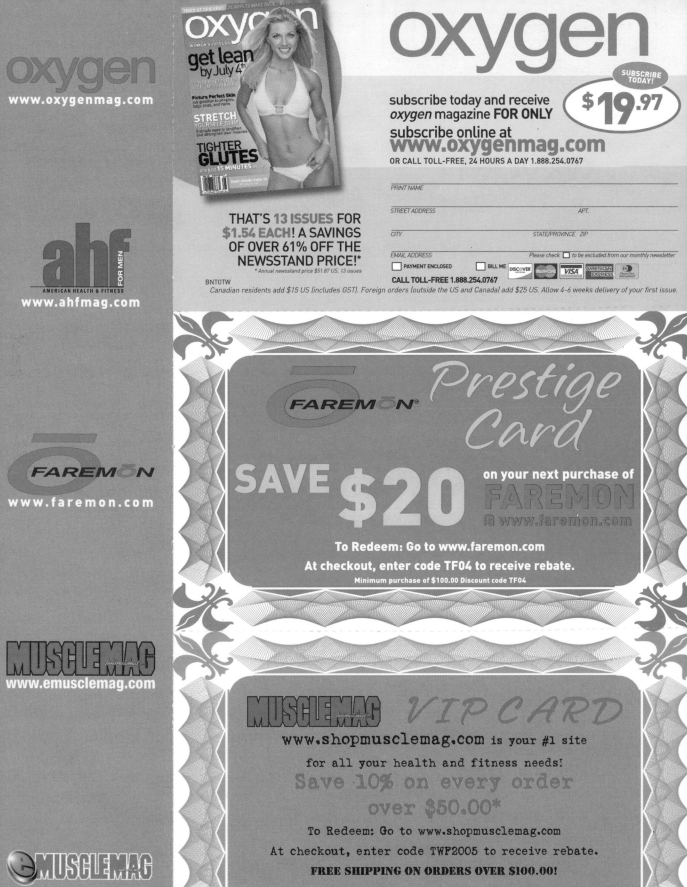